Hepatitis B and D Protocols
Volume 2

METHODS IN MOLECULAR MEDICINE™

John M. Walker, SERIES EDITOR

99. Pain Research: *Methods and Protocols,* edited by *David Z. Luo, 2004*

98. Tumor Necrosis Factor: *Methods and Protocols,* edited by *Angelo Corti and Pietro Ghezzi, 2004*

97. Molecular Diagnosis of Cancer: *Methods and Protocols, Second Edition,* edited by *Joseph E. Roulston and John M. S. Bartlett, 2004*

96. Hepatitis B and D Protocols: *Volume 2, Immunology, Model Systems, and Clinical Studies,* edited by *Robert K. Hamatake and Johnson Y. N. Lau, 2004*

95. Hepatitis B and D Protocols: *Volume 1, Detection, Genotypes, and Characterization,* edited by *Robert K. Hamatake and Johnson Y. N. Lau, 2004*

94. Molecular Diagnosis of Infectious Diseases, *Second Edition,* edited by *Jochen Decker and Udo Reischl, 2004*

93. Anticoagulants, Antiplatelets, and Thrombolytics, edited by *Shaker A. Mousa, 2004*

92. Molecular Diagnosis of Genetic Diseases, *Second Edition,* edited by *Rob Elles and Roger Mountford, 2004*

91. Pediatric Hematology: *Methods and Protocols,* edited by *Nicholas J. Goulden and Colin G. Steward, 2003*

90. Suicide Gene Therapy: *Methods and Reviews,* edited by *Caroline J. Springer, 2004*

89. The Blood–Brain Barrier: *Biology and Research Protocols,* edited by *Sukriti Nag, 2003*

88. Cancer Cell Culture: *Methods and Protocols,* edited by *Simon P. Langdon, 2003*

87. Vaccine Protocols, *Second Edition,* edited by *Andrew Robinson, Michael J. Hudson, and Martin P. Cranage, 2003*

86. Renal Disease: *Techniques and Protocols,* edited by *Michael S. Goligorsky, 2003*

85. Novel Anticancer Drug Protocols, edited by *John K. Buolamwini and Alex A. Adjei, 2003*

84. Opioid Research: *Methods and Protocols,* edited by *Zhizhong Z. Pan, 2003*

83. Diabetes Mellitus: *Methods and Protocols,* edited by *Sabire Özcan, 2003*

82. Hemoglobin Disorders: *Molecular Methods and Protocols,* edited by *Ronald L. Nagel, 2003*

81. Prostate Cancer Methods and Protocols, edited by *Pamela J. Russell, Paul Jackson, and Elizabeth A. Kingsley, 2003*

80. Bone Research Protocols, edited by *Miep H. Helfrich and Stuart H. Ralston, 2003*

79. Drugs of Abuse: *Neurological Reviews and Protocols,* edited by *John Q. Wang, 2003*

78. Wound Healing: *Methods and Protocols,* edited by *Luisa A. DiPietro and Aime L. Burns, 2003*

77. Psychiatric Genetics: *Methods and Reviews,* edited by *Marion Leboyer and Frank Bellivier, 2003*

76. Viral Vectors for Gene Therapy: *Methods and Protocols,* edited by *Curtis A. Machida, 2003*

75. Lung Cancer: *Volume 2, Diagnostic and Therapeutic Methods and Reviews,* edited by *Barbara Driscoll, 2003*

74. Lung Cancer: *Volume 1, Molecular Pathology Methods and Reviews,* edited by *Barbara Driscoll, 2003*

73. *E. coli*: *Shiga Toxin Methods and Protocols,* edited by *Dana Philpott and Frank Ebel, 2003*

72. Malaria Methods and Protocols, edited by *Denise L. Doolan,* 2002

71. *Haemophilus influenzae* Protocols, edited by *Mark A. Herbert, Derek Hood, and E. Richard Moxon,* 2002

70. Cystic Fibrosis Methods and Protocols, edited by *William R. Skach,* 2002

69. Gene Therapy Protocols, *Second Edition,* edited by *Jeffrey R. Morgan,* 2002

68. Molecular Analysis of Cancer, edited by *Jacqueline Boultwood and Carrie Fidler,* 2002

METHODS IN MOLECULAR MEDICINE™

Hepatitis B and D Protocols

Volume 2: Immunology, Model Systems, and Clinical Studies

Edited by

Robert K. Hamatake, PhD

Johnson Y. N. Lau, MD

Ribapharm Inc., Costa Mesa, CA

Forewords by

Timothy M. Block, PhD and Baruch S. Blumberg, MD, PhD

T. Jake Liang, MD

Humana Press Totowa, New Jersey

999 Riverview Drive, Suite 208
Totowa, New Jersey 07512

www.humanapress.com

This publication is printed on acid-free paper. ∞

ANSI Z39.48-1984 (American Standards Institute) Permanence of Paper for Printed Library Materials.

Cover design by Patricia F. Cleary.

Cover illustration: Figure 4, Chapter 34, R. G. Gish and S. Locarnini. Background: Figure 1, Chapter 13, Volume 1, K. Abid and F. Negro.

Printed in the United States of America. 10 9 8 7 6 5 4 3 2 1
ISSN 1543-1894

Library of Congress Cataloging in Publication Data
Hepatitis B and D protocols / edited by Robert K. Hamatake, Johnson Y. N. Lau
p. ; cm. —(methods in molecular medicine; 95-96)
Includes bibliographical references and indexes.
Contents: v. 1. Detection, genotypes, and characterization—v. 2. Immunology, model systems, and clinical studies.
ISBN 978-1-61737-363-3 e-ISBN 978-1-59259-670-6

1. Hepatitis B—Laboratory manuals. 2. Hepatitis B virus—Laboratory manuals. 3. Delta -associated agent—Laboratory manuals. 4. Delta infection—Laboratory manuals. I. Hamatake, Robert Kiyoshi, 1953– . II. Lau, Johnson Y. N. (Johnson Yiu-Nam). III. Series
[DNLM: 1. Hepatitis B. 2. Hepatitis D. WC 536 H53335 2004]
QR201.H46H43 2004
616.3'623-1–dc21 2003011624

To our wives, April T.G. Hamatake and Jane W.S. Fang-Lau, for their unfailing support, and our children, Kyle Hamatake, David Hamatake, Grace (Ling-Ling) Lau, Gillian (Gi-Gi) Lau, and Gabrielle (Ching-Ching) Lau, for keeping us rejuvenated.

Foreword

Despite the availability of an effective vaccine, there are still 400 million people, worldwide who are chronically infected with hepatitis B virus (HBV). For them, the vaccine, as currently applied, has no value. Given the possible consequences of HBV infection, the number of those chronically infected with HBV presents an enormous public health challenge. For example, the major etiology of hepatocellular carcinoma (HCC) is chronic infection with HBV. Although fifth in cancer incidence, worldwide, HCC/liver cancer is the third leading cause of cancer death. The high mortality associated with HCC arises because the disease is often detected late and is unresponsive to treatment. The number of deaths caused by PHCC is expected to rise over the next 20 years. Those chronically infected with HBV have a life risk of death to HCC of between 10 and 25%. Even the limited efficacy of drugs for the treatment of chronic HBV helps underscore the point that this disease is responsive to therapy. Drugs that target the polymerase (e.g., hepsera and lamivudine) and interferon alpha represent two distinct strategies and show that both conventional antiviral and immunotherapeutic approaches can be used in management. However, the current inventory of therapeutics is inadequate. Interferon alpha is of limited value, only parenterally available, and fraught with adverse reactions. The polymerase inhibitors are undermined by either a high frequency of resistance or, in the case of hepsera, additional concerns about toxicity. Other areas of concern also remain. There is still no reliable means of predicting disease outcome for chronic carriers, making early detection of liver disease and decisions about drug efficacy, as well as who should be treated and for how long, difficult. Moreover, tests for HBV DNA levels (and other markers) are often of dubious quantitative value. Because HBV patients are becoming more sophisticated and more demanding about these markers and many follow their viremia (DNA) levels like investors follow the Dow Jones Industrial values, it is essential that meaningful lab values be provided. The current vaccines are effective, but they are expensive, and escape mutants may be a problem waiting to happen.

Thus, without a doubt, more work needs to be done in all of the key areas of the management of HBV.

The good news is that there have been important advances. A clearer picture about the kinds of drugs that can be effective, their pathogenesis, and the development of research tools should facilitate the discovery process.

It is the matter of research tools that these volumes address. In an almost encyclopedic fashion, Hamatake and Lau have assembled a comprehensive, "how to" guide for the study of HBV. It is worth noting that many of the methods described will have value in the study of other viruses and liver diseases in general, despite being highly focused upon HBV.

This is a very practical resource, in every respect. In more than 40 chapters, leaders in the field who have "been there" have contributed step-by-step "programmed" approaches, telling the readers how to reproduce their findings. It is something of a users guide for do-it-yourselfers.

It is not an overstatement to write that nearly every aspect of HBV research is covered, section by section, virus detection through vaccine and drug development. Thus, *Hepatitis B and D Protocols* is likely to become as essential a resource to those studying HBV as was the fabled Maniatis series (published by Cold Spring Harbor Press) for Molecular Biology. It is certainly going to get a great deal of attention in the Hepatitis B Foundation labs, and, because of its value, we hope it is used in labs throughout the world. The more it is used, the more likely HBV research will be advanced.

***Timothy M. Block,* PhD**
Professor and Director of the Jefferson Center
and Hepatitis B Foundation Laboratory
Thomas Jefferson University
and President, Hepatitis B Foundation
Doylestown, PA

***Baruch S. Blumberg,* MD, PhD**
Nobel Laureate, 1976
Senior Adviser to the President of Fox Chase Cancer Center
and Professor of Medicine and Anthropology
University of Pennsylvania
Philadelphia, PA

Foreword

The identification of the "Australian antigen" by Dr. Blumberg, which was subsequently recognized to be the hepatitis B virus surface antigen, marks the discovery of an important pathogen for liver diseases. The virus was the first hepatitis virus discovered almost four decades ago. Despite the magnitude of the infection and the significant efforts by the scientific community, hepatitis B continues to be a global health problem affecting more than 350 million people worldwide. Many scientific milestones in basic and clinical research on hepatitis B had profound impact on this viral infection in the history of medicine: hepatitis B virus vaccine was introduced two decades ago; interferon alpha was approved for the treatment of chronic hepatitis B and two other antiviral drugs have also been approved; liver transplantation under high dose hepatitis B immunoglobulin coverage can now be offered to patients with end-stage hepatitis B related liver disease. These advances have also introduced new paradigms in our understanding of the fundamental concepts of viral infection in general. Certainly, more work looms ahead of us in order to ultimately conquer this viral infection. To equip the basic and clinical investigators with all the available tools is of utmost importance in this quest. As illustrated in this book, the marriage between basic science and clinical medicine is critical.

In the last few decades, we have witnessed the groundbreaking progress and the introduction of new clinical paradigms in hepatitis B virus infection. The next decade must underscore further application of our knowledge to translational research, bridging basic science and clinical medicine, and to capitalize on our understandings to conquer this viral infection. Undoubtedly, with all the scientific efforts contributed by many dedicated scientists and with our willingness to share knowledge, the common goal of improving human health by eradicating this virus can be achieved in this millennium.

T. Jake Liang, MD
Chief, Liver Diseases Section
NIDDK National Institutes of Health
Bethesda, MD

Preface

The 36 years since the identification of hepatitis B virus (HBV) in 1967 has seen the establishment of HBV virology as a rich and extensive field of science and the recognition of HBV as one of the top 10 leading causes of death in the world. There are an estimated 400 million people chronically infected with HBV worldwide, with 20–30% of these projected to die from complications of chronic liver disease, including cirrhosis and liver cancer. Hepatitis delta virus (HDV) was first identified in 1980 as a novel transmissible agent distinct from HBV that requires the HBV envelope protein for its infectivity. HDV co-infection in chronic HBV patients is associated with a more severe disease outcome than those not co-infected. HBV and HDV infections represent a significant health burden to the worldwide community.

Despite the lack of an inflectable cell culture system, an enormous amount of information has been obtained on the virology and immunology of HBV and HDV infections. Modern molecular biological techniques and research with related viruses have enabled much of the HBV and HDV life cycle to be elucidated, leading to a number of therapeutic approaches for treating chronically infected patients. Innovative detection methods based on these findings and techniques have led to diagnostic and clinical monitoring assays of increasing sensitivity. However, our understanding of the viral life cycle and virus–host interactions is incomplete and will require much more research for a complete comprehension of the pathogenesis of disease caused by viral infection. Hepatitis B and D Protocols contains a collection of research techniques, divided into two volumes, used in the study of HBV and HDV. The authors represent a number of scientific disciplines, but share in common their interest in hepatitis research and their expertise in their respective areas. Although most of these techniques have been described in peer-reviewed journals, these chapters provide far more detail and are written so that investigators can use them as manuals. A few reviews are included in some specialized areas such as antiviral testing and the design of clinical trials. We hope that this compilation of techniques used in the different areas of HBV and HDV research will prove useful to scientists and encourage multidisciplinary approaches to their research, so that clinical investigators will find it beneficial for their understanding of the current HBV and HDV research.

We would like to take this opportunity to extend our gratitude to our teachers and friends: Dr. Zhi Hong, Dr. Maria Seifer, Dr. David Standring, Professor P. C. Wu, Professor C. L. Lai, Dr. H. J. Lin, Professor Roger Williams, and Dr. Graeme J. M. Alexander. Without their guidance and support, we would not have the opportunity of presenting this highly practical manual to you today.

Robert K. Hamatake, PhD
Johnson Yiu-Nam Lau, MD

Contents

Dedication v
Foreword by Timothy M. Block and Baruch S. Blumberg vii
Foreword by T. Jake Liang ix
Preface xi
Contributors xvii
Contents for Volume 1 xxi

Part I. Viral-Specific Immunological and Other Host Responses

1 Studying Host Immune Responses Against Duck Hepatitis B Virus Infection
Darren S. Miller, Edward M. Bertram, Catherine A. Scougall, Ieva Kotlarski, and Allison R. Jilbert* *3

2 Measurement of Cell-Mediated Immune Response in Woodchucks
Stephan Menne and Paul J. Cote* *27

3 Study of Liver-Specific Expression of Cytokines During Woodchuck Hepatitis Virus Infection
Mengji Lu and Michael Roggendorf* *37

4 Induction of Anti-Hepatitis B Virus Immune Responses Through DNA Immunization
Michael Geissler, Robert Weth, Christian F. Grimm, Dörte Ortmann, and Hubert E. Blum* *43

5 Monitoring Gene Expression Using DNA Microarrays During Hepatitis B Virus Infection
Michael R. Beard and Stephen Locarnini* *55

6 Determination of Hepatitis B Virus-Specific CD8+ T-Cell Activity in the Liver
Michelina Nascimbeni and Barbara Rehermann* *65

7 Determining the Precursor Frequency of HBV Nucleocapsid Antigen-Specific T Cells
Jennifer A. Waters and Howard C. Thomas* *85

8 Detection and Characterization of Virus-Specific CD8+ T Cells Using the Tetramer Approach
Xiao-Song He and Harry B. Greenberg* *89

9 In Vitro Analysis of Hepatitis B Virus Specific CD4+ T Cells
Shilpa Chokshi and Nikolai V. Naoumov* *97

10 Induction of Humoral and Cellular Immune Responses to Hepatitis Delta Virus Through DNA Immunization in BALB/c Mice
Ren-Shiang Lee, Shih-Jer Hsu, Li-Rung Huang, Hui-Lin Wu, Shiou-Lin Lin, Ding-Shinn Chen, and Pei-Jer Chen ***111***

Part II. In Vitro and In Vivo Models

11 Infection of Primary Chimpanzee Hepatocytes with Recombinant Hepatitis D Virus Particles: *A Surrogate Model for Hepatitis B Virus*
Azeneth Barrera and Robert E. Lanford ***131***

12 Study of the Endocytosis and Intracellular Localization of Subviral Particles of Hepatitis B Virus in Primary Hepatocytes
Dieter Glebe and Wolfram H. Gerlich ***143***

13 The Tupaia Model for the Study of Hepatitis B Virus: *Direct Infection and HBV Genome Transduction of Primary Tupaia Hepatocytes*
Fritz von Weizsäcker, Josef Köck, Sabine MacNelly, Shaotang Ren, Hubert E. Blum, and Michael Nassal ***153***

14 Delivery of Hepatitis B Virus Therapeutic Agents Using Asialoglycoprotein Receptor–Based Liver-Specific Targeting
Masayoshi Konishi, Catherine H. Wu, and George Y. Wu ***163***

15 Woodchuck Hepatitis Virus Hepatocyte Culture Models
Norma D. Churchill and Tomasz I. Michalak ***175***

16 Duck Hepatitis B Virus Primary Hepatocyte Culture Model
Olivier Hantz and Fabien Zoulim ***189***

17 Enhancement of Infection of HepG2 Cells in Culture by Predigestion of Hepadnavirus with V8 Protease
Xuanyong Lu and Timothy M. Block ***199***

18 Construction of Recombinant Adenoviruses that Produce Infectious Hepatitis B Virus
Martin Sprinzl, Jérôme Dumortier, and Ulrike Protzer ***209***

19 Baculovirus-Mediated Gene Transfer for the Study of Hepatitis B Virus
Harriet C. Isom, Ayman M. Abdelhamed, John P. Bilello, and Thomas G. Miller ***219***

20 Transgenic Hepatitis B Virus Mouse Model in the Study of Chemotherapy
John D. Morrey ***239***

21 Transplantation of Human Hepatocytes in Immunodeficient UPA Mice: *A Model for the Study of Hepatitis B Virus*
Jörg Petersen, Martin R. Burda, Maura Dandri, and Charles E. Rogler ***253***

22 Duck Hepatitis B Virus Model in the Study of Hepatitis B Virus
Lucyna Cova and Fabien Zoulim ***261***

23 Hepatitis B Virus Transgenic Severe Combined Immunodeficient Mouse Model of Acute and Chronic Liver Disease
Mark A. Feitelson, Jonathan D. Larkin, and Raymond F. Schinazi ... ***269***

24 The Chimpanzee Model: *Contributions and Considerations for Studies of Hepatitis B Virus*
Pascal Gagneux and Elaine A. Muchmore ***289***

25 Hepatitis B in Liver Transplant Recipients as a Special Model of Antiviral Drug Development
Robert G. Gish and Adil Wakil ***319***

26 Hepatitis Delta Virus Transfection for the Mouse In Vivo Model
Jinhong Chang, Anthony Lerro, and John M. Taylor ***343***

27 Hepatitis Delta Virus RNA Transfection for the Cell Culture Model
Thomas B. Macnaughton and Michael M. C. Lai ***351***

PART III. ANTIVIRAL TESTING AND CLINICAL STUDIES

28 Analysis of Hepatitis B Virus Dynamics and Its Impact on Antiviral Development
Manuel Tsiang and Craig S. Gibbs ***361***

29 Genotyping Anti-Hepatitis B Virus Drug Resistance
Eric J. Bourne, Josée Gauthier, Vincent A. Lopez, and Lynn D. Condreay ***379***

30 A Parsimonious Method for Screening Drug Combinations for Antihepadnaviral Activity Using a Parametric Dose–Response Surface Approach
Tim Shaw and Stephen Locarnini ***387***

31 Hepatitis B Virus: *Where Are We and Where Are We Going?*
Michael P. Manns, Johannes Hadem, and Heiner Wedemeyer ***415***

32 Designing Studies to Evaluate Anti-Hepatitis B Virus Therapies: *From the Perspective of Studies for the Registration of Pharmaceutical Products*
Alison B. Murray ***445***

33 Specific Considerations in the Design of Hepatitis B Virus Clinical Studies in the Far East
Man-Fung Yuen and Ching-Lung Lai ***457***

34 Studying the Treatment of Chronic Hepatitis B Viral Infection in Special Populations
Robert G. Gish and Stephen Locarnini ***465***

35 Designing Clinical Development Programs for Anti-Hepatitis B Virus Drugs
Nathaniel A. Brown ***499***

36 Testing Antivirals Against Hepatitis Delta Virus: *Farnesyl Transferase Inhibitors*
Bruno B. Bordier and Jeffrey S. Glenn ***539***

Index ***555***

Contributors

AYMAN M. ABDELHAMED • *Department of Microbiology and Immunology, The Pennsylvania State College of Medicine, Hershey, PA*
AZENETH BARRERA • *Department of Virology and Immunology, Southwest Foundation for Biomedical Research, San Antonio, TX*
MICHAEL R. BEARD • *Royal Adelaide Hospital Florey Fellow, Infectious Diseases Laboratories, IMVS, Adelaide, Australia, and Adjunct Assistant Professor, Department of Microbiology & Immunology, University of Texas Medical Branch, Galveston, TX*
EDWARD M. BERTRAM • *Department of Immunology, University of Toronto, Toronto, ON M5S 1A8 Canada*
JOHN P. BILELLO • *Department of Microbiology and Immunology, The Pennsylvania State College of Medicine, Hershey, PA*
TIMOTHY M. BLOCK • *Department of Biochemistry and Molecular Pharmacology, Thomas Jefferson University, Doylestown, PA*
HUBERT E. BLUM • *Department of Internal Medicine II, University of Freiburg, Freiburg, Germany*
BRUNO B. BORDIER • *Division of Gastroenterology and Hepatology, Stanford University School of Medicine and Veterans Administration Medical Center, Palo Alto, CA*
ERIC J. BOURNE • *Department of Clinical Virology, GlaxoSmithKline, Research Triangle Park, NC*
NATHANIEL A. BROWN • *Hepatitis Clinical Research, Idenix Pharmaceuticals, Cambridge, MA*
MARTIN R. BURDA • *Heinrich-Pette-Institute for Experimental Virology and Immunology, University of Hamburg, Hamburg, Germany*
JINHONG CHANG • *Fox Chase Cancer Center, Philadelphia, PA*
DING-SHINN CHEN • *Hepatitis Research Center, National Taiwan University Hospital, Taipei, Taiwan*
PEI-JER CHEN • *Hepatitis Research Center, National Taiwan University Hospital, Taipei, Taiwan*
SHILPA CHOKSHI • *Institute of Hepatology, University College London, UK*
NORMA D. CHURCHILL • *Molecular Virology and Hepatology Research, Memorial University of Newfoundland, St. John's, Newfoundland, Canada*
LYNN D. CONDREAY • *Department of Clinical Virology, GlaxoSmithKline, Research Triangle Park, NC*
PAUL J. COTE • *Division of Molecular Virology and Immunology, Georgetown University Medical Center, Rockville, MD*
LUCYNA COVA • *INSERM U271, 151 Cours Albert Thomas, 69003, Lyon, France*
MAURA DANDRI • *Heinrich-Pette-Institute for Experimental Virology and Immunology, University of Hamburg, Hamburg, Germany*

JÉRÔME DUMORTIER • *Department of Virology, University of Heidelberg, Heidelberg, Germany*

MARK A. FEITELSON • *Department of Pathology, Anatomy and Cell Biology, Thomas Jefferson University, Philadelphia, PA*

PASCAL GAGNEUX • *Departments of Medicine and Cellular and Molecular Medicine, University of California San Diego, La Jolla, CA*

JOSÉE GAUTHIER • *Department of Clinical Virology, GlaxoSmithKline, Research Triangle Park, NC*

MICHAEL GEISSLER • *Department of Internal Medicine II, University of Freiburg, Freiburg, Germany*

WOLFRAM H. GERLICH • *Institute of Medical Virology, University of Giessen, Giessen, Germany*

CRAIG S. GIBBS • *Gilead Sciences, Foster City, CA*

ROBERT G. GISH • *Departments of Transplantation and Medicine, California Pacific Medical Center, San Francisco, CA*

DIETER GLEBE • *Institute of Medical Virology, University of Giessen, Giessen, Germany*

JEFFREY S. GLENN • *Division of Gastroenterology and Hepatology, Stanford University School of Medicine and Veterans Administration Medical Center, Palo Alto, CA*

HARRY B. GREENBERG • *Division of Gastroenterology and Hepatology, Stanford University School of Medicine and Veterans Administration Medical Center, Palo Alto, CA*

CHRISTIAN F. GRIMM • *Department of Internal Medicine II, University of Freiburg, Freiburg, Germany*

JOHANNES HADEM • *Department of Gastroenterology, Hepatology, and Endocrinology, Medical School of Hannover, Hannover, Germany*

OLIVIER HANTZ • *INSERM U271, 151 Cours Albert Thomas, 69003, Lyon, France*

XIAO-SONG HE • *Division of Gastroenterology, Stanford University School of Medicine, Stanford, CA*

SHIH-JER HSU • *Hepatitis Research Center, National Taiwan University Hospital, Taipei, Taiwan*

LI-RUNG HUANG • *Hepatitis Research Center, National Taiwan University Hospital, Taipei, Taiwan*

HARRIET C. ISOM • *Department of Microbiology and Immunology, The Pennsylvania State College of Medicine, Hershey, PA*

ALLISON R. JILBERT • *Department of Molecular Biosciences, Adelaide University, SA 5005, Australia*

JOSEF KÖCK • *Department of Internal Medicine II, University of Freiburg, Freiburg, Germany*

MASAYOSHI KONISHI • *Department of Medicine, Division of Gastroenterology-Hepatology, University of Connecticut Health Center, Farmington, CT*

IEVA KOTLARSKI • *Department of Molecular Biosciences, Adelaide University, SA 5005, Australia*

CHING-LUNG LAI • *Department of Medicine, The University of Hong Kong, Hong Kong*

Michael M. C. Lai • *Department of Molecular Microbiology and Immunology, University of Southern California, Keck School of Medicine, Los Angeles, CA*
Robert E. Lanford • *Department of Virology and Immunology, Southwest Foundation for Biomedical Research, San Antonio, Texas*
Jonathan D. Larkin • *Eli Lilly & Company, Indianapolis, IN*
Ren-Shiang Lee • *Hepatitis Research Center, National Taiwan University Hospital, Taipei, Taiwan*
Anthony Lerro • *Fox Chase Cancer Center, Philadelphia, PA*
Shiou-Lin Lin • *Hepatitis Research Center, National Taiwan University Hospital, Taipei, Taiwan*
Stephen Locarnini • *Victorian Infectious Diseases Reference Laboratory, North Melbourne, Australia*
Vincent A. Lopez • *Department of Clinical Virology, GlaxoSmithKline, Research Triangle Park, NC*
Mengji Lu • *Institut für Virologie, Universitätsklinikum Essen, Essen, Germany*
Xuanyong Lu • *Department of Biochemistry and Molecular Pharmacology, Thomas Jefferson University, Doylestown, PA*
Thomas B. Macnaughton • *Department of Molecular Microbiology and Immunology, University of Southern California, Keck School of Medicine, Los Angeles, CA*
Sabine MacNelly • *Department of Internal Medicine II, University of Freiburg, Freiburg, Germany*
Michael P. Manns • *Department of Gastroenterology, Hepatology, and Endocrinology, Medical School of Hannover, Hannover, Germany*
Stephan Menne • *Gastrointestinal Unit, Department of Clinical Sciences, College of Veterinary Medicine, Cornell University, Ithaca, NY*
Tomasz I. Michalak • *Molecular Virology and Hepatology Research, Memorial University of Newfoundland, St. John's, Newfoundland, Canada*
Darren S. Miller • *Department of Molecular Biosciences, Adelaide University, SA 5005, Australia*
Thomas G. Miller • *Department of Microbiology and Immunology, The Pennsylvania State College of Medicine, Hershey, PA*
John D. Morrey • *Institute for Antiviral Research, Department of Animal, Dairy and Veterinary Sciences, Utah State University, Logan, UT*
Elaine A. Muchmore • *San Diego Veterans Administration Medical Center and Department of Medicine, University of California, San Diego, La Jolla, CA*
Alison B. Murray • *Roche Molecular Systems, Oakland, CA*
Nikolai V. Naoumov • *Institute of Hepatology, University College London, UK*
Michelina Nascimbeni • *Liver Diseases Section, NIDDK, National Institutes of Health, Bethesda, MD*
Michael Nassal • *University Hospital Freiburg, Dept. of Internal Medicine II / Molecular Biology, Freiburg, Germany*
Dörte Ortmann • *Department of Internal Medicine II, University of Freiburg, Freiburg, Germany*

JÖRG PETERSEN • *Heinrich-Pette-Institute for Experimental Virology and Immunology, University of Hamburg, Hamburg, Germany*
ULRIKE PROTZER • *Molecular Infectiology at the Center for Molecular Medicine, University of Cologne, Cologne, Germany*
BARBARA REHERMANN • *Liver Diseases Section, NIDDK, National Institutes of Health, Bethesda, MD*
SHAOTANG REN • *Department of Internal Medicine II, University of Freiburg, Freiburg, Germany*
MICHAEL ROGGENDORF • *Institut für Virologie, Universitätsklinikum Essen, Essen, Germany*
CHARLES E. ROGLER • *Marion Bessin Liver Research Center, Department of Medicine, Albert Einstein College of Medicine, Bronx, NY*
RAYMOND F. SCHINAZI • *Department of Pediatrics, VA Medical Center, Emory University, Decatur, GA*
CATHERINE A. SCOUGALL • *Department of Molecular Biosciences, Adelaide University, Australia*
TIM SHAW • *Victorian Infectious Diseases Reference Laboratory, North Melbourne, Australia*
MARTIN SPRINZL • *Department of Internal Medicine I, University of Mainz, Mainz, Germany*
JOHN M. TAYLOR • *Fox Chase Cancer Center, Philadelphia, PA*
HOWARD C. THOMAS • *Imperial College of Science, Technology and Medicine, St. Mary's Campus, London, UK*
MANUEL TSIANG • *Gilead Sciences, Foster City, CA*
FRITZ VON WEIZSÄCKER • *Department of Internal Medicine II, University of Freiburg, Freiburg, Germany*
ADIL WAKIL • *Departments of Transplantation and Medicine, California Pacific Medical Center, San Francisco, CA*
JENNIFER A. WATERS • *Imperial College of Science, Technology and Medicine, St. Mary's Campus, London, UK*
HEINER WEDEMEYER • *Department of Gastroenterology, Hepatology, and Endocrinology, Medical School of Hannover, Hannover, Germany*
ROBERT WETH • *Department of Internal Medicine II, University of Freiburg, Freiburg, Germany*
HUI-LIN WU • *Hepatitis Research Center, National Taiwan University Hospital, Taipei, Taiwan*
CATHERINE H. WU • *Department of Medicine, Division of Gastroenterology-Hepatology, University of Connecticut Health Center, Farmington, CT*
GEORGE Y. WU • *Department of Medicine, Division of Gastroenterology-Hepatology, University of Connecticut Health Center, Farmington, CT*
MAN-FUNG YUEN • *Department of Medicine, The University of Hong Kong, Hong Kong*
FABIEN ZOULIM • *INSERM U271, 151 Cours Albert Thomas, 69003, Lyon, France*

Contents for Volume 1

Dedication v
Foreword by Timothy M. Block and Baruch S. Blumberg vii
Foreword by T. Jake Liang ix
Preface xi
Contributors xvii
Contents for Volume 2 xxi

Part I. Detection of Viral Markers

1 Overview of Commercial HBV Assay Systems
Stefan Zeuzem* *3

2 Detection of HBV DNA in Serum Using a PCR-Based Assay
Hau Tim Chung* *15

3 Detection of HBV DNA by Oligonucleotide Probing
Hsiang Ju Lin* *21

4 Detection of HBV RNA in Serum of Patients
Wei Zhang, Hans Jörg Hacker, Maria Mildenberger, Qin Su, and Claus H. Schröder* *29

5 Quantification of HBV Covalently Closed Circular DNA from Liver Tissue by Real-Time PCR
Scott Bowden, Kathy Jackson, Margaret Littlejohn, and Stephen Locarnini* *41

6 *In Situ* Hybridization for the Detection and Localization of HBV DNA in Liver Sections
Vicky C. H. Lai and Johnson Y. N. Lau* *51

7 Quantitative Assay of Hepatitis B Surface Antigen in Serum or Plasma Using Laurell Electrophoresis
Wolfram H. Gerlich, Ulrike Wend, and Dieter Glebe* *57

8 *In Situ* Detection of Hepatitis B Viral Antigens: *An Immunohistochemical Approach*
Jane W. S. Fang and Johnson Y. N. Lau* *65

9 Detection of Hepatitis B Virus X Antigen by Immunohistochemistry and Western Blotting
Jie Liu and Mark A. Feitelson* *71

10 Detection of Serum HDV RNA by RT-PCR
Antonina Smedile, Maria Grazia Niro, and Mario Rizzetto ***85***

11 Nonradioisotopic *In Situ* Hybridization for HDV RNA
Francesco Negro ***95***

12 Detection and Characterization of Small and Large HDV Antigens
Thomas B. Macnaughton and Michael M. C. Lai ***99***

13 Immunohistochemical Detection of Hepatitis Delta Antigen
Karim Abid and Francesco Negro ***107***

PART II. VIRAL GENOTYPES AND VARIANTS

14 HBV Vaccine-Escape Variants
Ashraf A. Basuni and William F. Carman ***115***

15 HBV Genotyping and Analysis for Unique Mutations
Anna Ayres, Stephan Locarnini, and Angeline Bartholomeusz ***125***

16 A One-Filter–Three-Probe Assay for Defective Interference (DI) Effects of Naturally Occurring Core Internal Deletion (CID) Variants of Human Hepatitis B Virus
Chiaho Shih and Ta-Tung Thomas Yuan ***151***

17 Detection of Hypermodified Middle-Envelope (M) Proteins Secreted from Naturally Occurring HBV Variants Containing a preS2 Internal Deletion
Chiaho Shih and Pei-Ching Tai ***165***

18 Hepatitis B Viral Genotyping with the Research INNO-LiPA HBV Genotyping Line Probe Assay
Sija De Gendt, Fred Shapiro, Jelena Juras, Els Van Assche, Geert Maertens, and Erwin Sablon ***175***

PART III. MOLECULAR BIOLOGICAL CHARACTERIZATION

19 Processing of Hepatitis B Virus Surface Proteins
Volker Bruss ***189***

20 Binding of Duck Carboxypeptidase D to Duck Hepatitis B Virus
Stephan Urban ***199***

21 Nucleoprotein Transport of HBV Capsid Particles
Michael Kann ***213***

22 Phosphorylation Analysis of Hepatitis B Virus Core Protein in Mammalian Cells
Jie Li, Yanyan Zheng, Jinah Choi, and Jing-hsiung Ou ***227***

23 Study of HBV Replication Capacity in Relation to Sequence Variation in the Precore and Core Promoter Regions
Fabien Zoulim, ShuPing Tong, and Christian Trépo ***235***

24 A *cis/trans* Genetic Test for Pleiotropic Phenotypes Associated with a Frequent Naturally Occurring Mutation at Amino Acid 97 of HBV Core Protein
Chiaho Shih and Ta-Tung Thomas Yuan ***247***

25 Studying DHBV Polymerase by In Vitro Transcription and Translation
Jianming Hu ***259***

26 Expression and Purification of Functional Hepatitis B Virus Polymerase in the Baculovirus Insect Cell System
Lisa Lott, Lena Notvall, and Robert E. Lanford ***271***

27 Localization of Duck Hepatitis B Virus Polymerase Within Cells
Ermei Yao and John E. Tavis ***281***

28 Endogenous Polymerase Assay for the Analysis of Hepatitis B Virus in Transgenic Mice
Zhenming Xu and Jing-hsiung Ou ***295***

29 Transcriptional Control of Hepatitis B Virus
Anneke K. Raney ***303***

30 In Vitro Reconstitution of ε-Dependent Duck Hepatitis B Virus Replication Initiation
Jürgen Beck and Michael Nassal ***315***

31 Hepatitis B Viruses: *A Triple Threat for Malignant Transformation of Hepatocytes*
Charles E. Rogler ***327***

Index ***339***

I

Viral-Specific Immunological and Other Host Responses

1

Studying Host Immune Responses Against Duck Hepatitis B Virus Infection

Darren S. Miller, Edward M. Bertram, Catherine A. Scougall, Ieva Kotlarski, and Allison R. Jilbert

1. Introduction

The duck hepatitis B virus (DHBV) is a species-specific virus that causes either transient (acute) or persistent infections, primarily in hepatocytes in the liver, with release of high titers of infectious virions and noninfectious "empty" surface antigen particles into the bloodstream.

Because hepadnavirus replication is noncytolytic, cell-mediated immune (CMI) responses to viral antigens are thought to be responsible for the clearance of virus from infected cells and for the liver damage seen in transient and persistent infections. This is presumed to occur via a direct, cytolytic effect of viral antigen-specific cytotoxic T lymphocytes (CTLs) on infected hepatocytes, or via the noncytopathic action of inflammatory cytokines. In addition, neutralizing antibodies have been shown to prevent infection by blocking the ability of virus particles to bind to receptors on target cells.

DHBV-infected ducks and woodchuck hepatitis virus (WHV)-infected woodchucks are the most widely accepted and frequently used animal models for the study of viral replication, infection outcomes, and the pathogenic mechanisms related to human hepatitis B virus (HBV) infection. Use of the DHBV model has allowed us to study the effects of viral dose, age, and inoculation route on the course of DHBV infection *(1–4)* and the effect of immunization with various forms of vaccine on all these parameters *(5)*. However, until recently, studies of the immune response to DHBV infection have been hampered by the relatively poor characterization of the duck lymphoid system and the lack of appropriate reagents. This chapter describes a number of assays that allow study of components of the duck immune system and the cellular and humoral immune responses to DHBV infection.

The chapter has been divided into three sections that include:

1. Purification and characterization of duck lymphocytes and thrombocytes from peripheral

From: *Methods in Molecular Medicine, vol. 96: Hepatitis B and D Protocols, volume 2*
Edited by: R. K. Hamatake and J. Y. N. Lau © Humana Press Inc., Totowa, NJ

blood *(6)* and conditions for in vitro growth and lectin stimulation of duck peripheral blood mononuclear cells (PBMCs; ***7,8***).
2. Histological methods for detection of cellular and viral antigens in duck tissues including identification of duck T lymphocytes using anti-human CD3ϵ antibodies ***(9)***, identification of Kupffer cells in the liver and phagocytic cells in the spleen, and detection of DHBV antigens in fixed tissues by immunoperoxidase staining.
3. Detection of viral antigens, DHBV-specific antibodies, and viral DNA in duck serum using enzyme-linked immunosorbent assays (ELISA) for DHBV surface antigen (DHBsAg), antibodies to DHBV surface antigen (anti-DHBs antibodies), antibodies to DHBV core antigen (anti-DHBc antibodies), and polymerase chain reaction (PCR) assays for detection of DHBV DNA.

These techniques provide the opportunity to study immune responses to DHBV but are by no means complete. For example, we have made numerous unsuccessful attempts to develop viral antigen-specific CTL assays but progress has been hampered by lack of suitable major histocompatibility class (MHC)-matched target cells. The recent cloning by Professor David Higgins and colleagues of a series of duck T-lymphocyte and cellular markers, that includes CD3, CD4, CD8, MHC I, and MHC II ***(10–13)***, should allow more comprehensive monitoring of immune responses to DHBV (*see* **Note 1**).

1.1. Purification and Characterization of Duck Lymphocytes and Thrombocytes from Peripheral Blood

Avian blood contains lymphocytes, monocytes, thrombocytes, red blood cells, heterophils, and eosinophils. Duck lymphocytes are round nongranular cells with large round nuclei and little cytoplasm and have a diameter of 4–8 μm ***(6)***. Duck monocytes are round cells with large, often indented, nuclei and with more cytoplasm than lymphocytes, although it can be difficult to distinguish one cell type from the other. Duck thrombocytes, which are essential for blood clotting, are of similar size to lymphocytes but are highly vacuolated, making it possible to distinguish them from lymphocytes using flow cytometry owing to their increased side scatter ***(6)***. Duck red blood cells (DRBCs) are nucleated and strictly ought to be considered as a subset of PBMCs. However, for the purposes of this chapter, duck PBMC preparations do not include DRBCs. They contain the mononuclear cells that can be separated from whole blood using Ficoll-Paque density gradients. DRBCs and heterophils pellet to the bottom of Ficoll-Paque gradients. Further information on avian hematology and photographs of the cell populations present in avian blood are available on the World Wide Web ***(14,15)***.

Most published reports of duck lymphocyte cultures have used PBMCs collected from Ficoll-Paque gradients including the cells present at the plasma–Ficoll-Paque interface and in the Ficoll-Paque above the DRBC pellet. PBMCs collected in this way include 22–26% T lymphocytes ***(9)*** and up to 60% thrombocytes, with the remainder not clearly identified, although most are likely to be B lymphocytes and monocytes.

Unlike the findings with mammalian and chicken lymphocytes, antibodies to duck immunoglobulins (Ig) bind to a large proportion of duck lymphocytes from blood, spleen, thymus, and bursa of Fabricius and therefore are not useful for identifying and isolating duck B lymphocytes ***(16)***. Moreover, monoclonal antibodies specific for determinants on mouse, rat, human, and chicken T lymphocytes do not react with duck lymphocytes (D. Higgins, personal communication). However, a rabbit antiserum that reacts with a conserved intracytoplasmic portion of the human CD3ε chain binds to duck lymphocytes with a staining pattern similar to that of mammalian T lymphocytes ***(6)***. These antibodies precipitate a 23-kDa protein from duck lymphoblast lysates, suggesting that duck lymphoid tissues contain lymphocytes functionally equivalent to mammalian and chicken T cells ***(6)***. Because the anti-human CD3ε antibodies are specific for an intracellular epitope, they cannot be used to identify and/or isolate viable cells. However, they have been used to identify a subset of duck lymphocytes by FACScan analysis (*see* **Subheading 3.1.2.** and **Fig. 1**). The CD3ε antibodies can also be used for immunostaining of lymphocytes in tissue sections (*see* **Subheading 3.2.1.**). Duck thrombocytes can be distinguished from lymphocytes by both flow cytometry (**Fig. 2A**) and FACScan analysis using the anti-duck thrombocyte BA3 monoclonal antibodies (subtype IgG2a; *see* **Subheading 3.1.3.**; **Fig. 2B**).

The methods described in **Subheading 3.1.4.** build on attempts in the 1980s to identify and separate duck lymphocytes into T and B cells ***(16)*** and to define conditions for the in vitro culture and optimization of responses to phytohemagglutinin (PHA) and concanavalin A (Con A) ***(17)***. We have further defined the in vitro culture conditions that support proliferation of duck lymphocytes. These include nylon wool fractionation of PBMCs, a technique that enriches for T lymphocytes in mammals and chickens, and coculturing nylon wool-fractionated duck PBMCs in the presence of homologous adherent cells (monocytes) and DRBC (***8,18***; **Subheading 3.1.4.**; **Fig. 3**).

Following culture of duck PBMCs large multinucleated syncytia are observed in approx 50% of cultures from 3–7 d of incubation. The presence of these syncytia often inhibits mitogen- and antigen-induced proliferation of the cells resulting in decreased incorporation of [^{3}H]thymidine. The syncytia are strikingly similar to osteoclasts that develop on culture of human ***(19)***, mouse ***(20)***, and chicken ***(21–23)*** PBMCs. Examples of duck syncytia are shown in **Fig. 4**.

Despite optimization of the in vitro proliferation assays described above, it is not yet possible to reproducibly detect proliferation of DHBV antigen-specific T lymphocytes from ducks immunized or infected with DHBV. Problems with reproducibility of the in vitro assays may, in part, be due to the development of syncytia and their inhibitory effects on lymphocyte proliferation. In any case, further efforts are required to standardize the assays before we can reliably measure CMI responses to DHBV infection.

Supernatants from PHA-stimulated duck PBMCs and spleen cells have also been shown to contain lymphokines capable of maintaining proliferation of duck lymphoblasts (*7*; *see* **Subheading 3.1.5.**). It is possible that supernatants from DHBV antigen-stimulated PBMCs from ducks previously infected with DHBV may contain cytokines equivalent to those released from mammalian and chicken T cells, which mediate CMI responses. Assays developed to detect such cytokines in culture supernatants may also prove to be useful in measuring CMI to DHBV.

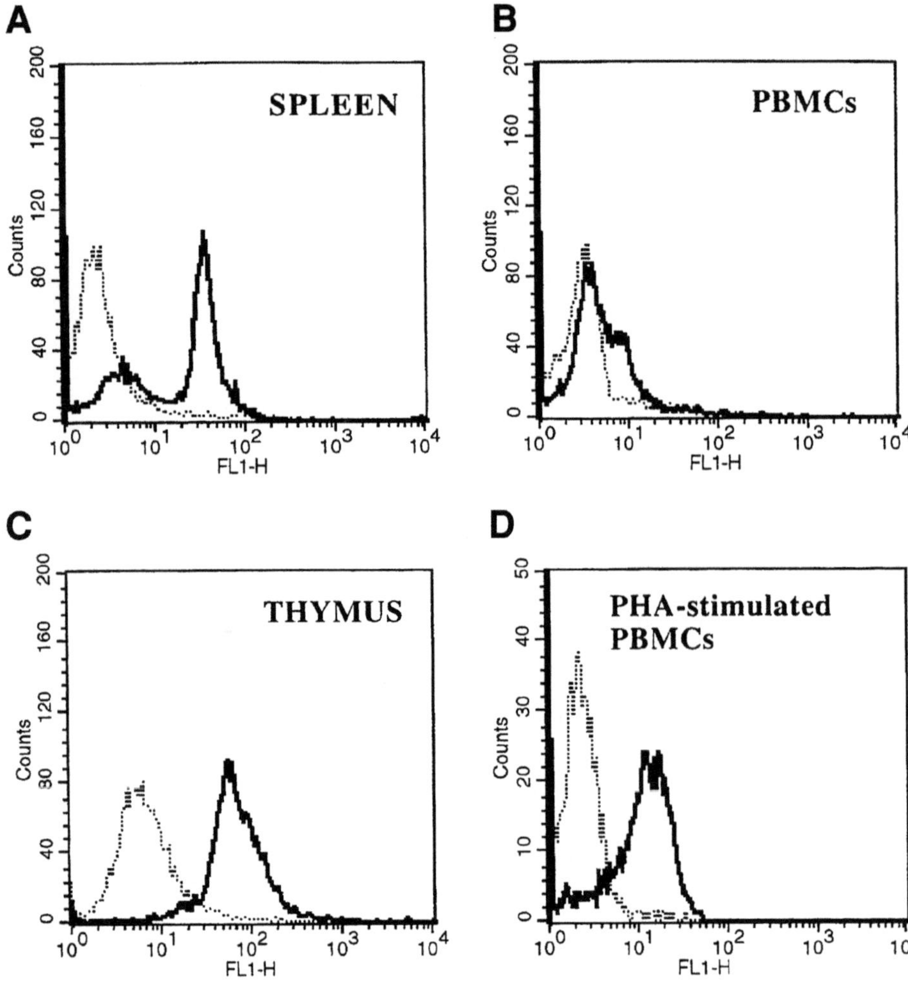

Fig. 1. FACScan analysis of single-cell suspensions of duck lymphoid organs. Cells were pretreated with acetone–paraformaldehyde and labeled with either rabbit anti-human CD3ε antiserum *(black line)* or the negative control rabbit anti-bovine myoglobin antiserum *(gray line)* before the addition of FITC-conjugated sheep anti-rabbit IgG as described in the text.

1.2. Histological Methods for Detection of Cellular and Viral Antigens in Duck Tissues

Histological and immunostaining techniques have been developed for the identification of duck T lymphocytes, Kupffer cells, and phagocytic cells in a range of tissues, and for the detection of DHBV antigens in liver, pancreas, kidney, and spleen. Using these techniques it is possible to monitor infected tissues for changes in cellular infiltra-

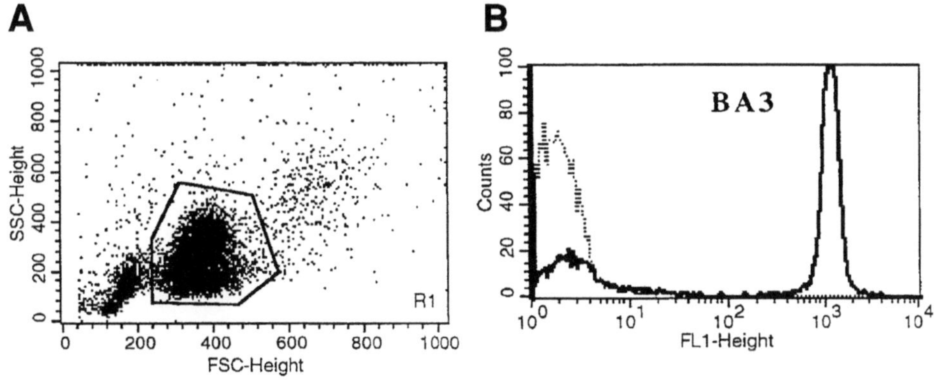

Fig. 2. FACScan analysis of duck PBMCs. Dot plot of duck PBMC (**A**). The gated region was analyzed further using the anti-duck thrombocyte BA3 monoclonal antibodies *(black line)* or a negative control monoclonal antibodies before the addition of FITC-conjugated sheep anti-mouse IgG (**B**). The cell populations in the gated region of **A** were also separated on a FACStar cell sorter *(data not shown)* and were morphologically identified as thrombocytes (with increased side scatter) and lymphocytes (with decreased side scatter).

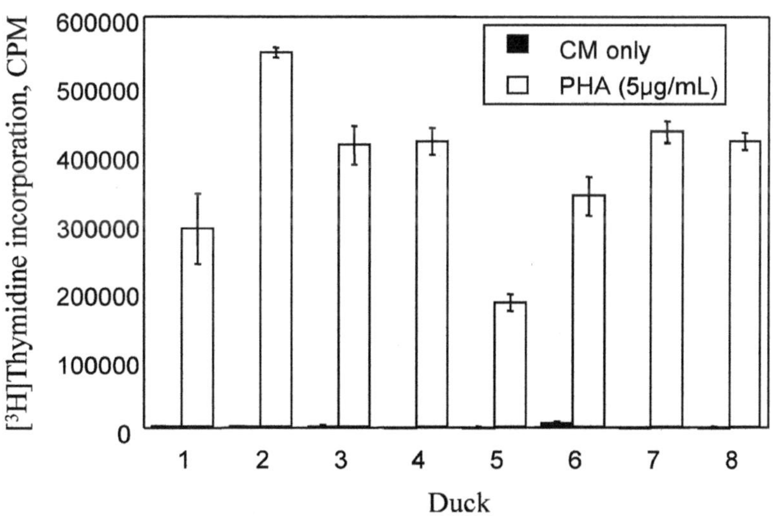

Fig. 3. Comparison of duck in vitro T-cell responses to PHA. Eight different ducks were bled and stimulation of their T lymphocytes by PHA (5 μg/mL) was measured following the method described in the text.

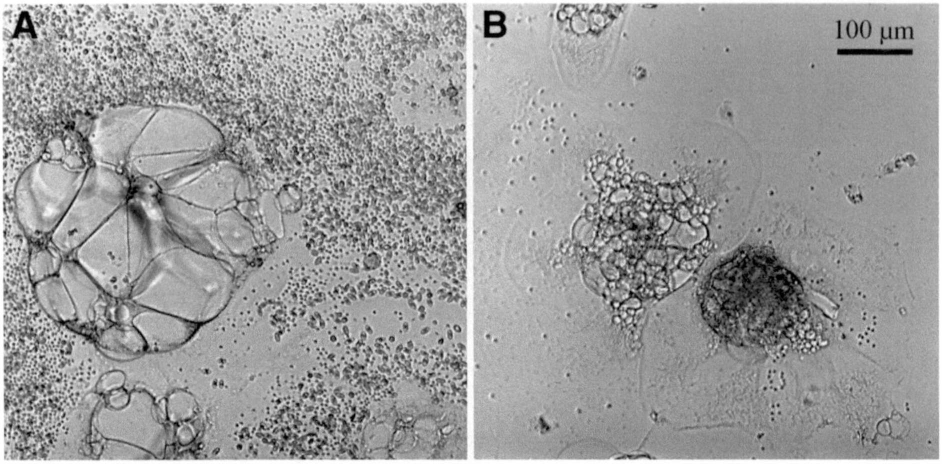

Fig. 4. Demonstration of giant cells (syncytia) in cultures of duck PBMCs (**A**) and adherent cells alone (**B**) following 5 d of culture as described in **Subheading 3.1.4.** and **Note 8.** In addition to the very large syncytia, DRBC and T lymphocytes can also be seen in **A.** Bar = 100 μm. Final magnification = × 90.5.

tion and viral expression, and relate these to the development of viraemia and antibody responses in the bloodstream ***(3)***.

Duck T lymphocytes can be detected in sections of formalin-fixed tissues using anti-human CD3ϵ antibodies (*see* **Subheading 3.2.2.**). Phagocytic cells can be identified in duck liver and spleen by intravenous inoculation of ducks with colloidal carbon followed by histological identification of carbon containing cells (*see* **Subheading 3.2.3.**). In the liver the phagocytic Kupffer cells are located within the hepatic sinusoids **(Fig. 5A)**, while the phagocytic cells present in the spleen are present around the periellipsoid sheath in a similar location to the ellipsoid-associated cells described in chicken spleen ***(24,25)***. Phagocytic cells in duck liver and spleen can also be identified in sections of ethanol-fixed tissues using mouse monoclonal antibodies, 2E.12, raised against duck liver and kindly supplied to us by Dr. John Pugh. This reagent identifies both Kupffer cells in the liver **(Fig. 5B)** and ellipsoid-associated cells in the spleen. Similar reagents that detect Kupffer and ellipsoid-associated cells have been described for the chicken ***(26,27)***. DHBV-infected cells can be identified in ethanol–acetic acid fixed tissues using polyclonal rabbit anti-recombinant DHBV core antigen (rDHBcAg; ***1***) and anti-DHBV pre-S/S monoclonal antibodies (1H.1; ***28***).

The primary cell type in the liver supporting DHBV replication is the hepatocyte, and high levels of viral antigens and viral DNA can readily be detected in the cytoplasm of infected cells within the liver lobule **(Fig. 5C)**. We have found no evidence that Kupffer or endothelial cells support DHBV replication ***(1–3)***; DHBV antigens and DHBV DNA have been detected within Kupffer cells only during the clearance phase of acute,

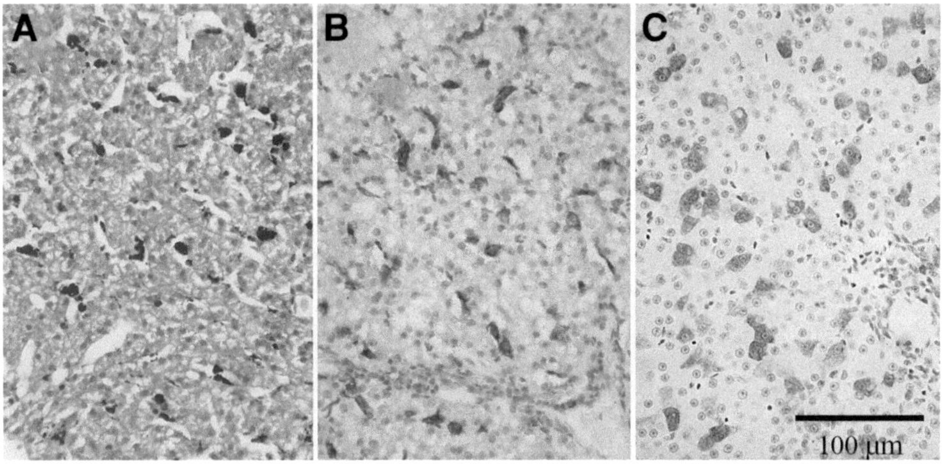

Fig. 5. **(A)** A section of formalin-fixed duck liver collected at autopsy 24 h after intravenous inoculation with 165 mg/kg body wt of colloidal carbon. Phagocytic (Kupffer) cells located within the hepatic sinusoids have taken up carbon. Counterstained with hematoxylin and eosin. **(B)**. Section of ethanol-fixed duck liver after immunostaining with the 2E.12 monoclonal antibodies specific for duck Kupffer and phagocytic cells. Stained cells are located within the hepatic sinusoids. Counterstained with hematoxylin. **(C)** A section of ethanol–acetic acid fixed duck liver collected from an adult duck (B47) 5 d following intravenous inoculation with a high dose of DHBV. Detection of DHBV pre-S/S antigen in the cytoplasm of hepatocytes using anti-DHBV pre-S/S monoclonal antibodies (1H.1). Counterstained with hematoxylin. Bar = 100 µm. Final magnification **A–C** = × 163.

transient DHBV infections or following challenge of immune ducks with high doses of DHBV (*3*; A. Jilbert, unpublished data).

1.3. Detection of Antigens, Antibodies, and Viral DNA in Duck Serum

Antibody responses to the HBV surface, core, and e antigens have been detected in the sera of humans following transient HBV infection. Anti-surface (anti-HBs) antibodies are a marker of resolution of transient HBV infection. In chronic HBV infection, antibodies to the viral surface proteins are generally not detected in serum, although it is possible their presence is masked by the formation of immune complexes with surface antigen particles. Antibodies to the HBV core protein (anti-HBc antibodies) can be readily detected in the sera of patients with chronic HBV infection as can antibodies to e antigen (anti-HBe antibodies) that develop following seroconversion from e antigenemia. Anti-HBe antibodies are unable to neutralize viral infectivity.

ELISAs have been developed for quantitation of DHBsAg **(Fig. 6)** and detection of anti-DHBs **(Fig. 7A)** and anti-DHBc **(Fig. 7B)** antibodies. In the DHBsAg ELISA rabbit anti-DHBs antibodies (*see* **Subheading 3.3.1.**) are used to coat the plates and capture DHBsAg from duck serum samples. Bound DHBsAg is then detected using anti-DHBV pre-S/S monoclonal antibodies (1H.1; *28*). In the anti-DHBs ELISA the

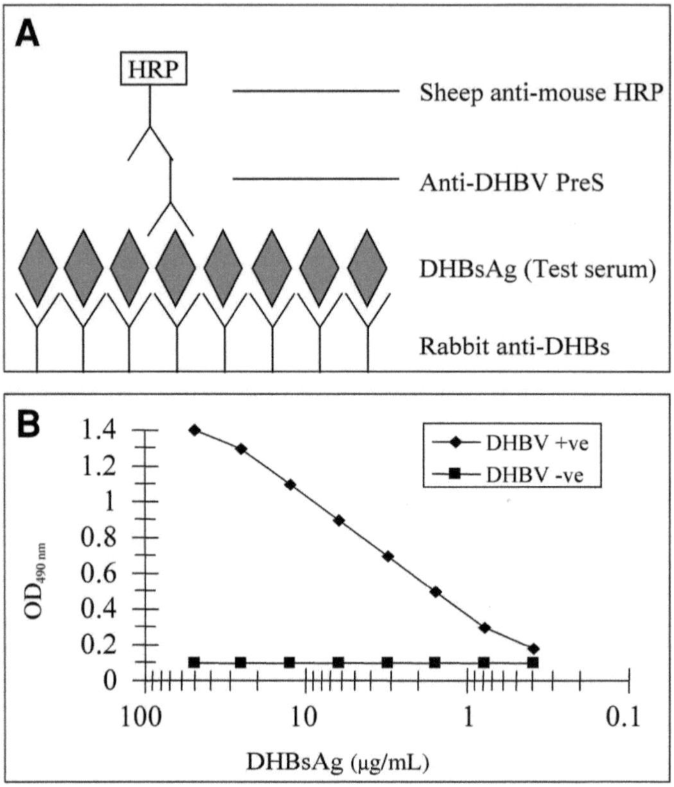

Fig. 6. (**A**) Diagrammatic representation of the quantitative ELISA used to detect DHBsAg in duck sera. (**B**) A typical standard curve for the quantitative DHBsAg ELISA generated using high titer DHBV-positive duck serum and NDS (negative control). The levels of DHBsAg in test samples are calculated using the standard curves. The cutoff for negative/positive results is set at three times the standard deviation from the mean value obtained with NDS.

plates are coated with 1H.1, followed by sucrose gradient purified DHBsAg to capture the antibodies, and bound antibodies are detected using rabbit anti-duck IgY. In the anti-DHBc ELISA plates are coated with rDHBcAg ***(1)***, and bound antibodies are again detected using rabbit anti-duck IgY antibodies. Rabbit anti-duck IgY antibodies are prepared by immunization of rabbits with duck IgY from egg yolk (***18***; *see* **Subheadings 3.3.2.** and **3.3.3.**). The ELISAs for detection of anti-DHBs and anti-DHBc antibodies thus detect total bound Ig and allow investigation of the overall humoral responses to DHBV infection ***(2–5)*** but do not distinguish between IgM, IgY, and IgY (ΔFc) ***(29)*** subtype antibodies.

In congenitally DHBV-infected ducks, anti-DHBc antibodies can be detected in the serum from approx 80 d post-hatch ***(4)***, while in experimentally DHBV-infected ducks anti-DHBc antibodies are detected from as early as 7–10 d post-inoculation and

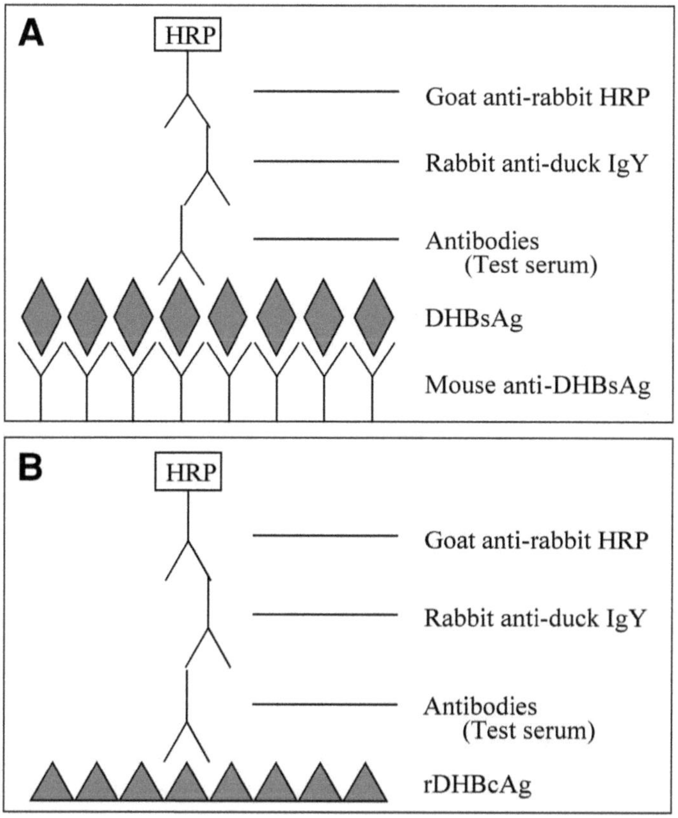

Fig. 7. (**A**) Diagrammatic representation of the ELISA used to detect anti-DHBs antibodies. Levels of anti-DHBs antibodies are expressed as the reciprocal of the log serum dilution that gives an OD of 0.4 at an absorbance of 490 nm. (**B**) Diagrammatic representation of the ELISA used to detect anti-DHBc antibodies. Levels of anti-DHBc antibodies are expressed as the reciprocal of the log serum dilution that gave an OD of 0.5 at an absorbance of 490 nm.

persist throughout the course of infection *(4)*. Anti-DHBs antibodies are detected at high levels only in the sera of ducks that have resolved their DHBV infection, but can also be detected at low levels in the sera of congenitally and experimentally DHBV-infected ducks with persistent DHBV infection (Wendy Foster, personal communication). In this case anti-DHBs antibodies may be masked by the formation of immune complexes between the anti-DHBs antibodies and circulating DHBsAg.

Detailed analyses of humoral immune responses to DHBV infection have been performed in 4-mo-old ducks inoculated with 1×10^3, 1×10^6, 1×10^9 or 2×10^{11} DHBV genomes *(3)*. In these studies increasing the dose of inoculated virus shortened the time to appearance and increased the levels of detectable antibodies. An increase in the inoculum from 1×10^9 to 2×10^{11} DHBV genomes resulted in >1 log increases in anti-

DHBc antibodies that reflected the extensive infection of the liver observed in these ducks on d 9–12 post-inoculation. Two of the three 4-mo-old ducks receiving the highest dose of virus were able to resolve their DHBV infection, and developed anti-DHBs antibodies.

2. Materials

2.1. Purification and Characterization of Duck Lymphocytes and Thrombocytes from Peripheral Blood

2.1.1. Solutions

1. Ficoll-Paque (Pharmacia, Uppsala, Sweden).
2. Hanks' balanced salt solution (HBSS), supplemented with 100 IU/mL of penicillin and 100 μg/mL of streptomycin, is used to prepare and wash cell suspensions.
3. Heat-inactivated (20 min at 56°C) normal duck serum (NDS): Each batch of NDS is tested to ensure that it does not stimulate or maintain proliferation of duck lymphocytes when added to culture medium.
4. Cell culture medium (CM): RPMI-1640 (Gibco Laboratories, Grand Island, NY) with 2 mmol/L of L-glutamine, 0.1 mmol/L of β-mercaptoethanol, 5 μg/mL of indomethacin, and 5% NDS (*see* **Note 2**).
5. PBS: 0.1 *M* phosphate-buffered saline, pH 7.2.
6. P/B/A: PBS with 0.1% bovine serum albumin (BSA), 0.1 % azide.
7. P/A: PBS with 0.1% azide.
8. Trypan blue for viable cell counting.
9. Phytohemagglutinin-P (PHA; Difco, Michigan, USA) is used for stimulation of duck lymphocytes and is made up as a stock of 1 mg/mL in PBS.
10. Rabbit anti-human CD3ε antiserum (DAKO, Denmark, cat. no. A 452) is an affinity-isolated polyclonal antiserum. It reacts to amino acids 156–168 (intracellular) of the human CD3ε chain and cross-reacts with duck T cells.
11. Intracellular staining solution: 45% acetone, 9.25% paraformaldehyde in PBS.
12. Normal sheep serum (NSS).
13. Fluorescein isothiocyanate (FITC)–anti-rabbit IgG and FITC–anti-mouse IgG (Silenus).
14. Cell culture supernatant from the cell line BA3, producing monoclonal antibodies specific for duck thrombocytes (the cell line is available from the authors on request).
15. 1% Paraformaldehyde in PBS.
16. [^{3}H]Thymidine, 1 μCi/50 μL of CM (Amersham).

2.1.2. Equipment

1. 10-mL syringes with 21-gauge needles.
2. Heparinized 10-mL blood collection tubes.
3. 10- and 50-mL centrifuge tubes.
4. Benchtop centrifuge (200–400*g*).
5. Biohazard hood.
6. Tissue culture quality pipets and pipettor (1 μL–10 mL volumes).
7. Hemocytometer and microscope.
8. Nylon wool columns: Each nylon wool (NW; Pacific Diagnostics) column consisted of 0.32 g of sterile NW in a 5-mL syringe wrapped in aluminum foil and autoclaved.
9. Parafilm.

10. 24-well tissue culture trays (Corning, cat. no. 25820).
11. 96-well tissue culture trays (Falcon, cat. no. 3072).
12. 25-cm^2 tissue culture flasks (Corning, cat. no. 25100-25).
13. Humidified incubator set at 37°C.
14. Flow cytometry tubes.
15. Flow cytometer (FACscan, Becton-Dickinson).
16. Tray shaker (Titertek).
17. Flow cell harvester (Flow Laboratories).
18. Glass fiber discs (Flow Laboratories).
19. β-counter (Beckman).

2.1.3. Samples for Study

Pekin-Aylesbury (*Anas platyrhynchos*) crossbred ducks were used for all experiments and were obtained at 1 d of age from commercial duck suppliers in Australia known to carry DHBV-negative or congenitally DHBV-infected ducks.

2.2. Histological Methods for Detection of Cellular and Viral Antigens in Duck Tissues

2.2.1. Solutions

1. 10% buffered formalin in PBS.
2. Glacial acetic acid (AR grade).
3. Xylene (AR grade—**toxic and must be used in a fume hood**).
4. Ethanol (AR grade; 100%) and diluted with distilled water to 95% and 70%.
5. PBS, pH 7.2.
6. Methanol (AR grade).
7. 10 m*M* Citrate buffer, pH 6.0.
8. Trypsin (grade II, 0.25 mg/mL) in PBS, pH 7.2.
9. Normal horse serum (NHS).
10. Rabbit anti-human CD3ϵ antiserum (DAKO, Denmark, cat. no. A 452).
11. Normal rabbit serum (NRS) for use as a negative control.
12. Monoclonal anti-duck DHBV pre-S/S antibodies (1H.1; *28*).
13. Monoclonal anti-duck Kupffer cell antibodies, 2E.12 (provided by Dr. John Pugh).
14. Polyclonal rabbit anti-recombinant DHBV core antigen (rDHBcAg) *(1)*.
15. Biotin–anti-rabbit Ig (Vectorstain ABC kit, Burlingame, CA, USA).
16. Streptavidin–horseradish peroxidase (HRP) (Vectorstain ABC kit, Burlingame, CA, USA).
17. Sheep anti-mouse HRP (Amersham, cat. no. NA 9310).
18. Goat anti-rabbit antiserum HRP (Kirkegaard and Perry Laboratories, Gaithersburg, MD).
19. 0.5 mg/mL of diaminobenzidine tetrahydrochloride (DAB; Sigma, cat. no. D-5637) in PBS. **Caution: DAB is toxic and the powder must be handled with care and dissolved and aliquoted in a fume hood.** Store frozen at –20°C.
20. H_2O_2.
21. Mayer's hematoxylin solution.
22. Methyl green.
23. DePeX mounting medium (Gurr Microscopy Products).

24. Colloidal carbon prepared from Indian ink (Educational Colours, Melbourne) should be dialyzed against saline and autoclaved, then mixed with 20 mg/mL of autoclaved gelatin in saline at 56°C. Finally, the carbon–gelatin mix should be filtered through a 0.8-μm filter to remove any clumps.
25. Fetal calf serum (FCS).

2.2.2. Equipment

1. Glass slides and coverslips.
2. Slide racks.
3. Slide staining chambers.
4. Magnetic stirrer and stirring rods.
5. Microwaves: Toshiba 1000 W and NEC (model 702).
6. "PAP pen" (Dakopatts, USA).
7. Humidified chamber.
8. Incubator set at 37°C.

2.3. Detection of Antigens, Antibodies, and Viral DNA in Duck Serum

2.3.1. Solutions

1. TBS: 10 m*M* Tris-HCl, pH 8.7; 140 m*M* NaCl, with 0.1% sodium azide.
2. 1% (w/v) dextran sulfate in TBS.
3. TN: 10 m*M* Tris-HCl, pH 7.4; 150 m*M* NaCl.
4. 66% (w/v) sucrose solutions in TN.
5. 1 *M* Tris-HCl, pH 9.0.
6. Saturated sodium sulfate solution.
7. Saturated ammonium sulfate solution.
8. PBS containing 0.05% Tween-20 (PBS/T).
9. 5% SM–PBS/T: 5% Skim milk in PBS/T.
10. *o*-Phenylenediamine (OPD) (Sigma, cat. no. P9187).
11. 0.1% BSA in PBS.
12. 2.5 *M* H_2SO_4.
13. Recombinant DHBV core antigen (rDHBcAg) ***(1)***.
14. Sheep anti-mouse HRP (Amersham, cat. no. NA 9310).
15. Anti-DHBV pre-S/S monoclonal antibodies (1H.1; ***28***).
16. Rabbit anti-duck IgY antibodies (*see* **Subheading 3.3.3.**).
17. Ammonium sulfate precipitated rabbit anti-DHBs antibodies (*see* **Subheading 3.3.4.**).
18. Goat anti-rabbit HRP (Kirkegaard and Perry Laboratories, Gaithsburg, MD).
19. 20% Polyethylene glycol 6000 (PEG) dissolved in 1 *M* NaCl.
20. 0.7% NaOH.
21. 3-Aminopropyl-triethoxysilane (Sigma, cat. no. A3648).
22. PCR reagents: 20 μ*M* of each primer, 10X PCR reaction buffer, 200 μ*M* dNTPs, 1.64 m*M* $MgCl_2$, *Taq* polymerase (Geneworks, Adelaide, cat. no. BTQ-1).
23. Forward PCR primer 2554: TTCGGAGCTGCCTGCCAAGG.
24. Reverse PCR primer 269c: GGAGCACCTGAGCTTGGATC.
25. 500 m*M* Tris-HCl, pH 6.8.
26. 0.06 *M* acetate buffer, pH 4.0. (Add 6.9 mL of glacial acetic acid to 2 L of distilled water. Add 0.756 g of NaOH).

2.3.2. Equipment

1. Dialysis tubing.
2. Whatman No. 1 paper.
3. Whatman No. 2 paper.
4. Beckman L8-80 centrifuge.
5. 50-mL polycarbonate Oakridge tubes.
6. Polypropylene centrifuge tubes (Beckman, cat. no. 331372).
7. Beckman SW-41 rotor and centrifuge.
8. 96-well flat-bottom ELISA trays (Corning Inc., cat. no. Costar 3590).
9. Dynatech MR 5000 plate reader set at a wavelength of 490 nm.
10. Microfuge.
11. Microfuge tubes.
12. Gene Amp 2400 PCR machine (Perkin Elmer).
13. Bicinchoninic acid protein assay kit (Sigma, cat. no. BCA-1).

3. Methods

3.1. Methods for Purification and Characterization of Duck Lymphocytes and Thrombocytes from Peripheral Blood

3.1.1. Purification of PBMCs

1. Using a 21-gauge needle and a 10-mL syringe collect 10–20 mL of blood from the jugular vein of a duck and dilute into an equal volume of HBSS in heparinized collection tubes. Mix well. (*See* **Note 3**.)
2. Carefully layer 3 mL of diluted blood over 3 mL of Ficoll-Paque at 4°C.
3. Centrifuge at 200*g* for 20 min at room temperature (RT) and collect the PBMCs present both at the plasma Ficoll-Paque interface and within the Ficoll-Paque layer above the red cell pellet. (*See* **Note 4**.)
4. Wash cells three times in HBSS and count cell numbers of the collected PBMCs using a hemocytometer and a microscope with a × 40 objective.
5. For nylon wool fractionated PBMCs, equilibrate each nylon wool column by adding CM, seal the ends with parafilm, and incubate for 1 h at 37°C. Make sure there are no air pockets in the column.
6. Load 5×10^7 duck PBMCs in 1.25 mL of CM warmed to 37°C onto each nylon wool column and incubate at 37°C in an atmosphere of 5% CO_2 in air. Collect the cells that do not adhere to nylon wool by washing each column with 6.5 mL of CM warmed to 37°C. Count the cells and resuspend in CM to the appropriate concentration. (*See* **Note 5**.)

3.1.2. Flow Cytometry Detection of T Lymphocytes by Intracellular Staining for CD3ε

1. Wash 10^7 PBMCs (from **Subheading 3.1.1., step 4**) two times in PBS by centrifuging at 200*g* for 8 min at 4°C, then remove the supernatant and carefully add a solution containing 45% acetone, 9.25% paraformaldehyde in PBS. Vortex-mix for 10 s, then wash three times with cold P/B/A. Treatment with this solution will make the cells permeable to antibodies; however, this process will also lead to some cell loss.
2. An indirect method is used to stain the cells. Incubate the cells with rabbit anti-human CD3ε antiserum (1:50 dilution) or NRS in P/B/A containing 10% NSS for 45 min at 4°C.

3. Wash the cells in P/B/A and incubate with FITC-conjugated sheep anti-rabbit IgG (1:100 dilution preadsorbed for 60 min by the addition of 10% NDS) for 45 min at 4°C.
4. Wash the cells once in P/B/A at 4°C, then once in P/A at 4°C, and then add 500 μL of 1% paraformaldehyde in PBS to the cell pellet. Paraformaldehyde-fixed cells can be stored for several weeks at 4°C or analyzed immediately by FACScan (Becton-Dickinson).
5. Examples of FACScan analysis of single cell suspensions of duck lymphoid organs and PHA-stimulated PBMCs stained with rabbit anti-human CD3ϵ antiserum are shown in **Fig. 1**.

3.1.3. Flow Cytometry Detection of Thrombocytes Using BA3 Monoclonal Antibodies

1. Wash 10^6 PBMCs two times in P/B/A and incubate with cell culture supernatant from the mouse hybridoma cell line BA3 containing 10% NSS for 45 min at 4°C.
2. Wash the cells two times in P/B/A and incubate with FITC-conjugated sheep anti-mouse Ig (1:100 dilution preadsorbed for 60 min by the addition of 10% NDS) for 45 min at 4°C and wash and fix in 1% paraformaldehyde before FACScan analysis as described above.
3. Alternatively, if BA3 monoclonal antibodies are not available, flow cytometry can be used to identify thrombocytes from lymphocytes by their increased side scatter. FACScan analysis of duck PBMCs and detection of thrombocytes with BA3 monoclonal antibodies is shown in **Fig. 2**.

3.1.4. Conditions for In Vitro Growth and Lectin Stimulation of Duck PBMCs

1. Purification of adherent cells (monocytes): Load 8×10^5 duck PBMCs in 50 μL of CM onto each well of a flat-bottomed 96-well tray and incubate for 1 h at 37°C in 5% CO_2. Shake trays for 30 s on a tray shaker and remove the nonadherent cells. Wash the wells two times with 200 μL of CM.
2. Purification of DRBC: Take 0.1 mL of DRBCs from the pellet beneath the Ficoll-Paque solution used to prepare duck PBMCs. Wash the DRBC three times in HBSS and resuspend in CM to 4×10^6 cells/mL for use in the in vitro proliferation assay. (*See* **Note 6**.)
3. Add 8×10^5 cells/well of nylon wool fractionated duck PBMCs in 100 μL of CM to the adherent monocytes in each well of a 96-well tray. Add 4×10^5 DRBCs/well in 50 μL and culture with 5 μg/mL of PHA in CM. (*See* **Note 7**.)
4. Culture cells for 4–6 d at 37°C in sealed boxes in a gas phase of 10% CO_2, 7% O_2, and 83% N_2. Proliferation is measured by addition of 50 μL of CM containing 1 μCi of [^{3}H]thymidine to each well and incubating for a further 4 h. (*See* **Note 8**.)
5. Harvest cells onto glass fiber discs using a flow cell harvester. The amount of radioactivity incorporated is measured using a β-counter. The results are expressed as counts per minute (cpm; mean ± SEM) for each quadruplicate set of cultures.
6. A comparison of the in vitro T cell responses of PBMCs from eight different ducks to 5 μg/mL of PHA is shown in **Fig. 3**.

3.1.5. Measurement of a Duck Interleukin-2 (IL-2)-Like Cytokine

1. Production of a duck IL-2-like cytokine: Take 10^8 Ficoll-Paque fractionated PBMCs prepared from individual ducks and resuspend in 5 mL of CM containing 20 μg/mL of PHA and incubate in 25-cm^2 flasks at 37°C in 10% CO_2 in air for 2.5 h. Duck PBMCs, in the presence of PHA, behave like mammalian PBMCs in that most of the cells readily adhere to the plastic surface after settling in the flask. Wash the cells that have attached to the flask three times in warm HBSS to remove unbound PHA and incubate them with 5 mL of fresh CM at 37°C in 10% CO_2 in air for a further 24 h. Harvest the supernatant from each culture and store at

−20°C to assay for the ability to maintain the proliferation of duck lymphoblasts (described in **step 3** below).

2. Production of duck T lymphoblasts: Culture 8 × 10^6 Ficoll-Paque fractionated duck PBMCs in each well of a 24-well tray in 2 mL of CM with 5 μg/mL of PHA. After 4 d in culture at 37°C in a sealed box in a gas phase of 10% CO_2, 7% O_2, and 83% N_2, pool lymphoblasts and wash four times in CM before resuspending at 2.5 × 10^5 cells/mL in CM.
3. Cytokine assay: Prepare duplicate 8 × twofold dilutions of each test supernatant in 100-μL volumes in CM in a 96-well tray. Add 100 μL of freshly prepared duck T lymphoblasts to each well and incubate for 20 h at 37°C in an atmosphere of 5% CO_2 in air. At this time pulse the tray for 4 h with [^{3}H]thymidine and measure cell proliferation as described above.

3.2. Histological Methods for Detection of Cellular and Viral Antigens in Duck Tissues

3.2.1. Tissue Sample Preparation for Histological and Immunoperoxidase Staining of T Lymphocytes, Kupffer Cells, and DHBV Antigens (*See* **Note 9**)

1. For routine histological examination and immunostaining of CD3ε antigens, fix tissue samples in 10% formalin in PBS overnight at RT.
2. For the immunostaining of Kupffer cells in the liver and phagocytic cells in the spleen, fix tissue samples in 95% AR ethanol for 1 h at RT then overnight at 4°C.
3. For the immunostaining of DHBV antigens in liver and other tissues, fix samples in ethanol–acetic acid (3:1) for 30 min at RT followed by a post-fixation in 70% AR ethanol overnight at 4°C.
4. Embed tissues, post-fixation, in paraffin wax using a short cycle on an automatic tissue processing machine (a representative short cycle is: 100% ethanol for 1 × 20 min, 1 × 10 min, 1 × 15 min, 1 × 30 min at 45°C with vacuum; 100% chloroform, 1 × 20 min, 1 × 10 min, 1 × 20 min at 45°C without vacuum; paraffin wax, 1 × 30 min, 1 × 20 min at 65°C with vacuum).
5. Section the embedded tissue at a thickness of 6 μm onto glass microscope slides previously coated with 3-aminopropyltriethoxysilane.
6. Dry the tissue sections on slides overnight at 37°C prior to use to help with adherence of the sections to the slides.

3.2.2. Identification of Duck T Lymphocytes in Tissue Sections Using Anti-human CD3ε Polyclonal Antibodies

1. Dewax sections of formalin-fixed, paraffin-wax-embedded tissues from duck liver, spleen, thymus, and bursa in AR xylene (2 × 5 min) and rehydrate through graded concentrations of AR ethanol (2 min each in 100%, 95%, 70%) followed by 2 min in PBS.
2. Treat sections for 30 min with 0.5% H_2O_2 in PBS to block endogenous peroxidase.
3. After air-drying, wash sections several times in deionized water and heat to just below boiling point in a microwave oven for 10 min in 10 m*M* citrate buffer, pH 6.0. (*See* **Note 10**.)
4. Cool sections to RT (approx 25 min) and treat with trypsin (grade II, 0.25 mg/mL in PBS) for 3 min.
5. "PAP" pen around the sections and place in PBS for 5 min
6. Block the sections with 3% NHS for 30 min at RT.
7. Drain excess NHS and add 100 μL per section of either rabbit anti-human CD3ε antiserum or rabbit control antiserum (each diluted in 3% NHS in PBS), and incubate under a coverslip and in a humidified chamber overnight at 4°C. (*See* **Note 11**.)

8. Wash sections 2 × 3 min in PBS and incubate with biotin-labeled anti-rabbit Ig for 30 min.
9. Wash sections 2 × 3 min in PBS and incubate with streptavidin-labeled HRP for 30 min.
10. Wash sections 2 × 3 min in PBS and develop with 0.5 mg/mL of DAB in PBS containing 0.03% H_2O_2.
11. Counterstain in Mayer's hematoxylin for liver and spleen and methyl green for thymus and bursa, then dehydrate through AR ethanol and AR xylene and mount with DePeX.

3.2.3. Identification of Kupffer Cells in the Liver and Phagocytic Cells in the Spleen Using Colloidal Carbon

1. Intravenously inoculate the duck with 165 mg/kg body wt of colloidal carbon in 20 mg/mL of gelatin saline.
2. Autopsy the duck 24 or 48 h after injection.
3. Sample liver and spleen tissues and fix in 10% formalin or 95% AR ethanol and embed and section onto glass slides as described above.
4. Cells that have taken up colloidal carbon can be identified in formalin-fixed hematoxylin and eosin stained sections as phagocytic Kupffer cells located in the sinusoids of the liver lobule **(Fig. 5A)** and as phagocytic cells located in the periellipsoid sheath region of the spleen. Phagocytic cells have been previously identified in chicken spleen as ellipsoid associated cells ***(24,25)***.

3.2.4. Immunoperoxidase Staining of DHBV Antigens and Kupffer Cells in Tissue Sections

1. Dewax tissue sections on slides with 2 × 5 min washes in AR xylene and then rehydrate with 2 × 2 min washes in AR ethanol (100%, 90%, 70%) followed by 2 × 5 min washes in PBS.
2. Inactivate endogenous peroxidase by incubation of the slides in 0.5% H_2O_2 in PBS for 15 min at RT.
3. Wash slides for 2 × 5 min in PBS and block with a 1:30 dilution of NSS in PBS. Incubate for 30 min at RT.
4. Primary antibodies: Monoclonal anti-DHBV pre-S/S (1H.1; ***28***), monoclonal anti-Kupffer cell, 2E.12 or polyclonal rabbit anti-rDHBcAg antibodies. Dilute each of the primary antibodies to 1:100 in PBS containing 10% FCS. Incubate each tissue section under a coverslip with 100 μL of the diluted antibodies for 1 h at 37°C and then at 4°C overnight. (*See* **Note 11**.) Wash slides 2 × 5 min in PBS.
5. Add the sheep anti-mouse HRP-conjugated secondary antibodies or the goat anti-rabbit HRP conjugated antibodies at a dilution of 1:40 in PBS containing 10% FCS. Incubate slides at 37°C for 1 h. Wash slides 2 × 5 min in PBS.
6. Develop the slides by the addition of DAB solution (1 mL or 0.5 mg/mL of DAB, 12.5 μL of 30% H_2O_2, 10 mL of PBS) for 9 min at RT in the dark.
7. Wash with PBS and counterstain with Mayer's hematoxylin for 1 min.
8. Remove excess hematoxylin from slides with 3 × 2 min washes in PBS.
9. Dehydrate slides with 2 × 2 min washes in AR ethanol (70%, 90%, 100%) and 2 × 5 min washes in xylene.
10. Finally, mount sections under coverslips in DePeX.
11. Cells that react with the 2E.12 monoclonal antibodies can be identified in ethanol-fixed and hematoxylin counterstained sections as Kupffer cells located in the hepatic sinusoids **(Fig. 5B)**.
12. DHBV-infected hepatocytes can be identified in ethanol–acetic acid fixed sections of duck liver using the 1H.1 monoclonal antibodies **(Fig. 5C)** or polyclonal anti-rDHBcAg antibod-

ies. Infected cells are randomly scattered throughout the liver lobule and viral surface and core antigens are detected in the cytoplasm but not in the nucleus of infected cells.

3.3. Methods for Detection of Antigens, Antibodies, and Viral DNA in Duck Serum

3.3.1. Preparation of DHBsAg for Immunization of Rabbits and as Capture Antigen for the Anti-DHBs ELISA

1. Load 5-mL samples of high-titer DHBV-positive duck sera onto 5 mL of a 20% (w/v) sucrose in TN that has been underlaid with a 500-μL cushion of 66% (w/v) sucrose in TN.
2. Place tubes in a SW-41 rotor and centrifuge at 190,000*g* for 4 h at 4°C.
3. Following centrifugation, collect 500-μL fractions from the bottom of the tubes.
4. When used as a capture antigen for detection of anti-DHBS antibodies, DHBsAg is prepared by pooling fractions 2–6 from the gradients and diluting to 5 mL with 0.1% BSA in PBS.
5. DHBsAg to be used as an immunogen for antibody production must be further purified; load 2 mL of fractions 2–6 containing DHBsAg onto a linear sucrose gradient consisting of 20–40% (w/v) sucrose in TN.
6. Centrifuge for 3 h at 190,000*g* at 4°C.
7. Following centrifugation, collect 500-μL fractions from the bottom of the gradient.
8. Electrophorese 50 μL from each fraction on a denaturing polyacrylamide gel to determine which fraction contains the most DHBsAg with the least amount of contaminating protein.
9. Use the purified DHBsAg for the immunization of rabbits by following the protocol for production of high-titer antibodies.

3.3.2. Preparation of Duck IgY from Duck Egg Yolk

1. Separate the yolks from 12 eggs and mix with 200 mL TBS and 30 mL of 1% (w/v) dextran sulfate in TBS.
2. Incubate for 30 min at RT and then add 75 mL of 1 *M* $CaCl_2$.
3. Centrifuge at 2000*g* for 30 min at 10°C.
4. Filter the supernatant through Whatman No.1 paper.
5. To this filtrate slowly add saturated ammonium sulfate, while constantly mixing, until a final concentration of 50% saturation is achieved.
6. Mix for 30 min at RT and then centrifuge the precipitate at 2500*g* for 30 min at 10°C.
7. Redissolve the precipitate in 50 mL of TBS and recentrifuge at 2500*g*. Collect the supernatant.
8. Slowly add saturated sodium sulfate until 50% saturation has been achieved and centrifuge at 2500*g* for 30 min at 10°C.
9. Redissolve the pellet in 50 mL of TBS and then add saturated sodium sulfate to a final concentration of 14%.
10. Mix for 2 h at RT. Centrifuge the precipitate at 5000*g* for 30 min at 10°C.
11. Repeat **steps 9** and **10** two more times.
12. Dialyze the resuspended pellet overnight against TBS.
13. Determine the protein concentration of the antigen using the bicinchoninic acid protein assay.
14. Determine the purity of the IgY using polyacrylamide gel electrophoresis (PAGE) analysis.

3.3.3. Protocol for the Production of High-Titer Antibodies Against DHBsAg and Duck IgY.

1. The purified protein (DHBsAg or IgY) should be diluted to 1 mg/mL in TBS.
2. Emulsify 100–200 μg of the protein in Freund's complete adjuvant.

3. Inject rabbits subcutaneously at 5–10 sites with the antigen–adjuvant mix.
4. Repeat the immunization two times at 1-mo intervals using 100–200 μg of protein in Freund's incomplete adjuvant.
5. Two weeks after each immunization a test bleed should be taken and tested for antibodies.
6. Euthanize and exsanguinate the animal when the antibody titer is sufficiently high.
7. Collect whole blood and incubate for 1 h at 37°C and then at 4°C overnight.
8. Centrifuge at 4000*g*, collect the serum, and add 0.05% sodium azide. Store at 4°C.

3.3.4. Ammonium Sulfate Precipitation of Rabbit Anti-DHBsAg Antibodies

1. Place 100 mL of rabbit serum into a beaker.
2. Add 200 mL of acetate buffer (0.06 *M*, pH 4.0).
3. Add 7.5 mL of octanoic acid and stir vigorously for 2 h.
4. Filter through Whatman No. 2.
5. To each 100 mL of filtrate add 4.0 mL of 1 *M* Tris-HCl, pH 9.0, and then 26 g of solid ammonium sulfate. Stir at 4°C for 2 h.
6. Centrifuge at 12,000*g* for 30 min.
7. Redissolve the precipitate in approx 25% of the original serum volume.
8. Dialyze overnight against TBS.
9. Centrifuge at 12,000*g* for 30 min.
10. Measure the protein concentration of the supernatant.
11. Dilute to 1 mg/mL in TBS. Store at –20°C.

3.3.5. Detection of DHBsAg Using a Quantitative ELISA (*See* **Notes 12–14**)

1. Coat trays with ammonium sulfate-precipitated rabbit anti-DHBsAg antibodies at a dilution of 1:500 in bicarbonate buffer, pH 9.6, and incubate at 37°C for 1 h and then at 4°C until use.
2. Block wells with 200 μL of 5% SM-PBS/T.
3. Set up standard curves at this stage. Use pooled serum from congenitally DHBV-infected ducks, diluted initially at a 1:1000 dilution in PBS and then twofold across the plate to a final dilution of 1:128,000 in PBS. To standardize the amount of serum proteins present in both test samples and in the standard curve, NDS is added to all dilutions at the same concentration as the sample being tested. That is, either a 1:100 dilution of NDS in PBS or 1:4000 dilution of NDS in PBS is also added to the appropriate standard curves. (*See* **Note 15**.)
4. Add test samples to the plate at a dilution of 1:100 in PBS for low-titer samples, and 1:4000 in PBS for high-titer samples. All samples and standards should be added to the plates in duplicate.
5. Add the 1H.1 monoclonal antibodies diluted to 1:1000. (*See* **Note 16**.)
6. Finally, add the sheep anti-mouse HRP conjugated antibodies. For serum samples tested at a 1:100 dilution, the conjugated antibodies are diluted 1:500 in 5% SM-PBS/T + 5% NSS + 5% NRS. For serum samples tested at a dilution of 1:4000, the conjugated antibodies are added to the plate at a dilution of 1:4000 in 5% SM-PBS/T alone.
7. The cutoff for negative/positive results is set at three times the standard deviation from the mean value obtained with NDS.
8. The levels of DHBsAg are then calculated by extrapolation from the standard curve from each individual plate assuming that the original pooled serum contained a previously calculated amount of DHBsAg. (*See* **Note 17**.)

3.3.6. Detection of Duck Anti-DHBs Antibodies by Indirect ELISA (See **Notes 12–14***)*

1. Coat the wells of a 96-well tray with 1:1000 dilution of the anti-DHBV pre-S/S 1H.1 monoclonal antibodies in bicarbonate buffer pH 9.6 for 1 h at 37°C and then at 4°C until use.
2. Block the wells of tray with 200 μL/well of 5% SM-PBS/T and incubate for 1 h at 37°C.
3. Add sucrose gradient purified DHBsAg (*see* **Subheading 3.3.1.4.**) diluted in 0.1% BSA to the wells of the plate.
4. The test duck serum is added at a dilution of 1:50 and titrated fivefold across the plate to a final dilution of 1:6250. (*See* **Note 16.**)
5. Add the rabbit anti-duck IgY antibodies at a dilution of 1:15,000.
6. Finally, add the goat anti-rabbit HRP-conjugated antibodies at a dilution of 1:5000.
7. Antibody titers should be expressed as the reciprocal of the log serum dilution that gave an OD of 0.4 at 490 nm. (*See* **Note 17**.)

3.3.7. Detection of Anti-DHBc Antibodies by Indirect ELISA (See **Notes 12–14***)*

1. Coat trays with 1 μg/mL rDHBcAg (*1*) diluted in PBS for 1 h at 37°C and then at 4°C until use.
2. Block wells with 200 μL of 5% SM-PBS/T.
3. Add the test duck serum to the plate at a dilution of 1:500 and serially dilute fivefold across the plate to a final dilution of 1:62,500.
4. Add the rabbit anti-duck IgY antibodies diluted to 1:15,000.
5. Finally, add the goat anti-rabbit HRP conjugated antibodies at a dilution of 1:5000.
6. Antibody titers should be expressed as the reciprocal of the log serum dilution that gave an OD of 0.5 at 490 nm. (*See* **Note 17**.)

3.3.8. PEG Precipitation of DHBV from Serum for PCR Analysis

1. Add 200 μL of serum to a microfuge tube with 100 μL of PEG diluted in 1 *M* NaCl.
2. Vortex the tube vigorously and then centrifuge at 14,000*g* in a microfuge for 10 min at RT.
3. Carefully remove the supernatant and discard.
4. Add 100 μL of 0.7% NaOH to the pellet and again vigorously vortex prior to incubation for 1 h at 60°C.
5. Following incubation, add 100 μL of 500 m*M* Tris-HCl, pH 6.8, and vortex the tube again.
6. Incubate for a further 15 min at 95°C.
7. Finally the sample should be centrifuged for 5 min, and the supernatant collected and used immediately in PCR or stored at –20°C.

3.3.9. PCR of Duck Serum to Detect DHBV DNA

1. A standard 50-μL PCR reaction mix is used containing 20 μ*M* of each oligonucleotide primer specific for the DHBV sequence, 1X reaction buffer, 200 μ*M* dNTPs, 1.64 m*M* $MgCl_2$, and 1 U of *Taq* polymerase for each reaction.
2. The program for the PCR reaction is set at 30 cycles of 95°C for 30 s, 55°C for 45 s, and 72°C for 45 s.
3. Ten microliters of duck serum that has been extracted via the PEG precipitation method is used as the template for each PCR reaction.
4. View products on agarose gels using ethidium bromide.
5. The lower limit of sensitivity of the assay is approx 150 DHBV genomes/mL of serum.

4. Notes

1. A range of cDNA clones for duck CD3ϵ; CD4; CD8α; CD44; CD58; IL-18; TCRα, β, γ, and δ; and MHC I and MHC II ***(10–13,30–39)*** were recently cloned by Professor David Higgins and colleagues in Hong Kong. The clones can be used in Northern blot hybridization and reverse transcription (RT)-PCR to monitor the relative levels of mRNA expression at the sites of DHBV infection and also provide the potential for development of antibody reagents for the duck immune system. Hence, they are likely to provide important insights into the different types of immune responses occurring in both acute and persistent DHBV infections, ultimately assisting in the development of vaccines for the treatment of persistent infections.
2. 5% NDS is optimal for duck cell culture.
3. For optimal separation of duck PBMCs from DRBCs and granulocytes using Ficoll-Paque solution, fast ducks for >3 h before bleeding, as this reduces the fat content in blood samples.
4. Thrombocytes are present both at the plasma–Ficoll-Paque interface and in the Ficoll-Paque layers between the interface and the red cell pellet. Collecting the clearly defined cell layer at, but not below, the plasma–Ficoll-Paque interface can decrease the proportion of thrombocytes in PBMC preparations.
5. The percentage of duck T lymphocytes in PBMCs recovered from Ficoll-Paque should be 22–26%, with enrichment of up to 50% after passing the cells through nylon wool columns.
6. Duck DRBCs are nucleated and they act as bystander or "filler" cells that enhance the level of proliferation of duck T lymphocytes in cultures in which activation is suboptimal.
7. Ducks vary in their ability to respond to lectins such as PHA; therefore, a range of concentrations may be needed to find the optimal dose. We have found 5 μg/mL of PHA to be optimal with most duck lymphocyte preparations. Owing to the lack of reagents to identify different duck cell types, it is not possible to determine why there is such variation.
8. Large syncytia form in some cultures of duck PBMCs and adherent cells, commonly occurring after 3–7 d of in vitro culture. Cells with similar morphology, often called osteoclasts, have been described in cultures of human ***(19)***, mouse ***(20)***, and chicken ***(21–23)*** PBMCs. We have observed syncytia that range in size from 200 to 500 μm in cultures of duck PBMCs (**Fig. 4A**) and also duck adherent cells (monocytes) alone (**Fig. 4B**). The syncytia are more commonly present in mitogen-stimulated cultures but are also observed in PBMC cultures without the addition of PHA or ConA and are observed in cultures from both male and female ducks. The presence of the syncytia often, but not always, heralds poor proliferation and low levels of thymidine incorporation in the cultures.
9. The effects of fixation on antigens within tissues can be drastic. Strict adherence to the suggested fixation regimen for each antigen is strongly advised.
10. For detection of duck T lymphocytes using microwave-mediated antigen detection, the slides are placed into two containers of citrate buffer solution (250 mL each) and then heated on full power using a Toshiba 1000-W microwave oven until the buffer solution begins to boil. The containers are then transferred to a NEC microwave oven (model 702) with the power setting on level 2 (magnetron cycle: 6 s ON, 16 s OFF) for 10 min. This will allow the solution to reach almost the boiling point in a cyclic manner, thereby minimizing damage to tissue sections during the heating process. Microwave-safe plastic jars and staining racks are recommended for the microwave procedure.
11. Sections should not be allowed to dry out, as this leads to nonspecific staining.

12. All serological assays should be performed in 96-well flat-bottom ELISA trays.
13. Incubations should be carried out for 1 h with 100 μL of reagent per well unless stated otherwise.
14. Following each step of the assay the ELISA plates should be washed three times with PBS containing 0.05% Tween-20 (PBS/T) except when antibodies conjugated with HRP are present. In this case the plates should be washed with PBS alone.
15. The actual concentration of DHBsAg is determined empirically for each pool of congenitally infected serum to be used as a standard in the DHBsAg ELISA.
16. Antibodies should be diluted in 5% skim milk in PBS containing 0.05% Tween-20 (5% SM-PBS/T).
17. Bound antibodies are visualized using 1 mg/mL of the substrate *o*-phenylenediamine (OPD) (Sigma) for 15 min at RT in the dark. The reaction is then stopped by addition of 50 μL of 2.5 M H_2SO_4 to each well. Read optical densities (ODs) on a Dynatech MR 5000 plate reader at a wavelength of 490 nm.

Acknowledgments

The techniques described in this chapter were developed in the Hepatitis Virus Research Laboratory at the Institute of Medical and Veterinary Science and the University of Adelaide and were funded by project grants from the National Health and Medical Research Council of Australia (NHMRC) and postgraduate research scholarship (EMB) from the University of Adelaide. We are indebted to our colleague Professor Chris Burrell and other staff and students from the laboratory who have contributed to the work. We are also indebted to Dr. John Pugh for supply of the anti-duck Kupffer cell (2E.12) and anti-DHBV pre-S/S (1H.1) monoclonal antibodies and to Professor David Higgins and colleagues for the supply of the duck cell marker cDNA clones.

References

1. Jilbert, A. R., Wu, T-T., England, J. M., et al. (1992) Rapid resolution of duck hepatitis B virus infections occurs after massive hepatocellular involvement. *J. Virol.* **66**, 1377–1388.
2. Jilbert, A. R., Miller, D. S., Scougall, C. A., Turnbull, H. T., and Burrell, C. J. (1996) Kinetics of duck hepatitis B virus infection following low dose virus inoculation: one virus DNA genome is infectious in neonatal ducks. *Virology* **226**, 338–345.
3. Jilbert, A. R., Botten, J. D., Miller, D. S., et al. (1998) Characterization of age- and dose-related outcomes of duck hepatitis B virus infection. *Virology* **244**, 273–282.
4. Jilbert, A. R. and Kotlarski, I. (2000) Immune responses to duck hepatitis B virus infection. *Dev. Comp. Immunol.* **24**, 285–302.
5. Triyatni, M., Jilbert, A. R., Qiao, M., Miller, D. S., and Burrell, C. J. (1998) Protective efficacy of DNA vaccines against duck hepatitis B virus infection. *J. Virol.* **72**, 84–94.
6. Bertram, E. M., Jilbert, A. R., and Kotlarski, I. (1998) Characterization of thrombocytes purified from peripheral blood mononuclear cells of the duck. *Res. Vet. Sci.* **64**, 267–270.
7. Bertram, E. M., Jilbert, A. R., and Kotlarski, I. (1997) An homologous *in vitro* assay to detect lymphokines released by PHA-activated duck peripheral blood leucocytes and spleen cells. *Vet. Immunol. Immunopathol.* **56**, 163–74.
8. Bertram, E. M., Jilbert, A. R., and Kotlarski, I. (1997) Optimization of an *in vitro* assay which measures the proliferation of duck T lymphocytes from peripheral blood in response to stimulation with PHA and ConA. *Dev. Comp. Immunol.* **21**, 299–310.

9. Bertram, E. M., Wilkinson, R. G., Lee, B. A., Jilbert, A. R., and Kotlarski, I. (1996) Identification of duck T lymphocytes using an anti-human T cell (CD3) antiserum. *Vet. Immunol. Immunopathol.* **51**, 353–363.
10. Chan, S. W. S., Middleton, D. L., Lundqvist, M. L., Warr, G. W., and Higgins, D. A. (2001) *Anas platyrhynchos* T-cell surface glycoprotein CD4 precursor mRNA complete cds. GenBank AF378701.
11. Chan, S. W. S., Middleton, D. L., Lundqvist, M. L., Warr, G. W., and Higgins, D. A. (2001) *Anas platyrhynchos* T cell antigen CD8 alpha mRNA. GenBank AF378373.
12. Chan, S. W. S., Middleton, D. L., Lundqvist, M. L., Warr, G. W., and Higgins, D. A. (2001) *Anas platyrhynchos* MHC class I antigen alpha chain mRNA, partial cds. GenBank AF393511.
13. Chan, S. W. S., Middleton, D. L., Lundqvist, M. L., Warr, G. W., and Higgins, D. A. (2001) *Anas platyrhynchos* MHC class II antigen beta chain mRNA, GenBank AF390589.
14. Avian hematology website: http://www.vet.utk.edu/path1/lesson1/ques1/ques1.html
15. Avian hematology website: http://www.lansdown-vets.co.uk/avian-clinical.htm
16. Higgins, D. A. and Chung, S-K. (1986) Duck lymphocytes I. Purification and preliminary observations on surface markers. *J. Immunol. Methods* **86**, 231–238.
17. Higgins, D. A. and Teoh, C. S. H. (1988) Duck lymphocytes II. Culture conditions for optimum transformation response to phytohaemagglutinin. *J. Immunol. Methods* **106**, 135–145.
18. Bertram, E. .M (1997) Characterization of duck lymphoid cell populations and their role in immunity to duck hepatitis B virus. Ph. D. thesis, University of Adelaide.
19. Most, J., Spotl, L., Mayr, G. Gasser, A., Sarti, A., and Dierich, M. P. (1997) Formation of multinucleated giant cells in vitro is dependent on the stage of monocyte to macrophage maturation. *Blood* **89**, 662–671.
20. Battaglino, R., Kim, D., Fu, J., Vaage, B., Fu, X. Y., and Stashenko, P. (2002) c-myc is required for osteoclast differentiation. *J. Bone Miner. Res.* **17**, 763–73.
21. Alvarez, J. I., Ross, F. P., Athanasou, N. A., Blair, H. C., Greenfield, E. M., and Teitelbaum, S. L. (1992) Osteoclast precursors circulate in avian blood. *Calcif. Tissue Int.* 51:48–53.
22. Machuca, I., Domenget, C., and Jurdic, P. (1999) Identification of avian sarcoplasmic reticulum Ca($^{2+}$)-ATPase (SERCA3) as a novel 1,25(OH)(2)D(3) target gene in the monocytic lineage. *Exp. Cell. Res.* **250**, 364–75.
23. Woods, C., Domenget, C., Solari, F., Gandrillon, O., Lazarides, E. and Jurdic, P. (1995) Antagonistic role of vitamin D3 and retinoic acid on the differentiation of chicken hematopoietic macrophages into osteoclast precursor cells. *Endocrinology* **136**, 85–95.
24. Olah, I. and Glick, B. (1982) Splenic white pulp and associated vascular channels in chicken spleen. *Am. J. Anat.* **165**, 445–480.
25. Del Cacho, E., Gallego, M., Arnal, C., and Bascuas, J. A. (1995) Localisation of splenic cells with antigen-transporting capability in the chicken. *Anat. Rec.* **241**, 105–112.
26. Mast, J., Goddeeris, B. M., Peeters, K., Vandesande, F., Berghman, L. R. (1998) Characterization of chicken monocytes, macrophages and interdigitating cells by the monoclonal antibody KUL01. *Vet. Immunol. Immunopathol.* **61**, 343–357.
27. Janse, E. M., and Jeurissen, S. H. (1991) Ontogeny and function of two non-lymphoid cell populations in the chicken embryo. *Immunobiology* **182**, 472–481.
28. Pugh, J. C., Di, Q. Mason, W. S., and Simmons, H. (1995) Susceptibility to duck hepatitis B virus infection is associated with the presence of cell surface receptor sites that efficiently bind viral particles. *J. Virol.* **69**, 4814–4822.
29. Magor, K. E., Higgins, D. A., Middleton, D. L., and Warr, G. W. (1994) One gene encodes the heavy chains for three different forms of IgY in the duck. *J. Immunol.* **153**, 5549–5555.

30. Chan, S. W. S., Warr, G. W., Middleton, D. L., Lundquist, M. L., and Higgins, D. A. (2000) *Anas platyrhynchos* T-cell receptor alpha mRNA, partial cds. GenBank AF323922.
31. Chan, S. W. S., and Higgins, D. A. (2001) *Anas platyrhynchos* T-cell receptor beta chain mRNA, complete cds. GenBank AY039002.
32. Chan, S. W. S. and Higgins, D. A. (2001) *Anas platyrhynchos* T-cell receptor delta chain precursor, mRNA, complete cds. GenBank AF415216.
33. Chan, S. W. S., Ko, O. K. H., and Higgins, D. A. (2001) *Anas platyrhynchos* T-cell receptor gamma mRNA, complete cds. GenBank AF378702.
34. Chan, S. W. S., Middleton, D. L., Lundqvist, M. L., Warr, G. W., and Higgins, D. A. (2001) *Anas platyrhynchos* T-cell receptor CD3 epsilon chain mRNA, complete cds. Genbank AF378704.
35. Chan, S. W. S., Middleton, D. L., Lundqvist, M., Warr, G. W., and Higgins, D. A. (2001) *Anas platyrhynchos* CD58 antigen mRNA, complete cds. GenBank AY032731.
36. Chan, S. W. S., Middleton, D. L., Warr, G. W., and Higgins, D. A. (2001) *Anas platyrhynchos* T cell antigen CD44 isoform a mRNA, complete cds. GenBank AY029553.
37. Chan, S. W. S., Middleton, D. L., Lundqvist, M., Warr, G. W., and Higgins, D. A. (2001) *Anas platyrhynchos* T-cell antigen CD44 isoform c mRNA, complete cds. GenBank AY032667
38. Chan, S. W. S., Warr, G. W., Middleton, D. L., and Higgins, D. A. (2001) *Anas platyrhynchos* T cell antigen CD44 isoform b mRNA, complete cds. GenBank AF332869.
39. Chan, S. W. S., Warr, G. W., Middleton, D. L., Lundquist, M. L., and Higgins, D. A. (2001) *Anas platyrhynchos* interleukin-18 (IL-18) mRNA, partial cds. GenBank AF336122.

2

Measurement of Cell-Mediated Immune Response in Woodchucks

Stephan Menne and Paul J. Cote

1. Introduction

Infection with hepatitis B virus (HBV) is a major health problem, with 350 million people chronically infected worldwide. Chronic HBV infection is characterized by severe hepatic disease sequelae, including chronic hepatitis, cirrhosis of the liver, and hepatocellular carcinoma *(1)*. The immunologic mechanisms that predispose to the development of chronic HBV infection are not completely understood. However, the cell-mediated immunity (CMI) to HBV is believed to play a crucial role in protection against viral infection, and development of efficient antiviral CMI is probably needed to avoid viral persistence and progression to chronic hepatitis *(1)*.

The woodchuck hepatitis virus (WHV) and its natural host, the Eastern woodchuck (*Marmota monax*), have been used extensively as an animal model for HBV infection, disease, and prevention (e.g., *2)*. This model is being applied further to study the immunopathogenesis, antiviral therapy, and immunotherapy of chronic WHV infection *(3–8)*. Such studies have demonstrated the need for more detailed investigation of the immune response of woodchucks, and to develop new molecular and cellular immunologic assays for measuring this response (**Table 1**). For example, in vitro proliferation assays for measuring the responses of woodchuck peripheral blood mononuclear cells (PBMCs) to viral antigens are a prerequisite for studying the CMI of woodchucks during WHV infection and therapy *(3,4–7)*. The use of a universal anti-CD3 antibody reagent indicated that woodchuck PBMCs that did not adhere to nylon wool and that proliferated after stimulation with WHV recombinant core antigen (rWHcAg) were CD3+ lymphocytes *(4)*. However, antibodies to woodchuck CD4 and CD8 positive lymphocytes are needed to enable more detailed lymphocyte phenotyping in PBMC cultures, and for applications of separation and depletion of such lymphocytes. Functionally active woodchuck cytokines and anti-cytokine antibodies are also needed to develop enzyme-linked immunosorbent assay (ELISA) methods for determining the responding cell type in PBMC cultures, for example, for differenti-

From: *Methods in Molecular Medicine, vol. 96: Hepatitis B and D Protocols, volume 2*
Edited by: R. K. Hamatake and J. Y. N. Lau © Humana Press Inc., Totowa, NJ

Table 1
Molecular and Cellular Immunologic Assays for Studying the Host Immune Response Against WHV in the Woodchuck Model

Assay/reagent	Method	Reference
Established for woodchuck model		
PBMC proliferation, Th epitopes, Th lines	Radiopurine, adenine	***3,4–7,9,10,11***
PBMC IL-2 production	IL-2 dependent murine NK cell bioassay	***3,12***
Macrophage, B cell, T cell staining	Immunostaining with anti-Lyz, anti-woodchuck IgG, anti-CD3 (Dako)	***4,8,13***
T cell cDNAs (CD3, 4, 8)	Endpoint/real-time RT-PCR	***9,13–16***
Cytokine cDNAs (IL-1β, 2, 4, 10, IFN-γ, TNF-α)	Endpoint/real-time RT-PCR	***8,9,13–19***
Cytokines/Antibodies (IL-6, IFN-γ, TNF-α)	Immunostaining, in vitro studies	***17,18***
MHC	PCR-based allotyping, antibodies	***19,20***
Needed for woodchuck model		
CTL assay/CTL epitopes/ CTL lines and clones	Autologous fibroblasts or PBMC blasts	
Anti-T cell antibodies (CD3, 4, 8)	Selection, depletion	
Anti-cytokine antibodies (IL-2, 4, 10, 12, IFN-γ, TNF-α)	Th1/Th2 ELISA	
Hepatocyte cDNAs	Libraries, host response	

Anti-Lyz, antibody against lysozyme; CD, cluster of differentiation; CTL, cytolytic T cells; ELISA, enzyme-linked immunosorbent assay; IFN-γ, interferon-γ; IgG, immunoglobuline G; IL, interleukin; NK, natural killer cells; MHC, major histocompatibility complex; PCR, polymerase chain reaction; RT, reverse transcription; Th, T-helper cells; TNF-α, tumor necrosis factor-α.

ation of type 1 and 2 responses. At present, the activation of woodchuck T helper 1 (Th1) cells can be measured by the production of interleukin-2 (IL-2) using an IL-2-dependent murine cell line ***(3)***. Th1 and Th2 cell responses can be differentiated, moreover, by recently developed real-time polymerase chain reaction (PCR) assay for mRNAs of woodchuck leukocyte CD markers and type 1/type 2 cytokines in PBMC cultures and tissues ***(9)***.

The CMI of woodchucks can be studied by in vitro proliferation of PBMCs using polyclonal activators (e.g., concanavalin A [Con A], lipopolysaccharide [LPS], phytohemagglutinin [PHA], human recombinant IL-2) and WHV antigens (e.g., rWHcAg, e antigen [WHeAg], surface antigen [WHsAg], x antigen [WHxAg], and antigen-derived peptides) for stimulation **(Fig. 1)**. Woodchuck PBMCs do not incorporate sufficient tri-

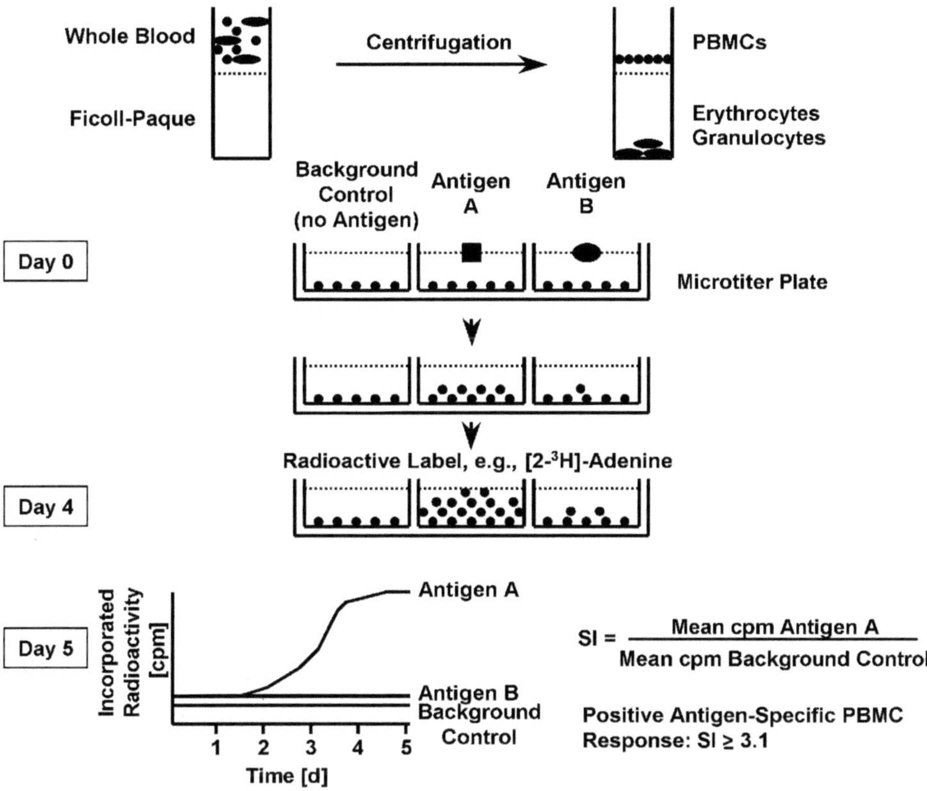

Fig. 1. Overview of the isolation of woodchuck PBMCs from whole blood and their use in the in vitro proliferation assay with radioactive labels (e.g., [2-^{3}H]adenine) for the detection of CMI against WHV in woodchucks.

tiated thymidine in proliferation responses to polyclonal stimulators **(Table 2)** and WHV antigens **(Table 3)**, which apparently relates to the inefficient transcription of the cytosolic thymidine kinase 1 gene ***(3,10,11)***. However, woodchuck PBMCs incorporate sufficient tritiated adenine, serine, adenosine, and deoxyadenosine ***(3,4–6,10,11)***, which enables the development of a meaningful proliferation assay (**Tables 2** and **3**).

This chapter describes a method for the isolation of woodchuck PBMCs from whole blood and their use in proliferation assays. The in vitro PBMC proliferation assay is optimized for woodchuck PBMCs and enables the high-throughput analyses of CMI from large numbers of woodchucks to many stimulators in a given experiment. This assay circumvents the problem of insufficient incorporation of tritiated thymidine mainly by the use of tritiated adenine (or other radioactive purine labels). The availability of this assay facilitates the characterization of host immune response kinetics in woodchucks with applications to the continued modeling of chronic HBV infection and therapy in humans.

Table 2

Incorporation of Tritiated Thymidine, Serine, Adenine, Adenosine, and Deoxyadenosine by Woodchuck PBMC Cultures After 4 D of Stimulation with Polyclonal Activators in the In Vitro PBMC Proliferation Assay

		SI (± SD)				
Stimulator	Outcome	[^{3}H]Thymidine	L-[3-^{3}H]Serine	[2-^{3}H]Adenine	[2-^{3}H]Adenosine	[8-^{3}H] Deoxyadenosine
ConA	Control	3.2 ± 0.2	47.3 ± 3.3	42.4 ± 3.2	37.8 ± 9.4	34.2
	Acute	3.2 ± 0.3	47.6 ± 4.5	42.6 ± 4.5	20.6	35.6
	Chronic	3.2 ± 0.2	48.0 ± 3.8	43.7 ± 3.6	nd	nd
PHA	Control	1.3 ± 0.1	6.9 ± 0.7	4.9 ± 0.6	nd	nd
	Acute	1.4 ± 0.1	7.1 ± 1.0	5.1 ± 0.8	nd	nd
	Chronic	1.4 ± 0.1	6.9 ± 0.9	5.0 ± 0.6	nd	nd

5×10^4 woodchuck PBMCs were cultured with ConA (8.0 μg/mL; 20 μg/mL for [2-^{3}H]adenosine and [8-^{3}H]deoxyadenosine) or PHA (2.4 μg/mL) in microtiter plates for 4 (3 d for [2-^{3}H]adenosine and [8-^{3}H]deoxyadenosine) including a 16- to 20-h pulse with 37 kBq of the respective ^{3}H labels. Stimulation indices (SI) represent the mean SI value of triplicate cultures from all woodchucks in each outcome group of infection. Four adult woodchucks per outcome group were tested (two control and one acute WHV-infected woodchucks for [2-^{3}H]adenosine, one control and one acute WHV-infected woodchuck for [8-^{3}H]deoxyadenosine). Control: WHV-uninfected woodchucks. Acute: Woodchucks with acute self-limited WHV infection (4–8 wk after experimental infection). Chronic: Woodchucks with chronic WHV infection. nd, not done. The mean cpm values of unstimulated PBMCs in medium alone (background control) of woodchucks in each outcome group were: [^{3}H]thymidine, control: 803 ± 39, acute: 812 ± 34, chronic: 795 ± 38; L-[3-^{3}H]serine, control: 1326 ± 62, acute: 1409 ± 95, chronic: 1357 ± 101; [2-^{3}H]adenine, control: 2857 ± 228, acute: 2956 ± 345, chronic: 3027 ± 287; [2-^{3}H]adenosine, control: 2107 ± 1061, acute: 2722; [8-^{3}H]deoxyadenosine, control: 2304, acute: 2223.

Table 3
Incorporation of Tritiated Thymidine, Serine, Adenine, and Adenosine by Woodchuck PBMC Cultures After 5 D of Stimulation with WHV Antigens in the In Vitro PBMC Proliferation Assay

		SI (± SD)			
Stimulator	Outcome	[^{3}H] Thymidine	L-[3-^{3}H] Serine	[2-^{3}H] Adenine	[2-^{3}H] Adenosine
Core	Control	1.1 ± 0.1	1.3 ± 0.1	1.6 ± 0.2	1.0
	Acute	1.4 ± 0.1	23.8 ± 8.1	11.9 ± 1.7	4.1 ± 0.7
	Chronic	1.1 ± 0.1	1.6 ± 0.6	1.3 ± 0.5	nd
Surface	Control	1.0 ± 0.1	1.0 ± 0.1	0.9 ± 0.1	1.2
	Acute	1.3 ± 0.1	11.0 ± 4.8	5.7 ± 2.2	3.5 ± 2.8
	Chronic	1.0 ± 0.1	1.2 ± 0.3	1.1 ± 0.3	nd

5×10^4 woodchuck PBMCs were cultured with recombinant WHV core antigen (core, 1.0 μg/mL; 0.75 μg/mL for [2-^{3}H]adenosine) or WHV surface antigen (surface, 2.0 μg/mL; 2.5 μg/mL for [2-^{3}H]adenosine) in microtiter plates for 5 d (7 d for [2-^{3}H]adenosine) including a 16- to 20-h pulse with 37 kBq of the respective ^{3}H labels. Stimulation indices (SI) represent the mean SI value of triplicate cultures from all woodchucks in each outcome group of infection. Seven adult woodchucks per outcome group were tested (three woodchucks per outcome group for [^{3}H]thymidine; one control and three acute WHV-infected woodchucks for [2-^{3}H]adenosine). Control: WHV-uninfected woodchucks. Acute: Woodchucks with acute self-limited WHV infection (4–8 wk after experimental infection). Chronic: Woodchucks with chronic WHV infection. nd, not done. The mean cpm values of unstimulated PBMCs in medium alone (background control) of woodchucks in each outcome group were: [^{3}H]thymidine, control: 763 ± 64, acute: 838 ± 22, chronic: 832 ± 108; L-[3-^{3}H]serine, control: 1110 ± 364, acute: 1279 ± 201, chronic: 1162 ± 543; [2-^{3}H]adenine, control: 2273 ± 952, acute: 2381 ± 458, chronic: 2365 ± 869; [2-^{3}H]adenosine, control: 2507, acute: 2621 ± 953.

2. Materials

2.1. Stimulators

1. Polyclonal activators: ConA (Sigma, St. Louis, MO, cat. no. C-2010); PHA (Sigma, cat. no. L-8902).
2. WHV antigens: rWHcAg and WHsAg are prepared as recently described ***(3–7)***.

2.2. Solutions

1. Isolation of PBMCs from blood: Ficoll-Paque (Amersham Pharmacia Biotech, Arlington Heights, IL, cat. no. 17-1440-03); 0.9%, NaCl (Baxter, Deerfield, IL, cat. no. 2F7124); glacial acetic acid (Fisher Scientific). Store all solutions at room temperature.
2. Medium for PBMC cultures: Complete medium contains AIM-V medium (*see* **Note 1**), supplemented with 10% heat-inactivated fetal bovine serum (FBS) and 5×10^{-5} m*M* β-mercaptoethanol ***(6,10,11)***. AIM-V medium (Gibco BRL, Rockville, MD, cat. no. 12055-09); FBS (Sigma, cat. no. F-2442); β-mercaptoethanol (Sigma, cat. no. M-6250). Complete medium is light sensitive. Store at 2–8°C (refrigerator temperature).
3. Radioactive labels: [2-^{3}H]adenine, specific activity = 703 GBq/mmol (Amersham Pharmacia Biotech, cat. no. TRK311); methyl[^{3}H]thymidine, specific activity = 925 GBq/mmol (Amersham Pharmacia Biotech cat. no. TRK120); L-[3-^{3}H]serine, specific activity = 999 GBq/m mol (Amersham Pharmacia Biotech, cat. no. TRK308); [2-^{3}H]adenosine, specific activity =

740–925 GBq/mmol (Amersham Pharmacia Biotech cat. no. TRK423); [8-^{3}H]deoxyadenosine, specific activity = 185–925 GBq/mmol (ICN Pharmaceuticals, Costa Mesa, CA, cat. no. 24053). All labels are radiation hazards. Store at 2–8°C (refrigerator temperature).
4. Liquid scintillation fluid: Betaplate Scint, Wallac, Gaithersburg, MD, cat. no. 1205–440. Store at room temperature.

2.3. Equipment

1. Isolation of PBMCs from blood: Sterile hood, for example, SterilGARD Hood (The Baker Company, Sanford, ME, cat. no. VBM-600); EDTA-containing vacutainer tubes (Becton Dickinson, Franklin Lakes, NJ, cat. no. 366454); conical tubes (Becton Dickinson, cat. no. 352070 for 50 mL, cat. no. 352196 for 15 mL); pipets (Becton Dickinson, cat. no. 357551 for 10 mL, cat. no. 357543 for 5 mL, cat. no. 357520 for 1 mL); Eppendorf tubes (1.5-mL), (Laboratory Product Sales, Rochester, NY, cat. no. L250502); hemocytometer (e.g., American Optical, Buffalo, NY).
2. In vitro proliferation assay: Microtiter plates (96-well round) (Becton Dickinson, cat. no. 353077); cell incubator (e.g., Forma Scientific, available through Fisher Scientific); automatic 96-well cell harvester, for example, MACH II 96 (Tomtec, Orange, CT); printed filtermat A (Wallac, cat. no. 1205-401); sample bag (Wallac, cat. no. 1205-411; liquid scintillation counter (e.g., 1205 Betaplate, Wallac).

2.4. PBMCs for In Vitro Assays

Woodchuck whole blood of a volume of 5 mL or greater drawn into EDTA-containing vacutainer tubes (*see* **Note 2**) are recommended for density gradient centrifugation with Ficoll-Paque in 50-mL conical tubes. PBMCs have also been successfully isolated from smaller volumes of blood using 15-mL conical tubes instead of 50-mL tubes. For best results, PBMCs should be isolated immediately after whole blood is drawn and blood should be transported and kept at room temperature (e.g., if shipped overnight). The effects of delay in isolation or storage of blood at temperatures below room temperature on the viability or yield of isolated PBMCs have not been completely studied. Before starting with the isolation of PBMCs, tubes and solutions should be prepared as follows:

1. Label three conical tubes for each woodchuck with the proper animal ID number. Furthermore, label one tube for NaCl and another one for Ficoll.
2. **The following steps should be carried out under a sterile hood and with good sterile handling practice.** Dependent on the whole blood volume add the same volume of 0.9% NaCl into the NaCl-labeled tube to ensure a 1:2 dilution.
3. Add Ficoll-Paque in the same volume as the 1:2 dilution of blood and NaCl into the Ficoll-labeled tube.

3. Methods

3.1. Isolation of Woodchuck PBMCs From Whole Blood

Precaution: Isolation of PBMCs must be performed under a sterile hood.

1. After opening and flaming the opening of the EDTA-containing vacutainer tubes under a sterile hood, draw the whole blood into a pipet and add it **slowly** to the bottom of the NaCl-containing conical tubes. Then remove 2 mL of NaCl from the top using the same pipet and

rinse the EDTA-containing vacutainer tubes to obtain all the blood. Add the NaCl back to the conical tube and mix the whole blood and the NaCl together gently by pipetting up and down. Finish the samples for all animals before going to **step 2**. **Critical parameter: Flaming the opening of the EDTA-containing vacutainer tubes and any of the bottles of solutions before use reduces the possibility of contamination. Furthermore, it is important to transfer whole blood and NaCl under sterile conditions without touching the outside surface of the EDTA-containing vacutainer tubes or the conical tubes with the pipet.**

2. Transfer the NaCl whole blood mixture with a pipet and lay it **carefully and slowly** on the top of the Ficoll-Paque without mixing. Finish the samples for all animals before going to **step 3**. By the time all the samples are finished, some erythrocytes may already migrate through the Ficoll in the earliest samples. **Critical parameter: The overlay of Ficoll with whole blood can be done easily by dropping the blood slowly at the wall of the conical tube. Avoid forceful addition of blood, which will destroy the Ficoll layer. If working with an autopipet, use the largest pipet as possible (e.g., 10 mL). This will allow easier control of the rate of adding blood.**
3. Centrifuge the conical tubes for 35–40 min at room temperature. For separation of lymphocytes from erythrocytes and granulocytes use approx 1700*g* for 15-mL conical tubes and approx 1300*g* for 50-mL conical tubes. **Critical parameter: It is important to run the centrifuge with the brake off, otherwise the gradient will be disrupted.**
4. Centrifugation will result in three layers. The top layer contains NaCl–plasma, the layer in the middle Ficoll, and the layer at the bottom erythrocytes and granulocytes. The phase between NaCl–plasma and Ficoll contains the mononuclear cells, composed mainly of lymphocytes and some monocytes (hereafter referred to as PBMCs). Using a fresh pipet, transfer the PBMCs to the third conical tube. Fill the conical tube up to the top with NaCl. Finish the samples of all animals before going to **step 5. Critical parameter: Pick up the majority of PBMCs first. Make sure to leave enough NaCl on top layer to cover the line of PBMCs adhering to the wall of the conical tube. To increase the yield of isolated PBMCs scrape the wall of the tube with the pipet to also recover attached cells. Be careful to avoid transfer of any erythrocytes and granulocytes.**
5. Wash PBMCs immediately by centrifuging the conical tubes at approx 300*g* for 10 min at room temperature to remove the Ficoll.
6. The centrifugation will result in a visible (white) pellet of PBMCs at the bottom of the conical tube. Carefully remove all the supernatant to avoid any loss of PBMCs. After vortexing the PBMCs to mix, refill the conical tubes up to the top with NaCl and centrifuge at 300*g* for 10 min at room temperature. Repeat this step one more time.
7. After the last wash carefully remove all the supernatant and vortex the PBMCs. Add 4 mL of complete medium and vortex again to mix.
8. For counting of cells, transfer 100 μL of PBMCs in complete medium from the conical tube into an Eppendorf tube by using a pipet. Dilute PBMCs 1:10 in 4% of glacial acetic acid using a fresh Eppendorf tube. After vortexing to mix, add approx 10 μL of PBMCs to a hematocytometer. Calculate the total number of cells in the original 4 mL of complete medium. This can be done by counting the cells in the 64 squares of the four corner areas under the coverslip of the hematocytometer in a total volume of 0.1 mm^3. Obtain the average cell number by dividing the total number of cells by 4. Multiply the average cell number by 10 to obtain the cell number per 1 mm^3. Multiply this by 1000 to obtain the cell number per 1 cm^3, which equals 1 mL of medium. Then account for the 10-fold dilution by multiplying the cell number by 10 to get the number of cells per 1 mL of medium. Multiply this number by 4 to achieve the total number of cells isolated. Add an appropriate volume of complete

medium to the conical tube to obtain a concentration of 2.5 × 10^6 cells/mL. If the cell concentration in the 4 mL of complete medium is lower, centrifuge the PBMCs again at 300*g* for 10 min at room temperature and remove all the supernatant. Then add the appropriate volume of complete medium to get the desired cell concentration. **Critical parameter: 4% of glacial acetic acid is used to destroy any contaminating erythrocytes in the PBMC samples to be counted. If the PBMC sample contains a higher number of erythrocytes, the use of 8% of glacial acetic acid and incubation for 10 min at room temperature is recommended.**

3.2. In Vitro *PBMC Proliferation Assay with Radioactive Labels*

Stimulators are added to the wells of a 96-well microtiter plate in a volume of 20 μL. This keeps the volume of stimulator preparation low (i.e., 1/10 of the final well volume), but easily dispersible by using a repeater pipet. Polyclonal activators and WHV antigens are used in triplicates at previously determined optimal concentrations ***(3,4,6)***: Con A (8.0 μg/mL), PHA (2.4 μg/mL), WHsAg (2.0 μg/mL), and rWHcAg (1.0 μg/mL). The desired concentrations of stimulators are achieved by diluting the stock solutions in an appropriate volume of 0.9% NaCl to obtain a 10-fold working solution. Controls may include irrelevant woodchuck serum protein as a control for WHsAg and irrelevant recombinant protein as a control for rWHcAg in the same concentration as above. For background control (unstimulated PBMCs in medium alone) add 20 μL of 0.9% NaCl into eight wells of the microtiter plate. For control of WHV antigens add 20 μL of irrelevant woodchuck protein into eight wells of the microtiter plate. Microtiter plates can be prepared in advance (and frozen) with all stimulators in the wells before transferring complete medium and freshly isolated PBMCs (*see* **Note 3**).

1. Add 160 μL of complete medium to each well of the previously prepared microtiter plate by using a multichannel pipet.
2. After vortexing to mix the PBMCs in complete medium, add 20 μL of PBMCs into each well of the microtiter plate by using a repeater pipet to reach the final concentration of 5 × 10^4 cells per well (i.e., in a total well volume of 200 μL).
3. Incubate cultured PBMCs for 5 d (*see* **Note 4**) at 37°C in a humidified atmosphere containing 5% CO_2.
4. Add 37 kBq (= 1 μCi) of a certain radioactive label (e.g., [2-^{3}H]adenine) to the PBMC cultures in each well of the microtiter plate on d 4 by using a repeater pipet. For transfer of 37 kBq of a radioactive label in a volume of 20 μL, dilute the stock solution with an appropriate volume of complete medium.
5. Place radioactively labeled microtiter plates back into the incubator for another 16–20 h, before harvesting the PBMC cultures on d 5.
6. After 5 d of culture, radioactively labeled PBMCs are harvested onto filtermats by using an automatic 96-well cell harvester. After air-drying overnight place one filtermat into a sample bag. Add 10 mL of liquid scintillation fluid to the filtermat and seal the sample bag. Incorporated radioactivity is then measured by counting in a liquid scintillation counter. Results for triplicate cultures are expressed as the stimulation index (SI), which is determined by dividing the total counts per minute (cpm) obtained in the presence of stimulator by that in the absence of stimulator (e.g., background control = unstimulated PBMCs in medium alone, PBMCs cultured with irrelevant woodchuck protein; *see* **Fig. 1**). **Critical parameter: For calculation of the SI value average the cpm derived from the eight wells containing the background control or the controls for WHV antigens by removing the highest and lowest cpm value** (*see* **Note 5**).

4. Notes

1. The use of AIM-V medium as main part of the complete medium for the culture of woodchuck PBMCs instead of RPMI 1640 (Gibco BRL) is recommended. AIM-V medium was demonstrated to significantly increase the uptake of radioactive label (i.e., [2-^{3}H]adenine) by woodchuck PBMCs in the in vitro proliferation assay ***(10)***.
2. The use of EDTA as an anticoagulant for blood sampling instead of heparin is critical. EDTA was shown to increase the uptake of radioactive label (i.e., [2-^{3}H]adenine) by woodchuck PBMCs in the in vitro proliferation assay ***(10)***.
3. For in vitro proliferation assays involving a large number of animals and many stimulators, plates can be prepared in advance for all test dates and stored at − 20°C until use. Allow frozen plates to thaw before adding complete medium and freshly isolated PBMCs.
4. The culture period of 5 d is optimized for WHV antigen-specific stimulations of woodchuck PBMCs. If only polyclonal activators are used, the culture period should be decreased to 4 d to get best proliferation results ***(10,11)***.
5. SI values of ⩾3.1 are considered positive for WHV antigen-specific PBMC responses of woodchucks. This positive cutoff is conservative in relationship to routine positive stimulations by WHV antigens; that is, the range of maximal antigen-specific SI values using [2-^{3}H]adenine is 7.0–12 (e.g., ***5,6***). The 3.1 cutoff level, therefore, represents at least 25–45% of the observed response range for positive stimulations induced by antigens. At the 3.1 SI cutoff, the positive sample cpm for antigens always is greater than two standard deviations (SDs) above the mean cpm of background control (i.e., unstimulated PBMCs in medium alone) from the same woodchuck, and is characteristically more than two SDs above the average cpm for antigen-stimulated PBMCs from uninfected control woodchucks.

Acknowledgments

S. M. and P. C. are supported by contract NO1-AI-05399 to the College of Veterinary Medicine, Cornell University with the National Institute of Allergy and Infectious Diseases (NIAID), and contract NO1-AI-45179 to the Division of Molecular Virology and Immunology, Georgetown University, School of Medicine with the NIAID. The authors thank Dr. Jan Maschke (University Hospital, Essen, Germany) for his contributions to the development and results of the in vitro PBMC proliferation assay.

References

1. Chang, K. M. and Chisari, F. V. (1999) Immunopathogenesis of hepatitis B virus infection. *Clin. Liver Dis.* **3,** 221–239.
2. Tennant, B. C. (1999) Animal models of hepatitis B virus infection. *Clin. Liver Dis.* **3,** 241–266.
3. Cote, P. J. and Gerin, J. L. (1995) In vitro activation of woodchuck lymphocytes measured by radiopurine incorporation and interleukin-2 production: implications for modeling immunity and therapy in hepatitis B virus infection. *Hepatology* **22,** 687–699.
4. Menne, S., Maschke, J., Tolle, T. K., Lu, M., and Roggendorf, M. (1997) Characterization of T-cell response to woodchuck hepatitis virus core protein and protection of woodchucks from infection by immunization with peptides containing a T-cell epitope. *J. Virol.* **71,** 65–74.
5. Menne, S., Maschke, J., Lu, M., Grosse-Wilde, H., and Roggendorf, M. (1998) T-cell response to woodchuck hepatitis virus (WHV) antigens during acute self-limited WHV infection and convalescence and after viral challenge. *J. Virol.* **72,** 6083–6091.

6. Menne, S., Roneker, C. A., Gerin, J. L., Cote, P. J., and Tennant, B. C. (2002) Deficiencies in the acute phase cell-mediated immune response to viral antigens are associated with development of chronic woodchuck hepatitis virus infection following neonatal inoculation. *J. Virol.* **76,** 1769–1780.
7. Menne, S., Roneker, C. A., Korba, B. E., Gerin, J. L., Tennant, B. C., and Cote, P. J. (2002) Immunization with surface antigen vaccine alone after treatment with L-FMAU breaks humoral and cell-mediated immune tolerance in chronic woodchuck hepatitis virus infection *J. Virol.* **76,** 5305–5314.
8. Nakamura, I., Nupp, J. T., Cowlen, M., et al. (2001) Pathogenesis of neonatal woodchuck hepatitis virus infection: chronicity as an outcome of infection is associated with a diminished acute hepatitis that is temporally deficient for the expression of interferon-gamma and tumor necrosis factor-alpha messenger RNAs. *Hepatology.* **33,** 439–447.
9. Menne, S., Wang, Y., Butler, S., Gerin, J. L., Cote, P. J., and Tennant, B. C. (2002) Real-time polymerase chain reaction assays for leucocyte CD and cytokine mRNAs of the Eastern woodchuck (*Marmota monax*). *Vet. Immunol. Immunopathol.* **87,** 97–105.
10. Kreuzfelder, E., Menne, S., Ferencik, S., Roggendorf, M., and Grosse-Wilde, H. (1996) Assessment of peripheral blood mononuclear cell proliferation by 2[^{3}H]adenine uptake in the woodchuck model. *Clin. Immunol. Immunopathol.* **78,** 223–227.
11. Maschke, J., Menne, S., Jacob, J. R., et al. (2001) Thymidine kinases and thymidine utilization in proliferating peripheral blood lymphocytes and hepatic cells of the woodchuck (Marmota monax). *Vet. Immun. Immunopathol.* **78,** 279–296.
12. Hervas-Stubbs, S., Lasarte, J. J., Sarobe, P., et al. (1997) Therapeutic vaccination of woodchucks against chronic woodchuck hepatitis virus infection. *J. Hepatol.* **27,** 726–737.
13. Guo, J. T., Zhou, H., Liu, C., et al. (2000) Apoptosis and regeneration of hepatocytes during recovery from transient hepadnavirus infections. *J. Virol.* **74,** 1495–1505.
14. Hodgson, P. D. and Michalak, T. I. (2001) Augmented hepatic interferon gamma expression and T-cell influx characterize acute hepatitis progressing to recovery and residual lifelong virus persistence in experimental adult woodchuck hepatitis virus infection. *Hepatology* **34,** 1049–1059.
15. Nakamura I., Nupp, J. T., Rao, B. S., et al. (1997) Cloning and characterization of partial cDNAs for woodchuck cytokines and CD3ε with applications for the detection of RNA expression in tissues by RT-PCR assay. *J. Med. Virol.* **53,** 85–95.
16. Wang, Y., Menne, S., Jacob, J. R., Tennant, B. C., Gerin, J. L., and Cote, P. J.(2003) Role of type 1 versus type 2 immune responses in liver during the onset of chronic woodchuck hepatitis virus infection. *Hepatology* **37,** 771–780.
17. Li, D. H., Havell, E. A., Brown, C. I., and Cullen, J. M. (2000) Woodchuck lymphotoxin-alpha,-beta, and tumor necrosis factor genes: structure, characterization and biologic activity. *Gene* **242,** 295–305.
18. Lohrengel, B., Lu, M., and Roggendorf, M. (1998) Molecular cloning of the woodchuck cytokines TNF-α, IFN-γ, and IL-6. *Immunogenetics* **47,** 332–335.
19. Lohrengel, B., Lu, M., Bauer, D., and Roggendorf, M. (2000) Expression and purification of woodchuck tumor necrosis factor alpha. *Cytokine* **12,** 573–577.
20. Michalak, T. I., Hodgson, P. D., and Churchill, N. D. (2000) Posttranscriptional inhibition of class I major histocompatibility complex presentation on hepatocytes and lymphoid cells in chronic woodchuck hepatitis virus infection. *J. Virol.* **74,** 4483–4494.
21. Yang, D. L, Lu, M., Hao, L. J., and Roggendorf, M. (2000) Molecular cloning and characterization of major histocompatibility complex class I cDNAs from woodchuck (Marmota monax). *Tissue Antigens* **55,** 548–557.

3

Study of Liver-Specific Expression of Cytokines During Woodchuck Hepatitis Virus Infection

Mengji Lu and Michael Roggendorf

1. Introduction

The woodchuck model has become a well-accepted animal system for the study of host immune responses to hepadnavirus infection. Recently, a series of woodchuck cytokines was characterized by molecular cloning ***(1–5)***. The availability of the sequence information and the essential reagents makes it possible to study the role of cytokines for the control of hepatitis B virus (HBV) infection and for immunopathogenesis in the woodchuck model.

The expression of cytokines in liver is of great interest in the context of HBV infection ***(6)***. First, the pattern of the intrahepatic cytokine expression reflects the host immune response to viral infection. Second, antiviral cytokines, especially interferon-γ (IFN-γ) and tumor necrosis factor-α (TNF-α), were found to suppress HBV gene expression and replication in the transgenic mouse model ***(7)***. Experimental data in the chimpanzee model indicate that the viral clearance in an acute self-limiting HBV infection occurs by a nonlytic mechanism, likely mediated by antiviral cytokines ***(8)***. Thus, studies of intrahepatic cytokine expression in the woodchuck model will contribute to our understanding of the role of cytokines for control of hepadnavirus infection.

There are a series of different methods used for the study of cytokine expression based on the detection of mRNA by reverse transcription-polymerase chain reaction (RT-PCR) and RNase protection assays ***(9–11)***. Northern blotting may be useful in particular cases if a specific mRNA species is analyzed. The sensitivity of Northern blot is not sufficient to detect the expression of the majority of relevant cytokines such as IFN-γ and TNF-α as only a small portion of cells in liver produce cytokines. RT-PCR can be used to detect low-level expression of cytokines. However, the quantification of a specific mRNA species requires real-time PCR analysis. The RNA protection assay may be a good choice in many cases, as it is a sensitive and quantitative assay. It is also possible to detect multiple species of mRNAs in a single reaction and thus allow the comparison of the relative levels

From: *Methods in Molecular Medicine, vol. 96: Hepatitis B and D Protocols, volume 2*
Edited by: R. K. Hamatake and J. Y. N. Lau © Humana Press Inc., Totowa, NJ

of gene expression with internal standards, preferably housekeeping genes such as β-actin and GAPDH. However, the RNase protection assay requires specific cloned cDNAs, which are transcribed into antisense RNA with labeled ribonucleotides.

2. Materials

2.1. Solutions

1. Sample buffer for agarose gel electrophoresis: Dissolve 25 mg of orange G (Sigma, Deisenhofen, Germany, cat. no. 01625) in 10 mL of 40% sucrose (Calbiochem Biosciences, La Jolla, CA, cat. no. 57313). Store at 4°C.
2. Tris–borate–EDTA (TBE) buffer: Prepare 10-fold concentrated stock with 540 g of Tris (molecular biology grade, Calbiochem Biosciences, cat. no. 648310), 275 g of boric acid (Merck, Darmstadt, Germany cat. no. 1.00160), and 200 mL of 0.5 *M* EDTA (Fluka Chemie AG, Bucks, Germany), fill up to 10 L with distilled water, store at room temperature, and dilute the stock 1:10 with distilled water for use.
3. Agarose gel: Weigh 1 g of agarose (molecular biology grade, Eurogentec, Seraing, Belgium, cat. no. EP-0010-10) in 100 mL of TBE buffer, heat to melt agarose completely in a microwave oven, add 5 μL of ethidium bromide (Carl Roth, Karlsruhe, Germany, cat. no. 2218.2, stock concentration 10 mg/mL), and cast the agarose gel in a gel chamber with a comb.
4. 5% Acrylamide/*bis*-acrylamide (19:1): Use prepared acrylamide-*bis* sequencing solution (Merck, cat. no. 100645) and dilute in sequencing diluent (Merck, cat. no. 100646).
5. 10% Ammonium persulfate (Sigma, cat. no. 7727-54-0): Dissolve 1 g of ammonium persulfate in 10 mL of distilled water, and store at 4°C.
6. *N, N, N', N'*-Tetramethylethylenediamine (TEMED) (Sigma, cat. no. 110-18-9): Store at 4°C.
7. 100% Ethanol (J. T. Baker, Deventer, Holland, cat. no. 8006): Store at –20°C.
8. 70% Ethanol: Add 30 mL of sterile water to 70 mL of ethanol. Store at –20°C.
9. Roti-Phenol (Carl Roth, cat. no.0038.1): Tris-saturated phenol, pH 7.5–8.
10. 3 *M* Sodium acetate, pH 5: Dissolve 40.81 g of sodium acetate $\cdot 3H_2O$ (Merck, cat. no. 106267) in 80 mL of distilled water, add glacial acetic acid with stirring until the pH reaches 5.2, adjust the volume to 100 mL with distilled water, and sterilize by autoclaving. Store at room temperature.

2.2. Kits and Enzymes

1. RNeasy Midikit (QIAGEN, Hilden, Germany, cat. no.75142) for RNA purification.
2. Multi-Probe RNA protection assay system: Riboquant™ (Pharmingen, San Diego, CA, cat. no. 45014K).
3. QIAshredder (QIAGEN, cat. no. 79654) for homogenizing samples.
4. MMLV reverse transcriptase (Promega, Madison, WI, cat. no. 1705).
5. *Taq* polymerase (Promega, cat. no. M1668).

2.3. Equipment

1. Pestle and mortar: Sterilize pestles and mortars at 200°C for 4 h; cool the devices with liquid nitrogen before use.
2. A microcentrifuge (Eppendorf 5415 C, Eppendorf, Hamburg, Germany).
3. GeneQuant pro RNA/DNA calculator and Microvolume spectrometer cells (Amersham Pharmacia Biotech UK, Buckinghamshire, England, cat. no. 80-2109-98 and cat. no. 80-2076-38): Use a volume as small as 50–100 μL to measure the concentrations of purified total RNAs.

4. Heat block: Preferred for RNase protection assay because it can be easily decontaminated.
5. Thermocycler (Thermocycler 60, Bachofer, Reutlingen, Germany).
6. Power supply: A low-voltage power supply (Power Pac25, Biometra, Gttigen, Germany) can be used for agarose gel electrophoresis. A high-voltage power supply (PowerPac 3000, Bio-Rad Laboratories, Hercules, CA, cat. no. 165-5057) is necessary for polyacrylamide gel electrophoresis.
7. Equipment for gel electrophoresis: Chambers for gel electrophoresis are available from many commercial suppliers. Sequi-Gen GT cells of a size of 38 × 50 cm (Bio-Rad, Laboratories, cat. no. 165-3863) are suitable for polyacrylamide gel electrophoresis.

2.4. Tissue Samples

Liver biopsies obtained by surgical laparotomy have to be frozen immediately in liquid nitrogen and stored at –80°C until use. A minimum of 25 mg of liver tissue should be processed to generate sufficient amounts of total RNAs for RNase protection assays (10–20 μg/assay).

Two types of positive controls are useful: woodchuck peripheral blood lymphocytes and cells transfected with expression plasmids for specific woodchuck cytokines. Woodchuck peripheral blood lymphocytes should be prepared and cultured for 2–3 d according to the protocol described by Menne et al. ***(12)***. Phytohemagglutinin (Sigma, cat. no. L9132) should be added at a final concentration of 5 μg/mL for stimulation of lymphocytes. Lymphocytes should be harvested by centrifugation and frozen immediately in liquid nitrogen until the preparation of total RNAs. Alternatively, permanent cell lines such as baby hamster kidney cells should be transfected with plasmids expressing woodchuck cytokines. The total RNAs from the transfected cells are suitable as standards in the RNase protection assay.

2.5. Specific Primers for Woodchuck Cytokines

Dissolve the primers for RT-PCR in TE buffer at a concentration of 100 m*M* and store at –20°C. Dilute the stock solutions of primers to concentrations of 50 m*M* and 10 m*M* for RT and PCR, respectively.

To detect the cDNA of woodchuck cytokines, the following primers are used:

IFN-γ: Sense primer 5'-TTTCTACCTCAGACTCTTTGAA-3', antisense primer 5'-AGTT TTAAATATTAATAAATAG-3' (accession number Y14138).

TNF-α: Sense primer 5'-AGAAAAGACACCATGAGCACAGAAAA-3', antisense primer 5'-ACCCATTCCCTTCACAGAGCAATGA-3' (accession number Y14137).

IL4: Sense primer 5'-AGAGCTATTGATGGGTCTCA-3', antisense primer 5'-TCTTTAGG CTTTCCAGGAAGTC-3' (accession number AF082495).

IL10: Sense primer 5'-GTGAAGATTTTCTTTCAAA-3', antisense primer 5'-GAGGTAT CAGAGGTAATAAATAT-3' (accession number AF01209).

IL15: Sense primer 5'-TGGATGGATGGCWGCTGGAA-3', antisense primer 5'-AAGAK TTCATSTGATCCAAG-3' (accession number MMU14332).

2.6. Cloned cDNAs for RNase Protection Assays

cDNA clones of woodchuck cytokines are needed for RNase protection assays. Typically, cDNA fragments between 200 and 500 basepairs (bp) in length are cloned into vectors containing a T7 promoter site such as pGEM-3Z (Promega, cat. no. P2151) for in vitro transcription. The in vitro-generated transcripts have to be antisense. If multiple probes are used in a single assay, they have to have different lengths, preferably within a close range. A difference of 20 bp between two probes is sufficient to be resolved by polyacrylamide gel electrophoresis. Probes with large differences in their lengths may make the gel electrophoresis difficult.

3. Methods

The general rule for handling RNA and inactivation of RNase should be followed as described in Sambrook et al. ***(13)***. A flow diagram of procedures to detect the specific mRNAs of woodchuck cytokines is depicted in **Fig. 1.**

3.1. Preparation of Total RNAs from Frozen Woodchuck Liver Samples

1. Grind frozen woodchuck liver samples to powder in liquid nitrogen with a pestle and mortar.
2. Dissolve the frozen powder in lysis buffer and homogenize the samples by continuous grinding. **Do not thaw liver samples without lysis buffer. RNAs are extremely unstable at this step.**
3. Shear the genomic DNA by passing the samples through the QIAShredder.
4. Apply the lysate to the column supplied with the RNeasy kit following the procedure described in the product manual. Use the Midi kit to generate sufficient amounts of total RNAs for RNase protection assays.
5. Dilute 5 μL of RNA preparation in 95 μL of distilled water. Measure the OD at UV wavelength 260 nm in the GeneQuant pro RNA/DNA calculator, calculate the concentrations of RNAs with the factor 1 OD = 40 μg of RNA/mL, and adjust the RNA preparations to a concentration approx 1 μg/μL. (*See* **Note 1**.)
6. Check the quality of RNA preparations on a freshly prepared agarose gel using at least 5 μg of total RNA. (*See* **Note 2**.)

3.2. *RT-PCR* (See Note 3)

1. Incubate 1–5 μg of purified total RNAs with 1 μL of antisense primer (50 m*M*) and 5 U of MMLV reverse transcriptase in the supplied buffer in a total volume of 10 μL at 37°C for 1 h.
2. Stop RT by heating the samples at 94°C for 5 min.
3. Run the PCR with 5 μL of RT reactions in a total volume of 50 μL. Use the following cycle parameter: 94°C for 1 min, 45°C for 1 min, and 72°C for 2 min over 30 cycles. (*See* **Note 4**.)
4. Add 2 μL of sample buffer to 10 μL of PCR, load the agarose gel, including an appropriate size marker (123-bp DNA ladder, Gibco BRL, cat. no. 15613-011), and run the gel at 80–100 V until the orange G dye reaches the end of agarose gel.
5. Visualize the DNA fragments under UV light. Identify the specific products for woodchuck cytokines according to their specific sizes: 345 bp for wIFN-γ, 731 bp for wTNF-α, 422 bp for IL4, 546 bp for IL10, and 715 bp for IL15. To verify the specificity of RT-PCR, the PCR products can be characterized by direct sequencing or cloning ***(9,13)***.

3.3. RNA Protection Assay

1. Cut 10 μg of the cDNA clones of woodchuck cytokines (*see* **Subheading 2.5.**) in a total volume of 20–50 μL with the appropriate buffer and 50 U of a single cut restriction enzyme at 37°C for 1 h. Add 100 μL of TE buffer to increase the volume, remove proteins by extraction with 100 μL of phenol, add 10 μL of 3 *M* calcium acetate, pH 5.2, and 250 μL of 100 ethanol to precipitate DNA, incubate at –70°C for 1 h or at –20°C overnight, sediment DNA

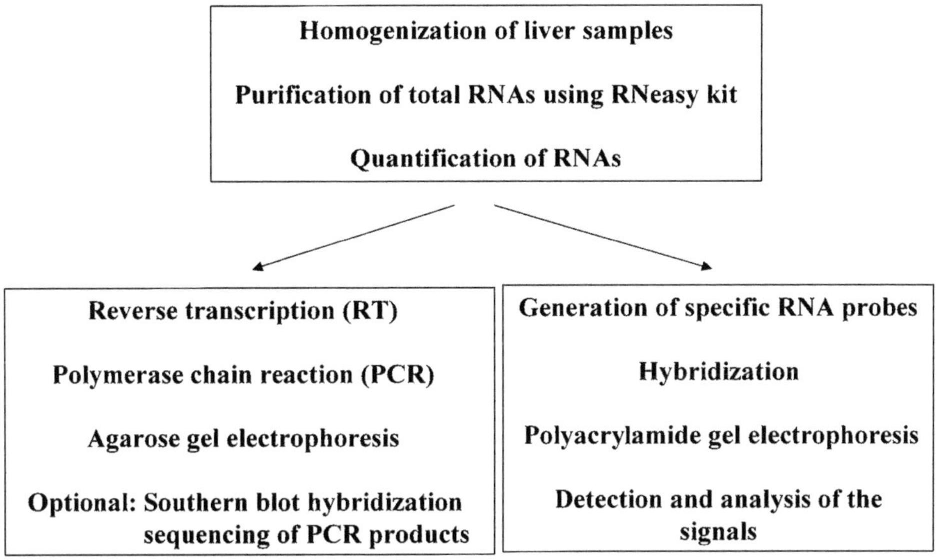

Fig. 1. Flow diagram: detection of woodchuck cytokine mRNAs in liver samples.

at full speed in a Eppendorf microcentrifuge for 15 min at 4°C, wash precipitated DNA once with 70% ethanol, air-dry DNA, and dissolve in TE buffer at a concentration of 0.5–1 µg/µL. (*See* **Note 5**.)

2. Follow the procedure described in the instruction manual of the RiboQuant™ for preparation of ^{32}P-labeled RNA probes, hybridization with total RNAs purified from liver, and RNase treatments using the kit.
3. Prepare 150 mL of 5% acrylamide in 1X TBE buffer, add 900 µL of ammonium persulfate and 60 µL of TEMED, pour the solution into the gel mold, and wait for 1 h. Assemble the polyacrylamide gel for electrophoresis and prerun the gel for at least 15–30 min at 2500 V. The amount of ammonium persulfate and TEMED may be changed to modulate the speed of polymerization.
4. Flush the wells and load the samples. Use duplicates to increase the accuracy of the assay. Run the gel at 50 W. The running time depends on the sizes of specific probes and may range between 2 and 4 h.
5. Disassemble the gel mold and transfer the polyacrylamide gel to a Whatman paper. Dry the gel in a vacuum dryer for 1 h at 80°C. (*See* **Note 6**.)
6. Visualize the protected RNAs by autoradiography, and identify the specific bands according to the positive controls. The quantification of signals can be done by using a Phosphorimager (Cyclon, Packard Instrument, Meridien, CT, cat. no. A431201). The relative level of mRNA may be calculated by normalization using internal controls such as β-actin or GAPDH mRNAs.

4. Notes

1. 10–20 µL of total RNA are necessary for an RNase protection assay.
2. RNA preparations should not show smears and contamination with genomic DNA.

3. A crucial point for RT-PCR is the elimination of possible contamination of samples by cDNA fragments, generated by previous RT-PCR or cloned into plasmids. Useful instructions can be found in **ref. *9***.
4. The annealing temperature may be increased to enhance the specificity of PCRs.
5. A large quantity of DNA templates can be generated and stored at –20°C. For multiple probe assays, different DNA templates can be mixed at this step. The ratio of these DNA templates needs to be optimized for specific experiments.
6. If the polyacrylamide gel sticks to the glass plates used for gel electrophoresis, treat the glass plates with Repel Silane.

References

1. Lohrengel, B., Lu, M., and Roggendorf, M. (1998) Molecular cloning of the woodchuck cytokines: TNF-alpha, IFN-gamma, and IL-6. *Immunogenetics* **47,** 332–335.
2. Guo, J.-T., Zhou, H., Liu, C., et al. (2000) Apoptosis and regeneration of hepatocytes during recovery from transient hepadnavirus infection. *J. Virol.* **74,** 1495–1505.
3. Zhou, T., Guo, J.-T., Nunes, F. A., et al. (2000) Combination therapy with lamivudine and adenovirus causes transient suppression of chronic woodchuck hepatitis virus infection. *J. Virol.* **74,** 11754–11763.
4. Nakamura, I., Nupp, J. T., Cowlen, B. M., et al. (2001) Pathogenesis of experimental neonatal woodchuck hepatitis virus infection: chronicity as an outcome of infection is associated with a diminished acute hepatitis that is temporally deficient for the expression of interferon gamma and tumor necrosis factor-alpha messenger RNAs. *Hepatology* **33,** 439–447.
5. Hogdson, P. D. and Michalak T. I. (2001) Augmented hepatic interferon gamma expression and T-cell influx characterize acute hepatitis progressing to recovery and residual lifelong virus persistence in experimental adult woodchuck hepatitis virus infection. *Hepatology* **34,** 1049–1059.
6. Chisari F. V. (2000) Viruses, immunity, and cancer: lessons from hepatitis B. *Am. J. Pathol.* **156,** 1118–1132.
7. Guidotti, L. G., Ishikawa, T., Hobbs, M. V., Matzke, B., Schreiber, R., and Chisari, F. V. (1996) Intracellular inactivation of the hepatitis B virus by cytotoxic T lymphocytes. *Immunity* **4,** 25–36.
8. Guidotti, L. G., Rochford, R., Chung, J., Shapiro, M., Purcell, R., and Chisari, F. V. (1999) Viral clearance without destruction of infected cells during acute HBV infection. *Science* **284,** 825–829.
9. Innis, M. A., Gelfand, D. H., Sninsky, J. J., and White, T. J. (1990) *PCR Protocols: A Guide to Methods and Applications*. Academic Press, San Diego, CA.
10. Gilman, M. (1993) Ribonuclease protection assay, in *Current Protocols in Molecular Biology,* Vol. 1 (Ausubel, F. M., Brent, R., Kingston, R. E., et al., eds.), John Wiley & Sons, New York, pp 4.7.1.–4.7.8.
11. Naylor, M. S., Relf, M., and Balkwill F. R. (1995) Northern analysis, ribonuclease protection, and in situ analysis of cytokine messenger RNA, in *Cytokines, a Practical Approach* (Balkwill, F. R., ed.), Oxford University Press, Oxford New York Tokyo, pp. 35–56.
12. Menne, S., Maschke, J., Lu, M., Grosse-Wilde, H., and Roggendorf, M. (1998) T-cell response to woodchuck hepatitis virus (WHV) antigens during acute self-limited WHV infection and convalescence and after viral challenge. *J. Virol.* **72,** 6083–6091.
13. Sambrook, J., Fritsch, E. F., and Maniatis, T. (1989) *Molecular Cloning: A Laboratory Manual*, 2nd edit. (Ford, N., Nolan, C., and Ferguson, M., eds.), Cold Springer Harbor Laboratory Press, Cold Spring Harbor, New York.

4

Induction of Anti-Hepatitis B Virus Immune Responses Through DNA Immunization

Michael Geissler, Robert Weth, Christian F. Grimm, Dörte Ortmann, and Hubert E. Blum

1. Introduction

Cellular and humoral immune responses to different hepatitis B virus (HBV) antigens are believed to play an essential role in the elimination of virus by the host. It is well established that the humoral immune response to HBV envelope antigens leads to protection against infection. By contrast, the activity of a broad-based cellular immune response to different HBV antigens has been shown to be one of the most important factors contributing to virus elimination from infected hepatocytes and may play an important role in the pathogenesis of the severity of hepatitis and the subsequent development of chronic liver disease *(1)*. More than 300 million people worldwide have persistent HBV infection and cytotoxic T-lymphocyte (CTL) activity against HBV structural proteins is not detectable in peripheral blood lymphocytes derived from these individuals. It is known that some chronic HBV-infected individuals spontaneously clear HBV DNA from serum each year, and this phenomenon is often accompanied by increased $CD4^+$ T-helper cell responses and acute exacerbation of the liver disease as manifested by increased alanine aminotransferase levels.

Enhanced liver injury is believed to be an in vivo correlate of viral specific $CD8^+$ CTL activity and cytokine-mediated nonspecific inflammatory responses against HBV-infected hepatocytes. An attractive hypothesis for the development of persistent viral infection is that HBV-specific CTLs are unable to clear virus from the liver because of substantially decreased intrahepatic levels or qualitative changes in CTL activity. The observation of spontaneous HBV clearance in some individuals implies that the suboptimal cellular immune response may be reversible. Therefore, strategies designed to boost the HBV-specific immune response or to alter the balance between the cytopathic and the regulatory components of the response may be able to terminate persistent infection.

From: *Methods in Molecular Medicine, vol. 96: Hepatitis B and D Protocols, volume 2*
Edited by: R. K. Hamatake and J. Y. N. Lau © Humana Press Inc., Totowa, NJ

From a theoretical point of view, DNA-based immunization presents many advantages *(2–7)*. In mice, a single intramuscular or intradermal injection of DNA is very efficient at inducing an immune response via an in vivo synthesis of the encoded antigens (**Fig. 1**) and a potent self-adjuvantation, probably through the CpG motifs *(8)*. The type of immune response is very similar to that induced by natural infection with respect to kinetics, antibody isotypes, and specificity of the humoral immune response. More important, it induces a very strong cellular immune response, predominantly T-helper-1 (Th1) and CTL responses. This response persists for several weeks. In addition, DNA-based vaccines have the advantage of low cost of production, ease of quality control, and the ability to be stored and transported at ambient temperatures.

It is of practical interest to note that a single intramuscular or subcutaneous injection of 100 μg of nonpackaged plasmid DNA and a single intradermal injection of a 100-fold lower dose of 1 μg of particle-coated plasmid DNA using the gene gun *(9–11)* prime similar serum antibody responses although the isotype profiles of these responses differ strikingly. These data indicate that "one-shot DNA vaccines" are feasible.

Several investigations have shown that humoral immune and CTL responses could be induced to viral structural and nonstructural proteins in both mice and chimpanzees *(12–24)*. In HBV transgenic mice, there are conflicting results whether DNA-based immunization against HBV envelope proteins is able to break tolerance against these structural proteins with a subsequent down-regulation of HBV replication and gene expression *(22,24–26)*. In the duck hepatitis B virus (DHBV) model, plasmids expressing DHBV large protein were able to induce a decrease in serum and liver viral DNA in chronic carriers *(27)*.

Codelivery of DNA vaccines with cytokines can modulate and enhance the cellular immune responses against viral antigens *(28,29)*. The strength of the immunomodulating effect of cytokines may depend on the nature of the expressed HBV antigen (e.g., intracellular vs secretion) *(13,30)*. The nature of the (intracellular or secreted) antigen expressed by a DNA vaccine (**Fig. 2**) can affect the levels of induced antibodies *(13,31)* and may affect the Th1 or Th2 bias of primed immune responses *(32,33)* (**Fig. 3**). The main factors that are under current investigation to improve the DNA-based vaccines include (1) the design of plasmid vectors; (2) the technique and route of DNA delivery (e.g., the optimization of in vivo transfection efficacy); (3) the enhancement/modulation of primed immune responses (e.g., characterization of adjuvants effects induced by codelivered cytokine, chemokine or costimulators); and (4) to combine the DNA-based vaccines with recombinant protein vaccines in prime/boost regimens.

If proven to be safe and immunogenic in humans, this approach is a promising candidate for both an effective prophylactic and therapeutic vaccine against HBV.

2. Materials

2.1. Plasmids

Expression plasmids used in DNA-based vaccination usually contain two units (**Fig. 4**): (1) the antigen expression (transcription) unit composed of promoter/enhancer sequences, followed by antigen-encoding and polyadenylation sequences, and (2) the

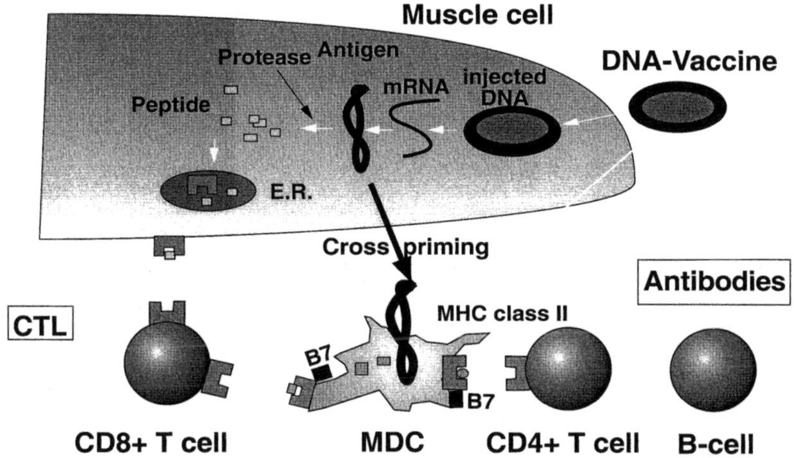

Fig. 1. Mechanism of induction of immune responses after im DNA immunization. Antigens encoded by DNA plasmids are either synthesized by muscle cells or antigen-presenting cells such as dendritic cells upon direct transfection or uptake of DNA resulting in priming of B- and T-cell responses against the encoded antigen. Alternatively, antigens already encoded are taken up by dendritic cells (cross-priming) and MHC class I restricted CD8+ T cell responses are initiated.

production unit composed of bacterial sequences necessary for plasmid amplification (origin of replication) and selection (bacterial antibiotic resistance genes such as the ampicillin- or the kanamycin-resistance genes). Different promoter/enhancer sequences have been used successfully to construct antigen-expressing vectors. These include viral promoter/enhancer sequences from human cytomegalovirus (HCMV) or the papovavirus SV40, or mammalian promoter/enhancer sequences, for example, from elongation factor-1α, desmin, or metallothionin ***(9,16,17,34–37)***.

Common CMV promotor-based vectors used for DNA-based immunization are pCI (Promega, Heidelberg, Germany) and pcDNA3 (Invitrogen, San Diego, CA, USA). Several investigators offer HBV antigen expressing plasmids via the Internet (http://www.dnavaccine.com).

Endotoxin-free plasmid DNA (*see* **Note 1**) should be created from bacterial lysates by anion-exchange chromatography resulting in highly purified, supercoiled (>90%) plasmid product (QIAGEN Plasmid Mega kit, Hilden, Germany). Plasmids for repetitive usage should be stored at 4°C; long-term storage should be performed at –20°C or –80°C.

2.2. Solutions

1. Phosphate-buffered saline (PBS): Dissolve 8 g of NaCl, 0.2 g of KCl, 1.44 g of Na_2HPO_4, and 0.24 g of KH_2PO_4 in 800 mL of distilled H_2O. Adjust the pH to 7.4 with HCl. Add H_2O to 1 L and sterilize. Store at 4°C.
2. 0.5% Bupivacaine (Aventis Pharma, Basel, Switzerland). Store at room temperature (RT).
3. 1 *M* calcium chloride: Dissolve 54 g of $CaCl_2 \cdot 6H_2O$ in 200 mL of pure distilled H_2O. Sterilize and store at –20°C.

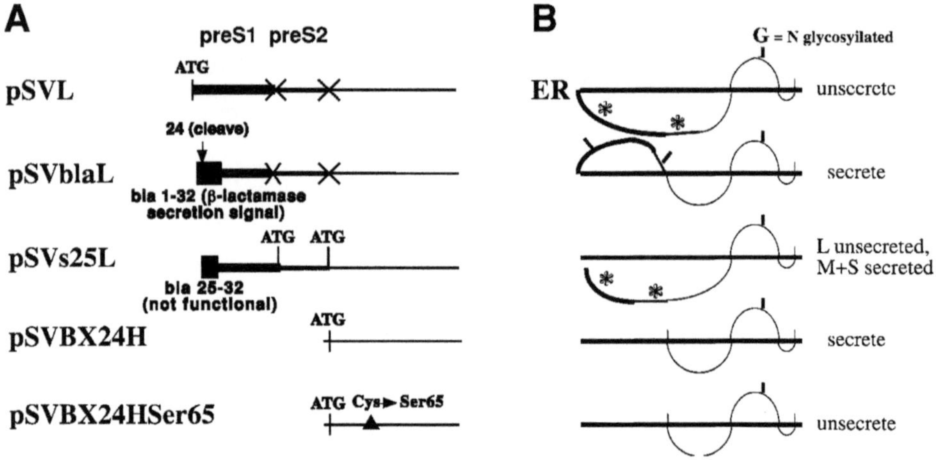

Fig. 2. Map of the transmembrane topology of HBV envelope proteins. DNA expression constructs. **A**: DNA expression constructs with the corresponding HBV surface encoding sequences (e.g., pre-S1, pre-S2, S) and the corresponding intact or deleted ATG translation initiation start codons. pSVL encodes wild-type HBV-LHBs and carries mutations of both the MHBs and SHBs start codons to the threonin codon ACG. pSVblaL carries a bacterial β-lactamase secretion signal sequence upstream from the LHBs coding sequence and encodes a secreted LHB protein. MHBs and SHBs start codons are mutated in the same manner as in pSVL. pSVs25L corresponds to pSVblaL but contains a truncated nonfunctional signal sequence as well as wild-type MHBs and SHBs and SHBs start codons. The pSVBX24H vector encodes HBV-SHBs. The pSVBX24HSer65 construct corresponds to plasmid pSVBX24H, except for codon 65 of the S-gene, which has been mutated from cysteine (TGT) to serine (TCT) by site directed mutagenesis. This mutated SHB protein is not secreted by the cell. **B**: Expected transmembrane topology at the ER of the different HBsAgs. Effective (G) and potential (*) glycosylation sites are marked. L, large envelope protein; M, middle envelope protein; S, small envelope protein.

2.3. Other Materials

1. 26-Gauge or 30-gauge × ½ needle (Sterican, Braun, Melsungen, Germany) for intramuscular injections.
2. Helios gene gun for intradermal application (Bio-Rad Life Science, Hercules, CA, USA).
3. Helium supply. Compressed helium of at least grade 4.5 should be used. The safety instructions provided by the supplier should be followed for installation. If the gun is to be used in more than one place, the user can have several helium cylinders and carry the gun between them.
4. Compressed nitrogen of at least grade 4.8 is required for cartridge preparation using the tubing prep station.
5. Nitrogen regulator. A single-stage regulator with an output gauge that registers a maximum of 30 psi is needed to produce the 0.4 L/min flow rate necessary for using the tubing prep station. A regulator is available from Bio-Rad (cat. no. 165–2425).

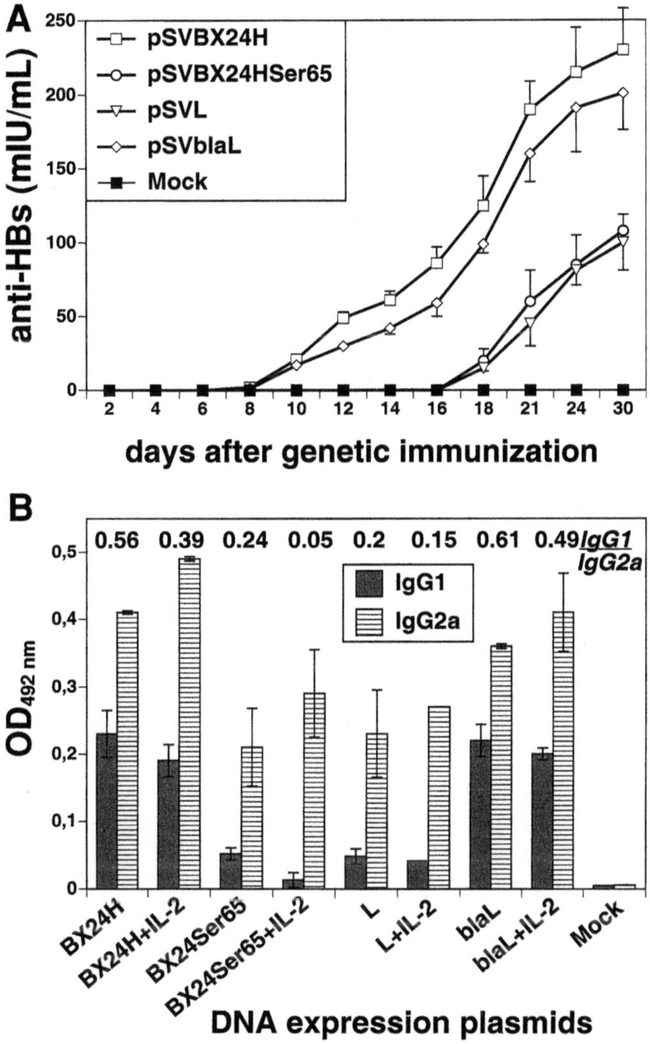

Fig. 3. Anti-HBs kinetics (**A**) and antibody subtype (**B**). **A**: Anti-HBs titers are expressed in mIU/mL and derived from bleedings of single mice at the indicated time points following immunization. Each group comprised five mice. **B**: Antibody IgG1 and IgG2a subtypes were determined by ELISA technique and derived from individual mouse sera diluted 1:50 on d 24 after genetic immunization. BX24H encodes secreted HBV small envelope protein; IL-2, DNAexpression construct encoding murine IL-2; BX24HSer65 encodes non-secreted HBV small envelope protein; L encodes non-secreted, blaL secreted HBV large envelope protein.

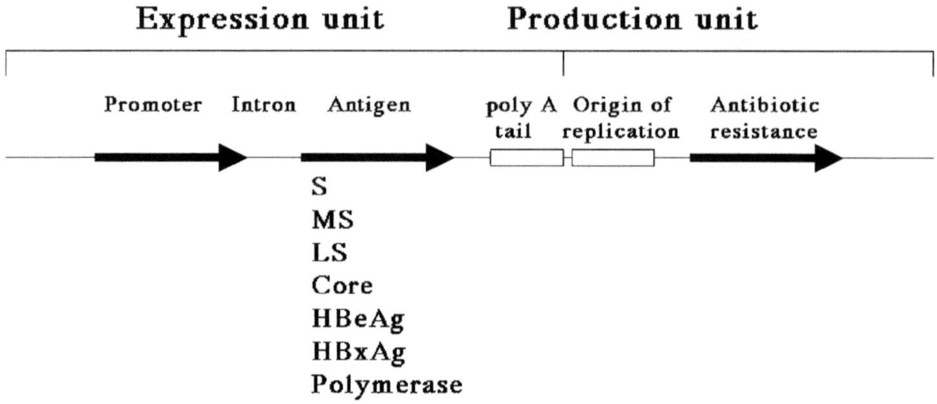

Fig. 4. Design of DNA expression plasmids. Expression plasmids used in DNA-based vaccination usually contain two units: the antigen expression (transcription) unit composed of promoter/enhancer sequences, followed by antigen-encoding and polyadenylation sequences, and the production unit composed of bacterial sequences necessary for plasmid amplification (origin of replication) and selection (bacterial antibiotic resistance genes). Plasmids examined in murine studies express all structural and non-structural HBV antigens.

2.4. Animal Maintenance

It is important to keep mice strictly under pathogen-free conditions in an appropriate animal facility. Ongoing infections by several microbial or viral agents may significantly decrease the efficacy of DNA vaccination.

2.5. Anesthesia

1. 10% ketamine hydrochloride (115.34 mg/mL; Essex Tierarznei, Munich, Germany).
2. 2% xylazine hydrochloride (23.32 mg/mL; Bayer Leverkusen, Germany).
3. 26-Gauge × ½ needle (Sterican, Braun, Melsungen, Germany).

3. Methods

3.1. DNA Intramuscular Vaccination

Mice are anesthetized with a single intraperitoneal injection (75 μL) of 100 mg/kg of Ketanest + 16 mg/kg of Rompun, which is a combination of an analgesic drug (ketamine) with a barbiturate (xylazine). For priming long-lasting, antiviral immunity by a single injection of an HBV expression DNA plasmid, the nonpackaged plasmid DNA is injected intramuscularly (into the M. tibialis anterior or M. quadriceps). However, large amounts of DNA (i.e., 50–100 μg/mouse) have to be injected to prime immune responses in mice (*see* **Note 2**). Increasing DNA amounts above 200 μg does not result in superior anti-HBV immune responses in mice. DNA should have a concentration of at least 2 mg/mL in PBS to inject 100 μg of DNA in a volume of 50 μL into the M. tibialis anterior using a 28-gauge or 30-gauge needle (*see* **Note 3**). If one targets the M.

quadriceps, a volume of 100 μL can be easily injected. In this case, we prefer to inject the 100-μL volume of plasmid DNA over five different sites into the quadriceps muscle of mice (*see* **Note 4**). Booster injections every 2 wk increase the antibody and helper T-cell responses to HBV core and surface antigens. They have, however, no significant effect on strength of CTL responses to those antigens. Immunized mice develop high antibody titers specific for HBsAg or HBcAg in the third week post-vaccination and persist at high levels for more than 9 mo ***(17)***. Anti-HBsAg titers may reach plateau levels of about 10,000 mIU/mL at 16–36 weeks post-vaccination. A single DNA-based vaccination induces long-lasting, HBsAg-specific CTL responses ***(16,24,38)***. A MHC-I (L^d)-restricted CTL reactivity specific for the well-known S 28-39 epitope (IPQSLDSWWTSL) of the HBsAg in HBV envelope immunized mice can be readily detected. CTL primed by a single intramuscular injection of HBsAg-encoding pCI/S plasmid DNA were first detected 6–8 d after vaccination, and remained detectable for at least 6 mo post-vaccination. (*See* **Note 5**.)

The intradermal application of plasmid DNA using the Helios Gene Gun (Bio-Rad, Munich, Germany, http://www.biorad.com, **Fig. 5A**) is an alternative vaccination technique for the induction of humoral and cellular immune responses against HBV antigens.

3.2. DNA Intradermal Vaccination Using the Gene Gun

If the gene gun is used for DNA vaccination, priming of Th2-biased immunity is observed, even if an identical antigen-encoding expression plasmid is used. Using this technique, 0.1–1 μg of plasmid DNA coated onto 0.5.- to 1.6.-mm gold particles are shot into the skin or surgically exposed muscle using the helium-driven gene gun with a defined pressure ***(9–11,39,40)***. Provided with the Bio-Rad system are the Helios gene gun, the helium regulator, the tubing cutter and 10 razor blades, an optimization kit, the Helios gene gun kit, the helium hose assembly, the tubing prep station, and gene shot cartridges.

Prior to the DNA application, gold particles have to be coated with plasmid DNA. For most systems, delivering 0.5 mg of gold per target is a good starting point. A 1-mL suspension of DNA–gold will fill an 8.5-inch length of tubing; therefore, 3 mL will be needed to fill 25-inch tubing, enough for 50 shots. To deliver 0.5 mg of microcarriers to each target (microcarrier loading quantities [MLQ] = 0.5), 25 mg of gold would need to be resuspended in a volume of 3 mL of ethanol, that is, 8.5 mg/mL. For many applications delivery of 1 mg of DNA per target is a good starting point. At a MLQ of 0.5 mg gold/cartridge, a DNA loading ratio (DLR) of 2 mg of DNA/mg of gold results in loading 1 mg of DNA per cartridge and therefore delivery of 1 mg of DNA per target. Therefore preparation of two lengths of tubing requires 100 mg of DNA and 50 mg of gold. Plasmid DNA coated gold particles are dissolved in 3 mL of a polyvinylpyrrolidone (PVP) solution in 100% ethanol (17.7 μg/mL). Often the concentration of PVP needs to be optimized for your application. A good starting point is 0.01 mg/mL. Prepare a stock solution of 20 mg/mL of PVP in ethanol. This stock solution can be diluted with ethanol to prepare PVP solutions at the desired concentration.

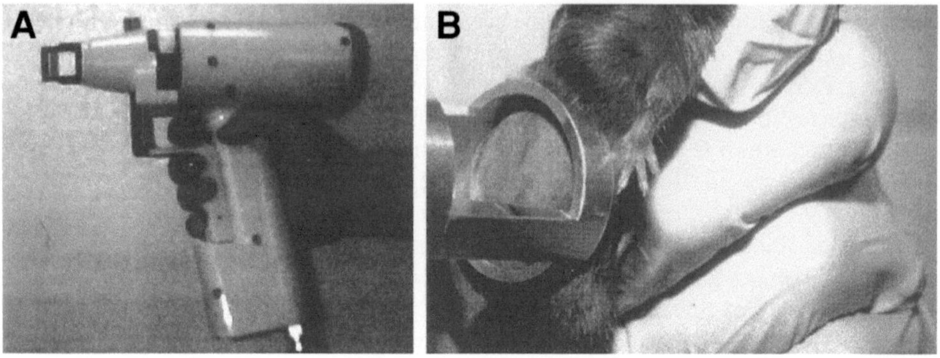

Fig. 5. Intradermal application of plasmid DNA using the Helios Gene Gun (**A**). Using this technique, 0.1–1 μg plasmid DNA coated onto 0.5–1.6 mm gold particles are shot into the abdominal skin using the helium-driven gene gun with a defined pressure. After removal of hair from the target site (usually abdomen of the mouse) the spacer is pressed directly against the target site (**B**) and the plasmid/gold particles are fired with about 400 psi.

3.3. Procedure

1. Weigh gold microcarriers into a 1.5-mL tube.
2. Add 100 μL of 0.05 *M* spermidine (Sigma, cat. no. S0266).
3. Briefly vortex-mix and sonicate the mixture to break up any gold clumps.
4. Add the required volume of plasmid (or plasmids) to achieve the desired DLR.
5. Mix DNA, spermidine, and gold by vortex-mixing for 5 s.
6. While vortex-mixing, add 100 μL of 1 *M* calcium chloride dropwise to the mixture.
7. Continue vortex-mixing for 5–10 s.
8. Allow the mixture to precipitate at room temperature for 10 min.
9. Microfuge for 15 s to pellet the gold.
10. Remove and discard the supernatant.
11. Resuspend and wash the pellet three times with fresh 100% ethanol.
12. Centrifuge briefly and discard the supernatant between each wash. (*See* **Note 6**.)
13. After the final ethanol wash, resuspend the pellet in 200 μL of the ethanol solution containing the appropriate concentration of PVP.
14. Transfer the gold–ethanol slurry into a 15-mL tube with a screw cap.
15. Rinse the microfuge tube once with the same ethanol–PVP solution to collect any remaining sample.
16. Add the required volume of ethanol–PVP solution to the centifuge tube to bring the DNA/microcarrier solution to the desired microcarrier loading ratio. The suspension is now ready for tube preparation.
17. The next step is the loading of the gene gun cartridge with the desired amounts of coated tubes. Then anesthetize the animal as described in **Subheading 3.1.** Remove hair from target site (usually abdomen of the mouse) (*see* **Note 7**) using a commercial depilatory (e.g., Veet, München, Germany) to expose the epidermis.
18. Clean with 70% ethanol and hold the spacer directly against the target site **(Fig. 5B)**. Discharge the gun. Fire the plasmid–gold particles with approx 400 $lb/in.^2$

A single intradermal inoculation of 0.1–1 μg particle-coated pCI/S plasmid DNA with the gene gun efficiently induces serum antibody responses to HBsAg ***(24)***. The kinetics of appearance and longevity of this antibody response are comparable to responses elicited by intramuscular injections of 100 μg of pCI/S plasmid DNA. The anti-HBsAg serum antibody titers induced by a single gene gun vaccination reaches plateau levels of approx 4000 mIU/mL. Gene gun–mediated injection of the pCI/S plasmid DNA selectively stimulates long-lasting Th2-biased antibody responses (IgG1/IgG2a ratio >60). In contrast to the efficient induction of antibody responses, the gene gun vaccination failed to prime HBsAg-specific CTL responses as we did not find reproducible evidence for major histocompatibility class (MHC)-I-restricted, HBsAg-specific CTL priming. We found low levels of CTL reactivity against HBsAg-expressing, syngeneic transfectants in only 3 out of 15 individual mice tested after primed cell populations were repeatedly restimulated in vitro. However, in other systems previous reports showed that gene gun mediated DNA immunization elicits CTL responses in mice, monkeys, or humans ***(33,39,41–45)***.

4. Notes

1. Plasmid DNA should be dissolved in PBS rather than TE buffer for optimal in vivo efficacy.
2. By reducing the amount of injected DNA to 10–20 μg/mouse, immunogenicity of the DNA vaccine rapidly declines. We never detected immune responses when mice were injected with 0.5–2 μg of plasmid DNA/mouse, even when the muscles were preconditioned by inflammation-inducing agents (e.g., cardiotoxin or bupivicaine) before DNA delivery to increase immune responses induced by DNA vaccination ***(12)***.
3. If several DNA plasmids are injected at the same time (e.g., cytokine and HBV plasmids), the concentration of the DNA plasmids should be high enough to result in a final volume of 50–100 μL injection volume.
4. It is important to place the needle in the center of the target muscle. If the penetration of the muscle is not deep enough, the DNA solution will flow out. By contrast, piercing through the muscle will result in weak or absent immune responses.
5. Usually, facilitator compounds are not necessary to achieve strong anti-HBV immune responses in mice. If necessary, 50–100 μL of bupivacaine (0.2–0.4%) diluted in PBS can be injected into the muscle 5 d prior to the injection of the HBV DNA. Alternatively, plasmid DNA can be dissolved directly in Bupivacaine in a final concentration of 0.25%.
6. This step is critical in the procedure: It is important that the ethanol does not absorb any water. The bottle should be kept closed between uses.
7. Using the gene gun, it is important to target the middle rather than the lower part of the abdomen to avoid damage or rupture of the urinary bladder.

References

1. Chisari, F. V. and Ferrari, C. (1995) Hepatitis B virus immunopathogenesis. *Annu. Rev. Immunol.* **13,** 29–60.
2. Lewis, P. J. and Babiuk, L. A. (1999) DNA vaccines: a review. *Adv. Virus Res.* **54,** 129–188.
3. Levitsky, H. I. (1997) Accessories for naked DNA vaccines. *Nat. Biotechnol.* **15,** 619–620.
4. McCarthy, M. (1996) DNA vaccination: a direct line to the immune system. *Lancet* **348,** 1232.

5. McDonnell, W. M. and Askari, F. K. (1996) DNA vaccines. *N. Engl. J. Med.* **334,** 42–45.
6. Ertl, H. C. and Xiang, Z. Q. (1996) Genetic immunization. *Viral Immunol.* **9,** 1–9.
7. Donnelly, J. J., Ulmer, J. B., Shiver, J. W., and Liu, M. A. (1997) DNA vaccines. *Annu. Rev. Immunol.* **15,** 617–648.
8. Krieg, A. M., Yi, A. K., Matson, S., et al. (1995) CpG motifs in bacterial DNA trigger direct B-cell activation. *Nature* **374,** 546–549.
9. Tang, D. C., De Vit, M., and Johnston, S. A. (1992) Genetic immunization is a simple method for eliciting an immune response. *Nature* **356,** 152–154.
10. Fynan, E. F., Webster, R. G., Fuller, D. H., Haynes, J. R., Santoro, J. C., and Robinson, H. L. (1993) DNA vaccines: protective immunizations by parenteral, mucosal, and gene-gun inoculations. *Proc. Natl. Acad. Sci. USA* **90,** 11478–11482.
11. Leitner, W. W., Seguin, M. C., Ballou, W. R., et al. (1997) Immune responses induced by intramuscular or gene gun injection of protective deoxyribonucleic acid vaccines that express the circumsporozoite protein from Plasmodium berghei malaria parasites. *J. Immunol.* **159,** 6112–6119.
12. Geissler, M., Tokushige, K., Chante, C. C., Zurawski, V. R., Jr., and Wands, J. R. (1997) Cellular and humoral immune response to hepatitis B virus structural proteins in mice after DNA-based immunization. *Gastroenterology* **112,** 1307–1320.
13. Geissler, M., Schirmbeck, R., Reimann, J., Blum, H. E., and Wands, J. R. (1998) Cytokine and hepatitis B virus DNA co-immunizations enhance cellular and humoral immune responses to the middle but not to the large hepatitis B virus surface antigen in mice. *Hepatology* **28,** 202–210.
14. Davis, H. L. (1998) DNA-based immunization against hepatitis B: experience with animal models. *Curr. Top. Microbiol. Immunol.* **226,** 57–68.
15. Davis, H. L., McCluskie, M. J., Gerin, J. L., and Purcell, R. H. (1996) DNA vaccine for hepatitis B: evidence for immunogenicity in chimpanzees and comparison with other vaccines. *Proc. Natl. Acad. Sci. USA* **93,** 7213–7218.
16. Davis, H. L., Schirmbeck, R., Reimann, J., and Whalen, R. G. (1995) DNA-mediated immunization in mice induces a potent MHC class I-restricted cytotoxic T lymphocyte response to the hepatitis B envelope protein. *Hum. Gene Ther.* **6,** 1447–1456.
17. Bohm, W., Mertens, T., Schirmbeck, R., and Reimann, J. (1998) Routes of plasmid DNA vaccination that prime murine humoral and cellular immune responses. *Vaccine* **16,** 949–954.
18. Davis, H. L., Michel, M. L., and Whalen, R. G. (1993) DNA-based immunization induces continuous secretion of hepatitis B surface antigen and high levels of circulating antibody. *Hum. Mol. Genet.* **2,** 1847–1851.
19. Chow, Y. H., Huang, W. L., Chi, W. K., Chu, Y. D., and Tao, M. H. (1997) Improvement of hepatitis B virus DNA vaccines by plasmids coexpressing hepatitis B surface antigen and interleukin-2. *J. Virol.* **71,** 169–178.
20. Kuhober, A., Pudollek, H. P., Reifenberg, K., et al. (1996) DNA immunization induces antibody and cytotoxic T cell responses to hepatitis B core antigen in H-2b mice. *J. Immunol.* **156,** 3687–3695.
21. Kuhrober, A., Wild, J., Pudollek, H. P., Chisari, F. V., and Reimann, J. (1997) DNA vaccination with plasmids encoding the intracellular (HBcAg) or secreted (HBeAg) form of the core protein of hepatitis B virus primes T cell responses to two overlapping Kb- and Kd-restricted epitopes. *Int. Immunol.* **9,** 1203–1212.
22. Mancini, M., Davis, H., Tiollais, P., and Michel, M. L. (1996) DNA-based immunization against the envelope proteins of the hepatitis B virus. *J. Biotechnol.* **44,** 47–57.

23. Michel, M. L., Davis, H. L., Schleef, M., Mancini, M., Tiollais, P., and Whalen, R. G. (1995) DNA-mediated immunization to the hepatitis B surface antigen in mice: aspects of the humoral response mimic hepatitis B viral infection in humans. *Proc. Natl. Acad. Sci. USA* **92,** 5307–5311.
24. Schirmbeck, R., Wild, J., Stober, D., et al. (2000) Ongoing murine T1 or T2 immune responses to the hepatitis B surface antigen are excluded from the liver that expresses transgene-encoded hepatitis B surface antigen. *J. Immunol.* **164,** 4235–4243.
25. Mancini, M., Hadchouel, M., Davis, H. L., Whalen, R. G., Tiollais, P., and Michel, M. L. (1996) DNA-mediated immunization in a transgenic mouse model of the hepatitis B surface antigen chronic carrier state. *Proc. Natl. Acad. Sci. USA* **93,** 12496–12501.
26. Shimizu, Y., Guidotti, L. G., Fowler, P., and Chisari, F. V. (1998) Dendritic cell immunization breaks cytotoxic T lymphocyte tolerance in hepatitis B virus transgenic mice. *J. Immunol* **161,** 4520–4529.
27. Triyatni, M., Jilbert, A. R., Qiao, M., Miller, D. S., and Burrell, C. J., (1998) Protective efficacy of DNA vaccines against duck hepatitis B virus infection. *J. Virol.* **72,** 84–94.
28. Xiang, Z. and Ertl, H. C. (1995) Manipulation of the immune response to a plasmid-encoded viral antigen by coinoculation with plasmids expressing cytokines. *Immunity* **2,** 129–135.
29. Geissler, M., Gesien, A., Tokushige, K., and Wands, J. R. (1997) Enhancement of cellular and humoral immune responses to hepatitis C virus core protein using DNA-based vaccines augmented with cytokine-expressing plasmids. *J. Immunol.* **158,** 1231–1237.
30. Geissler, M., Bruss, V., Michalak, S., et al. (1999) Intracellular retention of hepatitis B virus surface proteins reduces interleukin-2 augmentation after genetic immunizations. *J. Virol.* **73,** 4284–4292.
31. Inchauspe, G., Vitvitski, L., Major, M. E., et al. (1997) Plasmid DNA expressing a secreted or a nonsecreted form of hepatitis C virus nucleocapsid: comparative studies of antibody and T-helper responses following genetic immunization. *DNA Cell Biol.* **16,** 185–195.
32. Haddad, D., Liljeqvist, S., Stahl, S., et al. (1997) Comparative study of DNA-based immunization vectors: effect of secretion signals on the antibody responses in mice. *FEMS Immunol. Med. Microbiol.* **18,** 193–202.
33. Boyle, J. S., Koniaras, C., and Lew, A. M. (1997) Influence of cellular location of expressed antigen on the efficacy of DNA vaccination: cytotoxic T lymphocyte and antibody responses are suboptimal when antigen is cytoplasmic after intramuscular DNA immunization. *Int. Immunol.* **9,** 1897–1906.
34. Tokushige, K., Moradpour, D., T., W., Geissler, M., Hayashi, N., and Wands, J. R. (1997) Comparison between cytomegalovirus promoter and elongation factor-1a promoter-driven constructs in the establishment of cell lines expressing hepatitis C virus core protein. *J. Virol. Methods* **64,** 73–80.
35. Simon, M. M., Gern, L., Hauser, P., et al. (1996) Protective immunization with plasmid DNA containing the outer surface lipoprotein A gene of *Borrelia burgdorferi* is independent of an eukaryotic promoter. *Eur. J. Immunol.* **26,** 2831–2840.
36. Raz, E., Carson, D. A., Parker, S. E., et al. (1994) Intradermal gene immunization: the possible role of DNA uptake in the induction of cellular immunity to viruses. *Proc. Natl. Acad. Sci. USA* **91,** 9519–9523.
37. Kwissa, M., von Kampen v, K., Zurbriggen, R., Gluck, R. Reimann, J., and Schirmbeck, R., (2000) Efficient vaccination by intradermal or intramuscular inoculation of plasmid DNA expressing hepatitis B surface antigen under desmin promoter/enhancer control. *Vaccine* **18,** 2337–2344.

38. Geissler, M., Gesien, A., and Wands, J. R. (1997) Inhibitory effects of chronic ethanol consumption on cellular immune responses to hepatitis C virus core protein are reversed by genetic immunizations augmented with cytokine-expressing plasmids. *J. Immunol.* **159,** 5107–5113.
39. Pertmer, T. M., Roberts, T. R., and Haynes, J. R. (1996) Influenza virus nucleoprotein-specific immunoglobulin G subclass and cytokine responses elicited by DNA vaccination are dependent on the route of vector DNA delivery. *J. Virol.* **70,** 6119–6125.
40. Williams, R. S., Johnston, S. A., Riedy, M., De Vit, M. J., McElligott, S. G., and Sanford, J. C. (1991) Introduction of foreign genes into tissues of living mice by DNA-coated microprojectiles. *Proc. Natl. Acad. Sci. USA* **88,** 2726–2730.
41. Degano, P., Sarphie, D. F., and Bangham, C. R. (1998) Intradermal DNA immunization of mice against influenza A virus using the novel PowderJect system. *Vaccine* **16,** 394–398.
42. Mahvi, D. M., Burkholder, J. K., Turner, J., et al. (1996) Particle-mediated gene transfer of granulocyte-macrophage colony-stimulating factor cDNA to tumor cells: implications for a clinically relevant tumor vaccine. *Hum. Gene Ther.* **7,** 1535–1543.
43. Fuller, D. H., Murphey-Corb, M., Clements, J., Barnett, S., and Haynes, J. R. (1996) Induction of immunodeficiency virus-specific immune responses in rhesus monkeys following gene gun-mediated DNA vaccination. *J. Med. Primatol.* **25,** 236–241.
44. Sun, W. H., Burkholder, J. K., Sun, J., et al. (1995) In vivo cytokine gene transfer by gene gun reduces tumor growth in mice. *Proc. Natl. Acad. Sci. USA* **92,** 2889–2893.
45. Zarozinski, C. C., Fynan, E. F., Selin, L. K., Robinson, H. L., and Welsh, R. M. (1995) Protective CTL-dependent immunity and enhanced immunopathology in mice immunized by particle bombardment with DNA encoding an internal virion protein. *J. Immunol.* **154,** 4010–4017.

5

Monitoring Gene Expression Using DNA Microarrays During Hepatitis B Virus Infection

Michael R. Beard and Stephen Locarnini

1. Introduction

Under normal circumstances, hepatocyte infection with the hepatitis B virus (HBV) is noncytopathic. Hepatocellular damage is mediated by the cellular and humoral arms of the host's immune system *(1)*. The final clinical outcome of either clearance or persistence reflects a three-way interplay of hepatocyte, virus, and the host's immune response. Thus, an understanding of the impact of HBV replication on the "transcriptome" of hepatocytes would aid the understanding of the events that occur during active viral replication. Furthermore, such studies could also provide insights into the mechanism of HBV-associated hepatocarcinogenesis including the broader area of gene regulation following HBV infection.

The simplest approach in gene array studies is to perform a difference analysis, for example, active HBV replication in cells compared to no replication in the same cells. A number of in vivo and in vitro model systems are available for studying HBV *(2)*, including stable cell lines that express the virus. The recently developed HepAD38 cell line contains a tetracycline-regulatable wild-type HBV construct driven by the cytomegalovirus (CMV) immediate early promoter *(3)*, which allows for a convenient difference analysis of HBV replication. Essentially, in the absence of tetracycline, high-level productive replication occurs, while in the presence of the antibiotic HBV replication is essentially inhibited.

Hepatocellular carcinoma is one of the most common forms of primary liver cancer, with approx 1 million deaths annually. It is one of the few human tumors for which development is associated with infection with HBV or HCV. Despite these associations the precise mechanism of hepatocarcinogenesis remains unclear. Microarray analysis is well suited to investigate mRNA expression profiles in tumor and nontumor tissue, and numerous studies have identified novel genes associated with tumor development and progression, including hepatocellular carcinoma (HCC) *(4–8)*. Microarray analysis makes it possible to also investigate mRNA expression

From: *Methods in Molecular Medicine, vol. 96: Hepatitis B and D Protocols, volume 2*
Edited by: R. K. Hamatake and J. Y. N. Lau © Humana Press Inc., Totowa, NJ

profiles in HCC and compare directly with the corresponding nontumor profile from patients undergoing tumor resection. These studies have the ability to identify changes in mRNA expression that may elucidate potential pathogenic mechanisms and identify novel therapeutic targets and markers for molecular diagnosis and early detection.

In microarray technology, there are two main types of expression arrays:

1. cDNA spotted arrays configured as either (a) solid support glass arrays: up to 10,000 DNA probes, cDNA or oligonucleotides, usually produced in-house, or (b) membrane-based microarrays, for example, Clontech Atlas Arrays 1176 cDNAs
2. High-density oligonucleotide arrays: Affymetrix 12,626 oligos per array.

On cDNA spotted glass slide arrays, genes are generally represented by single DNA fragments (greater than several hundred basepairs in length) or oligonucleotides (50–80 mers) that are spotted onto specially prepared glass slides. The cDNA samples hybridized to the array are, in most cases, labeled by incorporating fluorescently tagged nucleotides during oligo-primed reverse transcription of mRNA ***(9)***. Different fluorophors (generally Cy3- and Cy5-dUTP) are used to label cDNAs from control and experimental test RNAs. The labeled cDNAs are then mixed together prior to hybridization to the array. Relative amounts of a particular gene transcript in the two samples are determined by measuring the signal intensities detected for both fluorophors and calculating signal ratios ***(10)***.

Membrane-based cDNA arrays such as the Clontech Atlas Array system (Clontech, Palo Alto, CA) are different from the solid support arrays in that cDNA fragments are printed directly onto nitrocellulose. This allows for standard hybridization and washing protocols and no requirement for any special equipment. cDNA is synthesized from total RNA and labeled with ^{32}P for both experimental and test RNA. These labeled cDNAs are then hybridized to identical but separate membranes and the mRNA expression profiles generated for each control and test are compared to determine changes in mRNA abundance.

On oligonucleotide arrays such as the Affymetrix system (Affymetrix, Santa Clara, CA), a given gene is represented by 15–20 different 25-mer oligonucleotides that serve as unique, sequence-specific detectors. An additional control element on Affymetrix arrays is the use of mismatch (MM) control oligonucleotides that are identical to their perfect match (PM) partners except for a single base difference in a central position. The presence of the mismatched oligonucleotide allows cross-hybridization and local background to be estimated and substracted from the PM signal ***(10)***. In the Affymetrix expression array system, eukaryotic mRNA is converted to biotinylated cRNA from oligo-dT-primed cDNA ***(11)***. Each sample is hybridized to a separate array. Transcript levels are calculated by reference to cRNA spikes of known concentration added to the hybridization mixture. Differences in mRNA levels between samples are determined by comparison of any two hybridization patterns produced on separate arrays of the same array type ***(10)***.

2. Materials

2.1. Starting Material and Typical Experimental Approach

DNA microarray technology allows investigation of gene expression profiles using a variety of sources as starting material. Using both membrane cDNA expression arrays (Clontech) and high-density oligonucleotide arrays (Affymetrix), the authors have investigated gene expression profiles in in vitro cell culture models of HBV replication such as the AD38 cell line *(3)* under conditions of conditional expression of HBV proteins using the tetracycline-inducible promoter system. In addition, this approach has also been used to examine differential gene expression in HBV-induced HCC where mRNA profiles from the HCC are compared to non-HCC liver surrounding the HCC. Fresh liver taken at biopsy or tumor resection is snap frozen in liquid nitrogen or stored at –80°C or at –20°C in RNAlater (Ambion) solution.

2.2. Membrane cDNA Microarrays

In this chapter, reagents for membrane-based cDNA expression arrays refer to the Atlas cDNA Arrays manufactured and distributed by Clontech. However, many manufacturers offer similar arrays in various formats. The authors have found these arrays to be reproducible and accurate. Furthermore, use of these arrays does not require the purchase of expensive equipment and any well-equipped molecular biology laboratory will have the necessary equipment.

1. RNAlater (Ambion, Austin TX).
2. RNAqueous, Total RNA isolation kit (Ambion, Austin, TX).
3. DNA-free, DNase 1 treatment and removal (Ambion, Austin, TX).
4. Diethylpyrocarbonate (DEPC)-treated RNase-free water.
5. RNase-free 1.5-mL microfuge tube with pestle (Kontes, Vineland, NJ).
6. Ceramic mortar and pestle.
7. 100% Ethanol.
8. Atlas cDNA microarray kit, contains labeling reagents (Clontech, Palo Alto, CA).
9. [α-^{32}P]dATP (10 μCi/μl: 3000 Ci/nmol; Amersham).
10. Sonicated salmon sperm DNA (Stratagene, La Jolla, CA).
11. 10X Denaturating solution: 1 *M* NaOH, 10 m*M* EDTA.
12. 2X Neutralization solution: 1 *M* NaH_2PO_4, pH 7.0.
13. Wash solution 1: 2X Saline sodium citrate (SSC), 1% sodium dodecyl sulfate (SDS).
14. Wash solution 2: 0.1% SSC, 0.5% SDS.
15. X-ray film (Kodak, BioMax) or Phosphorimage screen.
16. Hybridization oven.

2.3. High-Density Oligonucleotide Arrays

In contrast to the cDNA arrays discussed above the high-density oligonucleotide arrays consist of oligonucleotides that are chemically synthesized onto a silicon support through a process called photolithography *(10)*. While this method has a number of advantages over the cDNA membrane arrays, the main disadvantage is the cost of the arrays and the specialized equipment needed to probe and scan the arrays. The complete list of reagents and equipment is too large to list here and can be found at the University of Texas Medical Branch, Genomics Core Facility website (http://www.scms.utmb.edu/genomics/index.htm).

3. Methods

3.1. Preparation of RNA from Cell Lines and Tissue

1. The quality of RNA is essential for high-quality labeling and hybridization to both membrane-based cDNA arrays and oligonucleotide arrays. While in-house RNA isolation RNA preparation protocols are well established ***(12)***, the authors have found most consistent results using the RNAqueous total RNA isolation kit from Ambion. However, a number of phenol-free kits are available from other manufacturers that are also suitable. The Atlas Array system requires either total or poly(A) + purified RNA. The authors have found that total RNA works as well and in some cases better than poly(A) + isolated RNA.
2. Frozen liver specimens can be broken into small pieces or ground to a fine powder using a mortar and pestle sitting in liquid nitrogen. Specimens stored in RNAlater can be cut into 1-mm cubes with a scalpel. RNA is then extracted using the RNAqueous total RNA isolation kit by homogenizing the liver in a 1.5-mL microcentrifuge tube with a pestle according to the manufacturer's instructions. RNA from cells grown in 60-mm culture dishes is isolated in a similar manner using the RNAqueous total RNA isolation kit.
3. After elution of the RNA from the RNA isolation column, contaminating DNA is removed by treatment with DNase 1 for 15–30 min (*see* **Fig. 1**).
4. Concentrate the RNA by precipitation with 0.1 volume of 5 *M* ammonium acetate and 2.5 volumes of 100% ethanol. Place at –20°C for at least 30 min.
5. Recover the RNA by centrifugation at 14,000 rpm at 4°C for 15 min. Wash the RNA pellet in 70% ethanol. Remove all traces of ethanol and resuspend in 15–20 µL of DEPC-treated water.
6. Determine concentration and purity of RNA by reading the absorbance in a spectrophotometer at wavelengths 260 nm and 280 nm. Check quality of RNA (**Fig. 1**) by running 1 µg of RNA on a standard 1.5% TAE agarose gel.
7. Contaminating DNA can also be confirmed by using the RNA directly as a template in a polymerase chain reaction (PCR) for GAPDH.

3.2. Gene Expression Profiles Using Microarrays

Figure 2 is a summary of a typical microarray procedure.

3.2.1. Membrane cDNA Microarrays

The Atlas cDNA expression arrays contain cDNAs immobilized onto a nylon membrane. Each cDNA fragment is 200–600 basepairs and has been amplified from a region of the mRNA that lacks the poly(A) tail, repetitive sequence, or other homologous sequences. Broad coverage arrays are available that contain up to 1176 cDNAs representing various cellular functional groups while smaller arrays targeted to specific cellular functions are also available. Arrays are available to probe human, mouse, and rat mRNA populations. A summary of the procedure is outlined in **Fig. 2**.

1. In the author's laboratory, total RNA has been isolated from human liver tissue as described above from a number of HCCs and from liver surrounding the tumor and also from AD38

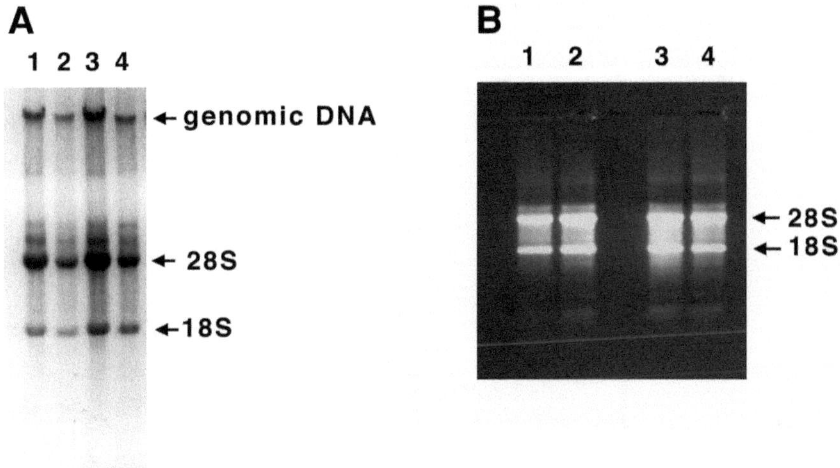

Fig. 1. Agarose gel electrophoresis of RNA extracted from AD38 cells treated in the presence (*lanes 1* and *2*) or the absence (*lanes 3* and *4*) of tetracycline for 10 days after seeding. **(A)** Initial extraction of total RNA from the cells using the Ambion RNAqueous Total RNA kit. The 18S and 28S ribosomal RNA as well as contaminating genomic DNA is marked. **(B)** The RNA samples from A after treatment with 1–2 U of DNase 1. All contaminating genomic DNA has been removed.

cells grown either in the presence (HBV replication suppressed) or absence (HBV replication positive) of tetracycline. As a control for the latter set of experiments HepG2 cells (parent cell line for AD38 cells) were cultured in the absence or presence of tetracycline and the RNA isolated.

2. All reagents and a detailed set of protocols are supplied with the microarrays and when followed correctly yield reproducible results. In brief, probes are synthesized from each RNA sample (test and control) using gene-specific primers by converting 2–5 μg of total RNA into ^{32}P-labeled first-strand cDNA using MMLV RT. Probes are then purified over a spin column (supplied) yielding probes in the range of $2–10 \times 10^6$ cpm. Equal probe concentrations in cpm are added to the matched membranes and allowed to hybridize overnight at 68°C in a hybridization oven. The membranes are then washed extensively as described, sealed in plastic film, and exposed to either X-ray film or Phosphorimage screen, and exposed for 2–3.

Figure 3 shows an example of a membrane array for an HBV related HCC.

3.2.2. High-Density Oligonucleotide Microarrays

The oligonucleotide arrays from Affymetrix contain 20-mer oligonucleotides that are chemically synthesized onto a silicon support. The advantage of this technology is that large numbers of oligonucleotides can be imprinted in a very small area.

1. Total RNA was isolated from human liver tissue and also from AD38 and HepG-2 cells as described above.

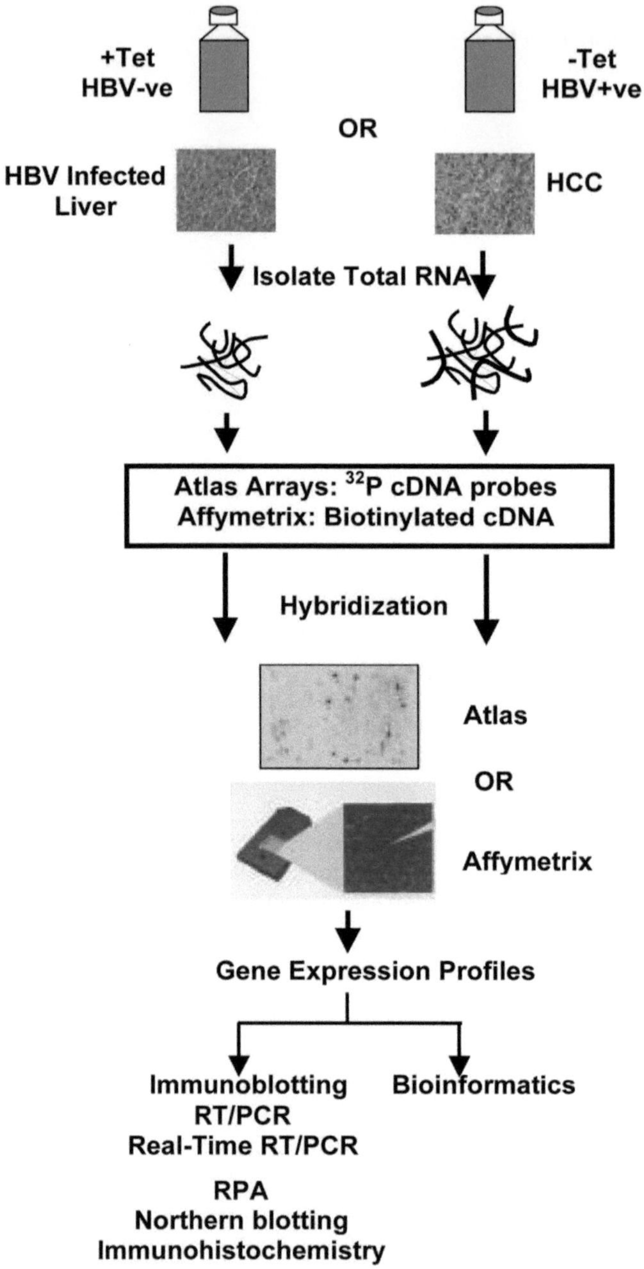

Fig. 2. Summary of a typical microarray procedure. The RNA from cell cultures actively expressing HBV (AD38 no tetracycline) or not (AD39 on tetracycline), or alternatively from tumor (HCC) or surrounding normal tissue is isolated as outlined in **Subheading 3**. The subsequent RNA is processed for Atlas arrays and/or Affymetrix chips and gene expression profiles determined. Differentially expressed genes so identified are confirmed by other techniques including immunoblot, immunohistochemistry, RT-PCR, real-time PCR, RNase protection assay (RPA), or Northern blot. The data can also be assimilated into databases.

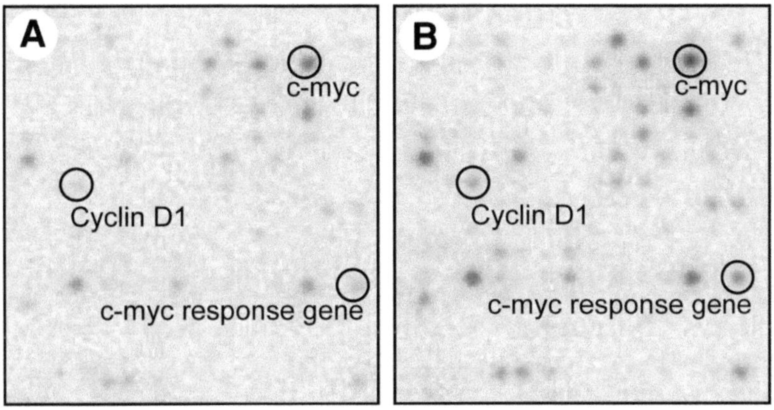

Fig. 3. The paired nylon membranes from an Atlas cDNA expression array. Membrane A was probed with labeled RNA isolated from surrounding tissue around the HCC, while membrane B was probed using the labeled RNA isolated from the tumor itself. In this analysis, the c-*myc* gene and the c-*myc* response gene are both up-regulated in the HCC.

2. All reagents required are listed and detailed protocols are supplied by the manufacturer and can be found at http://www.scms.utmb.edu/genomics/index.htm. At UTMB, 25 μg of total RNA is routinely used to produce biotinylated probes; however, as little as 8 μg can be used without a loss in sensitivity. Biotinylated, single-stranded antisense RNAs were prepared from total cellular RNA isolated using the RNAqueous RNA extraction kit (Ambion, Austin, TX). In brief, 25 μg of RNA was used as template for probe synthesis, and probes were hybridized to an Affymetrix human GeneChip® (Hu95A) containing 12,626 probe sets for known genes, according to the manufacturer's protocol (Affymetrix, Santa Clara, CA). The DNA arrays were scanned using an Affymetrix confocal scanner (Algient) and the data analyzed with Microarray GeneSuite software 4.0.1.

3.2.3. Analysis of mRNA Expression Profiles

Microarray experiments whether carried out using cDNA expression arrays or high-density oligonucleotide arrays typically generate thousands of data points and create significant challenges for data analysis and storage. Fortunately, both Clontech (AtlasImage) and Affymetrix (Microarray GeneSuite) provide useful software to analyze arrays. Both sets of analysis software generate mRNA expression profiles for a given RNA sample. These profiles can then be compared, after normalization to allow for differences in labeling efficiency and hybridization, with other related experiments to generate differential expression analysis. For example, using Affymetrix GeneChip analysis (Hu95A, 12,626 genes) it is possible to compare tumor and nontumor tissue in HBV-related HCC and 170 genes were differentially regulated: 86 up-regulated and 85 down-regulated by greater than twofold. While Affymetrix and Clontech claim a twofold change in mRNA abundance is significant, the authors routinely focus on mRNAs differentially regulated threefold and greater to exclude the possibility of inclusion of false positives and to make the data set more manageable.

Although differential mRNA expression profiles are useful, it is also important to identify patterns and groups in the data set that can be used to assign biological meaning to the expression profiles. It is possible to use sophisticated clustering and visualization programs such as hierarchial clustering developed by Eisen et al. ***(13)*** to group HBV- and HCV-related HCCs based on their gene expression profile and then correlate this with their histological classification, thereby identifying groups of genes similarly differentially regulated across tumors. The authors have found the Cluster and TreeView software (www. rana.Stanford.edu/software) available on the Web particularly useful for this type of analysis. However, there are a number of data and visualization programs suitable for analysis of microarray data (**Table 1**). It is impossible to analyze differentially expressed genes and expression profiles without using other databases. The public databases (GenBank, BLAST, and PubMed) and search engines provided by NCBI (National Center for Biotechnology Information, http://www.ncbi.nlm.nih.gov/) are essential while the KEGG (Kyoto Encyclopedia of Genes and Genomes, http://www.genome.ad.jp/keg/) allows one to assign a gene of interest to a specific biological pathway. Clontech (www.clontech.com) also maintains a website that provides functional information and selected references on genes present on their arrays.

3.2.4. Confirmation of Array Results

The large number of mRNAs probed by microarrays has the potential to generate false-positive mRNA expression profiles through random noise or non-specific experimental variation. This is particularly evident in cell culture studies in which experimental variation can result in mRNA expression profiles that are difficult to interpret. For these reasons the value of replicate experiments cannot be underestimated.

In the author's experience, mRNA abundance generated by arrays are generally a true reflection of the mRNA pools found within a population of cells. However, regardless of the type of array used it is essential that mRNAs of interest be confirmed by complementary methods. Abundance or lack of specific mRNAs can be determined by semiquantitative (RT)-PCR, real-time PCR, ribonuclease protection assay, or Northern blotting. These techniques are basic molecular tools and protocols are readily available in the literature. However, an increase in mRNA abundance may not necessarily correlate with increased protein expression, and Western blotting should be performed to correlate changes in mRNA levels with protein expression. Immunohistochemistry is also a useful complementary technique. This is particularly important when examining gene expression profiles in tumor tissue such as HCC in which the tumor is comprised of a complex population of cells. Immunohistochemistry not only allows identification of which cell type is expressing the particular protein of interest but also the intracellular distribution and the distribution within the tumor as a whole.

3.3. Conclusion

Microarray technology has many applications. It can define relationships between known genes, discover and define gene function and build quantitative databases. A

Table 1
Useful Software for Microarray Data Analysis

Spotfire Decision Site	www.spotfire.com
GeneCluster	www.genome.wi.mit.edu/MPR/software.html
Cluster and Tree View	www.rana.stanford.edu/software/
GeneSpring	www.sigenetics.com

number of investigators have begun applying this important technology to HBV ***(14)*** and different stages of liver disease ***(15)*** which, with appropriate interpretation ***(16)***, should provide important directions for future research activity.

References

1. Chisari, F. and Ferrari, C. (1995) Hepatitis B virus immunopathogenesis. *Annu. Rev. Immunol.* **13,** 29–60.
2. Delaney IV, W. E., Locarnini, S., and Shaw, T. (2001) Resistance of hepatitis B virus to antiviral drugs: current aspects and directions for future investigation. *Antivir. Chem. Chemother.* **12,** 1–35.
3. Ladner, S. K., Otto, M. J., Barker, C. S., et al. (1997) Inducible expression of human hepatitis B virus (HBV) in stably transfected hepatoblastoma cells: a novel system for screening potential inhibitors of HBV replication. *Antimicrob. Agents Chemother.* **41,** 1715–1720.
4. Lau, W. Y., Lai, P. B., Leung, M. F., et al. (2000) Differential gene expression of hepatocellular carcinoma using cDNA microarray analysis. *Oncol. Res.* **12,** 59–69.
5. Shirota, Y., Kaneko, S., Honda, M., Kawai, H. F., and Kobayashi, K. (2001) Identification of differentially expressed genes in hepatocellular carcinoma with cDNA microarrays. *Hepatology* **33,** 832–840.
6. Okabe, H., Satoh, S., Kato, T., et al. (2001) Genome-wide analysis of gene expression in human hepatocellular carcinomas using cDNA microarray: identification of genes involved in viral carcinogenesis and tumor progression. *Cancer Res.* **61,** 2129–2137.
7. Xu, L., Hui, L., Wang, S., (2001) Expression profiling suggested a regulatory role of liver-enriched transcription factors in human hepatocellular carcinoma. *Cancer Res.* **61,** 3176–3181.
8. Tackels-Horne, D., Goodman, M. D., Williams, A. J., et al. (2001) Identification of differentially expressed genes in hepatocellular carcinoma and metastatic liver tumors by oligonucleotide expression profiling. *Cancer* **92,** 395–405.
9. Eisen, M. B. and Brown, P. O. (1999) DNA arrays for analysis of gene expression. *Methods Enzymol.* **303,** 179–205.
10. Harrington, C. A., Rosenow, C., and Retief, J. (2000) Monitoring gene expression using DNA microarrays. *Curr. Opin. Microbiol.* **3,** 285–291.
11. Lockhart, D. J., Dong, H., Byrne, M. C., et al. (1996) Expression monitoring by hybridization to high-density oligonucleotide arrays. *Nat. Biotechnol.* **14,** 1675–1680.
12. Chomczynski, P.and Sacchi, N. (1987) Single-step method of RNA isolation by acid guanidinium thiocyanate–phenol–chloroform extraction. *Analyt. Biochem.* **162,** 156–159.
13. Eisen, M. B., Spellman, P. T., Brown, P. O., and Botstein, D. (1998) Cluster analysis and display of genome-wide expression patterns. *Proc. Natl. Acad. Sci. USA* **95,** 14863–14868.
14. Honda, M., Kaneko, S., Kawai, H., Shirota, Y., and Kobayashi, K. (2001) Differential gene expression between chronic hepatitis B and C hepatic lesion. *Gastroenterology* **120,** 955–966.

15. Kawai, H. F., Kaneko, S., Honda, M., Shirota, Y., and Kobayashi, K. (2001) alpha-fetoprotein-producing hepatoma cell lines share common expression profiles of genes in various categories demonstrated by cDNA microarray analysis. *Hepatology* **33,** 676–691.
16. McCaughan, G., Shackel, N., and Gorrell, M. (2001) Discussion on differential gene expression between chronic hepatitis B and C hepatic lesion. *Gastroenterology* **121,** 1263–1264.

6

Determination of Hepatitis B Virus-Specific CD8⁺ T-Cell Activity in the Liver

Michelina Nascimbeni and Barbara Rehermann

1. Introduction

The cellular, in particular the $CD8^+$ T-lymphocyte, response is thought to contribute to both viral clearance and liver cell injury in hepatitis B virus (HBV) infection *(1)*.

Acute, self-limited HBV infection is associated with a vigorous, polyclonal, and multispecific $CD4^+$ and $CD8^+$ T-lymphocyte response to epitopes within the HBV envelope, nucleocapsid, and polymerase proteins. This HBV-specific immune response is readily detectable in the peripheral blood, coincides with the maximum elevation of serum alanine aminotransferase (ALT) levels, and precedes clearance of HBV envelope (HBe) and surface (HBs) antigens and development of neutralizing antibodies *(2)*.

In contrast, the cellular immune response is weak and only rarely detectable in the blood of patients with chronic HBV infection. HBV-specific $CD4^+$ and $CD8^+$ T cells are not completely absent, however, because they have been isolated and expanded from liver biopsies *(3,4)* and exacerbations of disease activity, which often precede HBeAg clearance, have been attributed to an increase of the HBV-specific cellular immune response *(5)*. Thus, it has been postulated that in chronic hepatitis B, the HBV-specific immune response is too weak to eliminate HBV from all infected hepatocytes, but sufficiently strong to destroy continuously HBV-infected hepatocytes and to induce chronic inflammatory liver injury.

Different functions of $CD8^+$ T cells have been described that play a role in the antiviral immune response (**Table 1**). After recognition of virus-derived peptide antigens in the major histocompatibity complex (MHC) binding groove of HBV-infected cells, $CD8^+$ T cells become activated and lyse virus-infected hepatocytes by granzyme/perforin, tumor necrosis factor (TNF), and Fas/FasL-mediated pathways. In addition, $CD8^+$ T cells can also secrete cytokines such as interferon (IFN-γ) and TNF-α that downregulate HBV replication and gene expression without killing the infected cells *(1,6)*.

From: *Methods in Molecular Medicine, vol. 96: Hepatitis B and D Protocols, volume 2*
Edited by: R. K. Hamatake and J. Y. N. Lau © Humana Press Inc., Totowa, NJ

Table 1
CD8+ T Cell Responses in HBV Infection—A Double-Edged Sword

HBV-specific CD8+ T cells lyse virus-infected cells and contribute to liver injury

- HBV-specific T cells can be isolated from liver biopsies of patients with chronic hepatitis B *(3,7,8)* and lyse antigen-presenting cells in vitro.
- Acute, self-limited hepatitis B is associated with HBV-specific CD8+ T cells in the blood during the period of elevated liver enzymes *(2)*.
- Adoptive transfer of HBVenv-specific CTL into transgenic mice causes acute hepatitis B and liver injury *(24)*.

HBV-specific CD8+ T cells clear virus from infected cells via cytokine-mediated pathways.

- HBVcore, env, pol-specific CD8+ T cells persist for decades after recovery from hepatitis B and control minute amounts of persisting virus without causing liver injury *(25)*.
- HBV-specific CD8+ T cells are detectable in the liver of chronically infected patients who maintain low viral load and normal liver enzymes *(26)*.
- HBVenv-specific CD8+ T cells suppress HBV replication and gene expression and clear HBV nucleocapsid particles, replicative viral intermediates, and episomal closed circular (ccc) HBV DNA from infected cells without detectable liver injury *(6, 27)*.

To understand fully the role of different effector functions of HBV-specific T cells in the outcome of infection, it is therefore necessary to characterize these cells at the site of inflammation, the infected liver. This approach, however, is difficult because of the small number of lymphocytes that can be isolated from a standard fine-needle biopsy. Analysis of the CD8+ T-cell response has been proven to be technically even more difficult, as recombinant proteins generally cannot be introduced into the intracellular processing pathway that generates the peptides for presentation on MHC I molecules. To identify virus-specific CD8+ T cells within the intrahepatic cellular infiltrate, lymphocytes have therefore been cloned with antigen-specific and nonspecific stimuli *(3,7,8)* and tested for cytotoxic lysis of target cells infected with vaccinia viruses that express individual viral proteins. As an alternative approach, short 9- to 11-mer peptides with specific HLA binding motifs and high HLA binding affinity have been used to expand selectively peptide-specific T-cell precursors from the blood. Generally, one to two rounds of in vitro stimulation were required to expand HCV-specific T cells to a sufficient quantity to allow detection in cytotoxicity assays *(2)*.

While these techniques are useful to identify HBV epitopes recognized by CD8+ T cells, they also favor the outgrowth of certain T cells that are most compatible with the specific culture conditions. Thus, the obtained results reflect the antigen specificity, but not necessarily the in vivo frequency of antigen specific T cells.

Recently, new techniques have been developed that do not depend on in vitro expansion of specific T cells and therefore provide a more accurate assessment of the frequency of virus-specific T cells. FACS analysis, one of the most sensitive techniques to detect rare cells at frequencies of less than one cell per million *(9)*, can be used to quantitate virus-specific T cells that are stained with biotinylated MHC tetramers folded around individual HCV peptides. This technique is approx 100 to 1000-fold more sensitive than quantitation of T cells by limiting dilution analysis and can be combined with staining for additional cell surface markers such as DR, CD69, and CD38 to obtain information on the activation, effector, and/or memory status of antigen-specific cells. Two other techniques, intracellular cytokine analysis and cytokine Elispot, may also be used to quantitate precisely T cells of a given specificity. Both techniques require only short-term stimulation with antigen for 6 and 30 h, respectively, and therefore facilitate direct, ex vivo analysis of T-cell function.

In summary, it is recommended to employ several complementary techniques to assess quantitative as well as qualitative characteristics of the cellular immune response. This review focuses on protocols to isolate and analyze human HBV-specific $CD8^+$ T cells from fine-needle liver biopsies.

2. Materials

The following paragraphs list reagents and equipment under the main subheadings used in **Subheading 3.**

2.1. Isolation of Liver-Infiltrating Lymphocytes from Liver Resections and Fine-Needle Liver Biopsies

1. RPMI 1640 medium (Cellgro, VA): Supplemented with 10% fetal calf serum (FCS, Bio-Whittaker, Walkersville, MD), 2 m*M* L-glutamine (Cellgro, VA), 100 IU/mL of penicillin (Cellgro, VA), 100 μg/mL of streptomycin (Cellgro, VA), 10 m*M* 4-(2-hydroxyethyl) piperazine-1-ethanesulfonic acid (HEPES) (Cellgro, VA).
2. Hanks̀ balanced salt solution (HBSS, Gibco BRL, Rockville, MD): Supplemented with 0.5 mg/mL of type IV collagenase (Sigma, St. Louis, MO), 0.02 mg/mL of DNase I (Boehringer, Mannheim, Germany), 2% FCS, 0.6% bovine serum albumin (BSA).
3. 1X Phosphate-buffered saline (PBS, Cellgro, VA).
4. Ficoll Hypaque 1640 (Cellgro, VA).
5. Trypan blue solution diluted 1:3 in PBS (0.13% final concentration, Gibco BRL, Rockville, MD).
6. Cell freezing medium: 70% FCS, 20% RPMI 1640, and 10% dimethyl sulfoxide (DMSO) (Fisher Scientific, Pittsburg, PA).
7. Sterile razor blade, needle, sterile nylon mesh (100-μm-diameter pore size).
8. 2-mL glass grinder (PGC Scientific, Frederick, MD) with piston, hemocytometer.
9. Six-well cell culture plates, 15-mL tubes, 2-mL pipets (Costar).
10. Biological safety cabinet: Processing of liver tissue and isolation of liver-infiltrating lymphocytes should be performed in a certified biological safety cabinet under sterile conditions.
11. Centrifuge, liquid nitrogen cell storage tank, –70°C freezer.

2.2. Direct Ex Vivo *Analysis of Liver-Derived T Cells*

1. RPMI 1640 medium (Cellgro, VA): Supplemented with 10% FCS (Bio-Whittaker, Walkersville, MD), 2 m*M* L-glutamine (Cellgro, VA), 100 IU/mL of penicillin (Cellgro, VA), 100 μg/mL of streptomycin (Cellgro, VA), and 10 m*M* HEPES (Cellgro, VA).
2. 1X PBS; PBS–2% FCS; PBS–1%BSA; PBS–1% BSA–0.05% Tween-20 (Sigma, St. Louis, MO), PBS–20 m*M* EDTA, PBS–20% saponin.
3. 500 ng/mL of PMA and 10 μg/mL of ionomycin (Sigma, St. Louis, MO).
4. Brefeldin A or Monensin (Pharmingen, San Diego, CA). Cytofix/Cytoperm Plus™ with GolgiStop™ (Pharmingen, San Diego, CA).

5. 10×10^6 U/mL of DNase (Calbiochem, San Diego, CA).
6. 0.5% and 2% paraformaldehyde (Fisher Scientific, Pittsburg, PA).
7. Phycoerythrin (PE)-conjugated Annexin V (Pharmingen, San Diego, CA) stored at 4°C. 100 μg/mL of propidium iodide solution, stored at 4°C and protected from light. 1X Annexin buffer (Pharmingen, San Diego, CA) consisting of 10 m*M* HEPES/NaOH, pH 7.4; 140 m*M* NaCl; 2.5 m*M* $CaCl_2$ stored at 4°C.
8. PE-labeled mouse anti-human IFN-γ antibody, fluorescein isothiocyanate (FITC)-labeled mouse anti-human CD4 (Becton Dickinson, San Jose, CA), FITC-labeled mouse anti-human CD13 (Caltag, Burlingame, CA), FITC-labeled mouse anti-human CD19 (Caltag, Burlingame, CA), PerCP-labeled mouse anti-human CD8 (Becton Dickinson, San Jose, CA), FITC-labeled mouse-anti-human CD8 antibody (Becton Dickinson, San Jose, CA), PE-labeled HBV epitope MHC tetramers.
9. 96-Well round bottom plates. Yellow Sarstedt tubes and FACS tubes.
10. Biological safety cabinet: Processing of liver tissue and isolation of liver-infiltrating lymphocytes should be performed in a certified biological safety cabinet under sterile conditions.
11. Centrifuge, liquid nitrogen cell storage tank, –70°C freezer.
12. Flow cytometer.

2.3. In Vitro *Expansion of Intrahepatic T Cells and Generation of T-Cell Lines and Clones*

1. RPMI 1640 medium (Cellgro, VA): Supplemented with 10% FCS (Bio-Whittaker, Walkersville, MD), 2 m*M* L-glutamine (Cellgro, VA), 100 IU/mL of penicillin (Cellgro, VA), 100 μg/mL of streptomycin (Cellgro, VA), 10 m*M* HEPES (Cellgro, VA), and 100 U/mL of interleukin-2 (IL-2).
2. PBS–2% FCS.
3. 100 μg/mL of anti-CD3 antibody X35, stored at –20°C (Immunotech).
4. 100 U/mL of IL-2, 1 μg/mL of IL-7, 100 ng/mL of IL-12 (PeproTech, Rocky Hill, NJ).
5. HBV epitope peptides resuspended in DMSO at 20 mg/mL (stock solution, stored at –20°C) and diluted at 1 mg/mL with PBS (working solution, stored at 4°C).
6. Anti-CD8 Dynabeads (Dynal, Oslo, Norway).
7. Bispecific monoclonal antibody CD3,4B; CD3-specific monoclonal antibody X35 (Immunotech).
8. Biological safety cabinet: Processing of liver tissue and isolation of liver-infiltrating lymphocytes should be performed in a certified biological safety cabinet under sterile conditions.
9. Centrifuge, liquid nitrogen cell storage tank, –70°C freezer.
10. CO_2 incubator.
11. Multichannel pipet and combitips.
12. 96-Well round-bottom plates and 24-well flat bottom plates.
13. Microtiter plate carrier for centrifugation.
14. 1.5-mL tubes and polymerase chain reaction (PCR) tubes.
15. Magnet for 1.5-mL tubes.
16. End over end rotator.

2.4. *Functional In Vitro Analysis of $CD8^+$ T-Cell Lines and Clones*

1. RPMI 1640 medium (Cellgro, VA): Supplemented with 10% FCS (Bio-Whittaker, Walkersville, MD), 2 m*M* L-glutamine (Cellgro, VA), 100 IU/mL of penicillin (Cellgro, VA), 100 μg/mL of streptomycin (Cellgro, VA), and 10 m*M* HEPES (Cellgro, VA).

2. 1X PBS; PBS–2% FCS; PBS–1%BSA; PBS–1% BSA–0.05% Tween-20 (Sigma, St. Louis, MO).
3. Phytohemagglutinin (PHA, Sigma, St. Louis, MO).
4. 10% Triton X-100 diluted in water.
5. 1 mCi/mL Na_2 [^{51}Cr]O_4 (^{51}Cr; 300 mCi/mg; Amersham, Piscataway, NJ).
6. Target cells: Autologous Epstein–Barr virus (EBV)-transformed B lymphoblastoid cells or autologous PHA blasts.
7. Recombinant vaccinia viruses expressing individual HBV proteins, wild-type vaccinia virus, or HBV-derived peptides.
8. Biological safety cabinet: Processing of liver tissue and isolation of liver-infiltrating lymphocytes should be performed in a certified biological safety cabinet under sterile conditions.
9. Centrifuge, liquid nitrogen cell storage tank, –70°C freezer.
10. CO_2 incubator.
11. 96-Well round-bottom plates
12. β-counter.

3. Methods (*See* Note 1)

3.1. Isolation of Liver Infiltrating Lymphocytes from Liver Resections and Fine-Needle Liver Biopsies

3.1.1. Isolation of Lymphocytes from Liver Resections

Enzymatic digestion and pulverization with a syringe or a stainless-steel mesh can be used to isolate liver infiltrating lymphocytes from a larger piece of liver tissue. However, enzymatic digestion ***(10–12)*** appears to result in a higher cell yield and is described here.

1. Wash liver tissue extensively with 1X PBS to remove contaminating blood and place in a well of a six-well plate in a small amount of RPMI 1640 medium supplemented with 10% FCS, 2 m*M* L-glutamine, 100 IU/mL of penicillin, 100 μg/mL of streptomycin, and 10 m*M* HEPES (standard cell culture medium). Hold one part of the biopsy with a sterile needle and dissect the tissue in small pieces of 1 mm^3 with a sterile razor blade. The size of the small pieces is important; if they are too large, they will not be digested entirely by collagenase resulting in loss of lymphocyte recovery from the liver tissue.
2. Add 5 mL of HBSS containing 0.5 mg/mL of type IV collagenase, 0.02 mg/mL of DNase I, 2% FCS, and 0.6% BSA. Prepare the digesting solution fresh on the day of experiment. These quantities represent 100 U/mL of collagenase IV and 10 U/mL of DNase I. DNase prevents cell clumping.
3. Incubate at 37°C for 30 min with gentle agitation. Incubation of peripheral blood mononuclear cells (PBMCs) with enzymes for 30 min does not induce changes in cytokine production, cytotoxicity, and cell surface marker expression, except for CD56 ***(10)***. However, prolonged incubation with collagenase reduces cell viability.
4. Place a sterile 70- to 100-μm mesh on top of a 15-mL tube and filter the cell lysate to remove undissociated tissue.
5. Wash the mesh twice with 2 mL of HBSS and centrifuge the filtrate at 30*g* for 3 min. This should sediment a majority of the hepatocytes while most lymphocytes remain in the supernatant.
6. Collect the supernatant, suspend cells in HBSS and centrifuge at 400*g* for 10 min. This should sediment lymphocytes, Kupffer cells, and the remaining hepatocytes.

7. Resuspend the cell pellet in complete culture medium, then count cells in a 1:10 dilution with trypan blue and estimate cell viability. Yield is approx 1–6 × 10^6 cells per 200 mg of liver tissue with a cell viability of 70–80%.
8. Use liver-derived lymphocyte for direct ex vivo experiments (*see* **Subheading 3.2.**) or purify $CD8^+$ T cells as described in **Subheading 3.3.1.** Remaining lymphocytes can be cryopreserved in ice-cold 70% FCS, 20% RPMI 1640, and 10% DMSO, slowly cooled to –70°C and then store in liquid nitrogen for future use.

3.1.2. Isolation of Lymphocytes from Fine-Needle Liver Biopsies (See **Note 2**)

Mechanical disruption of liver tissue with a glass grinder is the easiest and fastest method to isolate liver-infiltrating lymphocytes from a fine needle biopsy of 1–2 cm length. Enzymatic digestion as described in **Subheading 3.1.1.** is also possible, but takes longer.

1. Place liver biopsy in a sterile tube containing RPMI 1640 medium supplemented with 10% FCS, 2 m*M* L-glutamine, 100 IU/mL of penicillin, 100 μg/mL of streptomycin, and 10 m*M* HEPES (complete culture medium). Wash biopsy in sufficient volume of medium (> 10 mL) to remove loosely attached, contaminating peripheral blood lymphocytes.
2. Harvest biopsy with a 2-mL sterile pipet and transfer to a 2-mL glass homogeneizer in 1 mL of complete culture medium. If the biopsy sticks to the wall of the pipet, quickly move the medium several times up and down the pipet until the biopsy is released.
3. Homogeneize the liver biopsy carefully by moving the piston in the homogenizer. Avoid generating bubbles, which affect cell viability. Remove fat or cirrhotic tissues that cannot be disrupted.
4. Harvest cell suspension with a 2-mL pipet and transfer to a 15-mL tube. Wash glass homogeneizer and piston with 2 mL of PBS, and transfer to the same 15-mL tube. Fill the tube with PBS and centrifuge at 400*g* for 10 min.
5. Remove supernatant carefully with a sterile Pasteur pipet attached to a vacuum pump. Leave approx 30 μL.
6. Resuspend cell pellet in 1 mL of complete culture medium and place on wet ice. This cell suspension can either be analyzed directly (*see* **Subheading 3.2.**) or subjected to a density gradient separation (*see* **steps 7–10** below). A clearer separation of lymphocytes and contaminating erythrocytes can be obtained by density gradient centrifugation, but results in a loss of up to 30% of cells because of the additional centrifugation steps.
7. For density gradient centrifugation, place 5 mL of Ficoll Hypaque 1640 (*see* **Note 3**) into a sterile 15-mL tube. Resuspend liver-derived lymphocytes in 9 mL of cell culture medium and carefully layer the cell suspension on top without mixing the two solutions. Centrifuge for 20 min at 1200*g* without brake.
8. With a sterile Pasteur pipet attached to a vacuum pump, carefully remove 8 mL of supernatant. Carefully aspirate lymphocytes at the interface of Ficoll and PBS into a 1-mL pipet. Note that the lymphocyte interphase can be almost invisible if the original liver biopsy is very small.
9. Transfer aspirate to a fresh 15-mL tube, repeat **step 8**, dilute aspirated cell suspension to 15 mL with PBS, and centrifuge once at 800*g* for 10 min with braking.
10. Aspirate the supernatant and resuspend the cell pellet in 500 μL of complete culture medium. Note that the additional wash and centrifugation that is generally performed after density gradient separation is omitted to avoid further loss of lymphocytes.

3.2. Direct Ex Vivo Analysis of Liver-Derived T Cells

One of the advantages of direct ex vivo phenotyping of liver-derived lymphocytes is that it does not require a large number of cells. The staining can be done either in 96-well round bottom plates or in FACS tubes. The use of 96-well plates facilitates the procedure, especially if many samples are included in the experiment.

3.2.1. Assessment of Cell Viability (see **Note 4**)

Dying cells experience changes in their cellular architecture that occur in two steps: an early loss of membrane asymmetry and a later step of membrane permeabilization.

During the first step, the membrane phospholipid phosphatidylserine (PS) is translocated from the inner part to the outer side of the plasma membrane, thereby exposing PS to the external environment. PS can be stained with fluorescently labeled annexin V, a Ca^{2+}-dependent phospholipid-binding protein to identify dying cells by flow cytometry.

During the second step, the permeabilized plasma membrane allows entry of soluble molecules, ions, and dyes such as propidium iodide (PI) into the cytoplasm. Thus, early and late steps of cell death can be distinguished by flow cytometry after staining with annexin V and PI. Cells that stain positive for both annexin V and PI are either in the end stage of apoptosis, undergoing necrosis, or are already dead. Cells that stain negative for both annexin V and PI are alive. As compared to trypan blue exclusion analysis and light microscopy, this method allows a more precise assessment of the early stages of apoptosis. It also allows exclusion of dying cells if analysis of cell function is performed by flow cytometry, as described in **Subheading 3.2.2. Figure 1** demonstrates the different cell populations isolated from liver biopsy and peripheral blood and **Fig. 2** demonstrates analysis of apoptosis and cell death with annexin and PI staining.

1. Place a small number of lymphocytes (50,000 cells) in a well of a 96-well round-bottom plate. If several samples are stained in different wells, they should be separated from each other by an empty well to avoid contamination. Centrifuge the plate for 5 min at 700*g*.
2. Quickly turn plate upside down on absorbant tissue to pour off the supernatant carefully (do not shake too much because the cell number is small and a substantial number of cells can easily be lost) and resuspend cell pellet in 80–100 μL of PBS supplemented with 2% FCS.
3. Add 2 μL of CD8-FITC antibody and incubate for 30 min at 4°C. If other cell surface markers have to be analyzed as well, additional antibodies should be included.
4. Wash once with 150 μL of PBS–2% FCS per well (*see* **steps 1** and **2**) and resuspend in 80–100 μL 1X annexin V buffer. This specific buffer (*see* **Subheading 2.2.**) contains Ca^{2+} required for binding of fluorescently labeled annexin to its ligand PS.
5. Add 5 μL of PE-labeled annexin V and incubate 15 min at 4°C in the dark.
6. Add 1 μL of PI solution to obtain a final concentration of 1 μg/mL. Because PI is extremely bright, a titration should be performed to confirm this recommended concentration. **Caution: PI is a potential carcinogen and mutagen and should be handled with extreme care**. Incubate 5–10 min at 4°C in the dark.
7. Wash the plate twice with 100 μL PBS–2% FCS at 4°C and resuspend cells in 100 μL of PBS containing 0.5% paraformaldehyde. Transfer cells into FACS tubes and analyze by flow cytometry within an hour. Note that annexin V binding can be disrupted very quickly.

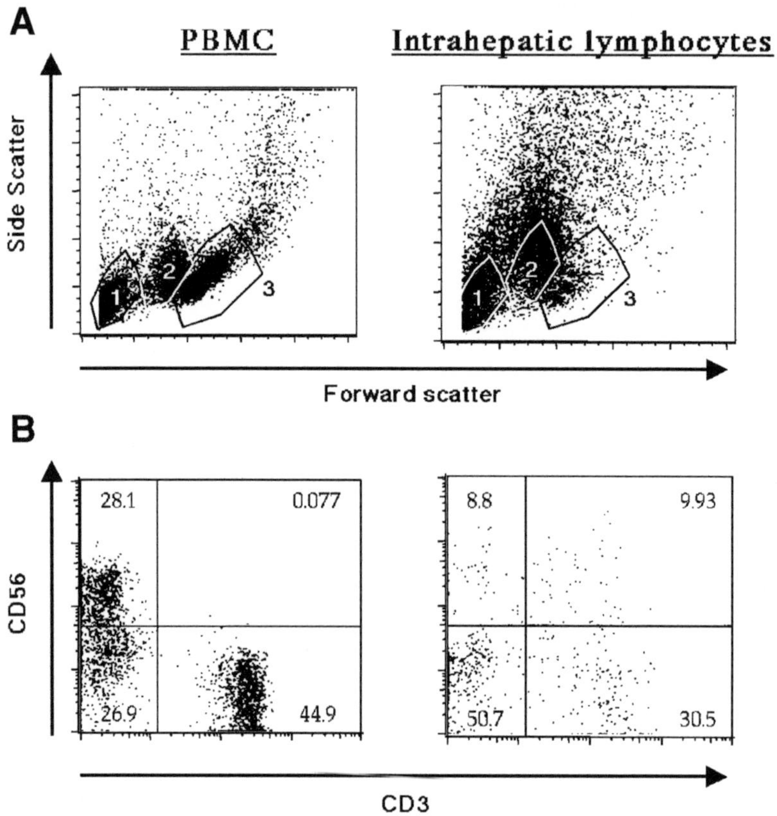

Fig. 1. Cell surface marker staining of circulating and liver-infiltrating lymphocytes. PBMCs were isolated from blood samples via density gradient centrifugation. Intrahepatic lymphocytes were isolated from a fine-needle liver biopsy as described in **Subheading 3.1.2.** and directly used for ex vivo analysis without any other purification step. **(A)** Forward scatter (FSC) vs side scatter (SSC) dot plots of peripheral blood and liver-derived lymphocytes. The three indicated regions distinguish the different cell populations. Region 1 contains debris or dead cells; region 2 contains red blood cells; region 3 contains lymphocytes. **(B)** Expression of CD56 and CD3 on lymphocytes detected in region 3. Cells located in the lower left quadrant do not express any of the two molecules. Cells located in the upper left quadrant express only CD56 while cells located in the lower right quadrant express only CD3. CD3 and CD56 double positive cells are predominantly found in the liver. The numbers in each quadrant indicate the percentage of cells stained with the respective antibodies. Note that in this case blood and liver biopsy were obtained from a chimpanzee infected with HCV. The same type of analysis can also be performed with samples of HBV-infected patients.

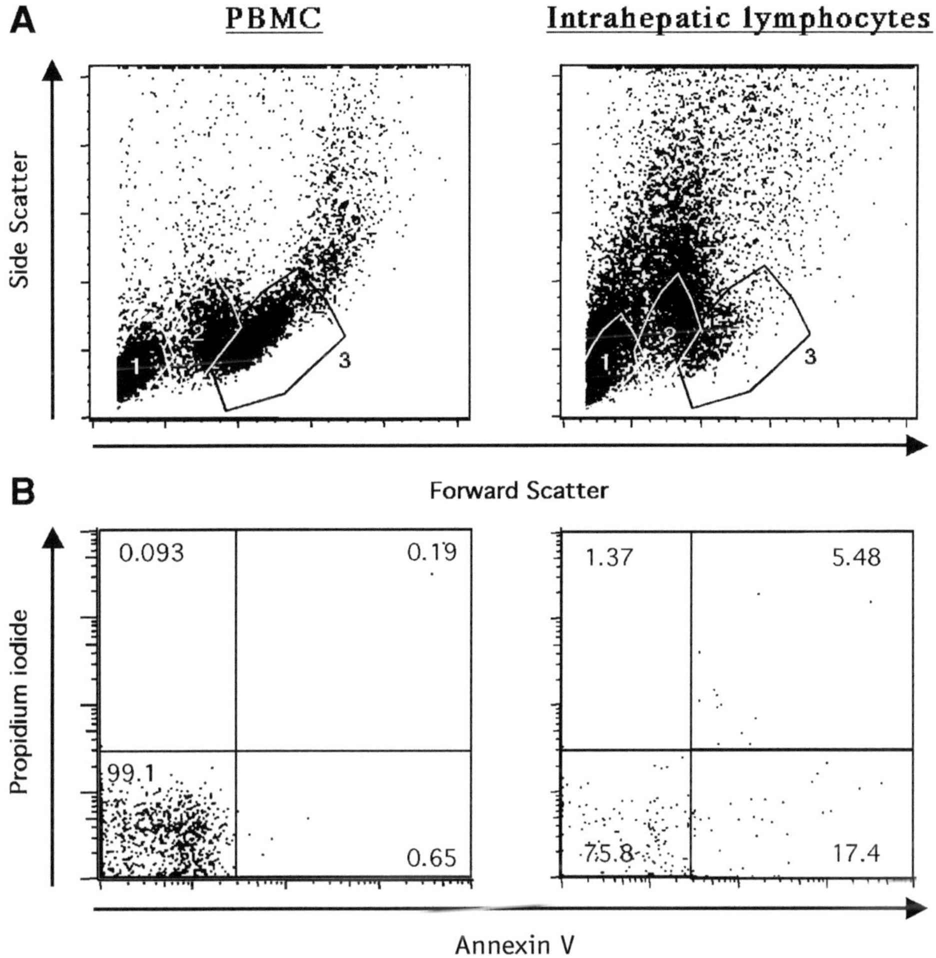

Fig. 2. Avnexin V staining of freshly isolated PBMCs and intrahepatic lymphocytes. Precise assessment of cell viability can be performed by flow cytometry using staining with annexin V as an early marker of apoptosis and PI as described in **Subheading 3.2.1.** In this experiment, freshly isolated PBMCs and intrahepatic lymphocytes were simultaneously stained with anti-CD3 antibody, annexin V and PI. **(A)** Forward scatter (FSC) vs side scatter (SSC) dot plot of freshly isolated PBMCs and lymphocytes isolated from a liver biopsy. The three regions define dead cells (region 1), red blood cells (region 2), and lymphocytes (region 3), respectively. **(B)** CD3 positive lymphocytes from peripheral blood and liver biopsy were analyzed for expression of annexin V and/or for incorporation of PI. Early apoptotic cells stain solely with annexin V and are located in the lower right quadrant. Late apoptotic, necrotic, or dead cells stain with both annexin V and PI and are in the upper right quadrant. The percentage of each population is indicated. Note that in this case blood and liver biopsy were obtained from a chimpanzee infected with HCV. The same type of analysis can also be performed with samples of HBV-infected patients.

8. Calculate the percentage of viable cells and exclude nonviable cells from further flow cytometric analysis by appropriate setting of gates.

3.2.2. Quantification of HBV-Specific $CD8^+$ T Cells

Virus-specific $CD8^+$ T cells recognize MHC class I–peptide complexes via engagement of their specific T-cell receptor. Therefore, the quantification of these $CD8^+$ virus-specific T cells can be achieved by staining with fluorescent-labeled complexes of four MHC class I molecules (tetramers) presenting the specific peptide of interest. While this method detects antigen-specific T cells regardless of their function, it can be combined with intracellular cytokine staining, CSFE labeling of proliferating cells, and other techniques that allow analysis of functionally active antigen-specific T cells.

The following protocol describes a three-color staining procedure for detection of tetramer-positive cells within the $CD8^+$ T-cell population; if detection of other specific surface molecules is necessary, antibodies against these molecules can be included in the mix.

1. Place $0.5–2 \times 10^6$ cells in a 5-mL FACS tube, add up to 3 mL PBS, and centrifuge 5 min at 700*g*. Because a large number of cells is required for analysis to detect the infrequent antigen-specific T cells, staining is performed in tubes rather than in 96-well plates.
2. Use a P-1000 pipet to remove 2.7 mL of supernatant. Then, use a P-200 pipet to remove the remaining supernatant carefully so that < 30 μL are left. When removing the supernatant, avoid touching the bottom of the tube with the tip because the number of cells might be so small that the pellet is not visible. Removal of supernatant should be performed rapidly to avoid spontaneous resuspension and subsequent loss of lymphocytes.
3. Resuspend cells in 10–20 μL of PBS–2% FCS (the final volume for staining should not exceed 30–35 μL), and store them at 4°C until tetramers and mix of antibodies are ready.
4. Centrifuge tetramers at 8000*g* for 10 min at 4°C to remove aggregates that will nonspecifically bind to the cells. MHC tetramers and HBV epitopes should be selected according to the HLA haplotype of the patient whose liver biopsy is analyzed.
5. Then, per sample to be stained, prepare a mix of 2 μL of anti-CD4 FITC, 2 μL of anti-CD13 FITC, 5 μL of CD19 FITC, and 2 μL of anti-CD8 PerCP antibody solution. All antibodies should be titered to determine the optimal concentration to stain PBMCs. If detection of other surface molecules is required, antibodies against these molecules can be included in the mix at this time. All antibodies should be titered before use. Add 0.5 μL of tetramer to the mix. Do not touch the bottom of the tetramer-containing tube with the tip to avoid aspiration of tetramer aggregates.
6. Add 11.5 μL of the antibody mix to the cells in the FACS tube and resuspend gently.
7. Incubate at room temperature for 45 min in the dark.
8. Wash once with PBS–2% FCS and resuspend cells in 100 μL of PBS–2% FCS.
9. Analyze immediately by flow cytometry or proceed to perform intracellular cytokine staining.

3.2.3. Cytokine Production of HBV-Specific $CD8^+$ T Cells (See **Note 5**)

Cytokine expression of HBV-specific T cells is highly relevant, because IFN-γ production of intrahepatic T cells has been associated with down-regulation of HBV replication. Because the level of T-cell receptor expression decreases during T-cell activation, staining with tetramers should be performed prior to stimulation. The following protocol can be used to detect Tc1 cytokines such as IFN-γ and TNF-α, Tc2 cytokines such as

IL-4, IL-5, IL-10; and to detect perforin. Because perforin is stored in intracellular vesicles, T-cell stimulation is not required to detect this protein. Therefore, **steps 1–4** of this protocol can be eliminated when intracellular staining for perforin is performed.

1. Resuspend 0.5–2 × 10^6 lymphocytes in 1 mL of RPMI–10% FCS in a yellow Sarstedt tube, add 50 ng/mL of PMA and 1 μg/mL of ionomycin, centrifuge 5 min at 65*g* without the brake, and incubate at 37°C for 2 h at a 20° angle so that the cell pellet rests horizontally.
2. Alternatively, lymphocytes can be stimulated with virus-specific antigens, for example, a mix of HBV epitope peptides, overlapping 15-mer peptides or with endogenously processed epitopes expressed by recombinant vaccinia viruses. For this antigen-specific stimulation, load autologous EBV transformed B cells with the specific peptide mix (1–10 μg/mL per peptide) or infect them with recombinant vaccinia viruses expressing HBV antigens (multiplicity of infection [MOI] = 10) 12–16 h prior to the lymphocyte stimulation. Incubate EBV-transformed B cells in complete medium at 37°C overnight. The next day, wash EBV-transformed B cells once in PBS, then resuspend them in 0.5 mL of complete medium, mix with 0.5 mL of liver-derived lymphocytes at a ratio of 1:1, and incubate the mix at 37°C for 2 h.
3. Add 10 μg/mL of Brefeldin A or Monensin and continue incubation for 4 h. During the stimulation procedure, some cells will die and DNA will be released leading to cell clumping. Following the incubation time, treat cells with 3000 U/mL of DNase for 10 min at 37°C which allows recovery of a higher number of viable cells.
4. Add 100 μL of EDTA at 2 m*M* final concentration, vortex gently for 20 s and incubate at room temperature for 15 min. Note that after several hours incubation at 37°C in plastic tubes, cells will stick to the plastic. This adhesion is mediated by cell surface adhesins, which act in the presence of Ca^{2+} and Mg^{2+}. EDTA inhibits adhesins by chelating Ca^{2+} and Mg^{2+} and therefore allows detachment of the cells.
5. Transfer cells to FACS tubes, wash yellow Sarstedt tubes with 3 mL of cold PBS, and transfer the washing solution into the same FACS tubes to increase the number of transferred cells. Centrifuge cells for 5 min at 700*g* and resuspend in Cytofix/Cytoperm™ (250 μL per 5 × 10^5 cells) for 20 min at 4°C. Alternatively, cells can be fixed with 2% paraformaldehyde for 20 min at 4°C, washed twice with cold PBS–1% BSA and permeabilized with 100 μL PBS–1% BSA–0.2% saponin for 20 min at 4°C. In this case, omit **step 6** and proceed directly to **step 7**.
6. Add 400 μL of 1X Perm/Wash™ solution and centrifuge at 800*g* for 10 min at 4°C; repeat this step once.
7. Dilute anti-IFN-γ antibodies in 100 μL of 1X Perm/Wash™ and stain cells with this solution for 30 min at 4°C.
8. Wash once with 400 μL of 1X Perm/Wash™, once with PBS–1% BSA, and resuspend in 100 μL of 2% paraformaldehyde.
9. Analyze samples immediately by flow cytometry.

3.3. In Vitro *Expansion of Intrahepatic T Cells and Generation of T-Cell Lines and Clones*

3.3.1. Positive Selection of CD8+ T Cells (See **Note 6**)

1. In a sterile 1.5-mL tube, place 10 times more magnetic beads than the expected number of CD8+ cells. Wash magnetic beads by adding 1 mL of cold PBS–2% FCS solution. Resuspend several times, then place the tube into the magnet. Let the beads attach to the magnet and remove supernatant. Repeat this washing step two times. After the last wash, resuspend the beads in 50 μL PBS–2% FCS and transfer them to a PCR tube.

2. Centrifuge liver-derived lymphocytes at 400*g* for 10 min, resuspend in 80 μL of PBS–2% FCS, and add them to the beads. Note that the cell concentration should be at least 10^6 cells/mL.
3. Place PCR tube on a rotating wheel and incubate for 30 min to 1 h at 4°C. Note that 80% of the tube should be filled with the cell suspension to allow optimal contact between beads and cells.
4. Transfer the cell suspension from the PCR tube to a sterile 1.5-mL tube. Wash the PCR tube with 100 μL of PBS–2% FCS and transfer the washing solution to the same 1.5-mL tube that already contains the cell suspension. Repeat this step one more time to ensure that all cells are transferred. Fill the 1.5-mL tube completely with PBS–2% FCS and resuspend cells and beads several times. Put the tube in the magnet, wait until beads separate, and remove the supernatant carefully. Repeat resuspension of $CD8^+$ T cells (sticking to the beads), magnetic separation, and removal of supernatant two times. Finally, resuspend cells in 100 μL of cell culture medium and count under a hemocytometer. It is not necessary to detach cells from beads.

3.3.2. In Vitro Expansion of Cell Lines and Clones (See **Note 7***)*

3.3.2.1. ANTIGEN-NONSPECIFIC CLONING OF LIVER-DERIVED LYMPHOCYTES

1. This protocol describes cloning of liver-derived lymphocytes at one cell per well and in 10 96-well plates. Liver-derived lymphocytes can also be cloned at 10, 50, and 100 cells per well. The procedure remains identical but the concentration of the lymphocyte suspension should then be adjusted at **step 3.**
2. Use either freshly isolated or thawed allogeneic PBMCs. 5×10^6 PBMCs are required for each 96-well round-bottom cloning plate, that is, 5×10^7 PBMCs for 10 plates. Resuspend PBMCs in 50-mL tubes at 2.5×10^6 cells/mL in complete cell culture and γ-irradiate cells at 7000 rad.
3. Dilute cell suspension to 10^6 cells/mL and supplement complete cell culture medium with 100 U/mL of recombinant IL-2. Pipet 50 μL of this cell suspension into each well of the 96-well round-bottom plates.
4. Dilute the suspension of liver-derived lymphocytes to be cloned to a concentration of 20 cells/mL in RPMI 1640 supplemented with 10% FCS, 2 m*M* L-glutamine, 100 IU/mL of penicillin, 100 μg/mL of streptomycin, and 100 U/mL of IL-2.
5. Add anti-CD3 at 0.02 μg/mL final concentration and pipet 50 μL of this cell suspension to each well of the cloning plates.
6. Centrifuge plates at 65*g* for 5 min without braking, then incubate at 37°C, 5% CO_2.
7. After 1 wk, add 100 μL of complete culture medium supplemented with 100 U/mL of IL-2. Then remove half of the culture medium every 3–4 d and replace with the same volume fresh, complete culture medium supplemented with 100 U/mL of IL-2.
8. Every 3 wk restimulate as follows: Remove 100 μL of medium from each well of the cloning plates, add 50 μL of fresh complete culture medium supplemented with 100 U/mL of IL-2 and 0.02 μg/mL of anti-CD3, and incubate the cultures for 10–15 min at 37°C.
9. Irradiate appropriate number of PBMCs from healthy donors as described in **step 2,** dilute to 2×10^6 cells/mL in complete culture medium containing 100 U/mL of IL-2, and add 50 μL of this cell suspension to each well. Note that anti-CD3 antibody is added to the cell cultures first followed by a short incubation time prior to addition of irradiated allogeneic PBMCs to allow binding of anti-CD3 to the liver-derived lymphocytes and to avoid absorption of most of the antibody by irradiated allogeneic PBMC.

3.3.2.2. Antigen-Specific Expansion of Liver-Derived Lymphocytes

Depending on the number of liver-derived lymphocytes recovered from liver biopsies, in vitro expansion of cell lines can either be performed with individual virus-derived peptides or with a pool of virus-derived peptides. This section describes these two procedures, which include 3 wk of in vitro culture with two rounds of stimulation in the presence of virus derived-peptides and feeder cells. This method can also be used to enrich the liver-derived lymphocyte population for HBV-specific T cells prior to antigen-nonspecific cloning (*see* **Subheading 3.3.2.1.**).

1. Use either freshly isolated or thawed autologous PBMCs, dilute to 10^6 cells/mL in complete cell culture medium, γ-irradiate cells at 3000 rad, and supplement the cell suspension with 20 U/mL of recombinant IL-2.
2. Separate autologous cells in as many 15-mL tubes as different stimulation conditions to be used, add peptides in a final concentration of 10 μ/mL, and distribute 50 μL of the cell suspensions in each well of a 96-well round-bottom plate.
3. Add 50–1000 liver-derived lymphocytes (depending on the frequency of HBV-specific T cells you expect within the suspension of liver-derived lymphocytes) in 50 μL of complete cell culture medium supplemented with 10 ng/mL of IL-7 and 300 pg/mL of IL-12 to each well and incubate the cells at 37°C, 5% CO_2 for 4 d.
4. At d 4, add 100 μL of complete cell culture medium containing 20 U/mL of IL-2 to each well. Note that IL-2 is not very stable when diluted in medium. Do not use medium containing IL-2 that is older than 2 wk. Restimulate weekly with 100,000 γ-irradiated (3000 rad) autologous lymphocytes, 10 μg/mL of each peptide, and 20 U/mL of IL-2. Perform functional assays (*see* below) as soon as the number of cells permits.

3.4. *Functional* In Vitro *Analysis of CD8+ T Cell Lines and Clones*

3.4.1. 51Cr-Release (Cytotoxicity) Assay

Measurement of antigen-specific cytotoxicity can be accomplished by incubation of liver-derived CD8+ T-cell lines and clones with target cells that present virus-specific antigens. Antigen-presenting cells (target cells) can either be infected with recombinant vaccinia viruses expressing viral proteins, loaded with overlapping peptides, or loaded with individual HBV-derived peptides that represent known epitopes.

This protocol uses two basic components: radiolabeled, antigen-presenting target cells and cytotoxic effector T cells. The cytotoxic activity of the effector T-cell population is quantitated based on the amount of radioactivity released by the target cells.

Caution: Follow standard radiation safety procedures when working with ^{51}Cr solution and ^{51}Cr-labeled target cells.

1. Different target cells can be used for the cytotoxicity assay: autologous EBV-B cells (B cells immortalized with EBV) and autologous PHA blasts. PBMCs stimulated with PHA have the advantage of a complete MHC match with the liver-derived lymphocytes. EBV-B cells are maintained in RPMI–10% FCS at a concentration of 10^5 cells/mL until the experiment is performed. PHA blasts are generated from autologous PBMCs by stimulation with 0.5 μg/mL of PHA and 40 U/mL of IL-2 at a concentration of 2×10^6 cells/mL per well in a 24-well plate in 1 mL of complete cell culture medium 6 d prior to the cytotoxicity assay and by adding 1 mL of complete medium containing 40 U/mL of IL-2 on d 4 of the culture.

2. For the purpose of epitope mapping, target cells are either infected with recombinant vaccinia viruses expressing different HBV proteins or loaded with HBV peptides that overlap by 5–10 amino acids. Sixteen hours before the experiment, calculate the number of target cells required for every condition tested. Place cell suspension in 15-mL tubes (one for each condition) and centrifuge for 10 min at 400*g*. Remove the supernatant so that approx 30–50 μL remain. Add the appropriate amount of recombinant vaccinia viruses or control virus to the cell pellet (for EBV-B cells use an MOI of 100, for PHA blasts use an MOI of 10) and incubate for 1 h at room temperature with gentle agitation. Wash cells with RPMI–10% FCS. Resuspend cells/mL at 1×10^6/mL in complete cell culture medium per well of a 24-well plate.

   If, alternatively, overlapping peptides are used, resuspend cells in complete cell culture medium to 1×10^6 cells/mL, add HBV-derived peptides at a final concentration of 10 μg/mL, and place 1 mL of the cell suspension into a well of a 24-well plate.
3. Incubate cells overnight at 37°C, 5% CO_2.
4. The next day, transfer target cells from each well into a separate 15-mL tube, add 2 mL of fresh medium, and centrifuge at 400*g* for 10 min.
5. Remove all but 50 μL of the supernatant. Add 100 μCi of ^{51}Cr with a filter tip and follow standard precautions while handling radioactive material. Resuspend cells gently and incubate at 37°C, 5% CO_2 for 1 h. Note that the uptake of ^{51}Cr may vary depending on the target used.
6. During the 1-h incubation phase of the target cells, transfer the effector cells from the culture plates in the incubator into separate 15-mL tubes, fill tubes with PBS, and centrifuge for 10 min at 400*g*.
7. Remove supernatant and resuspend each cell pellet in 200–500 μL of RPMI–10% FCS.
8. Count cells with trypan blue and dilute to 3.6×10^6 cells/mL in RPMI–10% FCS.
9. In the first column of a 96-well round bottom plate, add 100 μL of effector cell suspension in duplicates. This equals an effector to target cell (E:T) ratio of 120:1 provided that 3000 targets cells will be used. If different E:T ratios are needed (60:1, 30:1, 15:1, etc.), add 200 μL cell suspension in the first column of the plate; add 100 μL of RPMI–10% FCS to the other wells; then transfer 100 μL from the wells of the first column to the second one and proceed to the lowest E:T ratio.
10. Prepare triplicate wells for spontaneous and maximum ^{51}Cr release for each target cell condition. For spontaneous release, add RPMI–10% FCS to three wells, for maximum release add 100 μL of 10% Triton X to each well.
11. After incubation with ^{51}Cr, wash target cells from **step 5** twice with PBS and once with RPMI–10% FCS. **Caution: Follow standard radiation safety procedures when working with ^{51}Cr solution and ^{51}Cr-labeled target; use lead to shield against irradiation.**
12. After this last wash, carefully remove the supernatant with a filter tip.
13. Resuspend cells in 250 μL of RPMI–10% FCS, count and resuspend at 0.03×10^6 cells/mL. Add 100 μL of this cell suspension to each well that contains the corresponding effector cells and to the wells representing spontaneous and maximum release.
14. Centrifuge plate for 5 min at 65*g* without braking and incubate for 4 h at 37°C, 5% CO_2.
15. Transfer 80 μL of supernatant to a Lumaplate and dry at 56°C for 45 min. Seal the plate and count cpm.
16. Calculate antigen-specific cytotoxicity as [(percent cytotoxic activity in the presence of peptide) – (percent cytotoxic activity in the absence of peptide)]. Percent cytotoxicity can be determined from the formula 100 × [(experimental ^{51}Cr release – spontaneous release)/(maximum release – spontaneous release)].

3.4.2. Intracellular Cytokine Staining

Intracellular cytokine staining can be performed with cell lines in the same way as with freshly isolated liver-derived lymphocytes. To induce cytokine secretion, cell lines can either be stimulated in an antigen-nonspecific way using PMA–ionomycin or in an antigen-specific way using antigen-presenting cells pulsed with HBV-derived peptides or infected with recombinant vaccinia viruses encoding HBV antigens. An example for intracellular cytokine analysis of T-cell lines is provided in **Fig. 3**.

1. For antigen-nonspecific stimulation with PMA–ionomycin, resuspend 0.5–2 × 10^6 lymphocytes in 1 mL of RPMI–10% FCS in a yellow Sarstedt tube, add 50 μg/mL of PMA and 1 μg/mL of ionomycin, centrifuge 5 min at 65*g* without braking, and incubate the tube at a 20° angle so that the cell pellet rests horizontally at 37°C for 2 h. For antigen-specific stimulation, load autologous EBV-transformed B cells with the specific peptide mix (1–10 μg/mL/peptide) or infect them with recombinant vaccinia viruses expressing HBV antigens (MOI = 10) 12–16 h prior to the lymphocyte stimulation. Incubate EBV-transformed B cells in complete medium at 37°C overnight. The next day, wash EBV-transformed B cells once in PBS, then resuspend them in 0.5 mL of complete medium, mix with 0.5 mL of liver-derived lymphocytes at a ratio of 1:1, and incubate the mix at 37°C for 2 h.
2. Then proceed as described in **Subheading 3.2.3., step 3.** When performing intracellular cytokine staining with antigen-presenting cells, treatment with DNase is crucial, as many cell clumps are generated during the stimulation period because of cell death. DNase will digest DNA released by dead cells and allow individualization of cells. EBV-B cells can be identified and excluded from analysis based on size and granularity in the forward vs side scatter plot.

3.5. Summary

In summary, it is recommended to employ complementary techniques to assess quantitative as well as qualitative characteristics of the immune response. Because the size of available liver tissue and the number of lymphocytes that can be isolated are often limited, the methodological strategy needs to be devised according to the research question. This also implies, on the other hand, that care should be taken not to misinterpret results. For example, epitope specificities that are not detected in assays based on T-cell lines may still be present in vivo. Intrahepatic T cells with these epitope specificities may display a higher sensitivity to cell death upon in vitro restimulation.

4. Notes

1. Processing of liver tissue and isolation of liver-infiltrating lymphocytes should be performed in a certified biological safety cabinet under sterile conditions. Vaccination with HBsAg and standard laboratory safety techniques are recommended for all investigators handling human, specifically HBV-infected, samples and vaccination with vaccinia virus is recommended every 10 yr for investigators handling vaccinia virus expression constructs. Standard radiation safety guidelines should be followed when working with ^{51}Cr-labeled cells.
2. Glass grinders are used to homogenize small liver samples by mechanical disruption. This method is faster than the enzymatic digestion and gives a good yield of liver-derived lymphocytes. During this procedure, hepatocytes are destroyed while smaller lymphocytes pass between the piston and the wall of the grinder. Because some lymphocytes may be damaged during this process, it is recommended to check cell viability and integrity by staining with annexin V and PI followed by flow cytometry.

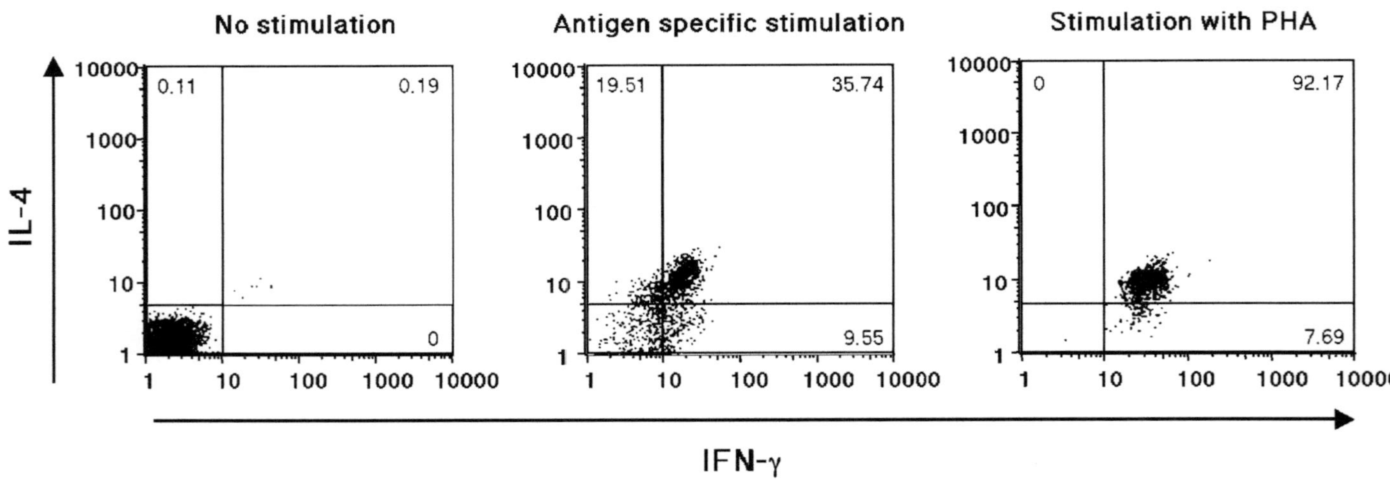

Fig. 3. Intracellular cytokine staining of liver-derived cell lines. Autologous EBV-transformed B cells were loaded with viral proteins overnight and subsequently used as antigen-presenting cells to stimulate liver-derived T cell lines as described in **Subheading 3.4.2.** After stimulation, cells were then stained with anti-CD4, anti-CD8, anti-IL-4, and anti-IFN-γ antibodies as described in **Subheadings 3.4.2.** and **3.2.3.** Results are presented for the gated, $CD4^+$ T-cell population. The graph on the left displays the results of unstimulated liver-derived cell lines. The middle graph demonstrates that approximately one third of the cell population produces IL-4 and IFN-γ in response to viral proteins. The graph on the right shows that 92% of the cell population express both IL-4 and IFN-γ antigen-nonspecific stimulation with PHA. Note that viral proteins stimulate predominantly $CD4^+$ T lymphocytes. If cytokine production of $CD8^+$ T lymphocytes is required, EBV-B cells should be loaded with virus-derived peptides. Note that in this case blood and liver biopsy were obtained from a chimpanzee infected with HCV. The same type of analysis can also be performed with samples of HBV-infected patients.

3. If lymphocytes are isolated from whole mouse liver, Percoll gradients or metrizamide gradients provide a better yield than Ficoll gradients ***(13–15)***. Cell populations isolated from large pieces of liver may contain a significant number of contaminating Kupffer cells which can be easily identified by flow cytometry and depleted by adherence to plastic. For this step, the cell suspension is placed into 10-cm Petri dishes at 1–2 × 10^6 cells/mL in RPMI–10%FCS and cultured for 90 min in a humidified 37°C, 5% CO_2 incubator. Nonadherent lymphocytes can be separated by gentle rocking of the Petri dish, washing with 37°C warm cell culture medium and aspiration with a pipet.
4. Trypan blue exclusion is a simple technique and can be performed rapidly. However, dye uptake varies depending on cell membrane integrity and small amounts of dye uptake can therefore remain unnoticed. If precise determination of the number of cells undergoing apoptosis is required, flow cytometric analysis of PI uptake and annexin V staining is recommended.
5. Flow cytometry is an invaluable tool to analyze intracellular cytokine contents and cell surface marker expression. This procedure, however, requires relatively large cell numbers (5 × 10^5) because of cell loss during stimulation and permeabilization process. In addition to intracellular cytokine staining, cytokine secretion assays are available in which cytokines are bound to the cell surface on secretion and stained for flow cytometry ***(16, 17)***.
6. In addition to positive selection of $CD8^+$ T cells with magnetic beads, an efficient approach uses negative selection with a bispecific antibody that crosslinks CD3 and the CD4 molecules on the cell surface and leads to the depletion of $CD4^+$ T cells ***(18–21)***.
7. In vitro expansion of cell lines and/or clones is useful to generate a homogeneous cell population for functional analysis and epitope mapping. Antigen-nonspecific cloning allows the growth of T cells regardless of their antigen specificity and their phenotype (CD4 or CD8). On the other hand, it may select for cells that are well adapted to tissue culture conditions, the concentration of IL-2, the type of serum used, and so forth and a selection bias cannot be avoided. Also, this approach may require at least 2 mo of cell growth, especially if cells are seeded at one cell per well. Generally, the cloning efficiency will be significantly higher if T cells are expanded with HBV-specific antigens. Although the number of lymphocytes recovered from a liver biopsy is generally too small to allow expansion of cell lines with individual viral peptides, it is possible to generate cell lines by bulk stimulation with a pool of virus-derived peptides ***(22, 23)***. If positive cytokine or cytotoxicity responses are observed against target cells pulsed with peptide pools, peptides can then be tested in smaller pools or individually to identify T-cell epitopes.

References

1. Guidotti, L. G. and Chisari, F. V. (1996) To kill or to cure: options in host defense against viral infection. *Curr. Opin. Immunol.* **8**, 478–483.
2. Rehermann, B., Fowler, P., Sidney, J., et al. (1995) The cytotoxic T lymphocyte response to multiple hepatitis B virus polymerase epitopes during and after acute viral hepatitis. *J. Exp. Med.* **181**, 1047–1058.
3. Barnaba, V., Franco, A., Alberti, A. B. C., Benvenuto, R., and Balsano, F. (1989) Recognition of hepatitis B envelope proteins by liver-infiltrating T lymphocytes in chronic HBV infection. *J. Immunol.* **143**, 2650–2655.

4. Ferrari, C., Penna, A., Mondelli, M., Fiaccadori, F., and Chisari, F. V. (1988) Intrahepatic HBcAg specific regulatory T cell networks in chronic active hepatitis B, in *Viral Hepatitis and Liver Disease* (Zuckerman, A. J., ed.), Alan R. Liss, New York, pp. 641–644.
5. Tsai, S. L., Chen, M. Y., Lai, M. Y., et al. (1992) Acute exacerbations of chronic type B hepatitis are accompanied by increased T cell responses to hepatitis B core and e antigens. *J. Clin. Invest.* **89**, 87–96.
6. Guidotti, L. G., Rochford, R., Chung, J., Shapiro, M., Purcell, R., and Chisari, F. V. (1999) Viral clearance without destruction of infected cells during acute HBV infection. *Science* **284**, 825–829.
7. Barnaba, V., Franco, A., Paroli, M., et al. (1994) Selective expansion of cytotoxic T lymphocytes with a CD4+CD56+ surface phenotype and a T helper type 1 profile of cytokine secretion in the liver of patients chronically infected with hepatitis B virus. *J. Immunol.* **64**, 5324–5332.
8. Ferrari, C., Penna, A., Giuberti, T., et al. (1987) Intrahepatic, nucleocapsid antigen-specific T cells in chronic active hepatitis B. *J. Immunol.* **139**, 2050–2058.
9. Radbruch, A. and Recktenwald, D. (1995) Detection and isolation of rare cells. *Curr. Opin. Immunol.* **7**, 270–273.
10. Curry, M. P., Norris, S., Golden-Mason, L., et al. (2000) Isolation of lymphocytes from normal adult human liver suitable for phenotypic and functional characterization. *J. Immunol. Methods* **242**, 21–31.
11. Norris, S., Collins, C., Doherty, D. G., et al. (1998) Resident human hepatic lymphocytes are phenotypically different from circulating lymphocytes. *J. Hepatol.* **28**, 84–90.
12. Norris, S., Doherty, D. G., Collins, C., et al. (1999) Natural T cells in the human liver: cytotoxic lymphocytes with dual T cell and natural killer cell phenotype and function are phenotypically heterogenous and include Valpha24-JalphaQ and gammadelta T cell receptor bearing cells. *Hum. Immunol.* **60**, 20–31.
13. Crispe, N. (1997) Isolation of mouse intrahepatic lymphocytes. *Curr. Protocol. Immunol.* 3.21.1–3.21.8.
14. Kakimi, K., Guidotti, L. G., Koezuka, Y., and Chisari, F. V. (2000) Natural killer T cell activation inhibits hepatitis B virus replication in vivo. *J. Exp. Med.* **192**, 921–930.
15. Liu, Z. X., Govindarajan, S., Okamoto, S., and Dennert, G. (2000) NK cells cause liver injury and facilitate the induction of T cell-mediated immunity to a viral liver infection. *J. Immunol.* **164**, 6480–6486.
16. Oelke, M., Moehrle, U., Chen, J. L., et al. (2000) Generation and purification of CD8+ melan-A-specific cytotoxic T lymphocytes for adoptive transfer in tumor immunotherapy. *Clin. Cancer Res.* **6**, 1997–2005.
17. Ouyang, W., Lohning, M., Gao, Z., et al. (2000) Stat6-independent GATA-3 autoactivation directs IL-4-independent Th2 development and commitment. *Immunity* **12**, 27–37.
18. Koziel, M. J., Dudley, D., Wong, J. T., et al. (1992) Intrahepatic cytotoxic T lymphocytes specific for hepatitis C virus in persons with chronic hepatitis. *J. Immunol.* **149**, 3339–3344.
19. Koziel, J. M., Dudley, D., Afdhal, N., et al. (1993) Hepatitis C virus (HCV)-specific cytotoxic T lymphocytes recognize epitopes in the core and envelope proteins of HCV. *J. Virol.* **67**, 7522–7532.
20. Koziel, M. J., Dudley, D., Afdhal, N., et al. (1995) HLA class I-restricted cytotoxic T lymphocytes specific for hepatitis C virus. Identification of multiple epitopes and characterization of patterns of cytokine release. *J. Clin. Invest.* **96**, 2311–2321.

21. Wong, D. K., Dudley, D. D., Afdhal, N. H., et al. (1998) Liver-derived CTL in hepatitis C virus infection: breadth and specificity of responses in a cohort of persons with chronic infection. *J. Immunol.* **160**, 1479–1488.
22. Penna, A., Chisari, F. V., Bertoletti, A., et al. (1991) Cytotoxic T lymphocytes recognize an HLA-A2 restricted epitope within the hepatitis B virus nucleocapsid antigen. *J. Exp. Med.* **174**, 1565–1570.
23. Prezzi, C., Casciaro, M. A., Francavilla, V., et al. (2001) Virus-specific CD8(+) T cells with type 1 or type 2 cytokine profile are related to different disease activity in chronic hepatitis C virus infection. *Eur. J. Immunol.* **31**, 894–906.
24. Moriyama, T., Guilhot, S., Klopchin, K., et al. (1990) Immunobiology and pathogenesis of hepatocellular injury in hepatitis B virus transgenic mice. *Science* **248**, 361–364.
25. Rehermann, B., Ferrari, C., Pasquinelli, C., and Chisari, F. V. (1996) The hepatitis B virus persists for decades after patients'recovery from acute viral hepatitis despite active maintenance of a cytotoxic T-lymphocyte response. *Nat. Med.* **2**, 1104–1108.
26. Maini, M. K., Boni, C., Lee, C. K., et al. (2000) The role of virus-specific CD8+ cells in liver damage and viral control during persistent hepatitis B virus (HBV) infection. *J. Exp. Med.* **191**, 1269–1280.
27. Guidotti, L. G., Ando, K., Hobbs, M. V., et al. (1994) Cytotoxic T lymphocytes inhibit hepatitis B virus gene expression by a noncytolytic mechanism in transgenic mice. *Proc. Natl. Acad. Sci. USA* **91**, 3764–3768.

7

Determining the Precursor Frequency of HBV Nucleocapsid Antigen-Specific T Cells

Jennifer A. Waters and Howard C. Thomas

1. Introduction

The measurement of the precursor frequency of cells present in a population that are participating in a given immune function has been widely done by limiting dilution assays (LDAs). These have been used for measuring proliferative and cytotoxic responses and cytokine production by lymphocytes in the peripheral blood population. They are particularly well suited to the identification of rare cells; bulk culture is not quantitative at the cellular level and, if a low frequency of responder cells is present, misleading negative results may be obtained. Another advantage of an LDA over conventional bulk culture is that it minimizes the cross-regulatory influence between cells. In this chapter a method for measuring the precursor frequency of T cells proliferating in response to nucleocapsid antigen is described.

LDAs require multiple replicate cultures set up at different cell concentrations *(1)*. It is important that the culture conditions are not limiting and that the addition of factors such as interleukin-2 ((IL-2) to the cultures does not produce nonspecific stimulation. To control for this and for the variation within each experiment it is important to also set up multiple cultures without antigen. An arbitrary upper limit of the negative response is set and the number of negative cultures at a given cell concentration is scored. The negative wells are scored, as a positive well could be caused by the clonal expansion of one or more precursors, whereas a negative means there are none *(2)*. The range of cell concentrations used must also be predetermined so as to yield an adequate number of points to give a titration curve; there are five suggested cell concentrations in this method.

For the enumeration of cytotoxic T lymphocytes (CTLs) the effector function has classically been measured using the chromium release assay. However, the development of major histocompatibility complex (MHC) tetramers has enabled sensitive detection of antigen-specific cells directly ex vivo. It has been shown that the frequency of antigen-specific $CD8^+$ cells, as opposed to the $CD8^+$ cells that cause lysis of the targets, during an

From: *Methods in Molecular Medicine, vol. 96: Hepatitis B and D Protocols, volume 2*
Edited by: R. K. Hamatake and J. Y. N. Lau © Humana Press Inc., Totowa, NJ

acute viral infection is higher than that estimated using the chromium release cytotoxic T-cell assay *(3)*. Tetramer labeling is useful only when an MHC I restricted peptide or peptides have been well defined. It does not allow the detection of responses restricted by those HLA class I alleles where epitope predictions are not available, so can be used only for a limited number of responses and in a population restricted by the MHC I allele. MHC tetramers have been used successfully when enumerating the $CD8^+$ response to HBV nucleocapsid antigen in patients acutely infected with HBV who are HLA-A2 positive *(4)*. In contrast, circulating tetramer positive CTL in hepatitis B e antigen (HBeAg)-positive persistent HBV infection were found only in a minority of patients *(5)*, consistent with the poorer cytotoxic responses in these patients.

It has also become possible to detect interferon-γ (IFN-γ) and interleukin-4 (IL-4) production in individual cells by intracellular staining *(6)* or by ELISPOT and this has introduced new and faster methods for enumeration of antigen-specific cells directly ex vivo. The detection of IFN-γ producing cells in response to nucleocapsid antigen has been estimated in patients with hepatitis B virus infection *(7)*, 61% of acutely infected patients and 25% of chronically infected patients had cells producing detectable IFN-γ. Neither acutely nor chronically infected patients had peripheral blood leukocytes (PBIs) producing detectable IL-4 by this method. In the same patients, bulk culture and the measurement of tritiated thymidine incorporation in a proliferation assay did not correlate with the ELISPOT results *(7)*. A high proliferative response occurred without a corresponding high number of IFN-γ producing cells; however, the ELISPOT assay was more frequently positive. A direct comparison of LDA by proliferation, a more sensitive technique than bulk culture when the number of responding cells is low, and the frequency of cells producing IFN-γ was not made.

This chapter describes the method for determining the precursor frequency of T cells that proliferate in response to nucleocapsid antigen. The proliferative response and production of IFN-γ by T cells are separate functions. No direct comparison between the two techniques and their relationship to the course of the disease, particularly in persistently infected patients, has been made. The use of either technique would depend on the reasons for the analysis.

LDA has the advantage of allowing a statistical analysis of the results obtained, which has been well discussed by Taswell *(8,9)*. Some assumptions must be made for the calculation of the precursor frequency. It is necessary to assume that only one cell of only one cell type is needed for a positive response, and this is termed the single-hit hypothesis. Statistical methods are applied to test the goodness of fit of the data points with the single-hit Poisson model by calculating chi-squared statistics and confidence intervals for the slope. Once it has been established that the dilution curve represents a single hit, then the frequency of the precursors can be calculated.

2. Materials

2.1. Reagents

1. Recombinant core antigen to give a final concentration of 5 mg/mL (Biogen, Cambridge, MA).
2. 5000 U/5 mL of preservative-free heparin (Leo Laboratories, Princes Risborough).
3. Ficoll-Paque™Plus (Amersham Pharmacia Biotech AB, Upsala, Sweden).

4. RPMI-1640 with glutamine (Sigma Chemical, St. Louis, MO).
5. Human AB serum (Sigma Chemical, St. Louis, MO).
6. 10,000 U/mL of penicillin, 10 mg/mL of streptomycin in 0.9% sodium chloride (Sigma Chemical,
7. 96-Well round bottom plates, sterile with a lid (Nunc Brand products, Denmark, available from Merck Eurolab).
8. 37 MBq /mL of tritiated thymidine ([*methyl*-^{3}H] thymidine), aqueous solution sterilized. (Amersham Pharmacia Biotech AB, Uppsala, Sweden, cat. no. TRA 120).
9. Glass fiber filters, self-aligning, RG, part no. 6005412 (Packard, Meriden, CT).
10. 200 U/mL of recombinant IL-2 (Roche).

2.2. Equipment

1. Certified class II cabinet vented to the outside, within a safety laboratory.
2. Incubator at 37°C with 5% CO_2.
3. 96-Well cell harvester (e.g. Matrix 96, Packard Instruments, UK.)
4. γ-Irradiator.

3. Methods

3.1. Separating Lymphocytes from Blood

1. Take the blood into preservative-free heparin, 100 U/10 mL of blood.
2. Dilute the blood with an equal volume of tissue culture medium (RPMI-1640) without added serum or with isotonic PBS.
3. Pipet 8 mL of Ficoll-Paque™Plus into 30-mL universal tubes. Pipet the diluted blood as a layer on top of the Ficoll, being careful that they do not mix. Any mixing at this stage will result in a poor recovery of PBLs.
4. After layering all of the blood, centrifuge the universal tubes in a benchtop centrifuge at 600*g* for 20 min at 20°C, with no brake.
5. The lymphocytes, monocytes, and macrophages form a layer at the interface between the two liquids, the red cells (and the majority of the polymorphonuclear cells) settle at the bottom of the universal tube. Remove the mononuclear cell layer into a fresh tube, taking this entire layer but with the minimum of Ficoll and tissue culture fluid.
6. Dilute out the PBLs with tissue culture medium and centrifuge at 550*g* for 5 min.
7. Wash the cells by resuspending the pellet in fresh medium and centrifuging at 125*g* for 5 min.
8. Wash the cells twice more, resuspending them in a known volume, and removing an aliquot for counting using a hemocytometer before the final centrifugation.
9. Resuspend the cells at 5×10^5 /mL in RPMI-1640 with 10% AB serum and penicillin–streptomycin (complete medium).

3.2. Limiting Dilution Assay

1. Dilute the lymphocytes to four more concentrations of cells in complete medium. Each dilution requires a minimum of 5 mL of cell suspension. The four other concentrations are 2.5×10^5, 1×10^5, 5×10^4, and 1×10^4/mL. (*See* **Note 1.**)
2. Pipet 48 replicate cultures of 100 μL for each of the cell concentrations into 96-well round-bottom tissue culture plates. Do not use the outer wells of the plate. Fill these wells with 200 μL of RPMI-1640 to help prevent evaporation in the culture wells. (*See* **Note 2.**)
3. Add hepatitis B core antigen (HBcAg) in 50 μL of complete medium to 24 of the wells to give a final concentration of 1 μg/well. To the other 24 wells add 50 μL of complete medium.

4. Add 1×10^4/well irradiated autologous PBMCs (3000 rad) to each well in 50 μL of complete medium.
5. Incubate the cultures in a humidified incubator with 5% CO_2 at 37°C for 7 d.
6. Add 2 U of recombinant IL-2 /well on d 4.
7. Pulse the cultures with 0.0375 MBq of tritiated thymidine ([^{3}H]Thy) (1 μ/Lwell diluted to 10 μL for more accurate pipetting) 16 h prior to harvesting. (*See* **Note 3.**)
8. Harvest the cultures on d 7 onto glass fiber filters using an automated cell harvester. (*See* **Note 4.**)
9. Count for 5 min on a scintillation counter.
10. Replicates with antigen are scored as negative if the counts incorporated are less than the mean plus three standard deviations of the counts incorporated in the controls. The frequency of responding cells and conformation to single hit kinetics are calculated using the Poisson distribution *(8,9)*.

4. Notes

1. It is important to mix the cell suspensions while pipetting. PBMC settle very quickly and any error in the number of cells added increases variability in the tritiated thymidine uptake.
2. It is very useful to use automatic multipipets as they decrease the pipetting errors.
3. When adding the tritiated thymidine, dilute so that a minimum of 10 μL is added to each well as this also reduces the error due to pipetting.
4. As with all tissue culture techniques it is important that there is no infection in the cultures. They should be examined carefully under the microscope before harvesting.

References

1. Quintans, J. and Lefkovits, I. (1973) Precursor cells specific to sheep red cells in nude mice. Estimation of frequency in the microculture system. *Eur. J. Immunol.* **3**, 392–397.
2. Sharrock, C. E., Kaminski, E., and Man, S. (1990) Limiting dilution analysis of human T cells: a useful clinical tool. *Immunol. Today* **11**, 281–286.
3. Murali-Krishna, K., Altman, J. D., Suresh, M., et al. (1998) Counting antigen-specific CD8 T cells: a reevaluation of bystander activation during viral infection. *Immunity* **8**, 177–187.
4. Webster, G. J., Reignat, S., Maini, M. K., et al. (2000) Incubation phase of acute hepatitis b in man: dynamic of cellular immune mechanisms. *Hepatology* **32**, 1117–1124.
5. Maini, M. K., Boni, C., Lee, C. K., et al. (2000) The role of virus-specific CD8(+) cells in liver damage and viral control during persistent hepatitis B virus infection. *J. Exp. Med.* **191**, 1269–1280.
6. Kumaraguru, U. and Rouse, B. T. (2000) Application of the intracellular gamma interferon assay to recalculate the potency of CD8(+) T-cell responses to herpes simplex virus. *J. Virol.* **74**, 5709–5711.
7. Jung, M. C., Hartmann, B., Gerlach, J. T., et al. (1999) Virus-specific lymphokine production differs quantitatively but not qualitatively in acute and chronic hepatitis B infection. *Virology* **261**, 165–172.
8. Taswell, C. (1981) Limiting dilution assays for the determination of immunocompetent cell frequencies. I. Data analysis. *J. Immunol.* **126**, 1614–1619.
9. Taswell, C. (1984) Limiting dilution assays for the determination of immunocompetent cell frequencies. III. Validity tests for the single-hit Poisson model. *J. Immunol. Methods* **72**, 29–40.

8

Detection and Characterization of Virus-Specific CD8+ T Cells Using the Tetramer Approach

Xiao-Song He and Harry B. Greenberg

1. Introduction

Hepatitis B virus (HBV)-specific CD8+ T cells, or cytotoxic T lymphocytes (CTLs), are believed to play an important role in the control of infection and development of liver injury *(1)*. Therefore the quantitative and qualitative analyses of such cells is important for understanding the mechanisms underlying the pathogenesis associated with the infection as well as the clearance or persistence of the infecting virus. Traditionally, HBV-specific CD8+ T cells were detected by cytotoxicity assay, while the frequency of such cells was estimated by limiting dilution assay (LDA). Both assays are based on the killing activity of CTLs. The number of virus-specific CTLs in clinical specimens (blood or liver samples) is usually very small. Therefore these assays require extensive in vitro expansion of virus-specific CD8+ T cells to generate CTL lines or clones, which is time consuming and labor intensive. As such assays can detect only CD8+ T cells that expand in vitro and kill specific target cells, they may not represent the characteristics of the overall CD8+ T cell responses against the virus.

The antigen specificity of T cells is determined by the T-cell receptor (TCR) expressed on each T cell, which recognizes peptide epitopes presented by major histocompatibility complex (MHC) molecules on the surface of antigen-presenting cells (APCs). The generation of tetrameric MHC–peptide complex *(2)*, which binds to specific TCRs with a reasonable affinity, allows direct identification of the CD8+ T cell subset with a unique antigen specificity. Hence, fluorescence-labeled peptide–MHC tetramers can be used to stain antigen-specific CD8+ T cells in peripheral blood mononuclear cells (PBMCs) or tissue-infiltrating lymphocytes. The tetramer-binding cells can then be directly detected on a single cell basis by flow cytometry (FACS analysis). The major advantage of the tetramer staining assay is its independence from any in vivo or in vitro function of CD8+ T cells, as well as its quantitative nature. Under optimal conditions antigen-specific CD8+ T cells in the peripheral blood at a level as low as 0.01% can be clearly detected *(3)*.

From: *Methods in Molecular Medicine, vol. 96: Hepatitis B and D Protocols, volume 2*
Edited by: R. K. Hamatake and J. Y. N. Lau © Humana Press Inc., Totowa, NJ

The sensitivity, or detection limit, of tetramer assay depends on the signal-to-noise ratio, or the background level of the assay. The background level of tetramer staining (as well as any antibody staining) depends largely on the condition of cells. Poorly prepared and/or preserved cells tend to generate more background signals than freshly prepared samples, while tissue-infiltrating lymphocytes and activated cells tend to generate more background signals than PBMCs and resting cells. Negative control samples should always be stained along with the experimental samples to assess the level of background noise. For example, if an HLA-A2 tetramer loaded with an HBV epitope is used to stain an HLA-A2$^+$ PBMC sample, PBMCs from HLA-A2$^+$ donors naive to HBV or HLA-A2$^-$ donors can be used as appropriate negative controls.

It is critical to minimize nonspecific background staining when the expected level of antigen-specific CD8$^+$ T cells is low (e.g., $< 0.1\%$). The background signals are often caused by dead or damaged cells that bind tetramers and antibodies nonspecifically. One solution for this problem is to use propidium iodide (PI), which selectively stains dead cells. Any cells stained by PI can then be gated out during analysis of FACS data. One of the channels of a three-color flow cytometer (e.g., FACScan) can be devoted to this purpose. The drawback of this method is that the potentially infectious samples (cells isolated from patients) cannot be fixed before being acquired on flow cytometer, because fixation kills all the cells and renders them stainable by PI. Alternately, antibodies against several markers not expressed by CD8$^+$ T cells can be added together with the tetramer. The stained samples can then be fixed with paraformaldehyde before being analyzed on flow cytometer. By gating on cells that are not stained with these antibodies, dead cells that nonspecifically bound the antibodies and the tetramer can be excluded. **Figure 1** shows an example of quantifying HCV-specific CD8$^+$ T cells from a frozen PBMC sample. Tc-labeled antibodies to CD4 (a marker for helper T cells), CD13 (a marker for monocytes), and CD19 (a marker for B cells) are used for negative gating at channel FL3, resulting in reduced nonspecific staining and a better separated tetramer-binding population.

Thanks to multicolor flow cytometric technology, tetramer staining can be combined with staining for other cellular markers to provide a multiparameter phenotypic analysis of an antigen-specific cell population. Depending on the researcher's interest, these could be markers indicating the activation status (CD69, CD25, CD38, HLA-DR, etc.), T-cell subset markers that have been associated with the memory/effector cell status (CD45RO, CD45RA, CD27, etc.), different TCR Vβ molecules, or other parameters. Intracellular markers, for example, perforin, can also be costained along with tetramer. In this case the cells are usually first stained with tetramer and antibodies for cell surface markers. After fixation and permeabilization of the cells, they are stained for the intracellular markers. A basic protocol for enumeration of tetramer-binding CD8$^+$ T cells and characterization of their surface phenotype is described in **Subheading 3.1.**

In addition to isolated PBMC samples, fresh whole blood samples can also be used for tetramer staining. In this case, tetramer and the antibodies are added to the whole blood directly. After staining, red blood cells are lysed before FACS analysis ***(4)***.

Tetramer staining can also be combined with any flow cytometry based functional analysis to directly assess the response of antigen-specific CD8$^+$ T cells to antigen stimulation on a single-cell basis. For example, when antigen-specific CD8$^+$ T cells are

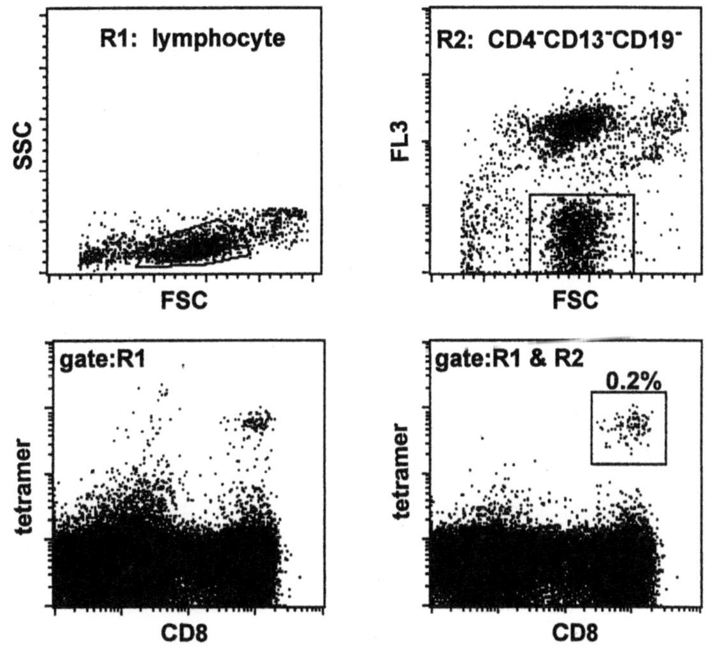

Fig. 1. Detection of CD8+ T cells specific for an HLA-A2 restricted epitope of the HCV protein NS3. PBMCs were stained with a PE-labeled HLA-A2 tetramer loaded with the NS3 peptide 1406–1415, APC-labeled anti-CD8, and Tc-labeled anti-CD4, CD13, and CD19. Displayed in the dot plots are cells gated on lymphocyte population only *(lower left panel)* or lymphocyte population and CD4−CD13−CD19− population *(lower right panel)*.

stimulated with their cognate antigen, they may respond by up-regulation of the activation marker CD69, as well as production of cytokines as interferon-γ (IFN-γ). A combined staining of the stimulated PBMCs with tetramer and anti-CD69, or tetramer and anti-IFN-γ, enables directly evaluating the functional status of antigen-specific CD8+ T cells. Such assays have been used to identify functional as well as anergic antigen-specific CD8+ T cells in different diseases ***(3–5)***. In this chapter we provide a protocol for the intracellular cytokine assay of antigen-specific CD8+ T cells (*see* **Subheading 3.2.**).

Tetramer staining is undoubtedly a powerful quantitative technique for analyzing antigen-specific CD8+ T cells, including those specific for HBV ***(6–8)***. This technique has greatly expanded opportunities for studying T-cell responses. However, simply comparing the results of tetramer staining to that of traditional assays such as LDA can be misleading. For example, studies have shown that the frequency of tetramer-binding cells to be 10–50 times greater than results of LDA for the same sample ***(9, 10)***. These results indicate only that LDA may underestimate the frequency of epitope-specific CD8+ T cells, but by no means suggest that tetramer assay is 50-fold more sensitive than

LDA. Actually these two assays are targeted at two distinct T-cell populations. Tetramer assays measure all $CD8^+$ T cells specific for an epitope, with a detection limit at the level of 0.01% of $CD8^+$ T cells, or approx 0.002% of PBMCs. On the other hand, LDA measures a subset of epitope-specific $CD8^+$ T cells that can be expanded in vitro. The detection limit for such cells by LDA could reach 0.0001%, which is 20-fold more sensitive than tetramer staining.

2. Materials

2.1. Tetramers

Tetramers can be synthesized using recombinant MHC I proteins and synthetic peptide epitopes following published methods *(2)*. They are also available at the NIH Tetramer Core Facility (http://www.niaid.nih.gov/reposit/tetramer/genguide.html), as well as a commercial source (http://www.ImmunomicsOnline.com). Most researchers use phosphatidyl ethanolamine (PE)-labeled tetramers, although APC-labeled tetramers have also been used. Every batch of tetramer needs to be validated and standardized by staining previously studied reference samples, for example, epitope-specific CTL lines or clones, or PBMC samples with known level of specific $CD8^+$ T cells. The shelf life of different tetramer preparations ranges from several weeks to several months. An increased nonspecific staining and decreased number and fluorescence intensity of positive cells usually indicate deterioration of the tetramer reagent. Therefore, tetramers should be tested periodically with known positive and negative samples to monitor their quality.

2.2. Antibodies

Fluorescence-labeled antibodies against T-cell subset markers can be obtained from BD Biosciences (San Jose, CA), BD Pharmingen (San Diego, CA), Caltag (South San Francisco, CA), and other vendors.

2.3. Solutions, Media, and Other Reagents

1. Phosphate-buffered saline without Ca^{2+}/Mg^{2+} (PBS).
2. FACS lysing solution: Add 10 mL of 10X stock solution (BD Biosciences) to 90 mL of distilled water to make a 1X working solution. Store at room temperature.
3. FACS permeabilizing solution: Add 10 mL of a 10X stock solution (BD Biosciences) to 90 mL of distilled water to make a 1X working solution. Store at room temperature.
4. FACS washing solution: Dissolve 2.5 g of bovine albumin fraction V and 0.25 g of sodium azide in 500 mL of PBS. Store at room temperature.
5. 1% Paraformaldehyde solution. Add 1 mL of 10% paraformaldehyde (Electron Microscopy Sciences, Ft. Washington, PA) and 1 mL of 10X PBS into 8 mL of distilled water. Store at 4°C.
6. Culture medium. RPMI 1640 medium supplemented with 10% heat-inactivated fetal calf serum, 100 U/mL of penicillin, and 100 μg/mL of streptomycin.
7. Brefeldin A (Sigma, St. Louis, MO). Prepare a 5 mg/mL solution in dimethyl sulfoxide (DMSO); this represents a 10X stock and should be stored at –20°C in aliquots of 20 μL. On the day of use add 180 μL of sterile PBS to one aliquot to make a 1X solution. The 1X solution may be stored at 4°C for up to 1 wk.
8. 20 m*M* EDTA solution: Dilute 500 m*M* EDTA stock solution, pH 8.0, 1:25 with PBS.

2.4. Equipment

1. Flow cytometer: FACScan (three-color), FACS Calibur (four-color), or equivalent instruments.
2. Benchtop centrifuge with a swing-bucket rotor (Beckman Allegra 6R or equivalent instruments).
3. Dounce tissue grinder, 7 mL (K885300-0007 from Fisher Scientific, Santa Clara, CA).

2.5. Preparation of Cell Samples

1. Blood samples. Depending on the type of assays to be carried out, venous blood can be drawn into standard Vacutainer tubes or CPT blood collection tubes (BD Biosciences) with different anticoagulants. **Critical parameters: For intracellular cytokine assay of whole blood, sodium heparin tubes (but not EDTA tubes) must be used for the blood drawing.** To isolate PBMCs, blood samples in standard Vacutainer tubes are processed with standard Ficoll-Hypaque gradient centrifugation method, while blood samples in CPT tubes should be processed following the manufacturer's instructions. PBMCs are used fresh or cryopreserved in 10% DMSO/90% fetal calf serum in liquid nitrogen.
2. Liver biopsy samples. Liver biopsy samples are placed in 10 mL of culture medium on ice and processed within 2 h. Transfer the tissue into a Dounce tissue grinder filled with 5 mL of fresh medium and gently grind the tissue with the small pestle to release the liver infiltrating lymphocytes (LILs). Transfer the cell suspension into a 15-mL centrifuge tube, use 5 mL of fresh medium to rinse the tissue grinder and the pestle, and combine the wash with the cell suspension. Stand the tube upright for 5 min to let the residual tissue settle to the bottom of the tube, then transfer the cell suspension into a new tube, avoiding carrying over the settled tissue. The cells are then pelleted at 300*g* for 10 min. Resuspend the cells in an appropriate volume of medium and count the cells. Up to 2×10^6 LILs can be recovered by this procedure from a biopsy tissue 10–20 mg in weight. However, the yield of LILs can vary greatly depending on the disease status. **Critical parameters: Do not attempt to purify LILs with Ficoll-Hypaque gradient, which can cause a significant loss of cells.**

3. Methods

3.1. Basic Protocol: Quantification and Phenotypic Characterization of Tetramer-Binding Cells in PBMCs and LILs

1. Either freshly isolated or cryopreserved cells can be used. Thaw the frozen cells at 37°C and wash once with 10 mL of FACS washing buffer. Resuspend cells in FACS washing buffer at a density up to 10×10^7 cells /100 μL. For each staining, aliquot 20 μL of the cell suspension that contains up to 2×10^6 cells into a 15-mL conical centrifuge tube.
2. Prepare the staining cocktail that contains tetramer and different antibodies (*see* **Note 1**), according to the design of experiment and flow cytometer available. **Critical parameters: Centrifuge the tetramers in an Eppendorf microfuge at top speed for 5 min to remove aggregates that may significantly increase nonspecific staining. This must be done every time before use.** The following are the recipes of three typical cocktails. All quantities are for one staining reaction with 20 μL of cell suspension. In each recipe, use FACS washing buffer to bring the volume to 10 μL for each staining.

   Recipe A. For quantification of tetramer-binding CD8+ T cells, using a FACScan flow cytometer (three-color):

PE-tetramer	1 μg
FITC-CD8 (Caltag)	0.7 μL

TC-CD4 (Caltag)	0.4 μL
TC-CD13 (Caltag)	0.4 μL
TC-CD19 (Caltag)	0.4 μL

Recipe B. For quantification and CD45RA phenotype analysis of tetramer-binding cells, using a FACScan flow cytometer (three-color):

PE-tetramer	1 μg
TC-CD8 (Caltag)	0.7 μL
FITC-CD45RA (Caltag)	1 μL

Recipe C. For quantification and CD45RA phenotype analysis of tetramer-binding cells, using a FACS Calibur flow cytometer (four-color):

PE-tetramer	1 μg
APC-CD8 (Caltag)	0.7 μL
FITC-CD45RA (Caltag)	1 μL
TC-CD4 (Caltag)	0.4 μL
TC-CD13 (Caltag)	0.4 μL
TC-CD19 (Caltag)	0.4 μL

3. Add the staining cocktail to the cells, mix by vortexing briefly.
4. Incubate at room temperature in the dark for 30 min.
5. Wash the cells with 5 mL of FACS washing buffer. Pellet the cells by centrifugation at 300*g* for 10 min.
6. Remove the supernatant by aspiration. Resuspend cells in 200 μL of 1% paraformaldehyde.
7. Acquire data on a flow cytometer within 24 h.
8. Data analysis: Set gates on small lymphocyte population based on forward scattering and side scattering, $CD8^+$ population, and $CD4^-CD13^-CD19^-$ population (if these antibodies are used for negative gating, recipes A and C).

3.2. Functional Analysis: Production of IFN-γ by Antigen-Specific $CD8^+$ T Cells

1. Aliquot 0.25 mL of freshly collected whole blood into 15-mL conical centrifuge tubes. The volume of blood and all the reagents used can be scaled up according to expected frequency of tetramer-binding cells. **Critical parameters: For the intracellular cytokine assay, blood can be collected only with heparin tubes but not EDTA or ACD tubes.** Alternately freshly isolated PBMCs can be used for this assay. In this case resuspend cells in culture medium at a density of 3×10^6/mL. Blood samples can be stored at room temperature for up to 24 h before antigen stimulation without significant loss of reactivity.
2. Add 5 μL of 1X BFA solution for every 0.25 mL of blood or cell suspension (final concentration of BFA is 10 μg/mL). Add specific peptide antigen or control peptide at selected concentration (usually 0.1–10 μg/mL). Mix by brief vortexing.
3. Incubate for 4 h with the tubes standing upright at 37°C (for whole blood), or in 5° slant at 37°C with 5% CO_2 (for PBMCs). After incubation, the samples can be processed immediately, or stored at 4°C overnight before proceeding to the next step.
4. Add 1/10 volume of 20 m*M* EDTA to the blood or cell cultures. Incubate at room temperature for 15 min. Vortex-mix for 10 s to detach cells from the tubes.
5. Add 2 mL of PBS and mix by vortexing to wash the cells. Pellet cells by centrifugation at 500*g* for 5 min. Carefully remove supernatant by aspiration without disturbing the cells. For

whole blood samples, leave minimum amount of supernatant over the blood cells; for PBMC samples, leave approx 20 μL of supernatant. Resuspend cells by vortexing.

6. Add 1 μg of tetramer. Mix by vortexing. Incubate at room temperature in the dark for 30 min.
7. Wash cells with 5 mL of FACS washing buffer. Pellet cells by centrifugation at 500*g* for 5 min. Remove supernatant by aspiration. Vortex-mix briefly to resuspend cells.
8. Add 2 mL of 1X FACS lysing solution for every 0.25 mL of whole blood, or 0.5 mL of 1X FACS lysing solution for PBMC samples. Mix by vortexing. **Critical parameters: Cells must be resuspended completely.** Incubate at room temperature in the dark for 10 min (*See* **Note 2.**)
9. Add 5 mL of FACS washing solution. Pellet the cells by centrifugation at 500*g* for 10 min. Remove supernatant by aspiration.
10. Add 0.5 mL of 1X FACS permeabilizing solution. Mix by vortexing. Incubate at room temperature in the dark for 10 min.
11. Add 5 mL of FACS washing solution. Pellet the cells by centrifugation at 500*g* for 10 min. Remove supernatant by aspiration, leaving approx 20 μL of supernatant. Resuspend cells by vortex-mixing.
12. Add the following staining cocktail to each tube:

FITC-IFN-γ (BD Biosciences)	6 μL
APC-CD8 (Caltag)	0.7 μL
TC-CD4 (Caltag)	0.4 μL
TC-CD13 (Caltag)	0.4 μL
TC-CD19 (Caltag)	0.4 μL

13. Incubate at room temperature in the dark for 30 min.
14. Wash cells with 5 mL of FACS washing solution. Pellet the cells by centrifugation at 500*g* for 10 min. Remove supernatant by aspiration.
15. Proceed to **steps 6–8** of the basic protocol (*see* **Subheading 3.1.**) for data acquisition. (*See* **Note 3.**)

4. Notes

1. Each tetramer and antibody from a different source must be titrated to determine the optimal staining condition, which should result in the highest specific staining and lowest background. The quantities listed in this chapter are supposed to serve as a reference for the titration. As shown in **Fig. 1**, the use of negative gating helps reduce background. This is especially important when the expected frequency of tetramer-binding cells is low. Therefore, it is always desirable to use negative staining antibodies and to dedicate one channel of the flow cytometer for negative gating.
2. Intracellular staining of cytokines (and other intracellular markers) requires fixation and permeabilization of cells. In the protocol described here the fixation of lymphocytes is achieved by treating samples with FACS lysing solution, which fixes the white cells while lysing the red cells. For some of the cell surface markers fixation does not affect their staining. These markers can be stained either after fixation and permeabilization, as the staining for CD8, CD4, CD13, and CD19 described in **Subheading 3.2.**, or be stained before fixation. In other words antibodies for these cell surface markers can be added together with anti-IFN-γ after fixation and permeabilization, as described in this protocol, or added with the tetramer before fixation. However, for many other markers fixation may affect staining.

Therefore whenever there is uncertainty, surface markers should be stained before fixation of cells.

3. TCRs on activated $CD8^+$ T cells can be down-modulated by stimulation of specific peptide–MHC complex ***(11)***. Down-modulation of TCRs have been shown to affect the staining intensity of activated $CD8^+$ T cells with tetramers ***(3,4)***. The extent of down-modulation depends on the amino acid sequence of the epitope, the concentration of peptide, as well as on how long the cells have been stimulated. Under extreme situations the tetramer staining of activated cells can be completely aborted. Although the TCR down-modulation affects the tetramer staining of activated T cells, it has no effect on the nonresponsive T cells that carry the specific TCR. Therefore it should not affect the use of tetramer/cytokine combination staining for the purpose of identifying nonfunctional or anergic $CD8^+$ T cells specific for the antigen.

Acknowledgments

The work on which this chapter is based was supported by NIH Grant AI40034, by funding from Eli Lilly/Stanford University Program of Excellence in Hepatitis Research, and by funds from the Hutchison Program in Translational Medicine at Stanford University. We thank Drs. M. M. Davis, L. J. Picker, and V. C. Maino for useful discussions, and M. M. Davis for supplying us with the tetramers.

References

1. Guidotti, L. G. and Chisari, F. V. (2001) Noncytolytic control of viral infections by the innate and adaptive immune response. *Annu. Rev. Immunol.* **19,** 65–91.
2. Altman, J. D., Moss, P., Goulder, P., et al. (1996) Phenotypic analysis of antigen-specific T lymphocytes (published erratum appears in *Science* [1998] **280**, 1821). *Science* **274,** 94–96.
3. He, X. S., Rehermann, B., Lopez-Labrador, F. X., et al. (1999) Quantitative analysis of hepatitis C virus-specific CD8(+) T cells in peripheral blood and liver using peptide-MHC tetramers. *Proc. Natl. Acad. Sci. USA* **96,** 5692–5697.
4. He, X. S., Rehermann, B., Boisvert, J., et al. (2001) Direct functional analysis of epitope-specific $CD8^+$ T cells in peripheral blood. *Viral Immunol* **14,** 59–69.
5. Lee, P. P., Yee, C., Savage, P. A., et al., (1999) Characterization of circulating T cells specific for tumor-associated antigens in melanoma patients. *Nat. Med.* **5,** 677–685.
6. Maini, M. K., Boni, C., Ogg, G. S., et al. (1999) Direct ex vivo analysis of hepatitis B virus-specific CD8(+) T cells associated with the control of infection. *Gastroenterology* **117,** 1386–1396.
7. Boni, C., Penna, A., Ogg, G. S., et al. (2001) Lamivudine treatment can overcome cytotoxic T-cell hyporesponsiveness in chronic hepatitis B: new perspectives for immune therapy. *Hepatology* **33,** 963–971.
8. Maini, M. K., Boni, C., Lee, C. K., et al., (2000) The role of virus-specific CD8(+) cells in liver damage and viral control during persistent hepatitis B virus infection. *J. Exp. Med.* **191,** 1269–1280.
9. Doherty, P. C. (1998) The new numerology of immunity mediated by virus-specific CD8(+) T cells. *Curr. Opin. Microbiol.* **1,** 419–422.
10. McMichael, A. J. and OCallaghan, C. A. (1998) A new look at T cells. *J. Exp. Med.* **187,** 1367–1371.
11. Valitutti, S., Muller, S., Cella, M., Padovan, E., and Lanzavecchia, A. (1995) Serial triggering of many T-cell receptors by a few peptide-MHC complexes (see comments). *Nature* **375,** 148–151.

9

In Vitro Analysis of Hepatitis B Virus Specific CD4+ T Cells

Shilpa Chokshi and Nikolai V. Naoumov

1. Introduction

Chronic infection with the hepatitis B virus (HBV) is estimated to affect 350 million persons worldwide and continues to be an important cause of morbidity and mortality *(1)*. It is generally accepted that the host immune response plays a key role in the course and outcome of HBV infection. In chronic HBV infection the immune responses are weak, narrowly focused, and impaired. In contrast, effective and long-term control over viral replication is associated with vigorous HBV-specific T-cell responses *(2)*. Studies of patients with spontaneous resolution of HBV infection have shown that the activation of hepatitis B nucleocapsid (HBcAg) specific $CD4^+$ T lymphocytes is a prerequisite for control over viral replication and hepatitis B surface antigen (HBsAg) clearance *(3,4)*. This HBcAg protein is the strongest immunogen for HLA class II restricted T-cell responses, and therefore most assays analyzing the CD4 immune responses in HBV have focused on this antigen *(2,5)*.

Understanding the heterogeneity of these immune responses in the natural history of HBV infection as well as differences in the response to antiviral treatment is essential for improving the management of this disease. This chapter describes four methods that are currently used for the analysis of HBV specific $CD4^+$ responses:

1. Proliferation assay.
2. ELISPOT assay.
3. Intracellular cytokine staining.
4. Cytokine secretion assay.

2. Materials

2.1. Proliferation Assay

2.1.1. Equipment

1. Swing-out centrifuge for cell separation.
2. Class II laminar flow cabinet.

From: *Methods in Molecular Medicine, vol. 96: Hepatitis B and D Protocols, volume 2*
Edited by: R. K. Hamatake and J. Y. N. Lau © Humana Press Inc., Totowa, NJ

3. 96-Well plate cell harvester.
4. 37°C/5% CO_2 incubator.
5. β-counter with 96-well format.

2.1.2. Reagents

1. Hepatitis B core antigen: Recombinant (American Reassert Products, MA, USA) (*see* **Note 1**).
2. Phytohemagluttinin: Mitogen used as a positive control (Sigma, Poole, UK).
3. Tetanus toxoid: Recall antigen as a positive control.
4. 96-Well tissue culture plates.
5. Human AB serum (*see* **Note 1**).
6. Buffered RPMI 1640 media: RPMI 1640 supplemented with 11.5 mL of 1 *M* 4-(2-hydroxyethyl)piperazine-1-ethanesulfonic acid (HEPES), 3 mL of 1 *M* sodium hydroxide, penicillin, and streptomycin.
7. 1 mCi/mL of [^{3}H]thymidine, aqueous solution.
8. Lymphoprep (Nygaard, Oslo, Norway).
9. Cell counting solution for freshly isolated peripheral blood mononuclear cells (PBMCs): 5 mL of acetic acid + 245 mL of distilled water + 100 μL of trypan blue. **Caution: Add acid to water**.
10. 1000 IU/mL heparin solution: Sterile pyrogen and preservative-free heparin sodium suitable for intravenous injection.
11. Normal saline: 0.9% Saline solution suitable for intravenous injection.

2.2. ELISPOT

2.2.1. Equipment

1. Class II laminar flow cabinet.
2. 37°C/5% CO_2 incubator.
3. Stereomicroscope or automated ELISPOT reader system.
4. Multichannel pipet.

2.2.2. Reagents

1. Hepatitis B core antigen: Recombinant (American Research Products, MA, USA) (*see* **Note 1**).
2. Phytohemagluttinin (Sigma, Poole, UK): Mitogen used as positive control.
3. 96-Well tissue culture plates.
4. Tetanus toxoid: Positive control.
5. ELISPOT kit for human interferon-γ (IFN-γ) (MabTech, Nacka, Sweden).
6. Polyvinylidene diflouride (PVDFP)-backed microplates (Millipore, MA, USA).
7. Human AB serum (*see* **Note 1**).
8. Buffered RPMI 1640 media: RPMI 1640 supplemented with 11.5 mL of 1 *M* HEPES, 3 mL of 1 *M* sodium hydroxide, penicillin, and streptomycin.
9. 5-Bromo-4-chloro-3-indoyl phosphate (BCIP)–nitrotetrazolium blue chloride (NBT) tablets (Roche, Lewes, UK).
10. Buffers:
    a. 70% Ethanol.
    b. Phosphate buffered saline (PBS).
    c. PBS–0.05% Tween.
    d. PBS–1% bovine serum albumin (BSA).

2.3. Flow Cytometry of Intracellular Cytokine Staining

2.3.1. Equipment

1. Class II laminar flow cabinet.
2. 37°C CO_2 incubator.
3. Flow cytometer.
4. Refrigerated swing-out centrifuge with plate holders.

2.3.2. Reagents

1. Hepatitis B core antigen: Recombinant (American Research Products, MA, USA).
2. Phorbol myristate acetate (PMA)/ionomycin (Sigma, Poole, UK): Mitogen used as positive control.
3. 96-Well tissue culture plates.
4. Human AB serum.
5. Brefeldin (Sigma, Poole, UK).
6. PBS.
7. Buffered RPMI 1640 media: RPMI 1640 supplemented with 11.5 mL of 1 *M* HEPES, 3 mL of 1 *M* sodium hydroxide, penicillin, and streptomycin.
8. IFN-γ (Pharmingen, CA, USA).
9. Anti-CD4 fluroescein isothiocyanate (FITC) (Pharmingen, CA, USA).
10. Cytofix/Cytoperm (Pharmingen, CA, USA).

2.4. Cytokine Secretion Assay

2.4.1. Equipment

1. Rotation device for tubes.
2. Class II laminar flow cabinet.
3. 37°C CO_2 incubator.
4. Flow cytometer.

2.4.2. Reagents

1. IFN-γ secretion detection kit (Miltentyi Biotech, UK).
2. C^{2+} and Mg^{2+}-free PBS supplemented with 0.5% BSA and 2 m*M* EDTA (referred to as buffer in **Subheading 3.**)
3. RPMI 1640 containing 5% human AB serum (referred to as media in **Subheading 3.**)
4. Staining reagents: Anti-CD4 FITC antibody (Pharmingen, CA, USA).
5. For each test prepare 10 mL of cold PBS, 100 μL of cold medium, and 1 mL of warm medium.

3. Methods

3.1. Proliferation Assay

The activation of $CD4^+$ T lymphocytes begins with the specific recognition of an antigen on the surface of antigen-presenting cells in association with HLA class II molecules. In response to the antigen, recognition-specific $CD4^+$ T cells undergo clonal expansion, which generates enough antigen-specific cells to handle the foreign antigen. The proliferation assay utilizes this pathway to assess the virus-specific T-cell responses. It measures the incorporation of radiolabeled tritiated thymidine ([^{3}H]thymidine) into newly synthesized DNA, which is directly proportional to the rate of cell division ***(6,7)***.

3.1.1. Preparation of the Tubes for Venipucture

1. Empty vacutainer tubes (10-mL volume) should be prepared by injecting 0.1 mL (100 U) of preservative-free sodium heparin (1000 IU/mL) through the cap of each tube with a sterile insulin syringe (*see* **Note 2**).
2. Tubes can be prepared up to 2 wk in advance if kept at 4°C after preparation.
3. Draw 10 mL of blood into each prepared vacutainer tube.

3.1.2. PBMC Separation (*See* Note 3)

1. Dilute the heparinized blood in a 1:1 ratio with normal saline solution.
2. Pour approx 15–20 mL of the blood–saline mixture over 10 mL of Ficoll gradient in a universal container.
3. First centrifugation at 750*g* for 20 min at 20°C. **Note**: Do not use brakes at this stage.
4. Because red blood cells are denser than Ficoll, they sediment to the bottom, while PBMC remain at the interface (**Fig. 1**).
5. Syphon off the top plasma layer and discard, then gently suction up the cloudy white PBMC interface with a sterile Pasteur pipet.
6. Wash the PBMC with buffered RPMI 1640 and centrifuge at 1000*g* for 10 min.
7. Discard the supernatant and resuspend the cell pellet in a small volume of buffered RPMI 1640 with vigorous pipetting (*see* **Note 4**). Add more media to fill the tube and centrifuge at 750*g* for 10 min.
8. Repeat **step 6**.
9. Final resuspension of the cell pellet in 3–4 mL of RPMI1640–10% human AB serum (v/v)
10. Count the freshly isolated cells by adding 25 μL of the cell suspension to 475 μL of the counting solution and counting with a hemocytometer (*see* **Note 5**).
11. Count cells in the four quadrants. Divide the total number of cells by 20 to give the concentration of the cells/mL of the suspension. Adjust the cell concentration to 2×10^6/mL in buffered RPMI–10% human AB serum.

3.1.3. Cryopreservation of PBMCs

1. Twenty minutes prior to use prepare the freezing mix: A solution of three volumes of buffered RPMI 1640 and two volumes of dimethyl sulfoxide. The mix should be left for at least 20 min at room temperature before use.
2. Count the cell suspension as described above and then pellet PBMCs by centrifugation at 1000*g* for 10 min.
3. Resuspend cells in 750 μL of heat-inactivated fetal calf serum per $5–10 \times 10^6$ PBMCs and add 250 μL of freezing mix. For example for 30×10^6 cells resuspend in 2.25 mL of fetal calf serum and 750 μL of freezing mix.
4. Add 1 mL per cryovial and place vials into a Nalgene freezing container (Mr. Frosty, Merck BDH, Leicestershire, UK), and freeze at –70°C. This is a specialized reusable freezing container for cooling samples at the recommended cooling rate of 1°C/min in preparation for long-term storage in liquid nitrogen.
5. After 24 h transfer the vials to liquid nitrogen.

3.1.4. Defrosting of Cryopreserved Cells

1. Prepare 20 mL of buffered RPMI supplemented with 20% fetal calf serum per vial of PBMCs to be defrosted and warm to 37°C in water bath.
2. Remove cells from liquid nitrogen and place on ice. **Note**: Vials should not be left on ice for longer than a few minutes.

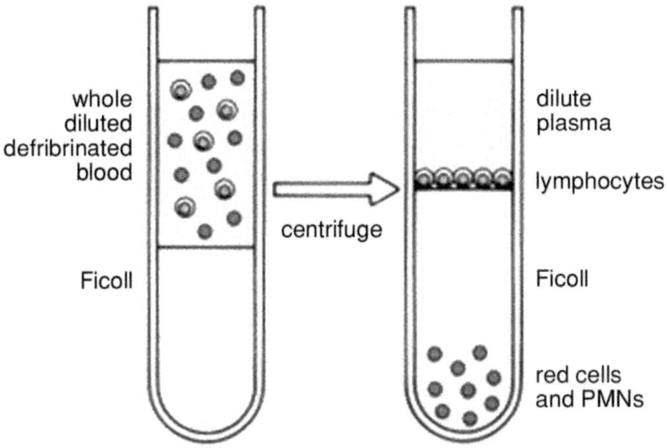

Fig. 1. Ficoll gradient separation of mononuclear cells from heparinized whole blood.

3. Defrost the vial by placing in the 37°C water bath for 1–2 min.
4. Quickly transfer contents into the supplemented RPMI and centrifuge at 1000*g* for 10 min.
5. Discard the supernatant and resuspend cells in media. Count cells by trypan blue exclusion (*see* **Note 6**).

3.1.5. Trypan Blue Exclusion

1. To 190 μL of trypan blue (0.1% solution) add 10 μL of cell suspension.
2. Load into a hemocytometer and count only the **white** cells in two diagonal quadrants. The blue cells are dead cells.
3. Multiply the number of cells in the two quadrants by 10^5 to give the number of cells per milliliter of cell suspension.

3.1.6. Proliferation Assay (*See* Note 7)

1. Adjust the cell concentration to 2×10^6 PBMCs/mL.
2. Prepare antigens at working concentrations in buffered RPMI–10% human AB serum as shown in **Table 1**.
3. Use the sterile 96-well, flat-bottomed microtiter tissue culture plates with lids (Merck BDH, Leicestershire, UK).
4. To 100 μL of antigen add 100 μL of the cell suspension (200,000 cells).
5. Incubate at 37°C/5% CO_2/100% humidified air for 5 d.

Table 1

Well	Antigen	Working concentration	Final concentration in well
1	No antigen	Medium only	Medium only
2	HBcAg	2 μg/mL	1 μg/mL
3	Tetanus toxoid	1 μg/mL	0.5 μg/mL
4	PHA	2 μg/mL	1 μg/mL

3.1.7. Thymidine Incorporation (*See* Note 8)

1. Following incubation of the plates add 0.5 mCi of [^{3}H]thymidine (in 50 µL of RPMI 10% human AB serum) to each well.
2. Prepare [^{3}H]thymidine at a concentration of 10 mCi/mL.
3. Reincubate for 16 h at 37°C/5% CO_2/100% humidified air.
4. The cells are washed and collected onto glass fiber filters using an automated 96-well format cell harvester (Tomtec, Wallac Oy, Turku, Finland).
5. The amount of radiolabel incorporated into the DNA is measured by a direct β-counter (TriLux, Wallac Oy, Turku, Finland) (*see* **Note 9**).

3.2. Frequency of Hepatitis B Core Specific CD4$^+$ T Cells (IFN-γ ELISPOT Assay)

The ELISPOT (enzyme-linked immunospot) assay is used for the detection and quantitation of individual cells secreting specific cytokines in response to an antigenic stimulus *(8)*. The ELISPOT assays are reproducible and sensitive and can be used to monitor antigen-specific CD4$^+$ or CD8$^+$ T cells with frequencies of well below 1:300,000.

This section describes the procedure for the detection of HBcAg-specific IFN-γ producing cells. The detection of interleukin-4 (IL-4), IL-5, and IL-10 can also be performed using the appropriate antibody kits (*see* **Note 10**).

3.2.1. Day 1: Stimulation of the Cells (*See* Note 11)

1. The PBMCs are prepared as described in **Subheading 3.1.** (*see* **Note 12**).
2. The protocol will be split over the 3 d required to perform the assay (**Fig. 2**).
3. Adjust cell concentration to 2 × 10^6 PBMC/mL.
4. Prepare antigens at working concentrations in buffered RPMI–10% human AB serum as shown in **Table 2.**
5. Add 100 µL of each antigen per well in triplicate to a round-bottom 96-well tissue culture plate (*see* **Note 13**).
6. Add 100 µL of PBMC suspension at 2 × 10^6/mL to each experimental well.
7. Incubate the plate(s) for 26 h at 37°C in a CO_2 incubator.

3.2.2. Day 2: Preparation of ELISPOT Plate

1. Add 100 µL of 70% ethanol to the required wells of the ELISPOT 96-well plate (*see* **Note 14**).
2. Incubate the plate for 15 min at room temperature.
3. Add 200 µL of sterile PBS to each well using a multichannel pipet, flick off PBS, and blot the plate on tissue thoroughly to remove all PBS. Repeat this wash step a further five times (*see* **Note 15**).
4. Add 100 µL of capture antibody to each experiment well.
5. Incubate at 4°C for 6 h in the dark
6. Wash each well with 200 µL of sterile PBS using a multichannel pipet. Perform six washes.
7. Add 100 µL of buffered RPMI/10% human AB serum to block the membrane and incubate plate(s) for 1 h at 37°C in a CO_2 incubator.
8. Flick off buffered RPMI/10% human AB serum and blot the plate.
9. Transfer PBMCs prepared on d 1 to corresponding wells on the ELISPOT plate (*see* **Note 16**).
10. Incubate the plate(s) for 20 h at 37°C in a CO_2 incubator (*see* Note **17**).

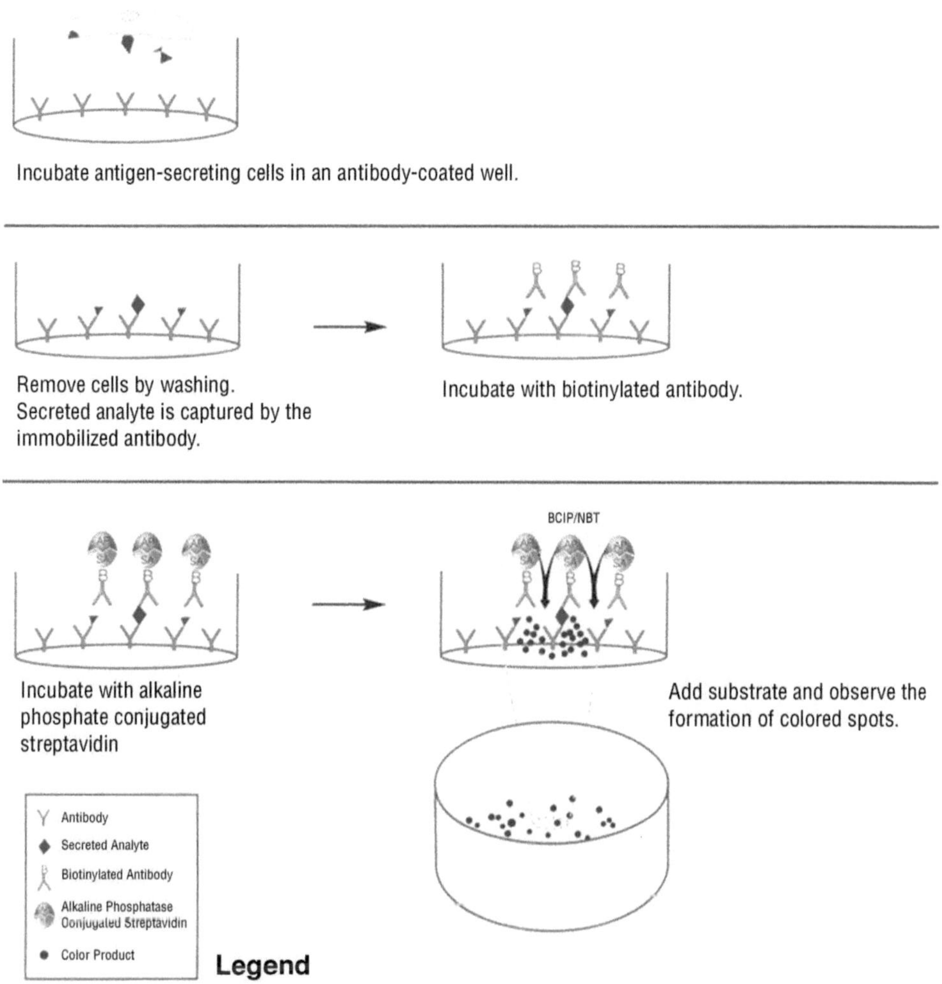

Fig. 2. A schematic representation of the principle of the ELISPOT assay and the stages involved.

Table 2

Well	Antigen	Working concentration	Final concentration in well
1	No antigen	Medium only	Medium only
2	HBcAg	4 μg/mL	2 μg/mL
3	Tetanus toxoid	1 μg/mL	0.5 μg/mL
4	PHA	2 μg/mL	1 μg/mL

3.2.3. Day 3: Development

1. Flick cells off and wash the ELISPOT plate with PBS/0.05% Tween; repeat.
2. Wash two times with PBS.
3. Wash two times with distilled water.
4. Prepare a 1 μg/mL concentration of biotinylated anti-IFN-γ antibody in PBS–1% BSA.
5. Add 100 μL of antibody to each experiment well of the ELISPOT plate.
6. Incubate for 2 h at room temperature.
7. Wash five times with PBS/ 0.05% Tween.
8. Wash two times with PBS.
9. Prepare 1:1000 dilution of the streptavidin–alkaline phosphatase conjugate in PBS/1% BSA.
10. Add 100 μL of streptavidin solution to each experiment well of the ELISPOT plate.
11. Incubate for 1.5 h at room temperature.
12. Wash six times with PBS.
13. Wash once with distilled water.
14. Prepare the BCIP/NBT tablet (Roche, Lewes, UK) solution by adding one tablet to 10 mL of distilled water.
15. Add 100 μL of BCIP/NBT solution to each experiment well of the ELISPOT plate.
16. Allow color to develop until either:

    a. Spots appear in PHA control wells or
    b. as soon as background staining appears.

    At this point flick off the BCIP/NBT solution and immerse in tray of tap water.
17. Flick off water and rinse thoroughly under running water. Ensure each well is filled and emptied at least five times.
18. Blot dry, remove plastic base, and dry inverted.
19. Read plate in automated ELISPOT reader or stereomicroscope **(Fig. 3)** (*see* **Notes 18** and **19**).

3.3. Frequency of Hepatitis B core specific CD4⁺ T Cells by Intracellular Cytokine Staining for IFN-γ

Recent advances have led to the development of immunofluorescent staining reagents and flow cytometric techniques that facilitate the study of individual cytokine-producing cells within a specific cell population. By using flow cytometry individual cells can be simultaneously analyzed for several parameters including cell size and granularity, as well as coexpressed levels of surface and intracellular markers defined by fluorescent antibodies.

1. Adjust concentration of PBMC to 3×10^6/mL in buffered RPM/10% heat-inactivated fetal calf serum (*see* **Note 20**).
2. Add 100 μL of cell suspension per well of a round-bottomed 96-well plate for each antigen.
3. Prepare antigens as shown in **Table 3**.
4. Add 100 μL of appropriate antigen or medium control (*see* **Notes 21** and **22**).
5. Add brefeldin a (10 μg/mL) to all wells (*see* **Note 23**).
6. Incubate plate for 6 h in a 37°C 5% CO_2 incubator.
7. Centrifuge the plate at 750*g* for 5 min.
8. Resuspend cells in 100 μL of cold PBS/1% FCS.

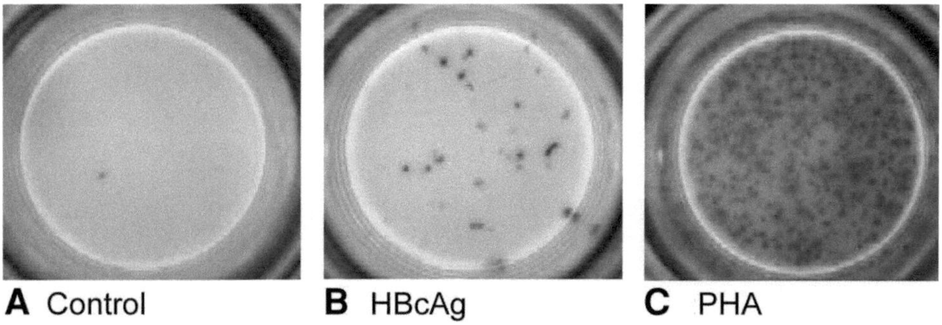

Fig. 3. Results of the ELISPOT assay, as analyzed with an automated ELISPOT reader (AID, Strasberg, Germany). Each spot represents a CD4+ T cell secreting IFN-γ in response to stimulation by medium alone (**A**), HBcAg (**B**), and PHA (**C**).

Table 3

Well	Antigen	Working concentration	Final concentration in well
1	No antigen	Medium only	Medium only
2	HBcAg	4 μg/mL	2 μg/mL
3	PMA	100 ng/mL	50 ng/mL
4	Ionomycin	2 μ*M*	1 μ*M*

9. Add 3 μL of anti-CD4 FITC antibody to each well.
10. Incubate on ice, in the dark for 20 min, and add 100 μL of PBS/1% FCS. Centrifuge at 750*g* for 5 min.
11. Resuspend in 100 μL of 1X Cytofix/Cytoperm (Pharmingen, CA, USA) and incubate on ice, in the dark for 20 min (*see* **Notes 24** and **25**).
12. Add 100 μL of 1X perm wash. Centrifuge at 750*g* for 5 min. Resuspend cells in a 1:5 dilution of anti-IFN-γ PE antibody (Pharmingen, CA, USA) or isotype control diluted in 1X perm wash.
13. Incubate on ice, in the dark for 30 min and add 100 μL of PBS–1% FCS.
14. Centrifuge at 1400 rpm (750*g*) for 5 min.
15. Resuspend cells in 50 μL of cold PBS–1% FCS. Repeat **steps 14** and **15.**
16. Collect cells on a flow cytometer.
17. Acquisition of 10,000–100,000 events is recommended.
18. A lymphocyte gate based on forward scatter and side scatter (FSC/SSC) properties should be activated prior to further gating to improve the sensitivity of the analysis.

3.4. Cytokine Secretion Assay

The cytokine secretion assay allows the detection, isolation, and analysis of live antigen-specific cytokine-secreting T cells. This assay allows the detection of very-low-frequency cells—up to 1 in 600,000 PBMCs. The kits involve the specific labeling of the cells followed by flow cytometric analysis. The advantage of using the cytokine

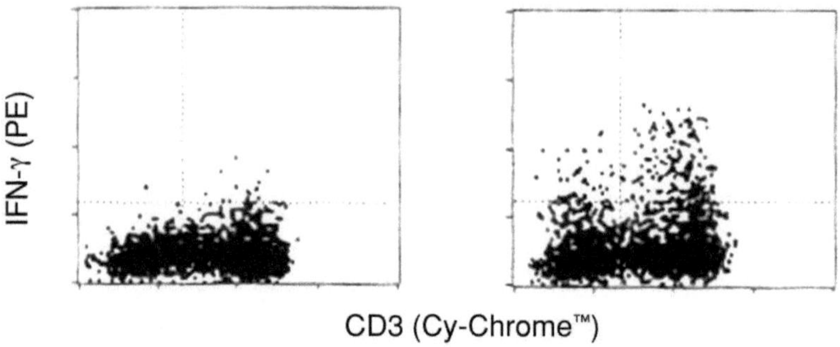

Fig. 4. Intracellular staining for IFN-γ producing T cells. PBMCs were stimulated with PMA (50 ng/mL) and calcium ionophore (250 ng/mL). **(Left)** Control; **(right)** in the presence of protein transport inhibitor (GolgiStop). Cells were stained with Cy-chrome labeled anti-CD3 and FITC-labeled anti-human IFN-γ and analyzed by flow cytometry.

secretion assay is that it allows the isolation of viable antigen-specific T cells post-analysis, which can be enriched and used for down-stream applications.

This section describes the procedure for the detection of HBcAg-specific IFN-γ producing cells. The detection of other cytokines may also be performed using the appropriate kits.

3.4.1. *Stimulation of the Cells (See* **Note 20***)*

1. Prepare antigens as shown in **Table 4** (*see* **Notes 26** and **27**).
2. Adjust the PBMC concentration to 1×10^7/mL and incubate 100 μL of cell suspension for each antigen in a 96-well tissue culture plate for 16–18 h; *see* **Table 4**.

3.4.2. *Labeling of Cells with IFN-γ Catch Matrix (See* **Note 28***)*

1. Transfer cells from 96-well tissue culture plate to Eppendorf tubes and wash cells by adding 1–2 mL of cold buffer.
2. Centrifuge at 300*g* for 10 min at 4–8°C, and remove supernatant completely.
3. Resuspend the cell pellet in 90 μL of cold medium.
4. Add 10 μL of IFN-γ Catch reagent provided in the kit, mix, and incubate on ice for 5 min.
5. Add 1 mL of warm (37°C) medium to cells.
6. Incubate cells for 45 min at 37°C under slow continuous rotation.

3.4.3. *Labeling of cells with IFN-γ Detection Antibodies*

1. Fill tubes with cold buffer.
2. Centrifuge at 300*g* for 10 min at 4–8°C and remove the supernatant completely.
3. Resuspend the cell pellet in 90 μL of cold medium.
4. Add 10 μL of IFN-γ detection antibody (PE) reagent provided in the kit, and add anti-CD4-FITC antibody.
5. Mix well and incubate for 10 min on ice.
6. Wash cells by adding 1 mL of cold buffer.
7. Centrifuge at 300*g* for 10 min at 4–8°C and remove supernatant completely.
8. Repeat **steps 6** and **7**.

Table 4

Well	Antigen	Working concentration	Final concentration in well
1	No antigen	Medium only	Medium only
2	HBcAg	20 μg/mL	10 μg/mL
3	Tetanus toxoid	20 μg/mL	10 μg/mL
4	SEB	2 μg/mL	1 μg/mL

9. Resuspend the cell pellet in 50 μL of cold buffer and transfer to FACS tubes for flow cytometric analysis.

3.4.4. Detection/Analysis of Antigen Specific Cells

1. Propidium iodide (PI) should be added just prior to flow cytometric analysis (*see* **Note 29**).
2. Acquisition of 10,000–100,000 events is recommended.
3. A lymphocyte gate based on forward scatter and side scatter (FSC/SSC) properties should be activated prior to further gating to improve the sensitivity of the analysis.
4. Upon activation of the lymphocyte gate, dead cells have to be gated out according to PI fluorescence in a FL2 vs FL3 plot.

4. Notes

4.1. Proliferation Assay

1. The AB serum and the recombinant HBcAg must be batch tested as they are prone to inherent variability. Both items can cause high background reactivities in normal patients. For the AB serum the company may provide a panel of human AB serum, which should be tested in a range of normal subjects to determine the lot that has the lowest background. The same is true for the antigen—in a recent study we tested a panel of recombinant HBcAg preparations from six different commercial sources and found that some induced a proliferative response in normal patients which may be due to very high levels of endotoxin in the preparation.
2. Only preservative-free sodium heparin should be used as the anticoagulant for the blood, as EDTA and other heparin preparations seem to affect the overall performance of the assay.
3. As with any tissue culture, particular care must be taken to ensure aseptic techniques are adhered to strictly.
4. The adequate resuspension of the cell pellets during the procedure of PBMC separation is vital to avoid clumps, which may mask any potential response.
5. Counting solution should only be used for freshly isolated PBMCs where the viability is always 100%. The advantage of using counting solution for freshly isolated PBMCs is that the acetic acid in the solution causes the rupture of red blood cells, allowing accurate counts of PBMCs. Counting solution should not be used for frozen cells for two reasons: First and most important, counting solution does not assess the viability of the cells. Second, during the freezing of the cells all contaminating red blood cells are lysed and therefore do not pose a problem during counting.
6. The assay can be performed on cryopreserved cells but trypan blue exclusion test must be performed on the cells. If the viability of the cells falls below 95%, the assay is not reliable.
7. This assay should be run with a minimum of three replicates to reduce variability.
8. Care must be taken when using radioactivity—gloves and laboratory coats should be worn. Local radioactive regulations should be adhered to.

9. Generally, the results of the proliferation assay are expressed as a Stimulation Index, which is calculated by dividing the mean counts per minute for the antigen-stimulated cultures by that of the control cultures (PBMCs with medium only). An SI greater than two times the mean plus two standard deviations for a group of healthy controls and patients with other liver diseases is considered significant.

4.2. ELISPOT Assay

10. Problems have been encountered with the performance of IL-10 ELISPOT kits. Very high backgrounds can be encountered in some healthy controls and patients, which is thought to be due to monocyte IL-10 production and/or to nonspecific activation of the T cells from the membrane. This variability in the background makes the analysis of the virus-specific production of IL-10 very difficult. Other assays such as the intracellular cytokine detection or the cytokine secretion assay may be more appropriate for the detection of IL-10.
11. As with any tissue culture, care must be taken to ensure aseptic techniques are adhered to strictly on d 1 and 2 of the protocol after which the assay can be performed on the bench.
12. The assay may perform better with cryopreserved cells (reduction of background spots in the medium-only wells) but trypan blue exclusion testing must be performed on the cells. If the viability of the cells falls below 95%, the assay is not reliable.
13. This assay should be run with a minimum of three replicates to reduce variability.
14. The soaking of the membrane with 70% ethanol for 15 min is very important to retain the integrity of the spots when trying to count.
15. The wash steps in this protocol are crucial and must be strictly adhered to.
16. Stimulation of the cells by the antigen in the ELISPOT plates on d 1 is not recommended as it leads to very high background in the medium-only wells.
17. Once the cells are plated care should be taken to not move the plate around, as this leads to fuzzy spots and trails of spots.
18. Counting of the spots is recommended to be done by using the automated ELISPOT reader. If this is not available, all plates must be counted by two independent observers, as there can be substantial interindividual variation when using the stereomicroscope.
19. Each spot represents an antigen-specific IFN-γ producing cell. Results are generally expressed as the number of spot forming cells (SFC) per million PBMCs. As there are 200,000 PBMCs in this assay, the number of SFC is multiplied by 5 to get the SFC/10^6 PBMCs.

4.3. Intracellular Cytokine Staining

20. As with any tissue culture, care must be taken to ensure sterile aseptic techniques are adhered to strictly.
21. For each test sample it is strongly recommended that a control (no antigen), a test peptide and a positive control are used.
22. It is also advised to use an isotype antibody as a control. This is a fluorochrome conjugated antibody of irrelevant specificity, which has an identical immunoglobulin (Ig) isotype to the anti-cytokine antibody being stained. The Ig isotype control shows the inherent staining background and thus can be used as a negative staining control.
23. Another factor that is very important is the use of a protein transport inhibitor—brefeldin. Without brefeldin the cells will not accumulate high levels of intracellular cytokine, and thus very little if any will be detected.

24. A common problem is the adequate permeabilization of cells. All antibodies for the intracellular staining must be diluted in solutions containing a permeabilization agent—saponin. Failure to do so results in reduced permeability and decreased staining.
25. Cell fixation prior to staining intracellularly is mandatory. If the cells are exposed to a staining buffer containing saponin prior to being fixed with paraformaldehyde, they will lyse and die.

4.4. Cytokine Secretion Assay

26. Mitogens such as phytohemagglutinin (PHA) or PMA/ionomycin are not recommended as positive controls as the resulting extremely high frequencies of IFN-γ secreting cells do not allow conclusions on the performance of the assay—tetanus toxoid or cytomegalovirus (CMV) antigen may be more suitable.
27. A control sample incubated without antigen should always be included.
28. Work fast, keep cells cold (exception during secretion period), precool and prewarm media or buffers prior to starting experiments.
29. Use PI to exclude dead cells.

References

1. Lee, W. M. (1997) Hepatitis B virus infection. *N. Engl. J. Med.* **337,** 1733–1745.
2. Chisari, F. V. and Ferrari, C. (1995) Hepatitis B virus immunopathogenesis. *Annu. Rev. Immunol.* **13,** 29–60.
3. Ferrari, C., Penna, A., Bertoletti, A., et al. (1990) Cellular immune responses to hepatitis B virus-encoded antigens in acute and chronic hepatitis B virus infections. *J. Immunol.* **145,** 3442–3449.
4. Jung, M. C., Diepolder, H. M., Spengler, U., et al. (1995) Activation of a heterogeneous hepatitis B (HB) core and e antigen specific CD4+ T cell population during seroconversion to anti-HBe and anti-HBs in hepatitis B virus infection. *J. Virol.* **69,** 3358–3368.
5. Lau, G. K., Suri, D., Liang, R., et al. (2002) Resolution of chronic hepatitis B and anti-HBs seroconversion in humans by adoptive transfer of immunity to hepatitis B core antigen. *Gastroenterology* **122,** 614–624.
6. Marinos, G., Torre, F., Chokshi, S., et al. (1995) Induction of T-helper cell responses to hepatitis B core antigen in chronic hepatitis B: a major factor in activation of the host immune response to hepatitis B virus. *Hepatology* **22,** 1040–1049.
7. Rossol, S., Marinos, G., Carucci, P., Singer, M. V., Williams, R., and Naoumov, N. V. (1997) Interleukin-12 induction of Th1 cytokines is important for viral clearance in chronic hepatitis B. *J. Clin. Invest.* **99,** 3025–3033.
8. Jung, M. C., Hartmann, B., Gerlach, J. T., et al. (1999) Virus-specific lymphokine production differs quantitatively but not qualitatively in acute and chronic hepatitis B infection. *Virology* **261,** 165–172.

10

Induction of Humoral and Cellular Immune Responses to Hepatitis Delta Virus Through DNA Immunization in BALB/c Mice

Ren-Shiang Lee, Shih-Jer Hsu, Li-Rung Huang, Hui-Lin Wu, Shiou-Lin Lin, Ding-Shinn Chen, and Pei-Jer Chen

1. Introduction

Current regimens (interferon) to treat hepatitis D patients have only transient but no lasting effects *(1)*."

Hepatitis delta virus (HDV) is a small-satellite single-stranded RNA virus that requires helper hepatitis B virus (HBV) to provide surface antigen (HBsAg) for assembly. The HDV virion particle can infect or superinfect in acute or chronic hepatitis B patients *(2)* and can cause acute hepatitis or rapidly progressive chronic disease *(3,4)*. The only current drug used to treat chronic HDV infection is interferon *(1)*, although it must be used at a high dosage for a long duration *(5)*. However, interferon benefits only a minority of patients and relapses often take place after discontinuation. Another drug, lamivudine, which is a potent inhibitor of HBV DNA replication, currently is used to treat chronic HBV patients. It has been used in clinical trail for HBV HDV chronic patients, but it does not effectively control disease activity *(6)*. Until now there has been no effective treatment or vaccine against acute or chronic HDV infection.

It has been reported that the immune response plays an important role in the pathogenesis of HDV infection *(7)*. HDV is not directly cytopathic, because expression of both large hepatitis delta antigen (L-HDAg) and small hepatitis delta antigen (S-HDAg) in cells is not cytopathic and in HDV transgenic mice does not cause liver disease *(8)*. Other studies showed that patients who recovered from HDV infection had a significant T-cell proliferation response to HDV synthetic peptides, suggesting that the cellular immune response of patients might determine disease activity after HDV infection *(9)*. A recent cohort study showed that HDV chronic patients with anti-HDV antibodies (Abs) have increased HBsAg clearance ability compared to HBsAg carriers without HDV infections *(10)*. It is conceivable that an alternative way to treat chronic HDV infection would be to augment patient's cellular and humoral immune responses to HDV or HBV.

From: *Methods in Molecular Medicine, vol. 96: Hepatitis B and D Protocols, volume 2*
Edited by: R. K. Hamatake and J. Y. N. Lau © Humana Press Inc., Totowa, NJ

Current available vaccines can be used successfully in the prevention of various infectious diseases by inducing long-lived Ab immune responses against these pathogens. However, for agents that infect intracellularly and require cell-mediated immunity, such as the pathogens of tuberculosis, malaria, leishmaniasis, and human immunodeficiency virus infection, Ab-mediated immune responses are not effective in protecting against these diseases. For HDV, the induction of anti-delta Ab is also not effective as the target antigen is inside the HBV envelope and not accessible. For these reasons, a new type of vaccination, using DNA that contains the gene encoding the antigen of interest for therapeutic applications, is under intensive investigation because of to its ability to induce long-lived immune responses, both humoral and cellular, against tumors and many viral infections in various animal models ***(11)***.

A plasmid DNA vaccine should include a minimum of five basic components: (1) an origin of replication to allow growth in bacteria (for this purpose the most commonly used is the *Escherichia coli* Co1EI origin of replication in pUC plasmids because it provides high copy numbers in bacteria); (2) a bacterial antibiotic resistance gene that allows for plasmid selection during bacterial culture (the ampicillin and kanamycin resistance genes are most commonly used in mice and human studies, respectively); (3) a strong promoter for optimal expression in mammalian cells (for this, virally derived promoters such as from cytomegalovirus [CMV] or simian virus 40 provide the greatest gene expression); (4) an antigenic sequence that is controlled by the strong promoter and expresses the antigen for inducing the immune response; and (5) stabilization of mRNA transcripts, achieved by incorporation of polyadenylation sequences such as that from bovine growth hormone (BGH) or simian virus 40 ***(11)***.

There are various routes to immunize an animal with DNA vaccines, and the most common way is to inject DNA into muscle ***(11)***. It has been shown recently that applying electric pulses (electroporation) to DNA-injected muscle greatly augments DNA uptake and gene expression ***(12)***. The induction of 100-fold antibody response was also observed in electroporation-treated mice compared with untreated mice after a single dose of 20–200 ng of DNA ***(13)***. In this chapter we focus on describing a protocol for DNA immunization in BALB/c through intramuscular injection with or without electric pulses. We also describe how to measure the cellular and the humoral immune responses after HDV cDNA vaccination. We used different plasmid DNA constructs encoding hepatitis delta antigen (HDAg) under the control of CMV early promoter or mutant HDV cDNA capable of persistent viral replication and small delta antigen expression as vaccines to induce immune responses against HDV in BALB/c mice. Recently, Huang et al. reported that immunization with the plasmid DNA, pD, encoding L-HDAg and the plasmid DNA, pS/pD encoding both HBV HBsAg and HDV L-HDAg, can induce humoral and T-helper-1 (Th1) cellular immune responses in BALB/c mice ***(14)***. We have obtained similar results with our plasmid DNA constructs (**Fig. 1**; *see* **Subheading 2.**).

1.1. Humoral Immunity Induced in HDV DNA Vaccine Immunized BALB/c Mice

There are great differences in immune responses elicited by current conventional protein vaccines (or live virus infection) compared to DNA vaccination in immunized

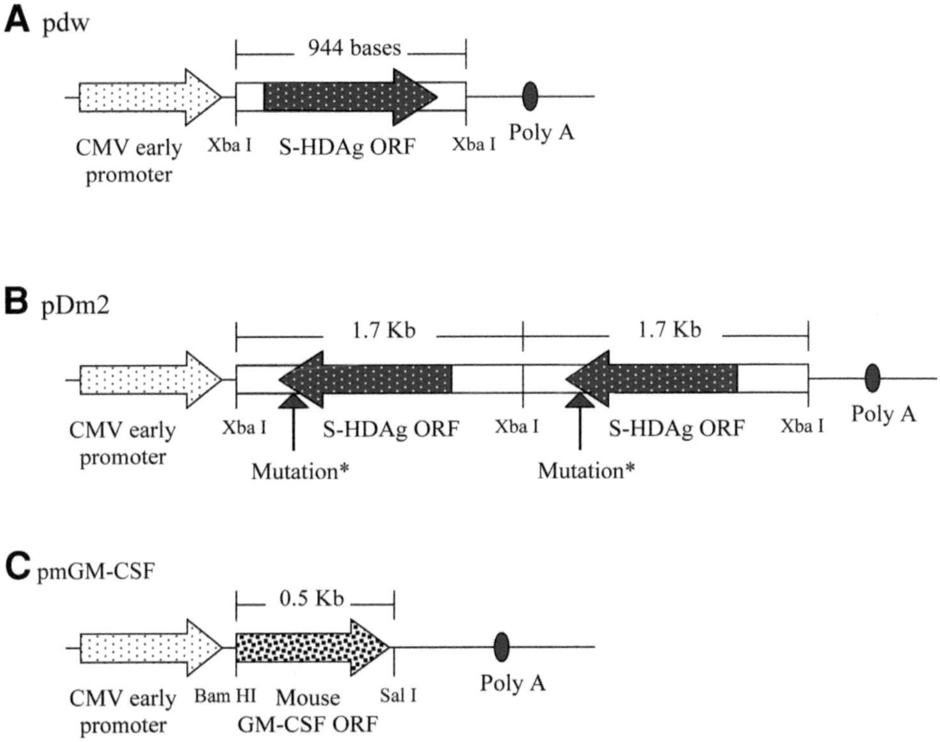

Fig. 1. Construction of DNA vaccines. All antigen coding sequences were subcloned with suitable restriction enzymes into multiple cloning sites of pcDNA3.1(+) vector under the control of the CMV early promoter. Two plasmid constructions for DNA vaccine against HDV and one plasmid for DNA adjuvant vaccine are described. **(A)** pdw contains an open reading frame (ORF) of wild-type small delta antigen (S-HDAg) sequence. **(B)** pDm2 contains a tandem dimer of small delta antigen (S-HDAg) ORF sequence with an insertion of adenine after the stop codon of S-HDAg sequence. The additional adenine creates another stop codon even if the original stop codon is mutated by RNA editing. This plasmid can synthesize a tandem dimer of HDV genomic RNA that is capable of self-replication in vivo, but it cannot form HDV particles with HBV surface antigen because of its inability to synthesize L-HDAg because of the additional stop codon ***(18)***. **(C)**, pmGM-CSF contains a mouse GM-CSF ORF sequence also under the control of the CMV early promoter in the pcDNA3.1(+) vector.

animal. Generally, an Ab response induced by DNA vaccine is less rapid, with lower titers and avidity ***(15–18)***. However, in a kinetic study comparing the induction of Ab response after intradermal (id) immunization with DNA encoding ovalbumin (OVA) and OVA protein, there was no difference in total OVA-specific Ab production at 2 or 4 wk post-vaccination. Moreover, the Ab induced by DNA immunization in this study had a higher avidity than that induced by OVA protein ***(19)***. The authors of this study had also shown that the routes of immunization could play an important role in directing different isotypes of Ab production. Intradermal immunization of DNA induced predominantly IgG1 with high avidity, whereas intramuscular (im) injection produced IgG2a of lower avidity *(19)*.

Plasmid DNA vaccination can induce different subtypes of Abs including IgG, IgM, and IgA. Cytokines such as interleukin-4 (IL-4) and interferon-γ (IFN-γ) favor IgG1 and IgG2a production, respectively. DNA vaccination generally enhances induction of Th1 cytokine IFN-γ, which is biased toward isotype IgG2a production. A general property of DNA vaccination in mice has been that DNA encoding secreted antigen generated higher levels of IgG1 than did membrane-bound antigen *(20)*. According to our observation, vaccination with the plasmid expressing only small delta antigen, pdw (*see* **Subheading 2.**) through im injection cannot induce any detectable anti-HDAg Ab response. In contrast, vaccination in the same way with another plasmid pDm2 (*see* **Subheading 2.**), which in addition to encoding for S-HDAg is also capable of replication in vivo, can induce different subtypes of anti-S-HDAg IgG Abs. The anti-HDAg Abs could be detected at wk 4 post-immunization and the Ab titer peaked at the 10th or 12th week post-immunization, then decreased slightly (**Fig. 2**). The Ab titer was maintained for a long duration (26 wk) (not shown). Moreover, when we analyzed IgG isotypes from total induced IgG, we found the isotype IgG2a to be dominant in most cases (**Fig. 3**). However, we did not directly compare the isotypes of Abs induced in mice immunized with DNA encoding HDAg or with recombinant HDAg protein at the same time. Nevertheless, we did make anti-HDV monoclonal Abs through intraperitoneal immunization with recombinant HDAg protein in BALB/c mice and we found that all of the selected monoclonal Abs were IgM and IgG (data not shown). Furthermore, in these high titer anti-S-HDAg Abs, the majority is isotype IgG2b and the minority is isotype IgG1, but there was not any isotype IgG2a Ab (P. Ou-Yang, P. J. Chen, and B. L. Chiang, unpublished data), which is very different from the Abs (IgG2a dominant) induced through DNA vaccination.

In addition, we also found that coimmunization with the adjuvant plasmid pmGM-CSF encoding mouse GM-CSF could enhance the production of anti-S-HDAg Ab in BALB/c mice in DNA immunization at low dose (1 μg/mouse), but there was no significant enhancement of the anti-S-HDAg Ab production with a high dose (100 μg/mouse) of pDm2 (**Fig. 4**).

1.2. Cellular Immunity Induced in HDV DNA Vaccine Immunized BALB/c Mice

Cellular immunity consists of $CD8^+$ cytotoxic T lymphocytes (CTL) and $CD4^+$ helper T lymphocytes. Activated $CD4^+$ T lymphocytes play a critical role in immune responses (1) by promoting B lymphocyte survival and inducing Ab production through CD40 ligand (CD40L)–CD40 interaction *(21)*; (2) by providing helper function to $CD8^+$ cytotoxic T lymphocytes through IL-2 production and/or through CD40L–CD40 costimulation *(22–24)*; and (3) through secreting different kinds of cytokines that have profound immunoregulatory effects in many disease states. In this regard, based on their production of certain cytokines, the activated $CD4^+$ T lymphocytes can be categorized into two distinct subsets: those that exclusively produce IFN-γ are Th1 lymphocytes and those

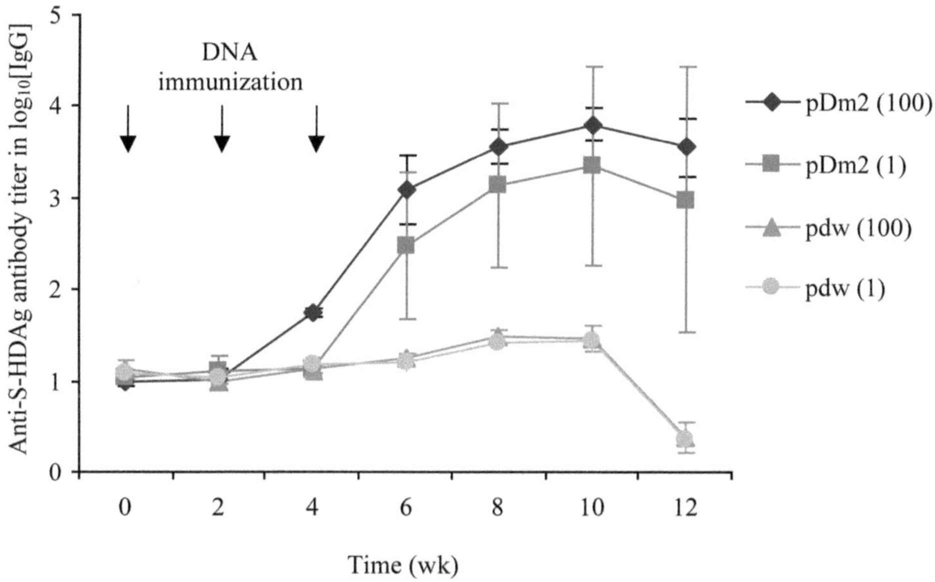

Fig. 2. Kinetics of anti-S-HDAg IgG antibody responses of BALB/c mice immunized with HDV small δ antigen expression vectors pdw and pDm2. BALB/c mice were pretreated with cardiotoxin 6 or 7 d before three consecutive intramuscular immunizations on d 0, 14, and 28 with a high dose (100 μg per mouse, 50 μg in 50 μL per injection) or a low dose (1 μg per mouse, 0.5 μg in 50 μL per injection) of plasmid DNA into quadriceps muscles of both hindlegs. Mice were bled every 2 wk after immunization. Anti-S-HDAg IgG antibody responses were analyzed by ELISA. Results, indicated as the mean ± standard error of individual $\log_{10}$ titers, are obtained from six mice per time point.

that exclusively produce IL-4, IL-5, and IL-13 are T-helper-2 (Th2) lymphocytes ***(25)***. Preferential induction of Th1 immune response by DNA vaccination has been demonstrated in several infectious disease models. For example, DNA vaccination with only CpG oligodeoxynucleotides could strikingly enhance IFN-γ and diminish IL-4 production in BALB/c mice that were already infected with *Leishmania major*, suggesting that Th1-type responses could be induced in the course of ongoing Th2 responses ***(26)***. Furthermore, in allergic or asthmatic diseases, an ongoing Th2 response could be prevented or limited by a Th1 response generated by DNA immunization ***(27)***. In a rat model of allergic hyperresponsiveness, it was shown that injection of plasmid DNA encoding a house dust mite allergen prevented the induction of IgE and reduced airway hyperreactivity ***(28)***. As noted previously, immunization with the plasmid DNA (pD) encoding L-HDAg or the pS/pD encoding defined previously and L-HDAg could induce T-cell proliferation response to HDAg ***(14)***. Moreover, pD or pS/pD immunized mice showed an increase of IL-2 and IFN-γ production from splenocytes stimulated with HDAg in comparison with pcDNA3 vector immunized mice, but there was no significant change in detectable IL-4 ***(14)***. However, in this study, the authors did not show whether immu-

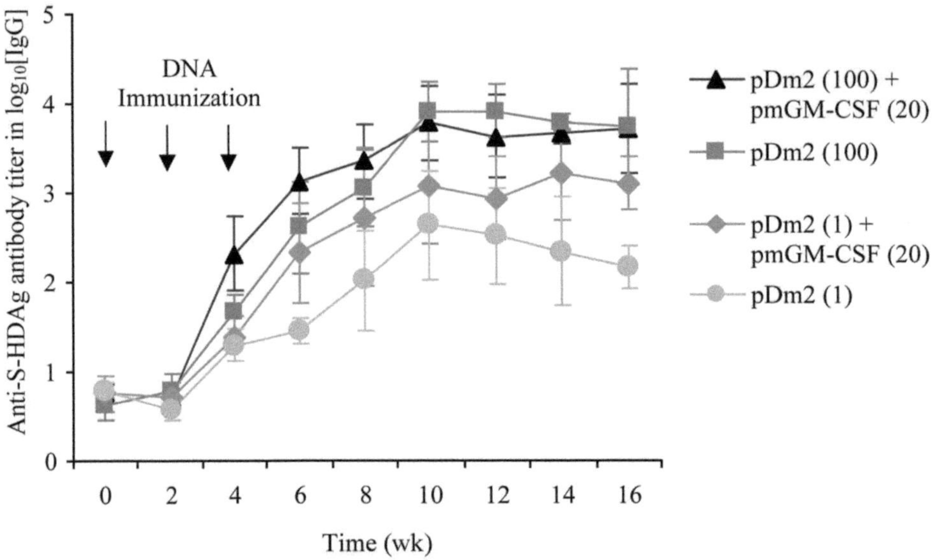

Fig. 3. Kinetics of anti-S-HDAg IgG antibody responses of BALB/c mice coimmunized with HDV small δ antigen expression vector pDm2 with or without mouse GM-CSF expression vector pmGM-CSF. BALB/c mice were immunized and bled as described in Fig. 2.

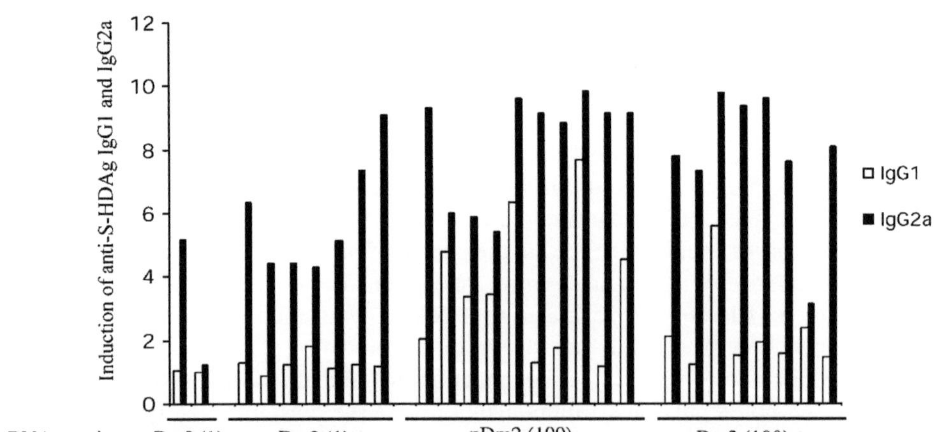

Fig. 4. Analysis of anti-S-HDAg IgG isotype antibodies induced in pDm2-pmGM-CSF coimmunized mice. Results shown were obtained from individual serum of the 12th week shown in the Fig. 3 and analyzed by IgG1 and IgG2a isotyping ELISA.

nization with plasmid DNA encoding only S-HDAg could induce an immune response. From our observation, immunization with pDm2, which can replicate in vivo and which contains a dimer of mutated L-HDAg gene encoding only S-HDAg, could induce humoral immune responses in all immunized mice and cellular immune responses in some immunized mice. But a simple plasmid, pdw, which contains only S-HDAg gene, could not induce any anti-HDAg immune response. Our results showed that vaccination with pDm2 could induce detectable anti-S-HDAg humoral responses 4 wk after the first injection (**Fig. 4**). In some immunized mice, T-cell proliferation (**Fig. 5**) and CTL responses (**Fig. 6**) to S-HDAg could also be demonstrated.

Many questions still remain with respect to the non-induction of T-cell immune responses, but anti-S-HDAg humoral responses occurred in all immunized mice. Generally, $CD4^+$ T-cell response should take place before Ab production in the T-dependent B cell immune response. In our experience, T-cell proliferation and CTL against S-HDAg could be detected only 1 or 2 wk after the first or the second booster (**Figs. 5** and **6**), but were never found later (*not shown*). The maximum induction of anti-S-HDAg Abs in immunized mice was always found 10–12 wk after the first plasmid DNA injection (**Figs. 2** and **3**). Moreover, in mice that had T-cell proliferation or CTL responses, we have never detected any anti-S-HDAg Ab in serum, and, vice versa, we have never found T-cell response in mice which already produced detectable anti-S-HDAg Ab in the serum. It seems that our data could correspond with the T-dependent B cell response in BALB/c mice immunized with plasmid DNA vaccine against HDV.

2. Materials

2.1. Special Equipment

1. Animal care-accredited facility.
2. Sterile laminar flow cabinet.
3. Microscope.
4. Scissors and forceps, kept in sterile beaker with 70% ethanol.
5. Electro Cell Manipulator (ECM 830, BTX, San Diego).
6. Genetrodes for in vivo electroporation (Model 508, BTX).
7. Low-speed centrifuge.
8. 37°C, 5% CO_2 humidified incubator.
9. Enzyme-linked immunosorbent assay (ELISA) reader (Emax, Molecular Devices).
10. ^{137}Cs 637 irradiator (No. IBL 637, CISBIO International).
11. Cobra 5003 γ-counter (Packard).
12. 96-Well cell harvester (Filtermate 196, Matrixfilter, Packard).
13. β-Counter (Matrix 96 direct β-counter, Packard).

2.2. Disposables

1. 25-mL and 75-mL cell culture flasks (Costar or Nunc).
2. 96-Well microtiter U-bottomed and flat-bottomed plates (Costar or Nunc).
3. 1.0-mL sterile syringe with 27-gauge needle (Terumo).
4. 10-mL sterile syringe without needle (Terumo).
5. 15-mL and 50-mL conical centrifuge tubes (Falcon, Becton-Dickinson).
6. ^{51}Cr counting tubes (No. 55.476, Sarstedt, Germany).

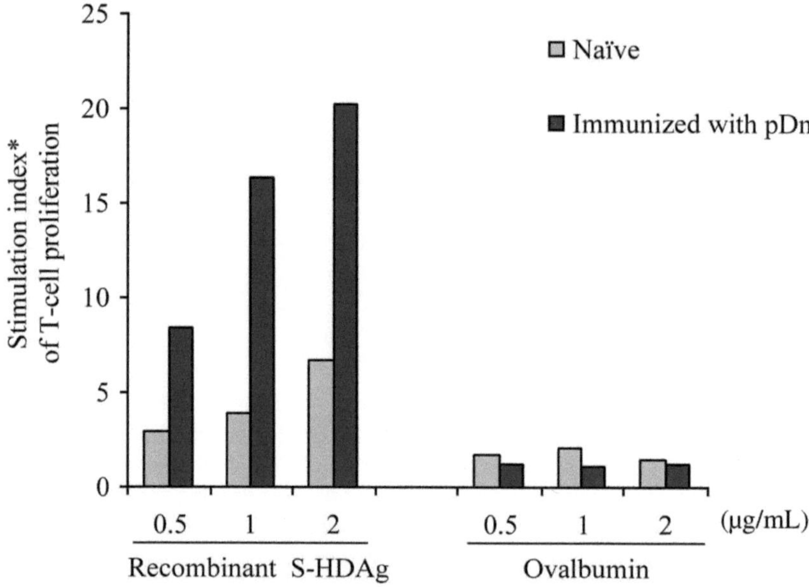

Fig. 5. Comparison of specific T-cell proliferative responses induced in pDm2 immunized mice and naïve mice. BALB/c mice, pretreated 7 d prior to immunization with cardiotoxin, were immunized intramuscularly with 100 μg of pDm2 on d 0 and d 14. On d 21, naïve and immunized mice were killed and spleens were ablated to isolate single-cell splenocytes. Splenocytes were counted and distributed into a 96-well microplate at a concentration of 2×10^5 cells/well and cultured with different concentrations of recombinant S-HDAg and ovalbumin as antigens. After 66-h culture, 1 μCi of [^{3}H]thymidine was added into each well and the plate was incubated for an additional 6 h, then cells were harvested on the membrane. The incorporation of [^{3}H]thymidine in proliferative cells was counted with a β-counter. The data expressed were obtained from one mouse of each group. The stimulation index* (SD) showed mean values (cpm) of triplicate cultures subtracted for background in the absence of antigen.

7. Sterile pipets.
8. 25-Gauge Teflon tube.

2.3. Animals

Female BALB/c mice, 5–6 wk old, are used and housed in an animal care accredited facility. Before manipulation, mice should be anesthetized by intraperitoneal injection with 100 μL of 2 mg/mL of Acepromazine-maleate (Fermenta Animal Health, USA). The skin overlying the quadriceps muscle of mice should be shaved before immunization.

2.4. Plasmid DNA

All antigen coding sequences in DNA vaccines used in this study were subcloned into multiple cloning sites of the pcDNA3.1(+) vector under the control of the CMV early promoter (**Fig. 1**).

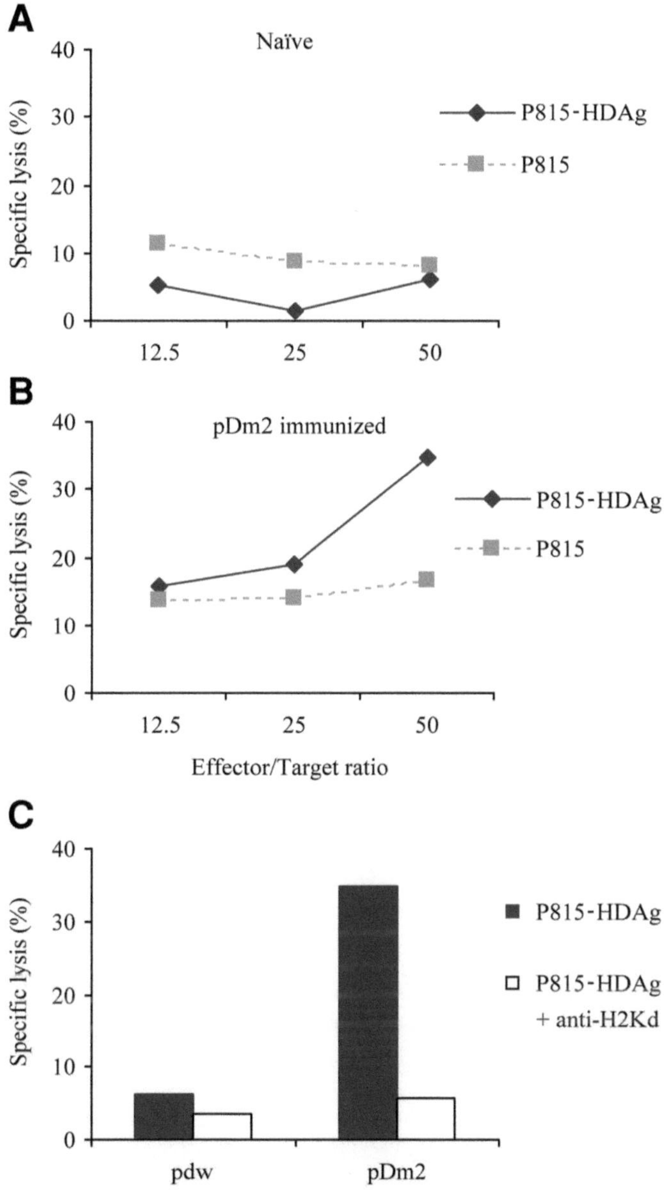

Fig. 6. Induction of CTL responses by pDm2 DNA vaccination. BALB/c mice, pretreated 7 d prior to immunization with cardiotoxin, were immunized intramuscularly with 100 μg of pDm2 on d 0 and d 14. On d 21 naïve and immunized mice were killed and spleens were ablated to isolate single-cell splenocytes. The splenocytes of naïve mice (**A**) and pDm2 immunized mice (**B**) were stimulated in vitro with P815-HDAg cells for 5 d and then tested on ^{51}Cr-labeled P815 and P815-HDAg target cells. The data expressed in the figure were obtained from one representive mouse of each group. For the inhibition of MHC I-restricted CTL activity assay shown in **C**, targets cells were incubated with medium alone or with anti-H-2 K^d (2 μg/mL) for 30 min before loading to mix with CTL at a 50:1 effector/target (E:T) ratio.

1. The plasmid pdw contains a wild-type small delta antigen (S-HDAg) open reading frame (ORF).
2. The plasmid pDm2, derived from pSVLDm2, contains a tandem dimer of mutated L-HDAg sequence encoding only S-HDAg. This plasmid is capable of self-replication in vivo but it cannot form HDV particle with HBV surface antigen, because the L-HDAg is essential for HDV virion assembly ***(29,30)***.
3. The plasmid pmGM-CSF containing mouse GM-CSF coding sequence was also used (**Fig. 1**).
4. The prokaryotic expression vector pET15a, which was used for cloning the S-HDAg coding sequence, was obtained from Novagen, and this vector contains an N-terminal His-Tag sequence allowing the purificaiton of the recombinant protein from a nickel-chelating resin affinity column (Ni-NTA Agarose, QIAGEN, cat. no. 30230, GmbH Germany).

2.5. Chemicals

1. Isopropyl β-D-thiogalactopyranoside (IPTG) (Sigma, cat. no. I6758), an inducer of *lac* promoter, is used to induce expression of recombinant protein in *E. coli* host.
2. Cardiotoxin, an agglutinin purified from the venom of the Naja snake (*Naja naja kaouthia*) (Sigma, cat. no. L8648), is used to induce a local inflammation in an animal.
3. Lectins such as Leukoagglutinin (PHA-L) (Sigma, cat. no. L4144) and concanavalin A (Con A) (Sigma, cat. no. C5275) are used to activate T-cell proliferation in vitro.
4. 2,2'-Azino-*bis*(3-ethylbenthiazoline-6-sulfonic acid) (ABTS) (Sigma, cat. no. A1888) is used as a soluble substrate for horseradish peroxidase (HRP) in ELISA applications.
5. Recombinant human IL-2 (PharMingen, cat. no. 19211T) is used to culture splenocytes in vitro.

2.6. Isotopes

1. 200–500 μCi/mL of $Na_2{}^{51}CrO_4$ (DuPont, New England Nuclear, or Amersham) is used to label target cells in CTL assay.
2. [Methyl-^{3}H]-thymidine (aqueous solution containing 2% ethanol, specific activity approx 5–7 Ci/mmol; DuPont, New England Nuclear, or Amersham) is used for DNA incorporation in proliferation of cells.

2.7. Cell Line

P815 mastocytoma cell line (ATCC TIB-64), derived from DBA-2 mouse, is used for its H-2^d genetic background that is the same as that of BALB/c mice. Because of the lack of information about major histocompatibility class (MHC) I antigenic peptides derived from S-HDAg, we expect that the MHC I antigenic peptides of S-HDAg can be processed and presented on the MHC I molecules of transformed cells when S-HDAg-transformed P815 cells express S-HDAg. Thus, these S-HDAg-transformed P815 cells can be used as target cells for detecting the CTLs induced in immunized BALB/c mice. The transfection of S-HDAg gene into P815 was performed by calcium-phosphate precipitating protocol with retrovirus particle containing the gene encoding S-HDAg ***(31)***. The expression of S-HDAg in transformed P815 cells can be demonstrated by Western blotting with anti-S-HDAg Ab D9-3 (*not shown*).

2.8. Culture Medium

Complete medium (CM) containing RPMI 1640 medium with 10% inactivated fetal calf serum (FCS), 1X penicillin–streptomycin–L-glutamine with 10 U/mL of penicillin-G sodium, 10 μg/mL of streptomycin sulfate, 29.2 μg/mL of L-glutamine (100X solution can be obtained from Gibco-BRL, cat. no. 10378-016), and 50 μ*M* 2-mercaptoethanol (2-ME) (Sigma, cat. no. M7522).

2.9. Solutions

1. ELISA coating buffer: Dissolve 10.4 g of $NaHCO_3$ in 900 mL of distilled H_2O and adjust pH to 8.2. Add distilled H_2O to a final volume of 1 L.
2. 10X phosphate-buffered saline (PBS) 2.3 g of NaH_2PO_4 (anhydrous); 11.5 g of Na_2HPO_4 (anhydrous); and 90 g of NaCl in 900 mL of distilled H_2O. Adjust pH to 7.2–7.4 using 1 *M* NaOH or 1 *M* HCl. Adjust the volume to 1 L with distilled H_2O. Store at room temperature and dilute to 1X PBS just before use.
3. Blocking buffer: 1X PBS + 1% bovine serum albumin (BSA) (Sigma, cat. no. A4503).
4. Washing buffer: 1X PBS + 0.5% Tween-20 (Merck, cat. no. 8.22184).
5. Substrate buffer: Dissolve 17.4 g of K_2HPO_4 and 21 g of citric acid–H_2O in 900 mL of distilled H_2O. Adjust pH to 4.3 with 10 *N* NaOH and add distilled H_2O to 1 L. Aliquot at 11 mL per vial and store at –20°C.
6. ACK buffer: Dissolve 8.29 g of NH_4Cl, 1 g of $KHCO_3$, 37.2 mg of Na_2EDTA in 800 mL of distilled H_2O and adjust pH to 7.2–7.4 with 1 *N* HCl. Adjust the volume to 1 L with distilled water. The ACK solution is sterilized through a 0.2-μm filter and stored at room temperature.
7. Hanks' balanced salt solution (HBSS, Gibco-BRL, cat. no. 14175-095).

2.10. Antibodies

1. Anti-S-HDAg Ab D9-3 is an IgG1 subtype monoclonal Ab, which was produced in our laboratory as described previously ***(32)***.
2. Purified mouse IgG1 (BD PharMingen, cat. no. 03011D) and mouse IgG2a (BD PharMingen, cat. no. 03021D).
3. Anti-mouse IgG1 (Clone A85-3, BD PharMingen, cat. no. 02241D) and anti-mouse IgG2a (Clone R12-4, BD PharMngen, cat. no. 02021D).
4. Peroxidase-conjugated AffiniPure rabbit anti-mouse IgG, Fcγ fragment specific (code no. 315-035-008, Jackson ImmunoResearch Laboratories).
5. Biotinylated anti-mouse IgG1 (Clone A85-1, BD PharMingen, cat. no. 03212C) and biotinylated anti-mouse IgG2a (BD PharMingen, cat. no. 03022C).
6. Horseradish peroxidase (HRP)-conjugated avidin (Pierce).
7. Anti-H-$2K^b$ (BD PharMingen, cat. no. 06101D) and anti-H-$2K^d$ (BD PharMingen, cat. no. 06091D) used for the inhibition of CTL.

2.11. Proteins

1. Hepatitis C virus (HCV) nonstructural protein 3 (NS3) used in T-cell proliferation assay for negative control antigen was obtained from Dr. W.-K. Chi at Development Center of Biotechnology, Taipei.
2. Ovalbumin (Sigma, cat. no. A7641).

2.12. Kits

1. EndoFree Plasmid Maxi Kits (QIAGEN, cat. no. 12362, GmbH Germany).
2. Nickel-chelating resin (Ni-NTA Agarose, QIAGEN, cat. no. 30230, GmbH Germany).

3. Methods

3.1. Purification of Plasmid DNA Vaccines

All plasmid DNA vaccines used in this study are purified with EndoFree Plasmid Maxi Kits (QIAGEN, cat. no. 12362) from *E. coli* DH5α host containing the designated plasmid DNA after overnight growth with vigorous shaking (200–300 rpm) in a 37°C incubator. The purification protocol follows the QIAGEN plasmid purification handbook with few modifications.

1. Harvest bacterial cells (200–400 mL) by centrifugation at 6000*g* for 15 min at 4°C.
2. Resuspend the bacterial pellet in 10 mL of buffer P1, then add 10 mL of buffer P2, mix gently but thoroughly by inverting four to six times, and incubate at room temperature for 5 min.
3. Add 10 mL of chilled buffer P3 to the lysate, and mix immediately but gently by inverting four to six times. Do not incubate the lysate on ice.
4. Centrifuge the lysate at 16,000*g* for 20 min and then pour the lysate supernatant into the barrel of the QIAfilter Cartridge. Incubate at room temperature for 10 min and remove the cap from the QIAfilter outlet nozzle. Gently insert the plunger into the QIAfilter Maxi Cartridge and filter the lysate supernatant into a 50-mL tube.
5. Add 2.5 mL of buffer ER (endotoxin-remove) to the filtered lysate supernatant, mix by inverting the tube approx 10 times, and incubate on ice for 30 min.
6. Equilibrate a QIAGEN tip 500 by applying 10 mL of buffer QBT, and allow the column to empty by gravity flow. Apply the filtered lysate supernatant to the QBT-equilibrated QIAGEN tip and allow it to enter the resin by gravity flow.
7. Wash the QIAGEN tip with 2 × 30 mL of buffer QC and elute DNA with 15 mL of buffer QN. Precipitate DNA by adding 10.5 mL (0.7 volume) of room-temperature isopropanol to the eluted DNA. Mix and centrifuge immediately at 16,000*g* for 30 min at 4°C. Carefully decant the supernatant.
8. Wash the DNA pellet with 5 mL of endotoxin-free 70% ethanol at room temperature and centrifuge at 16,000*g* for 10 min. Carefully decant the supernatant without disturbing the pellet. Air-dry the pellet for 5–10 min, and dissolve the DNA in a suitable volume of endotoxin-free buffer TE.

3.2. Recombinant S-HDAg Production and Purification

Recombinant S-HDAg was purified under denaturing condition from *E. coli* transformed with plasmid pET15-S-HDAg. The N-terminal His-Tag sequence of this recombinant protein allows the protein to be purified with a nickel-chelating resin (Ni-NTA Agarose) affinity column. The purification protocol follows the QIAGEN QIAexpressionist handbook for high-level expression and purification of 6xHis-Tagged proteins.

1. Briefly, *E. coli* BL21(DE3) and BL21(DE3)pLys strains were transformed with plasmid pET15-S-HDAg. The transformed bacterial cells (200–400 mL) are grown at 37°C with vigorous shaking.
2. When the OD_{600} reaches 0.5–0.7, a final concentration of 1 m*M* IPTG is added into the culture to induce expression of recombinant S-HDAg protein. The culture temperature is changed to 30°C and incubated for an additional 2.5–3 h. Harvest bacterial cells by centrifugation at 4000*g* for 20 min. Freeze the cells in dry ice–ethanol or liquid nitrogen, or store cell pellet overnight at –20°C.

3. Thaw the cell pellet for 15 min on ice and resuspend with 2 mL of urea–phosphate buffer (8 *M* urea; 0.1 *M* NaH_2PO_4; 0.01 *M* Tris-HCl, pH 8.0) for 50 mL of bacterial culture. Stir cells for 60 min at 4°C or lyse them by gently vortex-mixing, and then centrifuge lysate at 10,000*g* for 30 min at 4°C to pellet cellular debris.
4. Add 1 mL of the 50% Ni-NTA slurry to 4 mL of lysate and mix gently by shaking (e.g., 200 rpm on a rotary shaker) for 60 min at room temperature. Load the lysate–resin mixture carefully into an empty column with the bottom cap still attached. Remove the bottom cap and collect the flow-through. Wash resin twice with 4 mL of buffer C (8 *M* urea; 0.1 *M* NaH_2PO_4; 0.01 *M* Tris-HCl, pH 6.3). Elute the recombinant protein four times with 0.5 mL of buffer D (8 *M* urea; 0.1 *M* NaH_2PO_4; 0.01 *M* Tris-HCl, pH 5.9), followed by four times with 0.5 mL of buffer E (8 *M* urea; 0.1 *M* NaH_2PO_4; 0.01 *M* Tris-HCl, pH 4.5).
5. Add 5 μL of 2X sodium dodecyl sulfate-polyacrylamide gel electrophoresis (SDS-PAGE) sample buffer to 5 μL of different eluates for SDS-PAGE analysis.
6. Desalt the purified recombinant protein against gradient glycerol–PBS solution (from 10% glycerol to 0%). Concentrate the recombinant protein by a SpeedVac centrifugation and stop centrifugation when desired protein concentration is achieved. Do not dry the recombinant protein because dried recombinant protein powder can be insoluble for further use.

3.3. Preimmunization with Cardiotoxin and Immunization with Plasmid DNA

For immunization, a 1.0-mL syringe with 27-gauge needle is used for injection of plasmid DNA into the quadriceps muscles. The 27-gauge needle is encompassed with a 25-gauge Teflon tube except for 2 mm length of the needle tip (*see* **Note 1**). Use a Teflon-tube-encompassed 27-gauge needle 1.0-mL syringe to perform injection of cardiotoxin and plasmid DNA. The needle top should penetrate vertically into the quadriceps muscles to avoid the leakage of injection.

1. One week (6 or 7 d) before the first DNA immunization, each anesthetized BALB/c mouse is injected with 50 μL of cardiotoxin (10 μ*M*) into quadriceps muscles of each hindleg.
2. For the first immunization, plasmid DNA is injected into the cardiotoxin-treated quadriceps muscles with a low dose (0.5 μg in 50 μL of water/hindleg, 1 μg/mouse) or a high dose (50 μg in 50 μg of water/hindleg, 100 μg/mouse). The plasmid pmGM-CSF (20 μg/mouse) is used to coimmunize with pDm2 in mice. Two boosters are followed on the second week and on the fourth week.
3. For applying electric pulses after DNA injection, the two gold tips (placed 5 mm apart) of Genetrodes (Model 508) are put onto the skin of the DNA injection site and then electric pulses are generated by the Electro Cell Manipulator (ECM 830, BTX). Three pulses (100 V, 50 ms/pulse length, and the field strength at 200 V/cm) are applied then the polarity is reversed and three more pulses are applied.

3.4. Collection of Blood Serum from Mouse

There are many ways to collect blood serum from mouse and detailed methods are described clearly in *Current Protocols in Immunology* ***(33)***.

1. Briefly, obtain the blood from orbital sinus or plexus from immunized mice with microhematocrit capillary tube. Introduce the end of the microhematocrit capillary tube into the orbital sinus with axial rotation.
2. Slowly advance the tip of the microhematocrit capillary tube gently toward the rear of the socket until blood flows into the tube. If possible, let blood flow into a 1.5-mL microcen-

trifuge tube until 0.2–0.4 mL are collected and then remove the microhematocrit tube from the orbit.

3. Dab excess blood from site with a gauze sponge or swab moistened in saline or PBS. Let individual blood stand for about 30 min at room temperature and then centrifuge at 3000 rpm for 10 min. The serum is in the supernatant of blood after the centrifugation. Collect the individual serum into another microcentrifuge tube and store at –20°C.

3.5. ELISA

ELISA method is used for detecting the anti-HDV Ab induced in immunized mice.

1. Coat the wells of a 96-well microtiter plate with 2 μg/mL of recombinant S-HDAg in coating buffer overnight at 4°C.
2. Wash S-HDAg-coated plates with PBS three times and block with blocking buffer for 2 h at room temperature.
3. Add diluted sera of immunized mice and standard control samples into the wells of plates except two wells with PBS buffer as negative control.
4. A twofold serial dilution (from 1:200,000 to 1:12,800,000) of an anti-S-HDAg IgG1 monoclonal Ab, D9-3, can be used as the standard. Incubate the plates overnight at 4°C and then treat with horseradish-peroxidase-conjugated rabbit anti-mouse IgG Fcγ fragment (Jackson ImmunoResearch, USA) for 1 h at room temperature to detect total anti-HDV IgG.
5. After washing with PBS, develop the plates by addition of ABTS substrate and then read at 420 nm in an ELISA reader (Emax, Molecular Devices). The Ab titer can be calculated by linear regression analysis plotting dilution vs the absorbance at 420 nm of D9-3 at 1:640,000 dilution. The titers can be calculated to be the $\log_{10}$ highest dilution and be given as arithmetic mean ± standard error.
6. For analysis of anti-HDV IgG1 or IgG2a titer, use S-HDAg-coated plates except coat two columns of the 96-well plate with 2 μg/mL of anti-mouse IgG1 (cat. no. 02241D, PharMingen) or 2 μg/mL of anti-mouse IgG2a (cat. no. 02021D, PharMingen), respectively. A twofold serial dilution of purified mouse IgG1 or mouse IgG2a starting from 30 ng/mL are used as standards for quantification. After incubation with dilutions of individual serum and IgG1 or IgG2a standards, wash and then add biotinyated anti-mouse IgG1 or IgG2a Abs to the plates. Incubate for 2 h at room temperature, wash, and then add HRP conjugated avidin (Pierce) for 30 min. The development of the plates can be done the same way as for total IgG before. The negative control consists of pooled sera from non-immunized mice and the results can be shown as the ratio of the absorbance at 420 nm of samples to negative control.

3.6. Isolation of Spleen Cells from Immunized Mice

1. Carefully remove each spleen from immunized mouse with sterile scissors and forceps and place spleen in a 100 × 15-mm Petri dish containing about 10 mL of RPMI 1640 medium. Then press and crush the spleen directly against the bottom of the Petri dish with the plunger of a 10-mL syringe until mostly fibrous tissue remains.
2. Collect the single-cell suspension with a 10-mL pipet and put into a 15-mL conical centrifuge tube. Let the tube stand for 10 min and then withdrew the cell suspension into another 15-mL conical centrifuge tube without taking the last 2 mL with cell debris in the bottom of tube. The cell debris contain fibrous tissue and uncrushed small pieces of tissue.
3. Centrifuge the cell suspension for 5 min at 400*g* in a suitable centrifuge (such as Sorvall RT7 centrifuge with Sorvall RTH-250 rotor) and discard the supernatant.

4. Resuspend the pellet of spleen cells with 3 mL of ACK buffer and incubate for 2 min at room temperature with occasional shaking to lyse the red blood cells. Add HBSS buffer to fill the tube, centrifuge 10 min at 256*g*, and discard the supernatant. Wash the pellet again with HBSS and resuspend in a suitable volume of RPMI complete medium for counting the number of cells to further manipulation.

3.7. T-Cell Proliferation

1. After counting, adjust the spleen cells to 8×10^6 cells/mL with RPMI complete medium. Distribute cells into 96-well U-bottom microtiter plate with $2–8 \times 10^5$ cells/well. It is useful to compare 2, 4, and 8×10^5 cells/well in initial pilot experiments.
2. In the experiments, the wells contain recombinant S-HDAg (8 μg/mL, 4 μg/mL, 2 μg/mL, and 1 μg/mL) for measuring the response of S-HDAg-specific T cells. The positive control wells contain mitogens Con A (0.4 μg/mL or 2 μg/mL) or PHA-L (2 μg/mL or 10 μg/mL) (*see* **Note 2**). The negative control wells contain other recombinant proteins such as HCV NS3 or ovalbumin (OVA) (at 8, 4, 2, and 1 μg/mL).
3. Incubate the plates in 5% CO_2 incubator at 37°C for 72 h. Add 20 μL of [^{3}H]thymidine (50 μCi/mL) into each well and incubate 6 h before harvesting the cells on the membrane using the 96-well cell harvester. Dry the membrane in an 80°C oven for at least 1 h and then count the incorporated [^{3}H]thymidine with the Liquid Scintillation & Luminescence counter (1450 MICRO BETA, Wallac TRILUX). The T-cell proliferation response can be indicated by the stimulation index (SD) = (the number of counts of cells with antigens)/(the number of counts of cells without any antigen).

3.8. Measurement of CTL Activity in DNA Immunized Mice

Before measuring CTL activity of spleen cells of immunized mice, the spleen cell suspensions have to be cultured with γ-ray (10,000 rads) irradiated (by 637 irradiator) S-HDAg transformed P815 (P815-HDAg) cells. The optimal ratio is often at 10 (splenocytes) to 1 (P815-HDAg cell). Add human recombinant IL-2 (10–50 U/mL) into culture to amplify effector CTLs. After a 5-d in vitro stimulation, harvest the nonadherent CTL as effector cells in the standard chromium (^{51}Cr) release assay.

1. Centrifuge target cells (P815 and P815-HDAg) ($\leq 1 \times 10^6$ cells) in a 15-mL conical tube for 5 min at 200*g* at room temperature. Discard most of the supernatant, but leave approx 0.1 mL of medium with the cell pellet.
2. Resuspend the cells gently and add 0.2 mL of $Na_2{}^{51}CrO_4$ (approx 1 mCi/mL) solution into the tube. Mix the target cells gently and incubate in a loosely capped 15-mL conical tube for 1 h in a 5% CO_2 incubator at 37°C.
3. During the ^{51}Cr labeling of target cells, wash the stimulated effector CTLs with RPMI complete medium. Count and dilute the effector CTLs to designed effector/target ratios (50:1, 25:1, and 12.5:1), and add 100 μL/well of effector CTLs into 96-well conical bottom plates.
4. After extensive washing with RPMI complete medium, 100 μL/well of the ^{51}Cr-labeled target cells are added into wells containing different numbers of effector CTLs.
5. For the inhibition of MHC I-restricted CTL activity assay centrifuge the plate for 5 min at 400*g*, the target cells should be incubated with 2 μg/mL of anti-MHC I Ab, anti-H-2K^d in the case of P815, for 30 min before loading to mix with CTLs. After 4 h of incubation at 37°C, transfer 100 μL of culture supernatants to 51Cr counting tubes and count in a Cobra 5003 γ-counter (Packard) to determine the amount of ^{51}Cr released in each well. The percentage of specific lysis can be calculated by using the following formula: % specific lysis = 100 ×

(experimental release – spontaneous release)/(maximum release – spontaneous release). The maximum release represents the number of counts measured in 1 *N* HCl target cell lysate and the spontaneous release represents the number of counts in the presence of medium only.

4. Notes

1. The 2-mm length of needle tip not encompassed with the Teflon tube is suitable for just penetrating into the quadriceps muscles and allowing the injection liquid to stay in the quadriceps muscles. If the needle tip is longer than 2 mm, it will traverse the quadriceps muscles. And if the needle tip is shorter than 2 mm, there will be leakage of the injection liquid.
2. The use of different concentrations of mitogens (Con A or PHA-L) for the positive control is very important because T cells isolated from different mice do not have the same proliferation responses to the same concentration of mitogen. For example, the maximal incorporation of [^{3}H]thymidine of lymphocytes of mouse A is with 2 μg/mL of Con A and for lymphocytes of mouse B, the maximal incorporation of [^{3}H]thymidine could be with 0.4 μg/mL of Con A. The mitogen used in experiments is merely to test whether isolated lymphocytes are functional. If there is no or very little incorporation of [^{3}H]thymidine in the well containing isolated lymphocytes treated with the mitogens, we can consider that the isolated lymphocytes are not suitable for the experiment.

References

1. Chen, P. J., Wu, H. L., Wang, C. J., Chia, J. H., and Chen, D. S. (1997) Molecular biology of hepatitis D virus: research and potential for application. *J. Gastroenterol. Hepatol.* **12,** S188–192.
2. Rizzetto, M., Hoyer, B., Canese, M. G., Shih J. W., Purcell, R. H., and Gerin, J. L. (1980) delta Agent: association of delta antigen with hepatitis B surface antigen x and RNA in serum of delta-infected chimpanzees. *Proc. Natl. Acad. Sci. USA* **77,** 6124–6128.
3. Gerin, J. L. (2001) Animal models of hepatitis delta virus infection and disease. *ILAR J.* **42,** 103–110.
4. Smedile, A., Farci, P., Verme, G., et al. (1982) Influence of delta infection on severity of hepatitis B. *Lancet* **ii** 945–947.
5. Farci, P., Mandas, A., Colana, A., et al. (1994) Treatment of chronic hepatitis D with interferon alfa-2a. *N. Engl. J. Med.* **330,** 88–94.
6. Lau, D. T., Doo, E., Park, Y., et al. (1999) Lamivudine for chronic delta hepatitis. *Hepatology* **30,** 579–581.
7. Negro, F. and Rizzetto, M. (1993) Pathobiology of hepatitis delta virus. *J. Hepatol.* **17(Suppl. 3),** S149–S153.
8. Guilhot, S., Huang, S. N., Xia, X. P., La Minica, N., Lai, M. M. C., and Chisari, F. V. (1997) Expression of hepatitis delta virus large and small antigens in transgenic mice. *J. Virol.* **68,** 1052–1058.
9. Nisini, R., Paroli, M., Accapezzato, D., et al. (1997) Human CD4+ T-cell response to hepatitis delta virus: identification of multiple epitopes and characterization of T-helper cytokine profiles. *J. Virol.* **71,** 2241–2251.
10. Niro, G. A., Gravinese, E., Martini, E., et al. (2001) Clearance of hepatitis B surface antigen in chronic carriers of hepatitis delta antibodies. *Liver* **21,** 254–259.
11. Gurunathan, S., Klinman, D. M., and Seder, R. A. (2000) DNA vaccines: immunology, application, and optimization. *Annu. Rev. Immunol.* **18,** 927–974.

12. Mir, L. M., Bureau, M. F., Gehl, J., et al. (1999) High-efficiency gene transfer into skeletal muscle mediated by electric pulses. *Proc. Natl. Acad. Sci. USA* **96,** 4262–4267.
13. Widera, G., Austin, M., Rabussay, D., et al. (2000) Increased DNA vaccine delivery and immunogenicity by electroporation in vivo. *J. Immunol.* **164,** 4635–4640.
14. Huang, Y. H., Wu, J. C., Tao, M. H., et al. (2000) DNA-based immunization produces Th1 immune responses to hepatitis delta virus in mouse model. *Hepatology* **32,** 104–110.
15. Deck, R. R., DeWitt, C. M., Donnelly, J. J., Liu, M. A., and Ulmer, J. B. (1997) Characterization of humoral immune responses induced by an influenza hemagglutinin DNA vaccine. *Vaccine* **15,** 71–78.
16. Robinson, H. L., Boyle, C. A., Feltquate, D. M., Morin, M. J., Santoro, J. C., and Webster. R. G. (1997) DNA immunization for influenza virus: studies using hemagglutinin- and nucleoprotein-expressing DNA. *J. Infect. Dis.* **176(Suppl)**, S50–55.
17. Boyle, C. M., Morin, M., Webster, R. G., and Robinson, H. L. (1996) Role of different lymphoid tissues in the initiation and maintenance of DNA-raised antibody responses to the influenza virus H1 glycoprotein. *J. Virol.* **70,** 9074–9078.
18. Kang, Y., Calvo, P. A., Daly, T. M., and Long, C. A. (1998) Comparison of humoral immune responses elicited by DNA and protein vaccines based on merozoite surface protein-1 from *Plasmodium yoelli,* a rodent malaria parasite. *J. Immunol.* **161,** 4211–4219.
19. Boyle, J. S., Silva, A., Bardy, J. L., and Lew, A. M. (1997) DNA immunization: induction of higher avidity antibody and effect of route on T-cell cytotoxicity. *Proc. Natl. Acad. Sci. USA* **94,** 14626–14631.
20. Boyle, J. S., Koniaras, C., and Lew, A. M. (1997) Influence of cellular location of express antigen on the efficacy of DNA vaccination: cytotoxic T-lymphocyte and antibody responses are suboptimal when antigen is cytoplasmic after intramuscular DNA immunization. *Int. Immunol.* **9,** 1897–1906.
21. Banchereau, J., Bazan, F., Blanchard, D., et al. (1994) The CD40 antigen and its ligand. *Annu. Rev. Immunol.* **12,** 881–922.
22. Ridge, J. P., Di Rosa, F., and Matzinger, P. (1998) A conditioned dendritic cell can be a temporal bridge between a CD4+ T-helper and a T-killer cell. *Nature* **393,** 474–478.
23. Bennett, S. R. M., Carbone, F. R., Karamalis, F., Flavell, R. A., Miller, J., and Heath, W. R. (1998) Help for cytotoxic-T-cell responses is mediated by CD40 signalling. *Nature* **393,** 478–480.
24. Schoenberger, S. P., Toes, R. E. M., van der Voort, E. I. H., Offringa, R., and Melief, C. J. M. (1998) T-cell help for cytotoxic T lymphocytes is mediated by CD40-CD40L interaction. *Nature* **393,** 480–483.
25. Seder, R. A. and Paul, W. E. (1994) Acquisition of lymphokine-producing phenotype by $CD4^+$ T cells. *Annu. Rev. Immunol.* **12,** 635–673.
26. Zimmermann, S., Egeter, O., Hausmann, S., et al. (1998) CpG oligodeoxynucleotides trigger protective and curative Th1 responses in lethal murine leishmaniasis. *J. Immunol.* **160,** 3627–3630.
27. Raz, E., Tighe, H., Sato, Y., et al. (1996) Preferential induction of a Th1 immune response and inhibition of specific IgE antibody formation by plasmid DNA immunization. *Proc. Natl. Acad. Sci. USA* **93,** 5141–5145.
28. Hsu, C. H., Chua, K. Y., Tao, M. H., et al. (1996) Immunoprophylaxis of allergen-induced immunoglobulin E synthesis and airway hyperresponsiveness in vivo by genetic immunization. *Nat. Med.* **2,** 540–544.
29. Chang, F. L., Chen, P. J., Tu, S. J., Wang, C. J., and Chen, D. S. (1991) The large form of hepatitis δ antigen is crucial for assembly of hepatitis δ virus. *Proc. Natl. Acad. Sci. USA* **88,** 8490–8494.

30. Chao, M., Hsieh, S. Y., and Taylor, J. (1990) Role of two forms of hepatitis delta virus antigen: evidence for a mechanism of self-limiting genome replication. *J. Virol.* **64,** 5066–5069.
31. Wang, H. W., Chen, P. J., Lee, C. Z., Wu, H. L., and Chen, D. S. (1994) Packaging of hepatitis delta virus RNA via the RNA-binding domain of hepatitis delta antigens: different roles for the small and large delta antigens. *J. Virol.* **68,** 6363–6371.
32. Mu, J. J., Wu, H. L., Chiang, B. L., Chang, R. P., Chen, D. S., and Chen, P. J. (1999) Characterization of the phosphorylated forms and the phosphorylated residues of hepatitis delta virus delta antigens. *J. Virol.* **73,** 10540–10545.
33. Donovan, J. and Brown, P. (1995) Blood collection, in *Current Protocols in Immunology* (Coligan, J. E., Kruisbeek, A. M., Margulies, D. H., Shevach, E. M., and Strober W., eds), John Wiley & Sons, New York, pp. 1.7.1–1.7.5.

II

In Vitro and In Vivo Models

11

Infection of Primary Chimpanzee Hepatocytes with Recombinant Hepatitis D Virus Particles

A Surrogate Model for Hepatitis B Virus

Azeneth Barrera and Robert E. Lanford

1. Introduction

The discovery of hepatitis B virus (HBV) four decades ago initiated the progressive increase in knowledge of an important hepatotropic infectious agent that culminated in the design of the first successful recombinant vaccine for a human infectious disease. Despite this medical achievement, HBV infections continue to present a paramount health problem, which stems from the establishment of chronic infections of HBV that can progress to cirrhosis and hepatocellular carcinoma. There are over 350 million chronic carriers worldwide for which no cure exists, requiring the development of new and better treatments for this disease. The mechanisms of HBV replication and assembly have been well-characterized, owing to the advent of molecular biology techniques and the development of infectious HBV clones. However, two major experimental impediments that were recognized from the beginning continue to be obstacles in the illumination of the early steps of HBV infection. The narrow host range of HBV and the absence of cell lines susceptible to infection have hampered studies on the mechanisms of viral entry. More specifically, the cellular receptor for HBV has not been identified. The isolation of the HBV receptor would create a new target for drug interactions, expanding the limited choice of treatments that currently exists. Identifying viral receptors has often required several distinct approaches. At present, the only hepadnaviral infection system that has yielded promising results and may help identify all viral receptor components is the infection of primary duck hepatocytes with duck hepatitis B virus (DHBV) ***(1–10)***. DHBV is significantly diverse from HBV, however, and the human homolog of the putative receptor identified for DHBV has not been shown to be involved in HBV attachment or entry. One unique approach that has not been widely used is in vitro infections with hepatitis D virus (HDV) as a model for studying the early

From: *Methods in Molecular Medicine, vol. 96: Hepatitis B and D Protocols, volume 2*
Edited by: R. K. Hamatake and J. Y. N. Lau © Humana Press Inc., Totowa, NJ

steps of the HBV replication cycle. The requirement of HDV to exploit the HBV envelope proteins for assembly, secretion, and cellular transmission of particles raises the possibility that both viruses use the same receptor. This chapter describes the utility of primary chimpanzee hepatocyte cultures infected with recombinant HDV particles to study the early steps in the HBV infection process.

A key factor in the ability to successfully characterize hepatotropic viruses using primary hepatocytes was the generation of methods for isolating and cultivating cells in which differentiated cellular functions were preserved. Many different cultivation systems for primary hepatocytes have been described ***(11,12)***. Our laboratory developed methods for the cultivation of highly differentiated primate hepatocytes utilizing a serum-free medium supplemented with growth factors and hormones ***(13,14)***. Initial studies using this system demonstrated the *de novo* synthesis of lipoprotein(a) by hepatocytes ***(15)*** and characterized the effects of allelic variations on the biogenesis of lipoprotein(a) ***(16–20)***. Although studies on hepatitis C virus (HCV) infection using this cultivation system produced varied results, HCV replication was detectable using a strand-specific reverse transcriptase-polymerase chain reaction (RT-PCR) assay for the replicative negative strand of HCV RNA ***(13)***. This system has proven highly efficient, however, for studies on GBV-B infection of primary tamarin hepatocytes ***(21–23)***. Because GBV-B is the virus phylogenetically most closely related to HCV, it has been proposed as a potential surrogate model for the study of HCV infections of humans ***(23)***. Whereas this culture system supports HBV replication in chimpanzee hepatocytes ***(24)***, its use for the study of in vitro HBV infections is limited for reasons that remain unresolved. However, several published reports have described an in vitro HBV infection system using primary human hepatocytes ***(25–27)***. These studies demonstrated that in the presence of polyethylene glycol (PEG), cultures of primary human hepatocytes were susceptible to infection with HBV and could be utilized to characterize determinants of host specificity of HBV.

Although in vitro infections of primary chimpanzee hepatocytes with HBV are marginal, we found that this system is exceptionally well suited for the analysis of HDV infection. Initial studies conducted with HDV demonstrated that high levels of replicating HDV RNA were observed by Northern hybridization following exposure to HDV particles in vitro, and susceptibility to infection was shown to persist for several weeks in culture ***(24)***. A full cycle of HDV infection was observed when using cultures derived from an HBV-infected chimpanzee; the presence of HBV envelope proteins in the infected cultures promoted the assembly and secretion of high levels of HDV particles into the medium ***(24)***. Further studies demonstrated that infectious, recombinant HDV particles could be produced in vitro by cotransfection of the Huh7 cell line with two plasmids; one vector contains a cDNA copy of HDV, and the other plasmid expresses the HBV envelope proteins ***(28)***. Recombinant HDV particles were infectious in primary chimpanzee hepatocyte cultures, and infectivity could be neutralized using antibodies to the pre-S1 and pre-S2 domains of the HBV envelope ***(28)***. The effect of neutralizing antibodies on HDV infection confirmed that this culture system was capable of supporting the biological interaction of viral particles with the cellular membrane, indicating a powerful system for exploring determinants of infectivity. In a separate study, it was demonstrated that recombinant HDV particles could be produced with different combinations of HBV envelope proteins, including only small (S), S plus middle (M), and S plus M plus large (L) envelope proteins ***(29)***. All particles contained HDV RNA and had similar sedimentation profiles; however, only particles containing the L protein and thus the pre-S1 domain were infectious in chimpanzee hepatocytes. This observation permits the construction of a variety of pre-S1 variants to define the requirements for infectivity.

More recently, we have exploited the pseudotyping properties of HDV to make recombinant HDV particles with the woolly monkey hepatitis B (WMHBV) envelope (*unpublished data*). WMHBV is the only other known primate hepadnavirus aside from HBV, bridging the evolutionary gap between HBV and woodchuck hepatitis virus. Because woolly monkeys are endangered and are not available for experimental purposes, several directions have been undertaken to establish models for HBV using WMHBV. Host range analyses of WMHBV in animals available for experimental purposes have demonstrated that the newly isolated hepadnavirus exhibited the typical characteristic of a restricted host range ***(30)***. Black-handed spider monkeys, which are close relatives of woolly monkeys, were susceptible to infection with WMHBV, while chimpanzees were not. One of the experimental directions underway is the utilization of the primary hepatocyte cultivation method to develop a tissue culture system for WMHBV. Preliminary observations have shown that this method is ideal for the maintenance of primary spider monkey hepatocytes (*data not shown*) and therefore is a potential candidate for the establishment of the cultivation of WMHBV. Another experimental approach for the study of WMHBV is the HDV system, which is a useful model for the production of recombinant particles with variant envelopes. Because of the exceptionally high level of HDV RNA replication, HDV infection is easily documented by Northern blot analysis. The combination of this technology and the isolation of a primate hepadnavirus with a different host range than HBV provides the opportunity to define the determinants for host range and/or receptor binding, as well as identification of the receptor itself. This chapter details the method for the production of recombinant HDV particles and in vitro infection of primary chimpanzee hepatocytes with these particles.

2. Materials

2.1. Production of Recombinant HDV Particles

2.1.1. Cell Line and Plasmids

1. Huh7 hepatoma cell line ***(31)***.
2. For production of HDV proteins and HDV RNA, we use the recombinant plasmid pSVLD3, which contains a head-to-tail trimer of full-length HDV cDNA for expression of HDV genome RNA under the control of the simian virus 40 late promoter ***(32,33)***.
3. Production of HBV envelope proteins in Huh7 cells is achieved by using the expression vector pZHB2.7. The HBV insert, which contains the pre-S1–pre-S2-S gene, spans nucleotides 2425 through 1 to nucleotide 1987 (ayw subtype) and can direct the expression of the S, M, and L proteins. It includes the HBV promoter upstream of the pre-S1 region for expression of the mRNA for the L protein, the HBV promoter within the pre-S1 region for expression of

the M and S mRNAs, and the HBV polyadenylation signals. The HBV insert is cloned into the *Bam*H I site of the plasmid pZErO-1 (Invitrogen).

2.1.2. Transfection of Huh7 Cells

1. Dulbecco's modified Eagle's medium (DMEM)–Ham's F12 medium (Mediatech, Herndon, VA, cat. no. MT 15-090-CV) containing L-glutamine (Mediatech, cat. no. MT 25-005-CI) at a final concentration of 2 m*M* and gentamicin sulfate at a final concentration of 50 μg/mL.
2. DMEM–Ham's F12 medium as described in **item 1** and supplemented with 10% fetal bovine serum (FBS) (HyClone, Logan, UT, cat. no. SH30071.03).
3. *Trans*IT-LT1 lipid reagent; 1.33 mg/mL in 80% ethanol (Mirus, Madison, WI, cat. no. MIR2304).
4. Corning-brand treated polystyrene 100-mm tissue culture dishes (Fisher Scientific, cat. no. 08-772-23).
5. Cell culture incubator maintained at 37°C and infused with 10% CO_2.
6. 50-mL sterile disposable polystyrene conical tubes (Fisher Scientific, cat. no. 05-538-49).

2.2. Preparation of HDV Inoculum

1. PEG 8000 (Sigma, cat. no. P2139); 40% in phosphate-buffered saline (PBS) (Fisher Scientific, cat. no. BP399-20). Store solution at 4°C.
2. TRIzol Reagent (Life Technologies, cat. no. 15596-026).
3. Glycogen (Roche Diagnostics, cat. no. 901 393).
4. Isopropanol.
5. Diethylpyrocarbonate (DEPC)-treated H_2O (ICN Biomedicals, Aurora, OH, cat. no. 821739).
6. Beckman SW28 centrifuge tubes (Beckman Instruments, cat. no. 326823). Siliconize the tubes before using for PEG precipitation of HDV particles.
7. Acrodisc 0.45-μm syringe filters with HT Tuffryn membrane (Pall Life Sciences, cat. no. 4184).
8. Millex 0.22-μm syringe-driven filter units (Millipore, cat. no. SLGV 013 SL).

2.3. In Vitro Infection of Primary Hepatocyte Cultures

Hepatocytes are isolated by a two-step collagenase perfusion method and cultivated in a serum-free medium containing specific growth factors and hormones. Wells of a six-well tissue culture plate are coated with a collagen solution and dried before seeding the hepatocytes at a density of 3×10^6 cells per well. The thin collagen film utilized in our system is helpful in the initial attachment and establishment phase of the cultures. For a detailed list of materials needed for this procedure, refer to Chapter 48 of *Methods in Molecular Medicine, Vol 19: Hepatitis C Protocols* ***(13)***.

1. Williams' Medium E (WME) basal: WME (Life Technologies, (cat. no. 12551-032) containing 10 m*M* 4-(2-hydroxyethyl) piperazine-l-ethanesulfanic acid (HEPES), pH 7.4 (Sigma, cat. no. H6147), and 50 μg/mL gentamicin sulfate.
2. Serum-free medium formulated for primary hepatocytes (*see* **Note 1**).
3. BD Primaria six-well tissue culture plates (Becton, Dickinson and Co., Franklin Lakes, NJ, cat. no. 353846).
4. Rat tail collagen (Collaborative Biomedical, cat. no. 40236) diluted 1:5 in H_2O and filtered through a 0.22-μm syringe-driven filter unit.

2.4. Detection of HDV Replication by Northern Blot Hybridization

1. Formaldehyde gel running buffer, 10X (Eppendorf – 5 Prime, cat. no. 955 15 544-1). This is a 10X 3-(*N*-morpholino)-propanesulfonic acid (MOPS) buffer intended for use at 1X as electrophoresis buffer for formaldehyde–agarose gel electrophoresis of RNA. The buffer does not contain formaldehyde.
2. RNA loading buffer: For 20 mL: Add 2.5 mL of 10X formaldehyde gel running buffer, 12.5 mL of formamide, 4.25 mL of formaldehyde, 0.75 g of Ficoll 400, 12.5 mg of xylene cyanol FF, and 12.5 mg of bromophenol blue. Bring the volume to 20 mL with H_2O.
3. Water bath set at 70°C.
4. Horizontal gel electrophoresis unit with a water cooling coil.
5. Formaldehyde–agarose gel: For 300 mL: Dissolve 3 g of agarose in 200 mL of H_2O. Once the temperature of the solution has cooled enough to allow handling, add 30 mL of 10X formaldehyde gel running buffer and 54 mL of formaldehyde. Bring volume to 300 mL with H_2O for a 2.2 *M* formaldehyde–1% agarose gel solution.
6. GeneScreen Plus Hybridization Transfer Membrane (NEN Life Science Products, cat. no. NEF976).
7. Saline sodium citrate 20X (SSC): 3 *M* NaCl, 0.3 *M* sodium citrate (Eppendorf5 Prime, cat. no. 2-227160).
8. Capillary upward-transfer system ***(34)***.
9. Stratalinker UV Crosslinker 1800.
10. Glass dishes with lids.
11. Variable temperature water bath shaker.
12. HDV Riboprobe prepared using Riboprobe Combination SystemSP6/T7 RNA Polymerase (Fisher Scientific, cat. no. P1460). Genomic and antigenomic probes are prepared from a plasmid (pSP72, Promega) containing an HDV insert from nucleotides 330–1200 and opposing T7 and SP6 promoters. The Riboprobe is then passed through a Sephadex G-25 Quick Spin column (Roche Diagnostics Corp., cat. no. 1273-949) to remove unincorporated radiolabeled nucleotides.
13. Sodium dodecyl sulfate (SDS) hybridization solution: For 1 L: Add 10 mL of a 20 mg/mL stock solution of salmon sperm DNA heated at 70°C to 50 mL of H_2O. Add 300 mL of 20X SSPE; 0.01 *M* NaH_2PO_4, 0.15 *M* NaCl, 0.001 *M* EDTA (Fisher Scientific, cat. no. BP1328-1). Add 100 g of SDS, and mix on a stir plate. Add 500 mL of formamide heated at 70°C. If the SDS has not gone into solution, heat the solution at 70°C until the SDS dissolves. Bring the final volume to 1 L with H_2O, and store at – 20°C in 50-mL aliquots.
14. High-stringency wash buffer: 0.1X SSC, 0.1% SDS.
15. Low-stringency wash buffer: 1X SSC, 0.1% SDS.

3. Methods

3.1. Production of Recombinant HDV Particles

In vitro production of HDV has been optimized for maximum production and secretion of particles using the protocol described. A transfection efficiency of approx 40% of Huh7 cells is observed using *Trans*IT-LT1 lipid reagent and a DNA vector expressing green fluorescent protein. Production of HDV particles is performed in 100-mm tissue culture dishes, and culture medium containing approx 9 ng of HDV RNA or 1×10^9 HDV genome equivalents is normally used to infect one well of a six-well tissue culture plate of primary chimpanzee hepatocytes.

The production of recombinant HDV particles requires the cotransfection of two plasmids. One plasmid expresses a transcript that represents three head-to-tail copies of the HDV genome and initiates HDV RNA replication, and the other plasmid encodes the HBV envelope proteins. An approx 1: 4 molar ratio of the HDV to HBV plasmid yields maximum HDV particle secretion.

3.1.1. Preparation of Cultures for Transfection

1. Seed Huh7 cells in 100-mm tissue culture dishes at a density of 8.4×10^6 cells per dish.
2. Add 10 mL of prewarmed DMEM–Ham's F12 medium supplemented with 10% FBS.
3. Incubate the cultures overnight at 37°C.

3.1.2. Transfection of Huh7 Cells

This protocol is outlined for the transfection of one 100-mm tissue culture dish. If transfecting more than one dish with the same transfection mixture, multiply the volume of reagents by the total number of dishes not to exceed nine, which is the volume limit of a 50-mL polystyrene conical tube.

1. Warm DMEM–Ham's F12 medium containing FBS in a 37°C water bath.
2. Wash the cultures seeded the previous day one time with 9 mL of DMEM–Ham's F12 medium.
3. Add 4.5 mL of DMEM–Ham's F12 medium to each tissue culture dish. This volume represents half of the final volume that will be added during the transfection procedure. The other half will contain the DNA–lipid complexes.
4. Incubate the cultures at 37°C while preparing DNA–lipid complexes.
5. Preparation of DNA–lipid complexes requires 30 μg of DNA and 45 μL of *Trans*IT-LT1 lipid reagent per 100-mm tissue culture dish. For a 60-mm tissue culture dish, reagents can be decreased by a factor of 3, which represents the approximate decrease in growth area.
6. Add 4.5 mL of DMEM–Ham's F12 medium without FBS to a 50-mL polystyrene conical tube.
7. Add 45 μL of *Trans*IT-LT1 lipid reagent.
8. Gently mix the solution by pipetting slowly or flicking the tube.
9. Incubate the solution at room temperature for 15 min.
10. Add 30 μg of DNA: 3.3 μg of pSVLD3 + 26.7 μg of pZHB2.7.
11. Gently mix the solution by pipetting slowly or flicking the tube.
12. Incubate the solution at room temperature for 15 min.
13. Retrieve the Huh7 cell cultures from the incubator, and add 4.5 mL of the transfection mixture per 100-mm tissue culture dish.
14. Incubate the cultures in the transfection mixture for 6 h at 37°C.
15. After 6 h of incubation, discard the transfection mixture, and add 15 mL of prewarmed DMEM–Ham's F12 medium supplemented with 10% FBS.
16. Incubate the transfected Huh7 cell cultures at 37°C.
17. Change the medium of the transfected cultures every 3 d.

3.2. Preparation of HDV Inoculum

1. Harvest the medium containing secreted HDV particles on 9, 12, 15, and 18 d post-transfection.

2. Pool the harvested medium, and save a 500-µL aliquot for Northern blot analysis of HDV RNA. When working with different HDV inocula, aliquots of the pooled culture medium are analyzed to adjust the inocula for comparable viral genome equivalents (*see* **Note 2**).
3. Harvested medium is stored at –80°C for future precipitation of viral particles for HDV RNA analysis or infection of primary hepatocyte cultures.
4. For Northern blot analysis of HDV RNA from a medium aliquot, clarify by centrifugation in a microfuge for 30 min.
5. Transfer the clarified medium to a fresh microcentrifuge tube, and precipitate virions with 9% PEG (0.500 mL of Huh7 culture medium + 0.225 mL of 40% PEG + 0.275 mL of PBS).
6. Mix well, and incubate on ice for 1 h.
7. Pellet precipitated viral particles in a microfuge for 20 min and 4°C. The PEG precipitate will appear as a cloudy smear on the side of the tube when using a fixed angle rotor.
8. Suspend the PEG precipitate with 1 mL of TRIzol Reagent.
9. Extract the RNA from HDV particles as described by the manufacturer of TRIzol Reagent, and precipitate the RNA with isopropanol. Add 10 µg of glycogen to the sample at the isopropanol precipitation step in order to visualize the RNA pellet.
10. Suspend the HDV RNA pellet in 5 µL of DEPC-treated H_2O, and analyze HDV RNA by Northern blot hybridization as detailed in **Subheading 3.4.** (*see* **Fig. 1**). For comparison of the infectivity of different inocula, adjust the inocula to contain comparable genome equivalents based on Northern blot and PhosphorImager analysis.
11. To prepare the inoculum, PEG-precipitate recombinant HDV particles comparable to 10^9 genome equivalents per well. Add 40% PEG solution to the clarified Huh7 culture medium for a final percentage of 9% PEG. Mix well and incubate on ice for 1 h. Pellet the precipitate by centrifugation in a Beckman SW28 rotor for 20 min at 10,000 *g* and 4°C.
12. Suspend PEG-precipitated HDV particles in 2 mL of serum-free medium.
13. Sonicate inoculum gently two times for 20 s, keeping it on ice between sonications. The inoculum is sonicated to break up PEG aggregates that may have formed and could bypass receptor-mediated entry of primary hepatocytes.
14. Filter the inoculum through a 0.22-µm syringe filter (*see* **Note 3**).

3.3. In Vitro Infection of Primary Hepatocyte Cultures

For a detailed methodology of the isolation and cultivation of primary hepatocytes, refer to Chapter 48 of *Methods in Molecular Medicine, Vol 19: Hepatitis C Protocols (13)*. Coat wells with collagen by adding sufficient collagen solution to each well to cover the bottom of the well, and then remove the excess solution. Dry plates with lids partially open overnight under a laminar flow hood with a UV light. Plate hepatocytes at 3×10^6 cells per well of a six-well culture dish.

3.3.1. Inoculation of Cultures with Recombinant HDV Particles

1. After approx 3 d post-seeding, wash primary hepatocytes three times with prewarmed WME basal.
2. Expose the hepatocytes to 2 mL of inoculum containing HDV particles for 16 h at 37°C.
3. Remove and discard the inoculum.
4. Wash the hepatocytes three times with prewarmed WME basal.
5. Add 2 mL of prewarmed serum-free medium.
6. Incubate the hepatocyte cultures at 37°C.

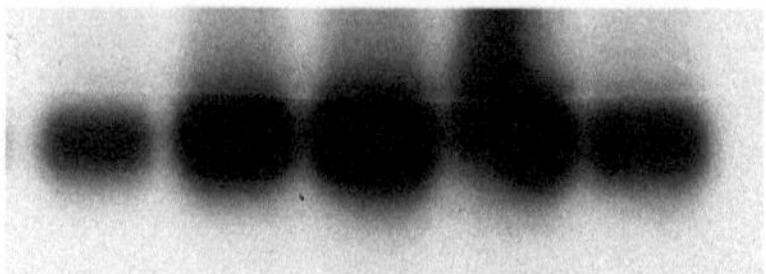

Fig. 1. Recombinant HDV particle production by Huh7 cells. Cultures of Huh7 cells were cotransfected with a plasmid containing a cDNA copy of the HDV genome and a plasmid that expresses the L, M, and S HBV envelope proteins. The culture medium containing secreted HDV particles was harvested on 9, 12, 15, and 18 d post-transfection. HDV RNA was analyzed by Northern hybridization as described in the text. A pool of equal amounts of the harvested medium was prepared as the inoculum for infection of primary hepatocyte cultures.

7. Change the medium every 2–3 d.
8. Harvest the hepatocytes on 3, 6, 9, and 12 d post-infection with 900 µL of TRIzol Reagent per well.

3.4. Detection of HDV RNA Replication by Northern Blot Hybridization (See *Fig. 2*)

1. Isolate total cellular RNA using TRIzol Reagent as specified by the manufacturer.
2. Suspend the RNA pellet in 25 µL of DEPC-treated H_2O.
3. Take the optical density (OD) reading of the total cellular RNA, and dilute the RNA to 1 µg/µL.
4. Transfer 5 µg of total cellular RNA to a fresh microcentrifuge tube, and add 20 µL of RNA loading buffer.
5. Heat the sample at 70°C for 10 min.
6. Chill on ice.
7. Analyze the RNA by horizontal agarose gel electrophoresis at 100 V and 16°C for 3 h.
8. Transfer the RNA onto a GeneScreen Plus membrane using traditional capillary upward transfer in 20X SSC overnight.
9. UV-crosslink the RNA to the membrane in a Stratagene UV Stratalinker at 120,000 µJ/cm^2 for about 30 s.
10. Prehybridize the membrane in a covered glass dish at 59°C in a water bath shaker for 5 h in SDS hybridization solution.
11. Hybridize the membrane at 59°C in a water bath shaker overnight in SDS hybridization solution containing 1×10^6 cpm/mL of an HDV RNA Riboprobe.
12. Wash the membrane two times in high-stringency wash buffer for 30 min at room temperature with shaking.
13. Wash the membrane two times in low-stringency wash buffer for 30 min at 65°C in a water bath shaker.
14. Allow the membrane to dry, and expose to film. The average exposure time for a good HDV RNA signal is overnight with one intensifying screen.

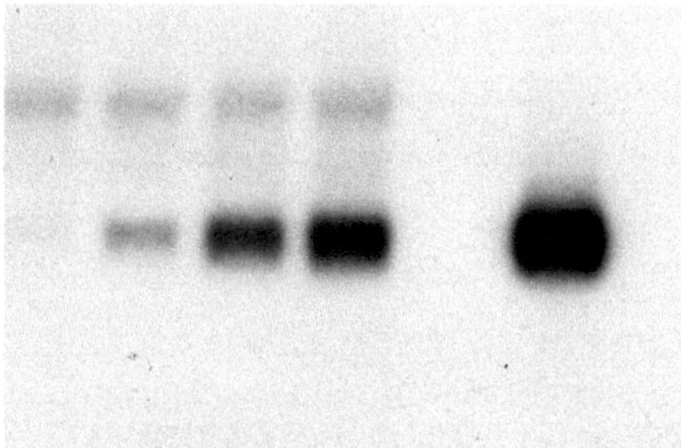

Fig. 2. HDV infection of primary chimpanzee hepatocyte cultures. Primary hepatocyte cultures were exposed to an inoculum containing recombinant HDV particles as described in the text. Cultures were washed to remove residual inoculum and maintained in serum-free medium. Lanes represent HDV RNA from 5 μg of total cellular RNA harvested on 3, 6, 9, and 12 d post-inoculation; and 5% of the inoculum (I).

4. Notes

1. Many different media formulations for liver cells have been described in the literature ***(12,35–40)***. Each has been developed for specific purposes. A medium developed working with rodent tissue will not necessarily perform well on primate tissue. Our medium was developed empirically by evaluating various concentrations and combinations of growth factors and hormones on cultures of baboon hepatocytes ***(14)***. The cultures were monitored for the maintenance of hepatocyte morphology, longevity, and the continued expression of highly stringent markers of hepatocyte differentiation. We have continued to experiment with the original formulation. Changes in the formulation may positively or negatively impact the expression of specific gene products, and thus the medium can often be simplified for a specific application.
2. Typically, HDV infections are performed with 2 mL of inoculum containing approx 9 ng of HDV RNA (1×10^9 HDV genome equivalents) per well of a six-well plate. This level of inoculum is generally obtained from 5 mL of the pooled medium from cultures of Huh7 cells. However, some HBV envelope variants affect the efficiency of HDV particle production. To standardize the inoculum, the appropriate volume of Huh7 culture medium is first precipitated with 9% PEG and suspended in 2 mL of medium. For variants that secrete poorly, the medium can be concentrated 10- to 20-fold by ultrafiltration (Amicon ultrafiltration unit with a 300,000 molecular weight cutoff ultrafiltration membrane; Fisher Scientific, cat. no. 14342) prior to PEG precipitation.
3. Dissolution of the PEG-precipitated pellet depends on several factors and can be problematic. The amount of serum protein present can greatly affect the ability of the PEG pellet to dissolve. Also, if the inoculum is stored at –80°C, some insoluble material will be present after thawing. The inoculum should be clarified before proceeding to in vitro infections. During the filtration of the inoculum, it is often necessary to filter the inoculum first through a 0.45-μm syringe-driven filter unit, followed by a 0.22-μm unit.

Acknowledgments

The authors would like to gratefully acknowledge C. Sureau, B. Guerra, and H. Lee for prior work on establishing the HDV model. This work was supported by NIH Grants RO1 A146609 and P51 RR13986.

References

1. Tong, S. P., Li, J. S., and Wands, J. R. (1995) Interaction between duck hepatitis B virus and a 170-kilodalton cellular protein is mediated through a neutralizing epitope of the pre-S region and occurs during viral infection. *J. Virol.* **69,** 7106–7112.
2. Kuroki, K., Cheung, R., Marion, P. L., and Ganem, D. (1994) A cell surface protein that binds avian hepatitis B virus particles. *J. Virol.* **68,** 2091–2096.
3. Ishikawa, T., Kuroki, K., Lenhoff, R., Summers, J., and Ganem, D. (1994) Analysis of the binding of a host cell surface glycoprotein to the preS protein of duck hepatitis B virus. *Virology* **202,** 1061–1064.
4. Kuroki, K., Eng, F., Ishikawa, T., Turck, C., Harada, F., and Ganem, D. (1995) gp180, a host cell glycoprotein that binds duck hepatitis B virus particles, is encoded by a member of the carboxypeptidase gene family. *J. Biol. Chem.* **270,** 15022–15028.
5. Breiner, K. M., Urban, S., and Schaller, H. (1998) Carboxypeptidase D (gp180), a Golgi-resident protein, functions in the attachment and entry of avian hepatitis B viruses. *J. Virol.* **72,** 8098–8104.
6. Li, J. S., Tong, S. P., and Wands, J. R. (1996) Characterization of a 120-kilodalton pre-S-binding protein as a candidate duck hepatitis B virus receptor.*J. Virol.* **70,** 6029–6035.
7. Tong, S. P., Li, J. S., and Wands, J. R. (1999) Carboxypeptidase D is an avian hepatitis B virus receptor. *J. Virol.* **73,** 8696–8702.
8. Li, J. S., Tong, S. P., and Wands, J. R. (1999) Identification and expression of glycine decarboxylase (p120) as a duck hepatitis B virus pre-S envelope-binding protein. *J. Biol. Chem.* **274,** 27658–27665.
9. Schaller, H. and Klingmuller, U. (1993) Hepadnavirus infection requires interaction between the viral pre-S domain and a specific hepatocellular receptor. *J. Virol.* **67,** 7414–7422.
10. Urban, S., Breiner, K. M., Fehler, F., Klingmüller, U., and Schaller, H. (1998) Avian hepatitis B virus infection is initiated by the interaction of a distinct pre-S subdomain with the cellular receptor gp180. *J. Virol.* **72,** 8089–8097.
11. Bayliss, M. K. and P. Skett. (1996) Isolation and culture of human hepatocytes, in *Methods in Molecular Medicine: Human Cell Culture Protocols* (Jones, E. J., ed.), Humana Press, Totowa, NJ, pp. 369–389.
12. Berry, M. N., Edwards, A. M., and Barritt, G. J. (1991) *Isolated Hepatocytes: Preparation, Properties and Applications.* Elsevier, New York.
13. Lanford, R. E. and Estlack, L. E. (1998) A cultivation method for highly differentiated primary chimpanzee hepatocytes permissive for hepatitis C virus replication, in J. Y. N. Lau, *Methods in Molecular Medicine: Hepatitis C* (Lau, J. Y. N., ed.), Humana Press, Totowa, NJ, pp. 501–516.
14. Lanford, R. E., Carey, K. D., Estlack, L. E., Smith, G. C., and Hay, R. V. (1989) Analysis of plasma protein and lipoprotein synthesis in long-term primary cultures of baboon hepatocytes maintained in serum-free medium. *In Vitro Cell. Dev. Biol.* **25,** 174–182.
15. Rainwater, D. L. and Lanford, R. E. (1989) Production of lipoprotein(a) by primary baboon hepatocytes. *Biochim. Biophys. Acta* **1003,** 30–35.

16. White, A. L., Rainwater, D. L., and Lanford, R. E. (1993) Intracellular maturation of apolipoprotein(a) and assembly of lipoprotein(a) in baboon hepatocytes. *J. Lipid. Res.* **34,** 509–517.
17. White, A. L., Hixson, J. E., Rainwater, D. L., and Lanford, R. E. (1994) Molecular basis for "null" lipoprotein(a) phenotypes and the influence of apolipoprotein(a) size on plasma lipoprotein(a) level in the baboon. *J. Biol. Chem.* **269,** 9060–9066.
18. White, A. L. and Lanford, R. E. (1994) Cell surface assembly of lipoprotein(a) in primary cultures of baboon hepatocytes. *J. Biol. Chem.* **269,** 28716–28723.
19. White, A. L. and Lanford, R. E. (1995) Biosynthesis and metabolism of lipoprotein(a). *Curr. Opin. Lipidol.* **6,** 75–80.
20. Lanford, R. E., Estlack, L., and White, A. L. (1996) Neomycin inhibits secretion of apolipoprotein[a] by increasing retention on the hepatocyte cell surface. *J. Lipid. Res.* **37,** 2055–2064.
21. Beames, B., Chavez, D., Guerra, B., Notvall, L., Brasky, K. M., and Lanford, R. E. (2000) Development of a primary tamarin hepatocyte culture system for GB virus-B: a surrogate model for hepatitis C virus. *J. Virol.* **74,** 11764–11772.
22. Lanford, R. E., Chavez, D., Guerra, B., et al. (2001) Ribavirin induces error-prone replication of GB virus B in primary tamarin hepatocytes. *J. Virol.* **75,** 8074–8081.
23. Beames, B., Chavez, D., and Lanford, R. E. (2001) GB virus B as a model for hepatitis C virus. *ILAR J.* **42,** 152–160.
24. Sureau, C., Jacob, J. R., Eichberg, J. W., and Lanford, R. E. (1991) Tissue culture system for infection with human hepatitis delta virus. *J. Virol.* **65,** 3443–3450.
25. Gripon, P., Diot, C., and Guguen-Guillouzo, C. (1993) Reproducible high level infection of cultured adult human hepatocytes by hepatitis B virus: effect of polyethylene glycol on adsorption and penetration. *Virology* **192,** 534–540.
26. Le Seyec, J., Chouteau, P., Cannie, I., Guguen-Guillouzo, C., and Gripon, P. (1999) Infection process of the hepatitis B virus depends on the presence of a defined sequence in the pre-S1 domain. *J. Virol.* **73,** 2052–2057.
27. Chouteau, P., LeSeyec, J., Cannie, I., Nassal, M., Guguen-Guillouzo, C., and Gripon, P. (2001) A short N-proximal region in the large envelope protein harbors a determinant that contributes to the species specificity of human hepatitis B virus. *J. Virol.* **75,** 11565–11572.
28. Sureau, C., Moriarty, A. M., Thornton, G. B., and Lanford, R. E. (1992) Production of infectious hepatitis delta virus *in vitro* and neutralization with antibodies directed against hepatitis B virus pre-S antigens. *J. Virol.* **66,** 1241–1245.
29. Sureau, C., Guerra, B., and Lanford, R. E. (1993) Role of the large hepatitis B virus surface envelope protein in infectivity of the hepatitis delta virion. *J. Virol.* **67,** 366–372.
30. Lanford, R. E., Chavez, D., Brasky, K. M., Burns, R. B., III, and Rico-Hesse, R. (1998) Isolation of a hepadnavirus from the woolly monkey, a New World primate. *Proc. Natl. Acad. Sci. USA* **95,** 5757–5761.
31. Nakabayashi, H., Taketa, K., Miyano, K., Yamane, T., and Sato, J. (1982) Growth of human hepatoma cells lines with differentiated functions in chemically defined medium. *Cancer Res.* **42,** 3858–3863.
32. Kuo, M. Y., Chao, M., and Taylor, J. (1989) Initiation of replication of the human hepatitis delta virus genome from cloned DNA: role of delta antigen. *J. Virol.* **63,** 1945–1950.
33. Sureau, C., Taylor, J., Chao, M., Eichberg, J. W., and Lanford, R. E. (1989) Cloned hepatitis delta virus cDNA is infectious in the chimpanzee. *J. Virol.* **63,** 4292–4297.

34. Sambrook, J., Fritsch, E. F., and Maniatis, T. (1989) *Molecular Cloning: A Laboratory Manual.* Cold Spring Harbor Press, Cold Spring Harbor, NY.
35. Edge, S. B., Hoeg, J. M., and Triche, T. (1986) Cultured human hepatocytes. Evidence for metabolism of low density lipoproteins by a pathway independent of the classical low density lipoprotein receptor. *J. Biol. Chem.* **261,** 3800–3806.
36. Enat, R., Jefferson, D. M., and Ruiz-Opazo, N. (1984) Hepatocyte proliferation in vitro: its dependence on the use of serum-free hormonally defined medium and substrata of extracellular matrix. *Proc. Natl. Acad. Sci. USA* **81,** 1411–1415.
37. Leffert, H. L. and Koch, K. S. (1982) Hepatocyte growth regulation by hormones in chemically defined media: a two-signal hypothesis, in *Growth of Cells in Hormonally Defined Media*, Vol. 9. (Sato, G. H. and Sirbasku A. A., eds.), Cold Spring Harbor Laboratory Press, Cold Spring Harbor, NY, pp. 597–613.
38. Reid, L. M. and Jefferson, D. M. (1984) Culturing hepatocytes and other differentiated cells. *Histopathology* **4,** 548–559.
39. Salas-Prato, M. (1982) Growth of fetal mouse liver cells in hormone-supplemented serum-free medium, (Sato, G. H. and Sirbasku, A. A. eds.), in *Growth of cells in hormonally Defined Media,* Vol. 9. Cold Spring Harbor Laboratory Press, Cold Spring Harbor, NY, pp. 615–624.
40. Sells, M. A., Chernoff, J., and Cerda, A. (1985) Long-term culture and passage of human fetal liver cells that synthesize albumin. *In Vitro Cell. Dev. Biol.* **21,** 216–220.

12

Study of the Endocytosis and Intracellular Localization of Subviral Particles of Hepatitis B Virus in Primary Hepatocytes

Dieter Glebe and Wolfram H. Gerlich

1. Introduction

Although our knowledge of the hepatitis B virus (HBV) life cycle has increased tremendously during the past 20 yr, the early steps of human HBV infection are still poorly understood. This is partly caused by the lack of a suitable cell culture system. Established hepatoma cell lines (e.g., HepG2 or Huh7) are not susceptible at all and proposed receptors for HBV have failed to support HBV entry to date. Because HBV is strictly hepatotropic, cultures of primary human hepatocytes are suitable for elucidation of the entry process of HBV, but very difficult to obtain and handle. Many insights into hepadnaviral uptake have come from the study of duck hepatitis B virus (DHBV) infection in primary duck hepatocytes. The characterization of a primary receptor of DHBV *(1)* and recombinant expression in nonsusceptible cell lines has shown that DHBV is taken up via endocytic vesicles *(2)*. Use of labeled DHBV virions from sera of infected ducks for uptake experiments using confocal microscopy has greatly improved the possibilities of studying the endocytic distribution of DHBV virions during infection.

Use of fluorescently labeled virions in the human system is hampered by the fact that purified HBV and primary human hepatocytes are not as easy to obtain as for the duck system. Instead of using HBV virions, we have fluorescently labeled highly purified subviral particles (HBsAg) from plasma of patients chronically infected with HBV, as subviral particles are present at 1000 times higher concentrations than virions in patients plasma and contain all three surface proteins of HBV.

Recombinant HBsAg has been used to investigate the binding of subviral particles to human hepatocytes by electron microscopy *(3)*. This group used recombinant HBsAg from yeast, consisting of only the small surface protein (SHBs). As the pre-S1 domain of the large surface protein (LHBs) is believed to contribute to initial binding to hepatocytes *(4)*, it is important to use subviral particles containing at least LHBs and SHBs. Recombinant HBV virions and subviral particles can also be obtained from

From: *Methods in Molecular Medicine, vol. 96: Hepatitis B and D Protocols, volume 2*
Edited by: R. K. Hamatake and J. Y. N. Lau © Humana Press Inc., Totowa, NJ

established hepatoma cell lines but require special cell culture conditions for optimal production *(5)*.

By using fluorescently labeled highly purified subviral particles from plasma of HBV-infected patients together with primary human hepatocytes, we could show by confocal microscopy that subviral particles of HBV are taken up by primary human hepatocytes but not by established human hepatoma cell lines (HepG2) and that they locate to distinct intracellular vesicles. The binding and uptake in primary human hepatocytes could be enhanced by desialylating subviral particles with a sialidase. On the other hand, HepG2 cells were not able to endocytose desialylated subviral particles but showed a massive binding (**Fig. 4**). This might be due to a loss of specific (co-) receptor(s) on HepG2 cells that are important for uptake of subviral particles and virus in this cell line.

In the following section we focus on the purification and labeling of subviral particles from HBV-containing plasma and preparation of primary human hepatocytes. The purification of HBV virions and subviral particles is a basic requirement for all further investigations on HBV entry. The described method for purification of subviral HBV particles from HBV-containing plasma using differential density gradient centrifugations are modern versions of established techniques that have proven to be successful for more than 25 yr *(6)*.

The preparation of primary human hepatocytes described here is an adaptation of the basic two-step collagenase method by Seglen *(7)*, which is straightforward and in our hands very reliable for isolation of primary hepatocytes from different species.

2. Materials

2.1. Solutions

1. TNE: 20 m*M* Tris-HCl, pH 7.4, 140 m*M* NaCl, 1 m*M* EDTA.

All sucrose solutions should be made as w/w.

2. To prepare a 60% (w/w) sucrose solution, dilute 60 g of sucrose with 40 g of TNE.
3. The density of the CsCl solutions (in TNE, pH 7.4) should be adjusted by use of a refractometer.
4. 0.2 *M* Sodium bicarbonate, pH 8.0: Dissolve 1.68 g of sodium bicarbonate in 100 mL of sterile double-distilled water and adjust the pH by the use of 1 *M* HCl.
5. 1.5 *M* Hydroxylamine, pH 8.0: Dissolve 1.04 g of hydroxylamine in 10 mL of sterile double-distilled water and adjust the pH with 5 *M* NaOH.

All media and supplements were purchased from Gibco/Invitrogen.

6. Hepatocyte dissociating medium: Dulbecco's modified Eagle's medium (DMEM) (with 4-(2-hydroxyethyl) piperazine-1-ethanesulfonic acid [HEPES], pH 7.4, without bicarbonate), supplemented with 0.05% collagenase (type II).
7. Hepatocyte washing medium: Hank's buffered salt solution (HBSS, with $CaCl_2$).
8. Hepatocyte plating medium: Williams E medium, supplemented with 10% fetal calf serum.
9. Hepatocyte cultivating medium: Williams E medium, supplemented with 0.1% bovine serum albumin (BSA) (crystallized), 5 µg/mL of insulin, 5 µ/mL of holo-transferrin, 5 ng/mL of sodium selenite, 100 IU/mL of penicillin, 0.1 mg/mL of streptomycin, 0.25 µg/mL of amphotericin B, 0.4 µg/mL of dexamethasone, and 1% dimethyl sulfoxide (DMSO).

10. Collagen-coated coverslips: coverslips were incubated with 0.5 mg/mL of collagen I (from rat tail, Falcon) for 2 h and washed two times with sterile phosphate-buffered saline (PBS).
11. Binding medium: DMEM (without phenol red, without bicarbonate, with 20 m*M* HEPES, pH 7.4) supplemented with 0.1% BSA (crystallized).
12. Fixative: 3% Paraformaldehyde (PFA) in PBS. Add 6 g of PFA to 180 mL of double-distilled water and incubate at 50°C with agitation. After the PFA has been dissolved, add 20 mL of 10X PBS (without calcium). The solution can be stored at 4°C for 14 d.
13. Permeabilization: 0.1% Triton X-100 in PBS.
14. Blocking buffer: 10% Normal goat serum in PBS
15. Embedding: Mowiol–DABCO: Dissolve 3.4 g of Mowiol with 6 g of glycerol for 1 h by gentle agitation. Add 6 mL of double-distilled water and stir for an additional 2 h. Add 12 mL of 0.2 *M* Tris-HCl, pH 8.5, and incubate at 50°C for 15 min. Centrifuge at 5000*g* for 15 min. Divide into aliquots of 1.0 mL in 1.5-mL tubes and store at –20°C. For use, dissolve 100 mg of 1.4-diazabicyclo(2.2.2)octan (DABCO), antifading agent, in 1 mL of Mowiol and store at 4°C in the dark for up to 14 d.

2.2. Equipment

1. Ultracentrifuge (e.g., Beckman Optima L-80) and SW 28 rotor with six tubes of 1 × 3½ in.
2. Cooled centrifuge for 50-mL tubes (e.g., Eppendorf).
3. Peristaltic pump (e.g., Masterflex).
4. Confocal laser-scanning microscope unit (Leica).

2.3. Tissues for Study

Fresh liver from surgery should be placed on ice immediately. The material has to contain at least 1 cm^3 tissue for isolation by two-step perfusion technique. The patient should be tested before partial hepatectomy for markers of HBV infection. Be sure to satisfy all ethical and safety requirements.

3. Methods

3.1. Purification of Subviral Particles from Plasma of HBV-Infected Patients

3.1.1. First Sucrose Density Gradient Centrifugation

1. Make a discontinuous sucrose gradient from 60–15% (w/w) in TNE. Pour the sucrose solutions (2 mL of 60%, 4 mL of 45%, 4 mL of 35%, 5 mL of 25%, 5 mL of 15%) slowly into a 38.5-mL polyallomer ultracentrifuge tube. Be careful not to disturb the different layers. Let the gradient rest for at least 4 h at 4°C.
2. Centrifuge the plasma in 50-mL tubes at 1700*g* for 15 min.
3. Take 19 mL of the clear supernatant and load it carefully onto the gradient. At least 4–5 mm of the tube should be free of plasma.
4. Centrifuge in a SW 28 rotor at 25,000 rpm (112,000*g*) for 15 h at 10°C.
5. After the run put a cannula from the top down into the tube and fractionate the gradient in 1.3-mL fractions from the bottom with the help of a pump.
6. Determine the sucrose density with a refractometer and the optical density at 280 nm (OD_{280}) in a photometer.
7. Characterize the fractions containing virus by dot blot or real time polymerase chain reaction (PCR) and the fractions containing subviral particles by sodium dodecyl sulfate-polyacrylamide gel electrophoresis (SDS-PAGE) or enzyme-linked immunosorbent assay (ELISA) (this requires appropriate dilution to avoid saturation of signals) against HBV sur-

face proteins (**Fig. 1**).. Usually the virus will concentrate at fractions 3 and 4, the HBV filaments at fractions 5 and 6 and the spheres at fractions 7–11. At fraction 12 the portion of contaminating serum proteins will be so high that these fractions are not suitable for the further preparation of subviral particles.

3.1.2. Cesium Chloride Flotation

1. For further purification using a CsCl gradient, pool the HBsAg containing fraction from **Subheading 3.1.1.** and adjust them with solid CsCl to a density of 1.31 g/cm^3.
2. Make a discontinuous CsCl gradient by placing 4 mL of CsCl solution (1.35 g/cm^3) into a 38.5-mL polyallomer ultracentrifuge tube.
3. Next overlay with the pooled samples (13 mL) with a density of 1.31 g/cm^3.
4. Continue with the next layers (6 mL of 1.27 g/cm^3, 6 mL of 1.24 g/cm^3, and 7 mL of 1.16 cm^3).
5. Centrifuge in a SW 28 rotor at 25,000 rpm (112,000*g*) for 36 h at 10°C.
6. After the run put a cannula from the top down into the tube and fractionate the gradient in 1.3-mL fractions from the bottom with the help of a pump.
7. Determine the CsCl density with a refractometer and the optical density at 280 nm (OD_{280}) in a photometer. The HBsAg will float to lower densities, whereas the serum proteins (except for lipoproteins) will remain at a density of 1.31 g/cm^3.
8. Determine the HBsAg-containing fractions as described in **Subheading 3.1.1.**
9. Pool the HBsAg containing fractions and desalt them by dialysis or ultrafiltration (*see* **Subheading 3.1.4.**).

3.1.3. Second Sucrose Density Gradient Centrifugation

1. Layer the pooled HBsAg fractions (9 mL) onto a second sucrose gradient ranging from 60% to 5% (w/w) sucrose (5 mL of 60%, 5 mL of 25%, 5 mL of 20%, 5 mL of 15%, 5 mL of 10%, and 5 mL of 5%).
2. Centrifuge in a SW 28 rotor at 25,000 rpm (112,000*g*) for 15 h at 10°C.
3. Take 1.3-mL fractions and determine the HBsAg-containing fractions as described in **Subheading 3.1.1.** The HBsAg will band at sucrose densities of 40% to 30%.
4. Pool the HBsAg containing fractions and proceed with ultrafiltration.

3.1.4. Ultrafiltration

For labeling the HBsAg with a fluorophore using succinimidyl ester, the buffer of the reaction must not contain primary amines, that is, Tris and so forth. The HBsAg fraction will be concentrated and desalted with ultrafiltration devices (membrane cutoff: 100 kDa Vivaspin 6).

1. Fill concentrator with HBsAg up to the maximum volume and centrifuge at 3000*g* until 0.3 mL remains in the retentate.
2. Fill the concentrator with 0.2 *M* sodium bicarbonate, pH 8.0, and centrifuge again.
3. Repeat these steps three times to remove completely the Tris-containing buffer.
4. Determine the concentration of purified HBsAg with a photometer at 280 nm using the formula: 4.3 OD_{280} = 1 mg/mL of HBsAg *(6)*. For a good labeling reaction the concentration should be not below 2 mg/mL (**Fig. 2**).

3.2. Labeling of Purified Subviral Particles with a Fluorophore

For labeling purified HBV subviral particles we use the water-soluble BODIPY-FL-CASE (Molecular Probes) with succinimydyl ester as reactive group. We selected the

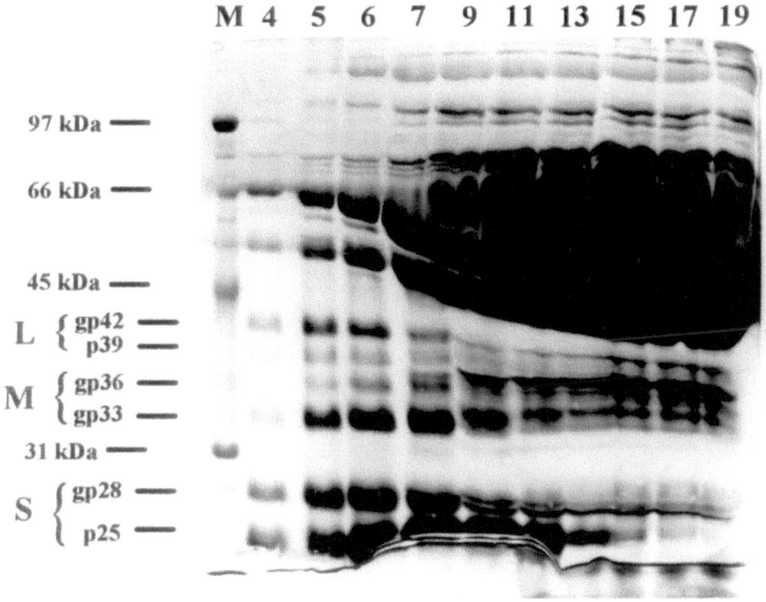

Fig. 1. Protein distribution of HBV-containing plasma after the first sucrose gradient. Ten microliters of fractions 4–19 were loaded onto a 12% SDS-PAGE-gel and visualized by silver-staining. Fraction 3 (not shown) is the virus peak, in fraction 4 virus is contaminated with filaments. Fraction 5 and 6 are filament rich, whereas the HBV spheres will concentrate at fractions 7–11. Fractions above 12 or 13 will be excluded from ongoing purification process, owing to the massive presence of plasma proteins.

amine-reactive BODIPY dyes from Molecular Probes because of their high fluorescence quantum yield and narrow emission bandwidth. BODIPY-FL-CASE has an excitation/emission maxima of 503/512 nm (fluorescein-like spectrum) but has a greater photostability than fluorescein.

1. Dissolve 0.5 mg of the fluorophore in 100 μL of 0.2 *M* sodium bicarbonate, pH 8.0, and immediately add the HBsAg from **Subheading 3.1.4.**
2. Vortex and incubate at 37°C in the dark for 1 h. Stop the reaction by adding 1/10 volume of 1.5 *M* hydroxylamine, pH 8.0.
3. Separate the conjugate from the unreacted labeling reagent using a Sephadex G-25 gel filtration column, equilibrated with PBS. The first eluted fluorescent fractions will be the labeled HBsAg.
4. If necessary, concentrate the labeled HBsAg by ultrafiltration.

3.3. Isolation of Primary Human Hepatocytes

Primary hepatocytes were purified by the modified two-step collagenase method first described by Seglen et al. *(7)*.

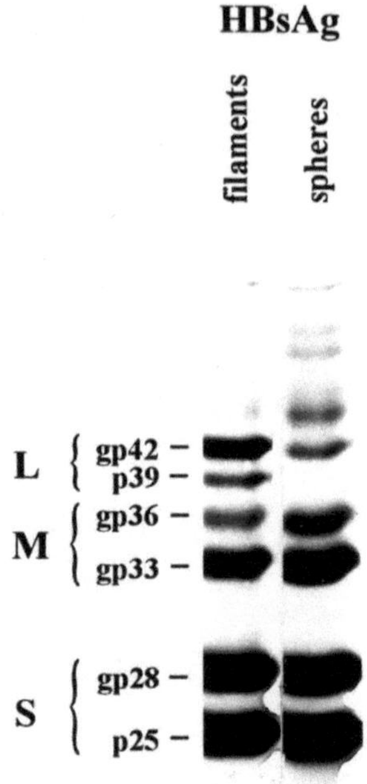

Fig. 2. Protein composition of highly purified HBsAg from HBV-containing plasma. Fractions containing filaments and spheres were divided after the first sucrose gradient and purified separately. Note that the filaments contain higher concentrations of LHBs, whereas spheres are rich in MHBs. The faint bands at higher molecular weight (> 42 kDa) are dimers.

1. Perfuse the liver section by placing the cannula tube connected to tubings filled with PBS directly into the largest visible blood vessel.
2. Turn on the pump and use a flow of approx 10–50 mL/min at room temperature (depending on the size of the section). Perfuse the liver tissue for 10–15 min. (*See* **Note 1**.)
3. Continue the perfusion with warm collagenase solution at 37°C for 15–40 min. Now the solution will be recirculated and after 15 min the consistency of the liver section will become soft with a speckled appearance. An exact perfusion time to obtain a good hepatocyte preparation cannot be given here because of the variation in the quality and batch-to-batch variability of the collagenase preparations.
4. At the end of the perfusion place the softened liver piece into a sterile culture dish and dissect the perfused parts from unperfused tissue with scalpels in 100 mL of collagenase solution.
5. Rinse, but do not press the cell homogenate through nylon mesh (pore size: 250 μm) and again through a nylon mesh of 75 μm pore size. This will yield isolated single or doublet hepatocytes.
6. Centrifuge the hepatocytes three times at 30*g* for 5 min at 4°C and aspirate the supernatants completely as they will contain mainly nonparenchymal cells and damaged hepatocytes.
7. Carefully resuspend the cells at each washing step with 4°C cold washing medium. After the last wash, resuspend the cells in plating medium and pour the cell suspension on collagen-coated coverslips (10^4 hepatocytes per coverslip) in 24-well plates.
8. After 2–8 h at 37°C, change medium to hepatocyte culture medium. The hepatocytes are now ready for uptake experiments (**Fig. 3**).

3.4. Binding and Endocytosis of Subviral Particles of HBV in Primary Hepatocytes Using Confocal Laser Scanning Microscopy

1. Dilute the BODIPY-labeled purified subviral particles in ice-cold binding medium at concentrations of 20–200 ng/mL.
2. Incubate for 60 min at 4°C for binding or for 15–30 min at 37°C for determining binding and uptake of labeled HBsAg. Because the asialoglycoprotein receptor (ASGPR), a liver-specific c-type lectin, induces endocytosis of desialylated glycoproteins ***(8)***, we desialylated the glycosylated HBsAg with neuraminidase from *Arthrobacter ureafaciens* ***(9)***. (*See* **Note 2.**)
3. Wash the coverslips five times with ice-cold binding medium. (Do not use PBS as this will result in detachment of the hepatocytes.)
4. Fix the cells in 3% PFA for 30 min at room temperature. If you do not plan to stain cell compartments with antibodies, the cells can now be mounted with Mowiol-DABCO.
5. For antibody staining, proceed with permeabilization of the cells with 0.1% Triton X-100 in PBS for 30 min, wash with PBS, and incubate the coverslips with blocking medium for 1 h at 37°C.
6. Incubate anti-endosome antibody (anti-early endosome antibody 1 [EEA1], Transduction/Pharmingen) at a dilution of 2 μg/mL in blocking buffer for 2 h at 37°C.
7. Wash cells intensively but not vigorously five times with PBS and proceed with the incubation of the second, anti-mouse-Cy5-labeled antibody (Amersham) at a concentration of 0.5 μg/mL for 1 h.
8. Wash again five times with PBS and use Mowiol-DABCO for mounting of the coverslips on the slide.
9. Let the slides dry overnight in the dark and seal the borders of the coverslips with clear nail polish.
10. Clean the coverslips with double-distilled water and proceed with microscopy or store them properly in special slide containers (Nalgene) at –20°C.

3.5. Confocal Laser Scanning Microscopy

We used a Leica DM IRBE microscope with a confocal scanning unit (Leica TCS NT, Heidelberg) and an argon–krypton laser with excitation wavelengths of 488 nm, 567 nm, and 648 nm. The excitation energy was set to 35–40% of maximum laser energy, which results in low unspecific background fluorescence of unlabeled hepatocytes. The far-red fluorescence of CY5 was corrected to blue to distinguish it from the red fluorescence of Texas red. For colocalization experiments **(Fig. 4)** we used electronic overlays of different channels, which were further processed with ADOBE Photoshop version 6.0 (ADOBE Systems).

4. Notes

1. Be sure that no air bubbles enter the liver as this will result in poor yield. The liver will change color from red-brown to light brown because of the loss of blood and this indicates the sections of the liver that are well perfused. Care has to be taken to not over-pressure the liver as this will damage the cells.
2. As a control for binding and uptake it is also possible to use Texas red-labeled holo-transferrin (Molecular Probes) which binds to the transferrin receptor and can be visualized after uptake in primary endosomes and recycling endosomes (data not shown).

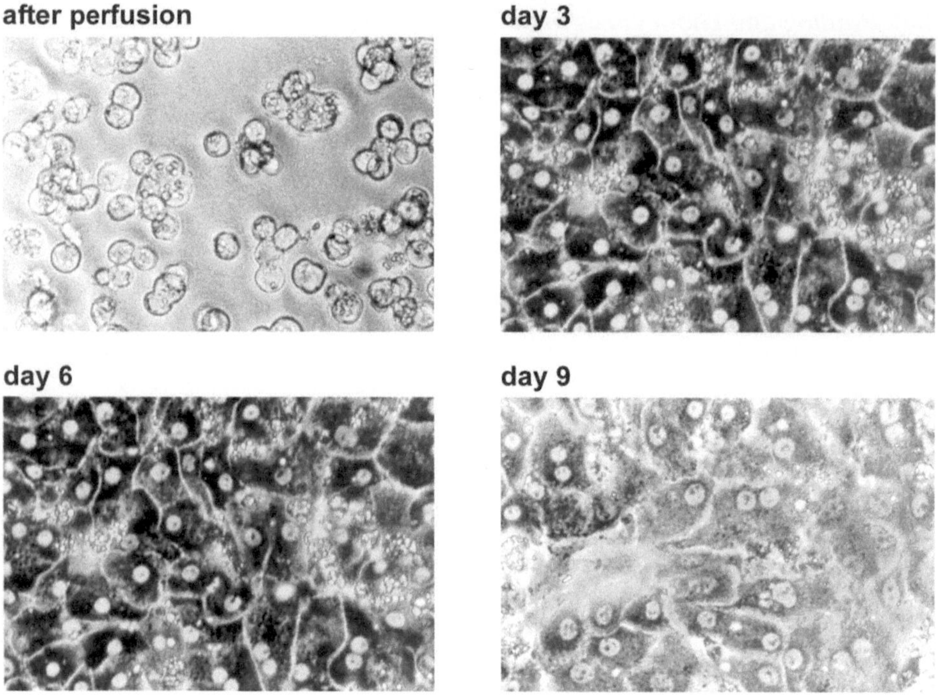

Fig. 3. Isolation and cultivation of primary human hepatocytes. Primary human hepatocytes were isolated by a two-step collagenase technique and cultivated on collagen coated coverslips. Hepatocytes preserve their shape and functionality for at least 10 d. Note the frequent presence of two nuclei and the bright borders between the cells, which are typical features of well-differentiated hepatocytes.

Acknowledgments

This work was supported by DFG SFB 535/A2. We thank Prof. Dr. Padberg for providing fresh liver tissue.

References

1. Kuroki, K., Cheung, R., Marion, P. L., and Ganem, D. (1994) A cell surface protein that binds avian hepatitis B virus particles. *J. Virol.* **68**, 2091–2096.
2. Breiner, K. M., Urban, S., and Schaller, H. (1998) Carboxypeptidase D (gp180), a Golgi-resident protein, functions in the attachment and entry of avian hepatitis B viruses. *J. Virol.* **72**, 8098–8104.
3. De Bruin, W., Leenders, W., Kos, T., Hertogs, K., Depla, E., and Yap, S. H. (1994). Hepatitis delta virus attaches to human hepatocytes via human liver endonexin II, a specific HBsAg binding protein. *J. Viral Hepat.* **1**, 33–38.
4. Chouteau, P., Le Seyec, J., Cannie, I., Nassal, M., Guguen-Guiouzo, C., and Gripon, P. (2001) A short N-proximal region in the large envelope protein harbors a determinant that contributes to the species specificity of human hepatitis B virus. *J. Virol.* **75**, 11565–11572.

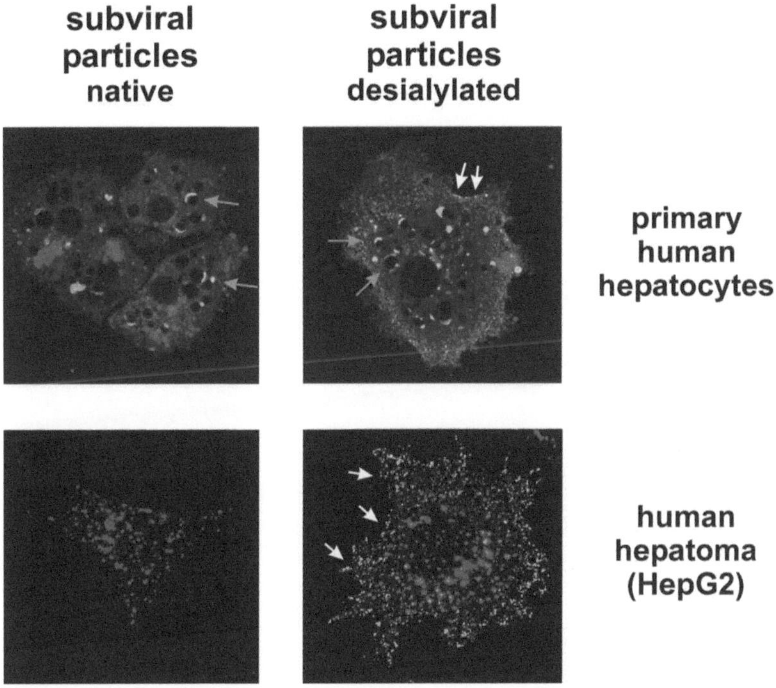

Fig. 4. Interaction of BODIPY-labeled subviral particles with primary human hepatocytes and human hepatoma cells (HepG2). Primary human hepatocytes and HepG2 cells were incubated with 200 ng/mL of BODIPY-labeled HBsAg at 37°C for 1 h, washed, and fixed. Primary endosomes were visualized using antibodies against EEA1 and a secondary Cy5-labeled antibody. Only with primary human hepatocytes do native and desialylated particles enter the cell and accumulate in round vesicles, possibly lipid storage vesicle *(gray arrows)*. Desialylated particles are located in primary endosomes only in primary human hepatocytes *(white arrows)*, indicating that they have been endocytized via the asialoglycoprotein-receptor (ASGPR). HepG2 cells are unable to bind native subviral particles, but binding could be induced by using desialylated subviral particles *(white arrows)*. However, uptake of both native and desialylated subviral particles by HepG2 cells is impaired.

5. Glebe, D., Berting, A., Broehl, S., et al. (2001) Optimised conditions for the production of hepatitis B virus from cell culture. *Intervirology* **44**, 370–378.
6. Gerlich, W. H. and Thomssen, R. (1975) Standardized detection of hepatitis B surface antigen: determination of its serum concentration in weight units per volume. *Dev. Biol. Standard.* **30**, 78–87.
7. Seglen, P. O. (1976) Preparation of isolated rat liver cells. *Methods Cell Biol.* **13**, 29–83.
8. Spiess, M. (1990) The asialoglycoprotein receptor: a model for endocytic transport receptors. *Biochemistry* **29**, 10009–10018.
9. Schmitt, S., Glebe, D., Alving, K., et al. (1999) Analysis of the PreS2 *N*- and *O*-linked glycans of the M surface protein from human hepatitis B virus. *J. Biol. Chem.* **274**, 476–482.

13

The Tupaia Model for the Study of Hepatitis B Virus

Direct Infection and HBV Genome Transduction of Primary Tupaia Hepatocytes

Fritz von Weizsäcker, Josef Köck, Sabine MacNelly, Shaotang Ren, Hubert E. Blum, and Michael Nassal

1. Introduction

With an estimated 350 million chronic carriers, hepatitis B virus (HBV) infection still represents a global health care problem. In particular, HBV is the most common cause of hepatocellular carcinoma worldwide. Replication of HBV has been extensively studied in transfected hepatoma cells, yet studies on early steps of viral infection are scarce. This is due to the fact that currently available permanent cell lines are not permissive for HBV infection, and human hepatocyte resources are limited. In this context the Asian tree shrew (*Tupaia belangeri*) has gained increasing interest. Tupaias are squirrel-sized animals closely related to primates (**Fig. 1**). Earlier studies suggested that they can be experimentally infected with human herpes simplex virus (HSV) ***(1)***, hepatitis B virus ***(2,3)***, and hepatitis C virus (HCV) ***(4)***. However, infection rates in vivo are generally very low for HBV and HCV.

To obtain a more robust model system for HBV infection, we have evaluated the use of primary tupaia hepatocytes (PTH). Using the protocols for culturing and infecting PTH described below, these cells can indeed be reproducibly infected with HBV ***(5)***. The experimental system offers a platform to study several of the unresolved problems related to binding, uptake, and uncoating of HBV in primary cells as well as antivirals. However, despite major improvements in controlling the factors determining the efficiency of HBV infection the level of HBV replication in PTH is still low.

An alternative to direct infection with HBV of PTH is the artificial introduction of HBV genomes using a gene transfer vehicle such as an adenovirus-derived vector (Ad-HBV). In this way, the limited efficiency of the HBV receptor-mediated entry process is bypassed, and essentially all PTH cells can be transduced ***(6,7)***. The rationales for using

From: *Methods in Molecular Medicine, vol. 96: Hepatitis B and D Protocols, volume 2*
Edited by: R. K. Hamatake and J. Y. N. Lau © Humana Press Inc., Totowa, NJ

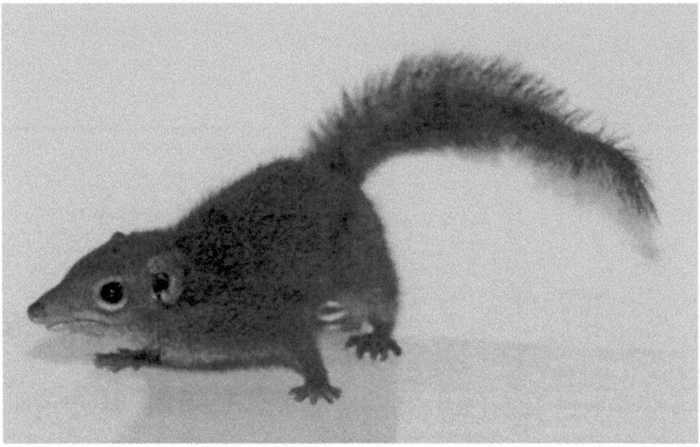

Fig. 1. An adult *Tupaia belangeri* from the colony held at the author's institution. The actual size of the animal's body is approx 15 cm.

Ad-HBV, including their potential for in vivo applications as well as protocols on their generation and characterization, are given in the chapter by Sprinzl et al. (Chapter 18). While Ad-HBV may be used to transduce HBV genomes into cells from various species, their application to PTH offers the possibility to study formation of nuclear covalently closed circular HBV DNA (cccDNA). This is not trivial because, for instance, in HBV-transgenic mice no evidence for the generation of this central intracellular intermediate of the HBV replication cycle could be obtained ***(8)***, except in a rather specific knockout background ***(9)***. By contrast, Ad-HBV transduced PTH are clearly capable of cccDNA formation ***(6)*** although the establishment of a true persistent HBV infection by this route is not yet established.

A potential problem for unambiguous proof of cccDNA formation, and particularly for quantitative determinations, for example, in therapeutic studies, is the presence of Ad-HBV DNA in the transduced cultures, especially when applied at high multiplicities of infection (MOI). Although these molecules do not support vector replication in the absence of complementation, they usually persist for the duration of the experiment, giving background signals that might interfere with HBV cccDNA detection. Similarly, cccDNA detection may be obscured by products generated from replicative HBV intermediates. The protocol given below is based on previously published procedures for cccDNA enrichment ***(6)*** but further optimized for maximal removal of non-cccDNA molecules. Essential aspects are (1) the use of isolated nuclei rather than whole cells as starting material; (2) two denaturing treatments (NaOH–SDS and NaOH, respectively) followed by neutralization/precipitation with potassium acetate and phenol extraction for removal of large DNA fragments; (3) treatment with nucleases that do not affect cccDNA but digest RNA and linear DNA, that is, RNase, a restriction enzyme that has no recognition site in HBV but several in the Ad-HBV vector, and Plasmid-Safe ATP-dependent DNase ***(10)***. The latter enzyme is virtually inactive on circular double-stranded DNA but digests linear DNAs; its original application is the removal of chromosomal DNA fragments frequently contaminating plasmid DNA preparations. Because it is an exonuclease, simultaneous treatment with a suitable restriction enzyme speeds up digestion of the Ad-vector DNA. Once the nuclear HBV cccDNA preparation is obtained, it can be processed for Southern blotting by any standard procedure.

At present both direct HBV infection of PTH and their vector-mediated transduction with HBV genomes offer new opportunities to address several, but not all, significant aspects of HBV biology. It is therefore important that our previous work has shown that the recently discovered woolly monkey hepatitis B virus (WMHBV), although less infectious for human primary hepatocytes ***(11)***, replicates much more efficiently in PTH ***(5)***. This allows the systematic analysis of the viral factors that determine the level of HBV replication in this cell culture system and should help generate HBV mutants with enhanced replication competence in tupaia cells. The same goal might be achieved by selecting for adaptive HBV mutations via serial passage in PTH, or possibly in vivo after an initial transduction using Ad-HBV. Ultimately, PTH-adapted HBV variants may prove to be useful tools for turning tupais into a general and practical small animal model of HBV infection.

2. Materials

2.1. Animal Care and Anesthesia

2.1.1. Animal Maintenance

See **Subheading 3**.

2.1.2. Anesthesia

1. 10 % Ketamine hydrochloride (115.34 mg/mL; Essex Tierarznei, Munich, Germany).
2. 2 % Xylazine hydrochloride (23.32 mg/mL; Bayer Leverkusen).
3. 26-Gauge × 1/2 needle (Sterican, Braun, Melsungen, Germany).

2.2. Liver Perfusion and Cell Culture

2.2.1. Stock Solutions and Reagents

1. 10 % Glucose dissolved in 0.9 % NaCl.
2. 0.5 *M* $CaCl_2$ dissolved in 0.9 % NaCl.
3. 15 m*M* 4-(2-Hydroxyethyl) piperazine-l-ethanesulfonic acid (HEPES).
4. 1 *M* EGTA (ethylene glycol tetraacetic acid; Titriplex VI; Merck, Darmstadt, Germany).
5. 200 m*M* Glutamine (Life Technologies, Karlsruhe, Germany).
6. 10,000 U/mL of penicillin, 10 mg/mL of streptomycin (Gibco, Karlsruhe, Germany).
7. 10 m*M* L-Hydrocortisone (water soluble; H-0390; Sigma, Munich, Germany).
8. 1 m*M* Insulin (Sigma, Munich, Germany).
9. Trypan blue (Sigma, Munich, Germany).
10. 229 U/mg of Collagenase CLSII, (Biochrom, Berlin, Germany) (*see* **Note 1**).

2.2.2. Buffers and Cell Culture Media

1. Hank's solution: 8 g of NaCl, 0.4 g of KCl, 3.57 g of HEPES, 0.06 g of $Na_2HPO_4 \cdot 2H_2O$, and 0.06 g of KH_2PO_4. Add H_2O to 1 L, adjust pH to 7.4, sterilize, and tightly close the flask.

2. Hank's solution I: Hank's solution supplemented with 5 m*M* EGTA, 1 % glucose, and penicillin–streptomycin at a dilution of 1:100.
3. Hank's solution II: Hank's solution I supplemented with 0.5 mg/mL of collagenase CLSII and 5 m*M* $CaCl_2$.
4. Williams Medium without glutamine (Biochrom, Berlin, Germany), supplemented with 10 μ*M* L-hydrocortisone, 20 μ*M* insulin, 15 m*M* HEPES, 2 m*M* glutamine, and penicillin–streptomycin at a dilution of 1:100.
5. Hepato-STIM Biocoat medium (Becton-Dickinson, Bedford, MA), supplemented with 2 m*M* glutamine, 15 m*M* HEPES, and penicillin–streptomycin at a dilution of 1:100.

2.2.3. Other Materials

1. Scalpel (no. 11; Feather PFM, Cologne, Germany).
2. Abbocath-T 18G (Venisystems, Abbott, Ireland).
3. Peristaltic pump (Reglo Digital; Isamtech, Zürich, Switzerland).
4. 70-μm mesh cell strainer (Becton-Dickinson).
5. Collagen I coated six-well plates (Becton-Dickinson).
6. Tissue culture centrifuge (Labofuge M, Heraeus, Stuttgart, Germany).

2.3. Purification of HBV Inoculum

1. Nycodenz (Nycomed Pharma AS, Oslo, Norway).
2. 11 × 34 mm polycarbonate centrifuge tubes (Beckman Instruments, Palo Alto, CA).
3. TLS55 swing-out rotor (Beckman Instruments).

2.4. Preparation of Ad-HBV Stocks

General methods for the generation of Ad-HBV vectors and characterization of the vector stocks are given by Sprinzl et al. (Chapter 18). Because of the rather broad host range and tissue tropism of adenoviruses, all work has to comply with appropriate biosafety regulations. Used equipment should be autoclaved and properly disposed of.

2.5. Infection of PTH with Ad-HBV

1. Titered stock of Ad-HBV vector (usually containing approx 10^{11} pfu/mL).
2. Primary tupaia hepatocytes cultured as described below.

2.6. Isolation and Detection of Nuclear HBV cccDNA

1. TNE buffer: 10 m*M* Tris-HCl, pH 8; 1 m*M* EDTA, 150 m*M* NaCl.
2. P1-1 buffer: 10 m*M* Tris-HCl, pH 8; 1 m*M* EDTA; 150 m*M* NaCl; 0.2% (v/v) Nonidet P-40 (NP-40).
3. P1-2 buffer: 10 m*M* Tris-HCl, pH 8; 1 m*M* EDTA; 0.2% (v/v) NP-40.
4. P2 buffer: 0.15 *M* NaOH, 6.2% sodium dodecyl sulfate (SDS).
5. P3 buffer: 3 *M* potassium acetate (adjusted to pH 4.8–5.0 using glacial acetic acid).
6. Buffer D: 1× NewEngland Biolabs restriction buffer 4, containing 1 m*M* ATP, 40 μg/mL of RNase A, 50 U/mL of *Hpa*I, and 300 U/mL of Plasmid-Safe ATP-dependent DNase.
7. Water-saturated phenol (AppliChem).
8. Glycogen (20 mg/mL; Roche).
9. RNase A (Roche).
10. Plasmid-Safe ATP-dependent DNase (Epicentre Technologies).
11. Standard equipment for agarose gel electrophoresis and Southern blotting.

3. Methods

3.1. Animal Care

3.1.1. Animal Maintenance and Breeding

Animals are kept pairwise in cages 1.50 m in height and 1 m in width. The cages are equipped with small sleeping boxes and wood. An automated light source generates a 12-h circadian rhythm. The animal facility is maintained at 70% air humidity and a temperature of 28°C. Nutrition includes fruit, vegetables, cheese, eggs, chicken-meat, and regular baby food. The animals have free access to drinking water.

The duration of pregnancy is 44 d yielding two or three newborns on average. Breast-feeding takes place once in 48 h. The offspring may be removed from the mothers and be placed on regular nutrition at the age of 5–6 wk. Adulthood is reached at the age of 12 wk and the average life expectancy of tupaias in captivity is 10 yr.

Immediately after giving birth, females are ready to conceive again. Thus, under optimal conditions a pair will produce about 25 new animals per year (*see* **Note 2**).

3.2. Preparation of Primary Hepatocytes

1. To anesthetize the animals, 5 mg/100 g body wt ketamine hydrochloride and 1 mg/100 g body wt xylazine hydrochloride are injected intramuscularly. Expect full anesthesia within 5 min.
2. Hank's solutions I and II are prewarmed in a 42°C water bath. The collagenase is added immediately prior to liver perfusion.
3. After shaving and cleaning the abdomen under sterile conditions, the abdominal cavity is opened and the portal vein is cannulated with a 18-gauge catheter. A silicon tube (2.4 mm diameter) is connected to the catheter and Hank's solution I is infused via a peristaltic pump at a flow rate of 20 mL/min. After starting the peristaltic pump, the vena cava and the right heart ventricle are incised to permit sufficient outflow. The liver is perfused with solution I for 5 min, followed by Hank's solution II for 13–15 min. Correct placement of the portal vein catheter is evidenced during perfusion by the steady and even color change in all liver lobes (*see* **Note 3**).
4. Following perfusion the liver and the gall bladder are removed, and the liver is transferred to a sterile crystal dish.
5. All of the following steps are performed in a sterile hood.
6. The liver capsule is carefully removed with a pincette. Gentle shaking will then disintegrate the perfused liver, yielding a suspension of single cells, some cell clumps, and cell debris.
7. The suspension is placed onto a 70-μg cell strainer and is filtered through the mesh by gravity flow.
8. The suspension is transferred to a 50-mL Falcon tube and washed twice with Williams medium (room temperature).
9. Cells are centrifuged at room temperature at 37.5*g* for 2 min in a cell culture centrifuge (*see* **Note 4**).
10. The cells are resuspended in Williams medium and the percentage of intact cells is determined by staining an aliquot with trypan blue. On average 80–90% of the cells will be viable.
11. The cells are seeded onto collagen-coated six-well plates at a density of 1–1.25 million cells per well and kept in a cell culture incubator at 37°C and 5% CO_2. After 4 h the cells are carefully rinsed in Williams medium, which is then replaced by Hepato-STIM medium.

3.3. Purification of the HBV Inoculum and Infection of PTH

We have previously observed that a human serum component inhibits binding of HBV particles to PTH, thus strongly limiting the efficiency of infection. The precise nature of the inhibitory factor is unclear at present. Fortunately, however, the factor can be easily separated from infectious HBV virions by gradient sedimentation using the iodinated benzoic acid derivate Nycodenz (*see* **Note 5**).

1. A 50% (w/v) Nycodenz stock solution is prepared in Hepato-STIM medium and is diluted in Hepato-STIM medium to generate solutions containing 42, 33, 25, 16, and 8% Nycodenz, respectively. Two hundred microliters of each solution is layered stepwise in 11 × 34 mm polycarbonate centrifuge tubes.
2. Two hundred microliters of infectious serum (*see* **Note 6**) is loaded onto the top of the gradient and the samples are centrifuged for 40 min at 55,000 rpm at 20°C in a TLS55 swing-out rotor (200,000*g*).
3. Subsequently, 155-μL aliquots are removed, beginning at the top. Fractions 1–4 contain the inhibitory factor and are discharged. Infectious HBV virions are present in fractions 5–8.
4. These fractions are added to PTH 1 d after seeding in 1 mL of Hepato-STIM medium. The inoculum remains on the cells overnight and the culture medium is replaced daily afterward.
5. Extraction of total DNA from infected PTH, agarose gel electrophoresis, and Southern blot analysis are performed according to previously published standard protocols. In a typical experiment cccDNA can be detected 5–7 d post-inoculation and single-stranded DNA is visible about 14 d post-inoculation. Compared with transfected hepatoma cells, the replication level of HBV in PTH is low.

3.4. Infection of PTH with Ad-HBV (See *Note 7*)

The following procedure refers to infection of PTHs seeded in 10 cm diameter dishes at a density of approx 5×10^6 cells.

1. Mix an aliquot of virus stock solution containing the appropriate number of plaque-forming units (pfu) with 2 mL/10 cm dish of Biocoat medium and add to the cells. Keep at 37°C in a CO_2 incubator for 1.5 h with occasional rocking.
2. Add supplemented Biocoat Hepato-STIM medium (*see* **Subheading 2.2.**). Add a 10-mL volume and continue incubation for the desired time; media should be changed every 2 d.
3. Conditioned media may be stored at 4°C for later analysis of secreted gene products (HBsAg, HBeAg, virions).

3.5. Isolation of Nuclear cccDNA

1. For maximal levels of cccDNA, harvest the cells 4–8 d post-infection. Wash the cell layer once with 10 mL of TNE buffer, then add 2 mL of P1-1 buffer per 10-cm dish, incubate briefly, and scrape all material off the plate using a rubber policeman. Collect the suspension in suitably sized centrifugation tubes, for example, equally distributed into two 2-mL Eppendorf tubes.
2. Centrifuge for 10 min at about 11,000*g*, and separate the supernatant (containing cores; *see* **Note 8**) from the pellet (nuclei).
3. To the nuclear pellet (*see* **Note 9**) add 1–2 mL of ice-cold P1-2 buffer (*see* **Note 10**); keep on ice to proceed immediately, or store at –80°C for later use.

4. Add the same volume of P2 buffer as P1-2 used in **step 3**, mix vigorously by vortexing; then incubate for 15–30 min at 37°C, mix occasionally.
5. Add 0.7 the volume of ice-cold P3 buffer as P1-2 used in **step 3** and mix immediately by inverting the tube several times; vortex-mix until the solution is no longer viscous. Keep on ice for 30 min with occasional mixing.
6. Centrifuge at 11,000*g* for 20 min at 4°C, and carefully transfer the supernatant (containing episomal DNA) into a fresh tube.
7. Extract the supernatant with an equal volume of water-saturated phenol and recover the aqueous phase.
8. Add glyogen to 20 μg/mL (*see* **Note 11**) and precipitate nucleic acids by adding 0.7 volume of isopropanol; centrifuge at 15,000*g* for 30 min at 4°C.
9. Carefully remove the liquid phase, then wash the nucleic acid pellet with 1 mL of 70% ethanol; recover nucleic acids by centrifugation, remove the liquid phase, and let air-dry.
10. To remove RNA and linear DNAs resuspend the nucleic acid pellet in 500 μL of buffer D and incubate for at least 2 h at 37°C (*see* **Note 12**).
11. Add 80 μL of 0.4 *M* NaOH and incubate at 37°C for 5 min.
12. Add 160 μL of buffer P3 and mix immediately; extract the solution once or twice with 750 μL of cold water-saturated phenol, and recover the aqueous phase.
13. Precipitate the DNA by adding an equal volume of isopropanol plus glycogen to 1 μg/mL (*see* **Note 11**), wash the pellet with 70% ethanol
14. Resuspend the pellet in 20 μL of TE buffer; one half of the preparation may be used for restriction digestion with a single-cutting enzyme, for example, *Xho*I; HBV-containing fragments originating from remaining Ad-HBV vector DNA will have a different size that can easily be distinguished from the 3.2-kb fragment generated from HBV cccDNA.
15. Perform Southern blotting by any standard procedure using a radioactively or otherwise labeled probe specific for HBV; on a standard 1% agarose gel (*see* **Note 13**) run in TAE buffer containing 0.5 μg/mL of ethidium bromide. HBV cccDNA will typically migrate at a position equivalent to that of a 1.8- to 1.9-kb linear double-stranded DNA.

4. Notes

1. Collagenase is the essential component for liver perfusion. Importantly, there are considerable variations between batches. Therefore, it is recommended to test a variety of batches and then order a large stock of the selected batch.
2. For successful breeding of tupaias several factors should be taken into account. (1) Not every pair will "match." If no offspring are produced within 4–6 mo, new pair formations should be tested. (2) Cannibalism is a notorious problem in tupaia colonies. It is known that tupaias are exquisitely sensitive toward a variety of changes in their environment, most notably noise. Indeed, tupaias are commonly used in stress research. Any kind of stress will greatly enhance the likelihood of cannibalism. To overcome this problem, conditions for animal maintenance should be kept as stable as possible. Another approach is to isolate newborns from their mothers as early as 1–2 d after birth and to raise them by hand-feeding. Obviously, however, this cumbersome procedure does not seem suitable for large-scale breeding. The easiest way to overcome both the matching-pair problem and cannibalism is to start up with as many animals as possible.
3. Depending on the length of the silicon tube and the flow rate, the actual temperature of solutions at the end of the tube may drop sharply thus greatly diminishing the collagenase activity. Therefore, it is recommended to measure the temperature at the end of the tube (outflow) and adjust the temperature of the water bath so that the outflow temperature is 37°C.

4. Primary hepatocytes are sensitive to physical stress. Therefore, all manipulations (in particular resuspensions) should be performed with great care.
5. Nycodenz can probably be substituted for by other density gradient media, but this has not been systematically analyzed by the authors. Nycodenz may also be dissolved in phosphate-buffered saline, but occasionally a precipitate entrapping most HBV virions may form in the gradient resulting in greatly reduced infectivity. This effect can be avoided by dissolving Nycodenz in Hepato-STIM medium.
6. Ideally, the titer of the inoculum should be $\geqslant 10^8$ virus genome equivalents per millimeter. Importantly, however, not all HBV-positive sera are equally effective, despite equal DNA titers (J. Kök and F. von Weizsäker, *unpublished observations*). The reasons accounting for this observation are unclear at present.
7. In numerous infection experiments with Ad-HBV vectors carrying a GFP marker gene in the vector, we never observed a spread or plaque formation, in keeping with the expected dependence of these vectors on complementation. Nonetheless, all operations should be performed with great care under a laminar flow hood in an approved facility; all personnel involved should be vaccinated against HBV.
8. The supernatant obtained in this way is suitable for analyzing core particle associated HBV DNA.
9. When establishing the protocol, we found it useful to add, at this step, a known amount of plasmid DNA to a nuclear pellet from nontransduced cells and take it through the entire procedure. In this way, the recovery yield, potential nicking of the cccDNA during the treatments, as well as the performance of the individual batch of agarose used in Southern blotting (*see* **Note 13**) can be assessed.
10. Keeping the volume of initially added buffer P1-2 small will make the preparation more convenient because of the smaller tubes/fewer centrifugation steps required. Particularly at higher cell densities, however, using the larger volume is recommended. The volume ratios of buffers P2 and P3 to P1-2 must be kept constant.
11. Glycogen acts as an inert carrier that increases the efficiency of DNA precipitation; this is especially of concern for the second precipitation because the total concentration of nucleic acids will be drastically reduced by the enzymatic treatment.
12. Because Plasmid-Safe DNAse is an exonuclease, digestion of large DNA fragments takes time; the incubation period can be extended to overnight digestion without negative effects on HBV cccDNA.
13. We have found that some batches of agarose used for gel electrophoresis give relatively fuzzy bands with the small amounts of cccDNA, although this effect may not be obvious with larger amounts of plasmid DNA that are detectable by ethidium bromide staining. Electrophoresis grade agarose from Bio-Rad usually works well but, if problems are encountered with cccDNA detection, performance of the individual agarose batch in use may be tested as described in **Note 9**.

References

1. Darai, G., Schwaier, A., Komitowski, D., and Munk, K. (1978) Experimental infection of *Tupaia belangeri* (tree shrews) with herpes simplex virus types 1 and 2. *J. Infect. Dis.* **137**, 221–226.
2. Yan, R. Q., Su, J. J., Huang, D. R., Gan, Y. C., Yang, C., and Huang, G. H. (1996) Human hepatitis B virus and hepatocellular carcinoma. I. Experimental infection of tree shrews with hepatitis B virus. *J. Cancer Res. Clin. Oncol.* **122**, 283–238.

3. Walter, E., Keist, R., Niederost, B., Pult, I., and Blum, H. E. (1996) Hepatitis B virus infection of tupaia hepatocytes in vitro and in vivo. *Hepatology* **24**, 1–5.
4. Xie, Z. C., Riezu-Boj, J. I., Lasarte, J. J., et al. (1998) Transmission of hepatitis C virus infection to tree shrews. *Virology* **244**, 513–520.
5. Kök, J., Nassal, M., MacNelly, S., Baumert, T. F., Blum, H. E., and von Weizsäker, F. (2001) Efficient infection of primary tupaia hepatocytes with purified human and woolly monkey hepatitis B virus. *J. Virol.* **75**, 5084–5089.
6. Ren, S. and Nassal, M. (2001) Hepatitis B virus (HBV) virion and covalently closed circular DNA formation in primary tupaia hepatocytes and human hepatoma cell lines upon HBV genome transduction with replication-defective adenovirus vectors. *J. Virol.* **75**, 1104–1116.
7. Sprinzl, M. F., Oberwinkler, H., Schaller, H., and Protzer, U. (2001) Transfer of hepatitis B virus genome by adenovirus vectors into cultured cells and mice: crossing the species barrier. *J. Virol.* **75**, 5108–5118.
8. Chisari, F. V. (1996) Hepatitis B virus transgenic mice: models of viral immunobiology and pathogenesis. *Curr. Top. Microbiol. Immunol.* **206**, 149–73.
9. Raney, A. K., Eggers, C. M., Kline, E. F., et al. (2001) Nuclear covalently closed circular viral genomic DNA in the liver of hepatocyte nuclear factor 1 alpha-null hepatitis B virus transgenic mice. *J. Virol.* **75**, 2900–2911.
10. Delaney, IV, W. E. and Isom, H. C. (1998) Hepatitis B virus replication in human HepG2 cells mediated by hepatitis B virus recombinant baculovirus. *Hepatology* **28**, 1134–1146.
11. Chouteau, P., Le Seyec, J., Cannie, I., Nassal, M., Guguen-Guillouzo, C., and Gripon, P. (2001) A short N-proximal region in the large envelope protein harbors a determinant that contributes to the species specificity of human hepatitis B virus. *J. Virol.* **75**, 11565–11572.

14

Delivery of Hepatitis B Virus Therapeutic Agents Using Asialoglycoprotein Receptor–Based Liver-Specific Targeting

Masayoshi Konishi, Catherine H. Wu, and George Y. Wu

1. Introduction

Many kinds of vectors for gene transfer have been developed in the last 20 yr. These include viral vectors such retroviruses ***(1,2)***, adenoviruses ***(3,4)***, and adeno-associated viruses ***(5)***; nonviral vectors utilizing cell-specific recognizing components ***(6,7)***; and lipid-mediated liposomes ***(8)***. Some of these gene-transfer methods have reached Phase I and II clinical trials, while others are still in the laboratory. This chapter focuses on protocols for the use of asialoglycoprotein receptor–based carriers to alter hepatitis B virus (HBV) viral replication in cell culture and animal models.

We have demonstrated previously that foreign genes can be targeted to hepatocytes in vitro ***(9)*** and in vivo ***(7)*** using a nucleic acid carrier system based on recognition by asialoglycoprotein receptor (ASGPR). The ASGPR is a receptor that can recognize and internalize galactose-terminal (asialoglycoproteins) through receptor-mediated endocytosis. Furthermore, this receptor is present in large numbers only on the surface of adult mammalian hepatocytes. The nucleic acid carrier system is composed of: (1) a liver cell targeting component consisting of an asialoglycoprotein; (2) a DNA binding component, usually a polycation such as poly-L-lysine, which can bind DNA in a strong, but noncovalent manner based on electrostatic attraction; and (3) in some cases, addition of a membranolytic component can be advantageous. Mixing of this conjugate with DNA in the proper proportions resulted in complexes that allowed delivery of DNA, and foreign gene expression in hepatocytes. In addition to new gene expression due to introduction of double-stranded DNA, the ASGPR-mediated DNA carrier system has also been used to deliver single-stranded antisense oligonucleotides. We have successfully demonstrated the inhibitory effects of antisense oligonucleotides on HBV gene expression in an HBV-producing hepatoma cell line ***(10)***, and in a liver cell line, Huh7, transiently transfected with an HBV expression plasmid ***(11)***. Furthermore, the targeted delivery of antisense oligonucleotides based on this system was

From: *Methods in Molecular Medicine, vol. 96: Hepatitis B and D Protocols, volume 2*
Edited by: R. K. Hamatake and J. Y. N. Lau © Humana Press Inc., Totowa, NJ

used to inhibit viral gene expression and replication in woodchuck hepatitis virus-infected woodchucks *(12)*.

Glycoproteins such as fetuin *(13)*, orosomucoid purified from serum and desialylated in the laboratory *(14,15)*, have been used as natural ligands for ASGPR. Large-batch purification of human orosomucoid from serum and rapid and convenient desialyation to obtain asialoorosomucoid (ASOR) have been achieved. This makes ASOR an attractive ligand to be used for synthesizing liver-specific carriers. Other investigators have used artificially generated galactose-terminated neoglycoproteins as liver-specific delivery agents *(16)*. Detailed protocols for the purification of ASOR from serum, synthesis of asialoorosomucold–polylysine (ASOR–PL) conjugate and its purification have been published elsewhere *(15)*. In the following sections, protocols are provided for the preparation of ASOR–PL complexes with antisense oligonucleotides, and methods for assaying for the effectiveness of the complexes on HBV replication.

2. Materials

Unless otherwise specified all chemicals were obtained from Sigma-Aldrich, St. Louis, MO.

2.1. Cell and Cell Culture

1. Huh7, asialoglycoprotein receptor (+) human liver cell line (from Dr. T. Jake Liang, NIH, Bethesda, MD).
2. SK Hep1, asialoglycoprotein receptor (–) human liver cell line (from Dr. David Shafritz, Albert Einstein College of Medicine, Bronx, NY).
3. HepG2 2.2.15, asialoglycoprotein receptor (+) cells, that constitutively produce infectious HBV particles (from Dr. George Acs, Mt. Sinai Medical Center, NY).
4. Dulbecco's modified Eagle's medium (DMEM) (Gibco/BRL, Gaithersburg, MD).
5. Heat-inactivated fetal calf serum (FCS) (Gibco/BRL).
6. CoStar tissue culture dishes, 6-well and 48-well from Corning, Corning, NY.

2.2. Antisense DNA and Gel Retardation Assay

1. A 21-mer phosphorothioate-linked oligonucleotide (TTTATAAGGGTCAATGTCCAT) was prepared complementary to the polyadenylation signal, and sequences immediately upstream of the HBV genome.
2. A random sequence of the same length and linkage as a negative control. Both oligonucleotides were obtained from Midland Certified Reagent Company (Midland, TX). The antisense oligonucleotides were purified to homogeneity by reverse-phase high-pressure liquid chromatography, and their appropriate sizes determined by denaturing polyacrylamide gel electrophoresis by the company.
3. ASOR–PL carrier *(15)*.
4. Ultrapure agarose (Gibco/BRL).
5. Gel running buffer: 0.09 *M* Tris-phosphate–0.002 *M* ethylene diaminetetraacetic acid (TPE).
6. Horizontal gel electrophoresis apparatus, model H5 (Gibco/BRL).

2.3. Preparation of Antisense Oligonucleotide–ASOR–PL Complexes

1. 1.0-cm Spectropore dialysis tubing, 1-kDa exclusion limit (Fisher Scientific, Pittsburgh, PA).

2. NaCl solution with the following concentrations: 2.0 *M*, 1.5 *M*, 1.0 *M*, 0.5 *M*, 0.25 *M*, and 0.15 *M*.
3. 0.45-μm Acrodisc filter (Gelman Sciences, Ann Arbor, MI).

2.4. Uptake of Antisense DNA Complexes by Hepatocytes

1. [γ-^{32}P]ATP (Amersham, Piscataway, NJ).
2. T4 polynucleotide kinase (Invitrogen, Carlsbad, CA).
3. 10 m*M* Ethylene diaminetetraacetic acid–phosphate-buffered saline (EDTA–PBS), pH 6.0.
4. 10 mg/mL of ASOR, in 0.15 *M* NaCl.

2.5. Assay for Hepatitis B

1. Hepatitis B surface antigen enzyme-linked immunosorbent assay (ELISA) kits (Abbott Labs, North Chicago, IL).
2. Hepatitis B e antigen ELISA kits (Abbott Labs).

2.6. Isolation of Core-Associated HBV DNA from Huh7 Cells

1. 10 m*M* Tris-HCl, pH 7.5; 10 m*M* EDTA.
2. RNase A.
3. Proteinase K (Gibco/BRL).
4. Tris-saturated phenol (Invitrogen).
5. Chloroform.
6. Lysis buffer: 20 m*M* Tris-HCl, pH 7.5, 100 m*M* NaCl, 0.5 % Nonidet P-40 (NP-40), 1 m*M* EDTA
7. $MgCl_2$.
8. DNase I (Invitrogen).
9. Sucrose.
10. Proteinase K–SDS solution: 10 m*M* Tris-HCl, pH 7.6, 10 m*M* EDTA, 1% sodium dodecyl sulfate (SDS), 1 mg/mL of proteinase K.
11. Sorvall RC5 centrifuge, SS-34 rotor.
12. Beckman L5 centrifuge, SW41 rotor.

2.7. Long Polymerase Chain Reaction (PCR) for HBV DNA

1. Primer from nucleotides 2936–2956 in the adw 2 HBV genome, at 20 m*M*.
2. Primer from nucleotides 2957–2977 in the adw 2 HBV genome, at 20 m*M*.
3. Klentaq DNA polymerase 5 U/μL (Ab Peptides, St. Louis, MO).
4. Exo$^-$*Pfu* DNA polymerase 2–3 U/μL (Promega, Madison, WI).
5. Bovine serum albumin (BSA) (Gibco/BRL).
6. dNTP 10 m*M* stock solution (Gibco/BRL).
7. 10X PCR buffer mix: 200 m*M* Tris-HCl, pH 8.55, at 25°C, 1.5 mg/mL of BSA, 160 m*M* ammonium sulfate, 35 m*M* magnesium sulfate, 0.4% (w/v) Triton X-100.
8. PCR reaction mixture: 10.0 μL of 10X PCR buffer, 1.25 m*M* dNTP stock, 1.0 m*M* sense primer, 1.0 m*M* antisense primer, and 1.2 mL of KlenTaq/*Pfu* enzyme mix.
9. DNA template-core associated HBV DNA isolated from medium or cells at 2 mg/mL.

2.8. RNase Protection Assay

1. pGEM-HBs plasmid containing nt 28–248 of adw HBV genome in pGEM-5Zf(+) vector.
2. Sal 1 (Gibco/BRL).
3. T7 RNA polymerase (Invitrogen).

4. 5X T7/T3 RNA polymerase buffer (Invitrogen).
5. RNase-free DNase I (Boehringer-Mannheim, Indianapolis, IN).
6. RPA II kit (Ambion, Austin, TX).
7. RNase A and T1 (Ambion).
8. 10 m*M* Dithiothreitol (DTT).
9. rNTP (minus UTP), 2.5 m*M* each (Promega).
10. RNasin Ribonuclease Inhibitor (Promega).
11. Water-saturated phenol (Gibco/BR).
12. XAR film (Kodak, Rochester, NY).
13. Bio-Rad Video Densitometer model 260 (Bio-Rad Labs, Hercules, CA).

3. Methods

3.1. Cell Culture

Huh7 [ASGP receptor (+) cells], SK Hep1 cells [ASGP receptor (–) cells], and HepG2 2.2.15 are cultured in DMEM containing 10% FCS at 37°C, 5% CO_2.

3.2. Gel Retardation Assay

This assay is used to determine the minimum amount of ASOR–PL protein carrier needed to bind antisense oligonucleotide to retard the mobility of antisense oligonucleotide in a 1% agarose gel electrophoresis.

1. Dissolve antisense oligonucleotide making a solution of 1 mg/mL in 0.15 *M* NaCl.
2. Dissolve ASOR-PL carrier making a solution of 1.0 mg/mL in 0.15 *M* NaCl.
3. Prepare a series of samples by adding 20-μL aliquots of ASOR–PL solutions to 20 μL of antisense oligonucleotide or plasmid DNA to give ASOR–PL/DNA mass ratios of 4.0:1, 3.0:1, 2.5:1, 2.0:1, 1.0:1, 0.5:1, 0.1:1, and 0:1. Mix the samples and leave at 25°C for 15 min.
4. Apply the samples onto 1% agarose gel using 1X Tris-phosphate–EDTA as running solution, run electrophoresis at 50 V for 30 min (*see* **Note 1**).
5. A representative gel retardation assay of ASOR–PL carrier bound to varying ratios of antisense oligonucleotide DNA is shown in **Fig. 1**.

3.3. Preparation of HBV Antisense-ASOR–PL Complexes

1. Using the weight ratio of antisense to ASOR–PL carrier determined in **Subheading 3.2.**, add antisense oligonucleotide DNA at 1 mg/mL of 2 *M* NaCl to 600 μL of ASOR–PL carrier at 0.50 mg/mL in 2 *M* NaCl at 25°C.
2. Put the mixture in 1.0-cm (flat width) dialysis tubing with an exclusion limit of 1 kDa.
3. Dialyze stepwise at 4°C for 0.5 h against 1 L of 1.5 *M*, 1.0 *M*, 0.5 *M*, 0.25 *M*, and 0.15 *M* successively.
4. Filter complex through 0.45-μm membranes.
5. Run an aliquot on 1% agarose gel (*see* **Subheading 3.2.**) to determine antisense DNA–ASOR–PL complex formation. No free DNA should be present on gel.

3.4. Assay for Liver-Specific Uptake of ASOR–PL-Antisense DNA Complex

1. Label antisense oligonucleotide with [γ-^{32}P]ATP using T4-polynucleotide kinase using standard end-labeling protocol *(17)*. The specific activity of labeled antisense oligonucleotide will be made up to 10^5 cpm/ng of DNA.

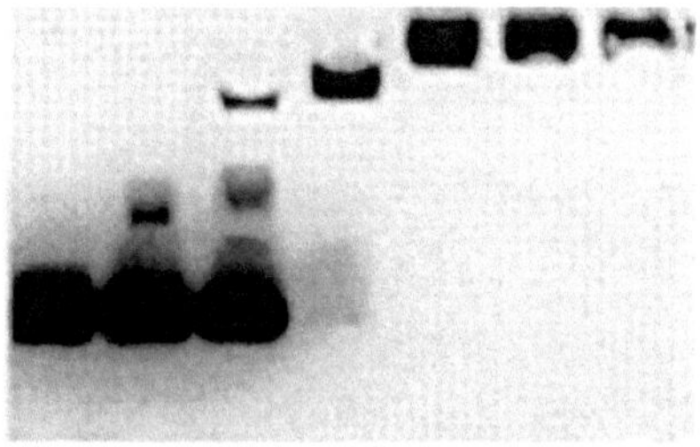

0 0.5 1 5 10 15 20

ASOR-PL (μg)

Fig.1. Effect of increasing proportion of ASOR–PL carrier on 21-mer antisense oligonucleotide DNA electrophoretic migration through a 1.0% agarose gel. ASOR–PL–antisense oligonucleotides complexes were made according to the method described in **Subheading 3.2.** and stained with ethidium bromide. Increasing amounts of ASOR-PL carrier, 0–20 μg, mixed with 2 μg of 12-mer antisense oligonucleotide DNA in each of the lanes resulted in progressive reduction of migration of the antisense oligonucleotide DNA in the complex.

2. Make a complex of ASOR–PL–^{32}P-antisense oligonucleotide DNA (*see* **Subheading 3.3.**). Adjust final specific activity to match that of ^{32}P-antisense oligonucleotide alone.
3. Make 100 mL of labeling medium ("hot medium") containing ^{32}P-antisense oligonucleotide–ASOR–PL complexes at concentration of 2.5 μ*M* with respect to antisense DNA. Take 50 mL of labeling medium and add 100X weight excess of ASOR. Label this medium "cold competitor" (*see* **Note 2**).
4. Seed 1 × 10^6 cells into 35-mm cell culture dishes. Make a set of Huh7 cells and one set of SK Hep1 cells.
5. Twenty-four hours after seeding cells, remove medium, and to one third of the dishes add 1 mL/dish of "hot medium," to the other third of dishes add 1 mL/dish of "cold competitor medium," and medium containing ^{32}P-antisense oligonucleotide alone to the last third of dishes. Put the cells back into 37°C, 5% CO_2 incubator.
6. At 30 min, 1 h, and 2 h remove three dishes of cells from each experimental group. Discard labeling medium, chill cells on ice, and wash cell surface with ice-cold 10 m*M* EDTA-PBS at pH 5.0 (*see* **Note 3**).
7. Wash cell surface quickly, three times, with ice-cold PBS, pH 7.2.
8. Add 0.5 mL of 0.01 *N* NaOH to each dish for 10 min at 25°C.
9. Collect solubilized cells into scintillation vials and save a 50 μL aliquot for protein determination using the standard Bradford assay protocol ***(18)***. To the remainder, add scintillation fluid and determine the total cellular uptake of labeled antisense oligonucleotide alone and labeled antisense oligonucleotide–ASOR–PL. Trypsinize three remaining dishes of cells and count number of cells. Express uptake as cpm per milligram of total cellular protein or cpm per number of cells. Alternatively, cpm can be converted to nanograms of labeled antisense oligonucleotide in the complex by using the initial specific activity of labeled antisense oligonucleotide and the result expressed as nanograms per milligram of total protein or nanograms per million cells.

A representative uptake of labeled antisense oligonucleotide–ASOR–PL complex by Huh7 cells and SK Hep 1 cells is shown on **Fig. 2**.

3.5. Treatment of HBV Producing Cells with HBV Antisense Oligonucleotide–ASOR–PL Complex

1. Seed 10^4 HepG2 2.2.15 cells in six-well culture dishes with DMEM plus 10% FCS.
2. Make HBV antisense–ASOR–PL complexes using methods detailed in **Subheading 3.3.** Vary the amount of HBV antisense oligonucleotide from 1 to 100 μ*M* in the liver specific carrier complexes. Controls include random antisense oligonucleotide–ASOR–PL complexes or sense oligonucleotide–ASOR–PL complexes.
3. Remove medium and add fresh medium containing varying concentrations of antisense oligonucleotide–ASOR–PL (1–100 μ*M* with respect to antisense oligonucleotide).
4. Replace daily with fresh treatment medium containing antisense–ASOR–PL complexes for the number of treatment days. Save discarded medium for HBV surface and core antigen assay and HBV core-associated particles.
5. Assay for intracellular HBV replication and core associated HBV at the end of treatment (*see* **Note 4**).

3.6. EIA Assay for HBV Surface Antigen

1. Use Abbott Labs EIA assay kit for HBV surface antigen.
2. Use 50–100 μL of medium from cells following HBV antisense oligonucleotide–ASOR–PL and follow the manufacturer's protocol for HBV surface antigen assay.

3.7. EIA for HBe antigen

Collect 200 μL of medium from cells following HBV antisense oligonucleotide–ASOR–PL treatments and follow the manufacturer's protocol to assay for HBe antigen.

3.8. Assays for HBV Replication

The effect of HBV antisense oligonucleotide–ASOR–PL complex on HBV replication can be evaluated by extracting core-associated HBV particles from medium and cell layer.

3.8.1. Isolation of Core-Associated HBV Particles from Medium and Extraction of HBV DNA

1. Clarify treated cell medium by centrifugation at 3000*g* at 15 min at 4°C, using an SS-34 rotor in a Sorvall RC5 centrifuge.
2. Centrifuge clarified medium at 41,000*g* for 24 h using SW 41 rotor, at 4°C, Beckman L5 centrifuge.
3. Resuspend the pellet in 10 m*M* Tris-HCl, pH 7.5, 10 m*M* EDTA.
4. Digest the resuspended pellet with 20 mg/mL of RNase A for 1 h at 37°C, followed by digestion with 100 μg/mL of proteinase K for 3 h at 50°C.
5. Add equal volume of phenol–chloroform (1:1), vortex-mix, centrifuge at 2000*g* for 10 min at 25°C.
6. Reextract aqueous top layer with an equal volume of chloroform. Precipitate DNA with 70% ethanol.

3.8.2. Isolation of Core-Associated HBV Particles from Cytoplasm

1. Wash treated cells two times with PBS, pH 7.2. Lyse cells with 20 m*M* Tris-HCl, pH 7.5, 100 m*M* NaCl, 0.5% NP-40, 1 m*M* EDTA.

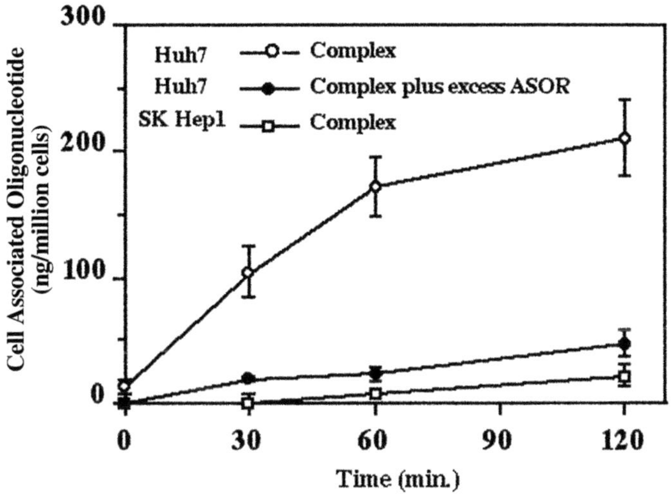

Fig. 2. Uptake of ^{32}P-21-mer HBV antisense oligonucleotide–ASOR–PL complexes in Huh7 cells and SK Hep 1 cells. Complexes were made according to the method detailed in **Subheading 3.3.** Uptake assay was performed as detailed in **Subheading 3.4.** (○) represented the uptake of labeled antisense oligonucleotide–ASOR–PL complex in Huh7 cells. Two hundred nanograms of labeled complex was taken up by 1 million Huh7 cells by 2 h. The uptake was mediated by ASGP receptors in Huh7 cells as the addition of 100-fold weight excess of unlabeled ASOR reduced uptake to minimal levels (●). The (■) represented uptake of labeled complex in SK Hep 1 cells. As expected, SK Hep 1 cells that do not have ASGP receptors took up minimal amount of antisense oligonucleotide–ASOR–PL complex.

2. Centrifuge cell lysate at 50,000*g* for 45 min at 20°C.
3. To supernatant add 1 *M* $MgCl_2$ to a final concentration of 10 m*M*.
4. Add 20 U/mL of DNase 1. Incubate for 2 h at 37°C. This step destroys noncore associated DNA.
5. Layer digest (typically 1 mL) over 9.0 mL of a 30% sucrose cushion. Centrifuge at 178,000*g* for 3 h at 20°C to collect core particles using a Beckman SW 41 rotor.
6. Digest pellet with 1 mg/mL of proteinase K in 10 m*M* Tris-HCl, pH 7.6, 10 m*M* EDTA, 1% SDS for 12 h at 37°C.
7. Extract DNA from digested material using phenol–chloroform (1:1) followed by precipitation with 2.5 volumes of ethanol.

3.8.3. Confirmation of Activity of Complexed Antisense on Viral DNA by Long PCR

To confirm the effect of antisense oligonucleotide–ASOR–PL complexes on HBV replication, full length 3.2 kb newly synthesized HBV DNA in core particles was amplified by the long PCR method ***(19)*** using the two primers detailed in **Subheading 2.2.** and a combination of KlenTaq 1 and exo$^-$*Pfu* DNA polymerases. Both enzymes are commercial heat-stable polymerases and exo⁻*Pfu* polymerase has high fidelity DNA polymerization properties.

1. Make up 10X PCR buffer mix (formula given in **Subheading 2.8.**).
2. Make up DNA polymerase mix consisting of 1/16 *Pfu* and 15/16 KlenTaq 1.
3. Adjust primer concentrations to 20 pmol/μL.
4. Make up reaction mixture.
5. Adjust template DNA to 2 mg/mL.
6. Add DNA template to reaction mixture.
7. Start PCR reaction at 68–72°C, 5 min.
8. Twenty-four cycles of 99°C, 30 s; 67°C, 30 s; 68°C, 11–24 min.
9. PCR products are analyzed by agarose gel electrophoresis stained by ethidium bromide. Look for full-length 3.2-kb HBV DNA.

3.9. Effects of Complexed Antisense on Viral RNA Levels

RNase protection assay is used to examine the effect of antisense–ASOR–PL complexes on cellular HBV RNA levels.

3.9.1. Preparation of Riboprobe

1. Linearize pGEM-HBS plasmid by digestion with Sal 1 for use as template for riboprobe.
2. Mix the following reagents at room temperature to avoid precipitation of spermidine in the T7/T3 polymerase buffer:

5X T7/T3 RNA polymerase buffer	4 μL
0.1 *M* DTT	1 μL
10 mg/mL of BSA	2 μL
rNTP (minus UTP), 2.5 m*M* each	4 μL
0.5 mg/mL of template DNA	1 μL
[α^{32}P]rUTP	6 μL
20–40 U/μL of RNasin	1 μL
50 U/μL of T7 RNA polymerase	1 μL
Total reaction volume	20 μL

3. Incubate at 37°C for 1 h.
4. Digest with 1 mL of RNase-free DNase I (15–30 U/μL) at 37°C for 15 min.
5. Add 150 μL of distilled water. Extract radiolabeled RNA once with an equal volume of phenol (water-saturated)–chloroform (1:1).
6. Extract once with equal volume of chloroform.
7. Add 0.1 volume of 5 *M* ammonium acetate to make a final concentration of 0.5 *M*.
8. Add 2.5 volumes of cold ethanol. Leave at –70°C for 10 min.
9. Precipitate RNA by centrifugation at 14,000 rpm, 4°C for 15 min. Discard the supernatant.
10. Resuspend pellet in 150 μL distilled water. Repeat **steps 5–9**.
11. Wash the RNA pellet with 75% ethanol.
12. Resuspend pellet in 50 μL of distilled water. Take a 2-μL aliquot for scintillation counting.
13. Adjust specific activity of probe to 1×10^5 cpm/ng.

3.9.2. Hybridization of Probe to RNA Sample from Treated Liver Cells

1. Extract RNA from liver cells using acid phenol method of Chomczynski and Sacci ***(20)***.
2. Measure 20 μg of cellular RNA in a 1.5-mL microfuge tube and evaporate aqueous solution.

3. Add 10 μL of solution A (RPA II kit, Ambion) and 1 μL of RNA probe (10^5 cpm) to the sample.
4. Heat 90°C for 3 min, cool on ice for 2 min and quick spin to bring all solution down.
5. Incubate at 42°C overnight (*see* **Note 5**).
6. Prepare dilute RNase solution by mixing 198 μL of RNase digestion buffer with 2 μL of RNase A/Rnase T1 mix
7. Add 200 μL of diluted RNase to sample and incubate at 37°C for 30 min.
8. Add 300 μL of the RNase inactivation/precipitation solution. Incubate at −20°C for 15 min (*see* **Note 6**).
9. Centrifuge sample at 14,000 rpm for 15 min. Remove the supernatant completely.
10. Resuspend the pellets in 8 μL of gel loading buffer II. Vortex-mix for 10 s and quick spin to pellet the sample.
11. Heat at 90°C for 3 min.
12. Apply sample onto 5% polyacrylamide/urea gel ***(21)***.
13. Run gel at 40 W until the dye is at the bottom.
14. Dry the gel.
15. Visualize bands on gel by exposure to XAR film.
16. Quantify gel bands by densitometry using a Bio-Rad Video Densitometer, Model 260. Express results as mean of the ratio of arbitrary densitometric units of HBV mRNA to β-actin mRNA signals in the same sample (*see* **Notes 7–9**).

4. Notes

1. The optimal ASOR–PL/DNA ratio for complex formation is determined from the migration of the samples with the lowest ratio that gives 80–90% DNA retardation.
2. Make up the labeling medium 1 h before commencement of uptake experiment and keep at 37°C.
3. Chilling the cells to 4°C will stop active uptake of complexes. Washing cell surface with 10 m*M* EDTA–PBS, pH 6.0, will remove cell surface bound complex.
4. HBV antisense–ASOR–PL complexes can also be used to pretreat liver cells prior to HBV infection resulting in inhibition of HBV replication, and decrease in HBV surface antigen production by the cells ***(11)***. For such experiments, cells are pretreated for 48 h with HBV antisense–ASOR–PL complexes followed by transfection with an HBV expression plasmid adwR9 or with a control expression plasmid, pTRI β-actin, not containing HBV DNA. Transfection medium is removed after 24 h, fresh medium added, and cells and cell medium assayed for HBV surface antigen and core-associated HBV DNA.
5. For quantitative detection, the labeled probe should be 3- to 10-fold molar excess over target RNA.
6. For short RNA (< 150 bp), add 100 μL of ethanol in addition to RNase inactivation/precipitation solution. For very short RNA (< 50 bp), add 200 μL of ethanol in addition to RNase inactivation/precipitation solution.
7. Bands that stay at the top of the lanes may be due to poorly purified probe, or due to residue left on the inside of microfuge tubes by manufacturing process. To avoid this problem, probe should be further purified by phenol–chloroform extraction.
8. A self-complementary probe is more likely to 'protect itself' resulting in smaller than expected, fairly intense bands in all lanes.
9. AU-rich region of the probe may locally denature (breathing) resulting in RNase degradation. In that case, RNase digestion should be carried out at lower temperature (ex. room temperature, 15°C or 4°C), or use solution T (RNase T1 only), that allow cleavage of 3'-G only.

References

1. Mulligan, R. C. (1991) Gene transfer and gene therapy: principles, prospects, and perspective, in *Etiology of Human Disease at the DNA Level* (Lindsten, J. and Peterson, U., eds.), Raven Press, New York, pp. 143–189.
2. Jolly, D. J., Yee, J.-K., and Friedmann, T. (1987) High-efficiency gene transfer into cells. *Methods Enzymol.* **149,** 10–25.
3. Rosenfeld, M. A., Yoshimura, K., Trapnell, B. C., et al. (1992) In vivo transfer of human cystic fibrosis transmenbrane conductance regulator gene to the air way epithelium. *Cell* **68,** 143–155.
4. Herz, J. and Gerald, R. D. (1993) Adenovirus-mediated transfer of low density lipoprotein receptor gene acutely accelerates cholesterol clearance in normal mice. *Proc. Natl. Acad. Sci. USA* **90,** 2812–2816.
5. Samulski, R. J., Zhu, X., Xiao, X., et al. (1991) Targeted integration of adeno-associated virus (AAV) into human chromosome 19. *EMBO J.* **10,** 3941–3950.
6. Wagner, E., Zenke, M., Cotton, M., Beug, H., and Birnstiel, M. L. (1990) Transferrin-polycation conjugates as carriers for DNA uptake into cells. *Proc. Natl. Acad. Sci. USA* **87,** 3410–3414.
7. Wu, G. Y. and Wu, C. H. (1988) Receptor-mediated gene delivery and expression in vivo. *J. Biol. Chem.* **264,** 16985–16987.
8. Felgner, P. L. and Ringold, G. M. (1989) Cationic liposome-mediated transfection. *Nature* **337,** 387–388.
9. Wu, G. Y. and Wu, C. H. (1987) Targeted gene delivery *in vitro* by soluble asialoglycoprotein–DNA complex. *J. Biol. Chem.* **262,** 4429–4432.
10. Wu, G. Y. and Wu, C. H. (1992) Specific inhibition of hepatitis B viral gene expression in vitro by targeted antisense oligonucleotides. *J. Biol. Chem.* **267,** 14236–14239.
11. Nakazono, K., Ito, Y., Wu, C. H., and Wu, G. Y. (1996) Inhibition of hepatitis B Virus replication by targeted pretreatment of complexed antisense DNA in vitro. *Hepatology* **23,** 1297–1303.
12. Bartholomew, R. M., Carmichael, E. P., Findeis, M. A., Wu, C. H., and Wu, G. Y. (1995) Targeted delivery of antisense DNA in woodchuck hepatitis virus-infected woodchucks. *J. Viral Hepat.* **2,** 273–278.
13. Wu, G. Y., Wu, C. H., and Stockert, R. J. (1985) Model for specific rescue of normal hepatocytes during methotrexate treatment of hepatic malignancy. *Proc. Natl. Acad. Sci. USA* **80,** 3078–3080.
14. Wu, G. Y., Keegan-Rogers, V., Franklin, S., Midford, S., and Wu, C. H. (1988) Targeted antagonism of galactosamine toxicity in normal rat hepatocytes in vitro. *J. Biol. Chem.* **263,** 4719–4723.
15. Findeis, M. A., Wu, C. H., and Wu, G. Y. (1994) Ligand-based carrier systems for delivery of DNA to hepatocytes. *Methods Enzymol.* 341–350.
16. Fiume, L., Busi, C., Mattioli, A., Balboni, P. G., and Barbanti-Brodano, G. (1981) Hepatocyte targeting of adenine-9-β-D-arabinofuranoside 5'-monophosphate (ara-AMP) coupled to lactosaminated albumin. *FEBS Lett.* **129,** 261–264.
17. Sambrook, J., Fritch, E. F., and Maniatis, T. (1989) *Molecular Cloning: A Laboratory Manual,* 2nd edit., Vol. 2, Cold Spring Harbor Laboratory Press, Cold Spring Harbor, NY, pp. 10.59–10.63.
18. Bradford, M. M. (1976) A refined and sensitive method for the quantitation of microgram quantities of protein utilizing the principle of protein-dye binding. *Analyt. Biochem.* **72,** 248.

19. Barnes, W. M. (1994) PCR amplification of up to 35-kb DNA with high fidelity and high yield from 1 bacteriophage templates. *Proc. Natl. Acad. Sci. USA* **91,** 2216–2220.
20. Chomczynski, P. and Sacci, N. (1987) Single-step method of RNA isolation by acid guanidinium thiocyanate–phenol–chloroform extraction. *Analyt. Biochem.* **162,** 156–159.
21. Sambrook, J., Fritch, E. F., and Maniatis, T. (1989) *Molecular cloning: A laboratory Manual,* 2nd edit., Vol. 2. Cold Spring Harbor Laboratory Press, Cold Spring Harbor, NY, pp. 11.23–11.28.

15

Woodchuck Hepatitis Virus Hepatocyte Culture Models

Norma D. Churchill and Tomasz I. Michalak

1. Introduction

Hepatocytes are the site of the most vigorous replication and virion assembly in the course of a serologically evident hepadnavirus infection. They also support persistent propagation of small quantities of hepadnavirus that continues as a serologically unapparent (occult) infection long after resolution of hepatitis or due to a primary silent invasion, as it was documented for woodchuck hepatitis virus (WHV) in the woodchuck model of hepatitis B ***(1–3)***. The lack of validated cultures of normal human hepatocytes susceptible to hepatitis B virus (HBV) and capable of supporting efficient propagation of the virus in vitro had an adverse impact in the past and continues to hamper studies on HBV pathobiology, vaccine development, and preclinical evaluation of anti-HBV agents. A number of important issues, including delineation of the nature of HBV hepatotropism, the molecular basis of HBV persistence in the liver, the mechanisms of HBV oncogenesis, and the virus effect on hepatocyte survival and function, await elucidation in the appropriate culture models. The natural occurrence of viruses similar to HBV in some lower mammals provides an opportunity to establish hepatocyte cultures permissive to *ortho*-hepadnavirus infection and to circumvent, at least to some degree, problems posed by the absence of appropriate human hepatocyte cultures. Among mammalian hepadnaviruses, WHV infection in the eastern American woodchuck (*Marmota monax*) has been validated as a valuable experimental paradigm of virologic, immunologic, and pathologic events occurring in HBV infection and hepatitis B in humans ***(3–5)***. In this laboratory, we have undertaken the task of developing primary hepatocyte cultures from both normal and WHV-infected woodchucks and lines of woodchuck hepatocytes prone to WHV in vitro ***(6,7)***. This chapter describes our experience with generation and maintenance of these cultures, and with in vitro infection and detection of WHV in these hepatocytes.

From: *Methods in Molecular Medicine, vol. 96: Hepatitis B and D Protocols, volume 2*
Edited by: R. K. Hamatake and J. Y. N. Lau © Humana Press Inc., Totowa, NJ

2. Materials

2.1. Liver Perfusion and Hepatocyte Isolation

2.1.1. Buffers and Solutions

Unless otherwise indicated all buffers are sterilized by autoclaving.

1. Calcium-free perfusion buffer: 9 m*M* 4-(2-hydroxyethyl)piperazine-1-ethanesulfonic acid (HEPES) (Calbiochem, La Jolla, CA; cat. no. 391338), pH 7.4, supplemented with 142 m*M* NaCl, 5 m*M* KCl, and 1 m*M* EGTA (Sigma Chemical, St. Louis, MO; cat. no. E4378).
2. Collagenase perfusion buffer: 90 m*M* HEPES, pH 7.6, 67 m*M* NaCl, 7 m*M* KCl, 3.8 m*M* $CaCl_2$ and 50 μg/mL of collagenase (type IV from Sigma; cat. no. C5138 or grade B from Boehringer Mannheim, Indianapolis, IN; cat. no. 1088 831). First, prepare the buffer without $CaCl_2$ and collagenase and sterilize by autoclaving in a 500-mL bottle. Prior to use, add collagenase and stir gently until dissolved. Immediately before perfusion, add $CaCl_2$ in 0.1 *M* solution filtered through a 0.2-μm syringe filter (Pall, Ann Arbor, MI; cat. no. 6224192 or equivalent).
3. Hank's balanced salt solution (HBSS) without calcium or magnesium (Gibco-BRL, Grand Island, NY; cat. no. 14170-112) or phosphate-buffered saline (PBS) (150 m*M* NaCl in 20 m*M* sodium phosphate buffer, pH 7.4) with 1 m*M* EDTA. These buffers are used for washing and final purification of hepatocytes.
4. Fetal calf serum (FCS) (US origin; Gibco-BRL; cat. no. 16000-044) treated for 30 min at 56°C and supplemented with 10% dimethyl sulfoxide (DMSO) for cryopreservation of hepatocytes.

2.1.2. Equipment and Supplies for Isolation of Hepatocytes by Whole Liver Perfusion

All items intended for contact with perfusion media, liver tissue, or hepatocytes are sterilized by autoclaving or purchased sterile from the suppliers.

1. Three sets of surgical instruments: Set 1 containing 14.5-cm forceps with teeth and 17.5-cm straight, dissecting scissors for cutting skin; set 2 with 14.5-cm forceps and 14.5-cm straight surgical scissors for opening the abdominal cavity; and set 3 containing two pairs of 14-cm hemostatic forceps, 14.5-cm curved blunt/blunt surgical scissors, 14.5-cm forceps, a ligation aid for blood vessels with a hole diameter of 0.8 mm (Fine Science Tools, Foster City, CA; cat. no. 18062-13), approx 25-cm long cotton thread, and one pair of very fine-point forceps for handling the liver blood vessels. All instruments available from Fine Science Tools.
2. Single-use polyethylene catheter with an 18-gauge, 5.1-cm (2-in.) needle unit with a hub for connecting to intravenous set adapter (Becton-Dickinson, Rutherford, NJ; cat. no. 3878181 or equivalent).
3. Disposable intravenous fluid infusion set with an air bubble trap chamber (Baxter Healthcare, Toronto, ON; cat. no. JC5401 or equivalent) for connecting the peristaltic pump tubing with the catheter.
4. Polyethylene tubing (approx 50-cm long with an inner diameter of 2.1 mm) connected, at one end, with a disposable 2-mL pipet to be submersed in perfusion media and, at the other end, with the peristaltic pump tubing.
5. Peristaltic pump with adjustable flow rate of 1–200 mL/min (type 49061, Sorvall, Newtown, CT equipped with pumphead model 7014 or equivalent pump) and silicone tubing. The tubing is flushed with 70% ethanol before and after each usage.

6. Glass tube with a sintered glass cap connected by tubing to a tank of medical O_2 (95%)–CO_2 (5%) gas mixture for oxygenation of perfusion media.
7. Water bath for maintaining perfusion media at 37°C.
8. Pyrex 500-mL Erlenmeyer flask for prewarming and oxygenation of collagenase perfusion medium.
9. Coors porcelain Büchner with 11.4-cm in diameter perforated plate (Fisher Scientific, cat. no. 10-356E) to support the liver during perfusion with collagenase medium.
10. Pyrex 1-L beaker for mincing collagenase-treated liver tissue.
11. Four layers of surgical gauze mounted in a polyethylene funnel for filtration of cells after the whole liver perfusion.
12. Pyrex Erlenmeyer 1-L flasks for waste liquids.
13. 50-mL conical centrifuge tubes with screw cups (Sarstedt, Newton, NC; cat. no. 62.547.205 or equivalent) for washing and pelleting of hepatocytes.
14. Low-speed centrifuge for cell sedimentation (type GS-6R; Beckman Instruments, Palo Alto, CA or equivalent).
15. Hemocytometer (Housser Scientific, Horsham, PA or equivalent).
16. Nalgene cryogenic 2-mL vials for hepatocyte storage.

2.1.3. Alternative Supplies Required for Hepatocyte Isolation by Microperfusion from Liver Biopsy or Autopsy Tissue Fragments

1. A 27-gauge needle connected to the perfusion circuit, as per **Subheading 2.1.2.**
2. Single use surgical blade (Becton Dickinson; No. 22, cat. no. 371122 or equivalent).
3. Stainless-steel cell dissociation sieve with 85-mL cup (Sigma; cat. no. CD-1) fitted with a 50-mesh screen (Sigma; cat. no. S0895).
4. Pestle of a 10-mL plastic syringe for pressing collagenase-treated liver tissue through the sieve.
5. Polystyrene 9-cm diameter Petri dishes for collection of hepatocytes after separation on the sieve.
6. 15-mL conical centrifuge tubes with screw cups (Sarstedt; cat. no. 62.554.205 or equivalent) for washing and pelleting of hepatocytes.

2.2. Hepatocyte Cultivation

2.2.1. Culture Medium

1. Hepato-STIM hepatocyte defined medium (Becton Dickinson; cat. no. 355056) with epidermal growth factor (10 ng/mL; Becton Dickinson), 2 m*M* glutamine, 0.4 μg/mL of glucagon (Sigma; cat. no. G3157), 50 IU of penicillin (ICN Biochemical, Horsham, PA), and 50 μg/mL of streptomycin (ICN).
2. Culture supernatant of HepG2 cells (American Type Culture Collection, Rockville, MD; cat. no. ATCC HB 8065) propagated in DMEM: Dulbecco's modified Eagle's medium supplemented with 10% heat-inactivated FCS, 1 m*M* sodium pyruvate, 0.1 m*M* nonessential amino acids, 50 IU/mL of penicillin, and 50 μg/mL of streptomycin (all from ICN). The supernatant is prepared when HepG2 monolayers become about 90% confluent. At this stage, the medium is replaced with fresh DMEM plus supplements and the cells are cultured for an additional 24 h. Then, the culture supernatant is poured off and filtered through a 0.2 μm pore size syringe filter.
3. Conditioned hepatocyte culture medium is composed of Hepato-STIM medium supplemented with 20% of HepG2 cell culture supernatant.

2.2.2. Gelatin-Coated Culture Dishes

Tissue culture flasks and multi-well plates used for woodchuck hepatocyte cultivation are coated with sterilized 0.1% gelatin (Difco Laboratories, Detroit, MI; cat. no. 0143-15-1) in PBS (*see* **Note 1**). The coated dishes are kept overnight at 4°C before use.

2.3. Hepatocyte Infection and Virus Detection

2.3.1. Elimination of Extracellular Viral Sequences

1. DNase digestion buffer: 100 m*M* $MgCl_2$ in 500 m*M* Tris-HCl, pH 8.0.
2. DNase, 1 μg/μL; activity 2 U/μg; deoxyribonuclease I; type IV from bovine pancreas (Sigma; cat. no. D-5025 or equivalent).
3. Trypsin, 10 mg/mL; activity 7300 U/mg; type XI from bovine pancreas (Sigma; cat. no. T-1005 or equivalent).
4. 0.1 *M* $CaCl_2$.
5. Trypsin inhibitor, 10 μg/mL; type II-O from chicken egg white (Sigma; cat. no. T-9253).

2.3.2. Dot-Blot Hybridization for WHV DNA Detection

1. Microcentrifuge 1.5-mL polypropylene tubes (Fisher Scientific; cat. no. 05-407-10 or equivalent) for freezing and thawing of hepatocytes.
2. Nylon membrane (Hybond-N; Amersham Life Science, Arlington Heights, IL; cat. no. RPN303N).
3. Microfiltration apparatus with vacuum manifold (Bio-Dot apparatus; Bio-Rad Laboratories, Richmond, CA; cat no. 170-3938).
4. Filter paper (3 MM chromatography paper; Whatman, Maldstone, UK; cat. no. 3030 917).
5. Denaturation solution: 1.5 *M* NaCl and 0.5 *M* NaOH.
6. Neutralizing solution: 1 *M* Tris-HCl buffer with 1.5 *M* NaCl, pH 7.4.
7. Vacuum oven with adjustable temperature.
8. 20X Saline sodium citrate (SSC): 3 *M* NaCl and 0.3 M citric acid trisodium salt (Sigma; cat. no. C-8532).
9. 50X Denhardt's solution: 0.5 g of Ficoll (type 400; Sigma; cat. no. F-4375), 0.5 g of polyvinylpyrrolidone (Sigma; cat. no. PVP-40T), and 0.5 g of bovine serum albumin (Sigma; cat. no. A-7030) in 50 mL of double-distilled, deionized water.
10. Hybridization solution: 1X SSC, 1% sodium dodecyl sulfate (SDS, Sigma; cat. no. L-4390), 16X Denhardt's solution, and 0.1 μg/mL of sonicated salmon sperm DNA (Sigma; cat. no. D-1626).
11. Hybridization oven with adjustable temperature (Isotemp; Fisher Scientific; cat. no. 13-247-10 or equivalent).

2.3.3. PCR Amplification of WHV DNA Sequences

1. PCR cocktail for amplification of WHV subgenomic sequences (per 100-μL reaction): 100 μ*M* of each oligonucleotide primer for either direct or nested amplification, 200 μ*M* of each deoxyribonucleoside triphosphate, 1.5 m*M* $MgCl_2$, 10 μL of reaction buffer (500 m*M* KCl, 200 m*M* Tris-HCl buffer, pH 8.4), and 1 U of heat-stable *Taq* DNA polymerase (GibcoBRL; cat. no. 18038-018).
2. PCR primers for detection of WHV core sequence: Primers for direct round of PCR: PCNV (5'-TTCAAGCCTCCAAGCTGTGCCTTGG; 1983–2007; numbers denote the position of the nucleotide sequence in WHV genome according to GenBank accession number M11082) and COR (5'-CTTCAATGGGTACATAA; 2586–2602), and primers for nested round of PCR:

PPCC (5'-CCCTATAAAGAATTTGG; 2033–2049) and CCOV (5'-TCTCGACTCTTCCGG AACATAC; 2439–2460).
3. PCR primers for detection of WHV envelope (surface) gene sequence: primers for direct round of PCR: PSW (5'-GGTAAACCATATTCTTGGGA; 2947–2966) and SUW (5'-CACTTCTGAGCATCTTACCGCCAT; 894–917), and primers for nested round of PCR: NSW (5'-CATCAAGTCTCCTAGGACTC; 303–322) and SSW (5'-CTTAGCCCGTTTCTC TTGGCTCA; 781–803).
4. PCR primers for detection of WHV X gene sequence: primers for direct round of PCR: PXO (5'-GCCAACTGGATCCTGCGCGGGACGTC; 1522–1547) and XPC (5'-TAGGAGGCTG TAGGCAT; 1891–1907), and primers for nested round of PCR: PXX (5'-CCTCAATCCAG CGGAC; 1568–1584) and XXC (5'-ATGGATTCCACCGTGAAC; 1742–1760).
5. PCR cocktail for amplification of full-length WHV genome (per 50 μL reaction): 300 μ*M* of each oligonucleotide primer, 200 μ*M* of each deoxyribonucleoside triphosphate, 5 μL of 10X Expand HF buffer with 1.5 m*M* $MgCl_2$ and 2.6 U of *Pwo-Taq* DNA polymerase mix (Expand High Fidelity PCR System; Boehringer Mannheim; cat. no. 1644955).
6. PCR primers for detection of the full-length WHV DNA: PPC1 (5'-AAATGCATGCGAC TTCTGT; 1908–1926) and XPC (5'-TAGGAGGCTGTAGGCAT; 1891–1907).
7. TE buffer: 10 m*M* Tris-HCl buffer, pH 8.0, and 1 m*M* EDTA, pH 8.0.

3. Methods

3.1. Isolation of Hepatocytes

Hepatocytes are isolated by the two-step collagenase perfusion procedure originally developed for preparation of parenchymal cells from the rat liver ***(8)***. This procedure was adopted in our laboratory to isolate woodchuck hepatocytes either by perfusion of the whole liver ***(9–12)*** or by microperfusion of a wide-edge liver biopsy acquired at laparotomy or liver tissue fragments collected during autopsy ***(6)***. The biochemical principles underlying this method has been previously described ***(13)***.

3.1.1. Preparation of Hepatocyte by Whole Liver Perfusion

1. Assemble the perfusion circuit and prime the pump and tubing with calcium-free perfusion buffer prewarmed to 37°C and saturated with a O_2–CO_2 mixture by bubbling the gas through a sintered glass tube at tension above 800 mm Hg. Carefully remove all air bubbles from the circuit because they may severely impair effectiveness of the intrahepatic perfusion. Prepare approx 500 mL of the buffer for a 3–4 kg animal (70–75 g of liver tissue) and have another 500-mL volume at hand when needed.
2. Anesthetize the woodchuck by intramuscular injection with an overdose of a 4:1 mixture of ketamine hydrochloride (Ketalean, 100 mg/mL; Biomeda-MTC, Cambridge, ON; cat. no. DIN 006123316) and xylazine (Xylazine HCl Injection, 100 mg/mL; Boehringer Ingelheim Canada, Burlington, ON; cat. no. DIN 022237528). Place the animal on the back on a stainless-steel sink drain or autopsy table that has been cleaned with antiseptic (e.g., clini-side). Shave abdomen and clean skin using 70% ethanol. Cut skin along the midline from sternum to the pubis and then horizontally from the vertical incision to both sides by using instruments from set 1. Flush the exposed abdominal wall with 70% ethanol and open the cavity using surgical instruments from set 2.
3. Move intestines to the right and expose the portal vein and the vena cava. Using a ligation aid instrument, place a ligation thread under the portal vein at approx 2–2.5 cm from the place of the vein entry into the liver and make a loose half-knot.

4. Carefully puncture the portal vein at the point no more than 0.5 cm proximally distant from the site where the ligation thread is located using the polyethylene catheter with an 18-gauge needle. The use of very fine forceps can be helpful to keep the vessel in place during piercing. Gently insert about three quarters (approx 4 cm) of the catheter length into the lumen without piercing the vessel wall. Quickly remove the needle from the catheter and tighten the ligature. Make an additional knot around the hub of the catheter to prevent its accidental withdrawal. If the cannula is correctly placed, blood should flow back from the liver and completely fill up the catheter.
5. Connect the hub of the catheter to the adapter of the intravenous set filled with calcium-free perfusion buffer. Take all care needed to avoid air bubbles in the system. Deliver the buffer initially at approx 10 mL/min. At this stage, close the portal vein with hemostatic forceps from instrument set 3 proximally to insertion of the catheter.
6. During the low-flow perfusion lasting for 2–3 min, the color of woodchuck liver should become noticeably pale yellow. Increase the flow rate to 40 mL/min and sever with scissors the inferior vena cava just above where the kidney veins enter. Perfusion is continued for at least 15 min until blood traces no longer are seen in the outgoing perfusate and the liver becomes completely blanched. Applying a very gentle massage of lobes between tips of fingers protected by a sterile glove may facilitate more effective perfusion and shorten its time. At this stage, the liver should retain its original size and firmness. The outgoing perfusion medium is drained by a deep cut in the wall on the right side of the abdominal cavity.
7. The liver should become uniformly blanched. Close the inferior vena cava with hemostatic forceps just below the diaphragm. Remove the liver together with the closed fragment of the inferior vena cava using curved surgical scissors from instrument set 3. Take particular care not to remove the catheter from the vena porta or to pierce the liver capsule.
8. Place the liver within a Coors porcelain funnel securely installed over a 500-mL Erlenmeyer flask containing prewarmed and oxygenated collagenase perfusion buffer. Carry on perfusion in a closed circuit at the rate of 40 mL/min for approx 20 min. The liver initially swells, but then becomes progressively softer and shrinks. Continue perfusion until the perfusate begins leaking through the liver capsule. At this stage, disconnect the liver from the perfusion circuit. Remove gall bladder, main vessels hanging outside the liver, and ligaments using instruments from set 3.
9. Transfer the liver into a 1-L beaker placed in a water bath at 37°C, add the collagenase buffer drained from the perfusion circuit, and gently mince tissue with fingers protected by a sterile glove. Hepatocytes should be readily released into the buffer. Incubate suspension for an additional 5–7 min, occasionally stirring the contents.
10. Pour the whole cell suspension onto four layers of surgical gauze mounted in a funnel and gently squeeze the contents by bringing together edges of the gauze filter. Collect filtrate to 50-mL conical centrifuge tubes and tighten screw caps.
11. Hepatocytes are purified from the resulting cell suspension by three rounds of centrifugation at 500 rpm (45*g*) for 5 min at ambient temperature. The cell pellet is suspended each time in 40 mL of HBSS or PBS. The final cell pellet is suspended in a small volume of HBSS or PBS and cells are counted using a hemocytometer. The cells obtained are diluted to concentration of 1×10^6/mL in oxygenated hepatocyte culture medium for further culture (*see* **Subheading 2.2.1.**) or suspended in FCS with 10% DMSO if intended for cryopreservation (see **Subheading 3.5.**)

3.1.2. Isolation of Hepatocytes by Microperfusion of Biopsy or Autopsy Tissue Fragments

1. A liver biopsy is obtained by surgical laparotomy using a 7-mm wide edge Schmeden triangular punch (No. 2; Almedic Canada, Montreal, Quebec; cat. no. A21-332 or equivalent). The laparotomy is performed in an operating room under aseptic conditions and general inhalant anesthesia induced by either halothane or isoflurane: 1-chloro-2,2,2-trifluoroethyl difluoromethyl.
2. Alternatively, liver tissue fragments are obtained during autopsy immediately after opening the abdominal cavity, using approach described in **Subheading 3.1.1.** If hepatocytes need to be isolated from the neoplastic parenchyma of the liver with hepatocellular carcinoma, a tumor nodule is separated from surrounding non-neoplastic tissue by delicate manual preparation under sterile conditions. Then, approx 5-mm^3 fragment from a middle part of the tumor nodule that does not show macroscopically evident necroses and hemorrhages is taken and extensively washed with HBSS until the blood is removed.
3. In the following step, a tissue fragment of 3–5 mm^3 (approx 100–150 mg) is placed in a sterile Petri dish and immediately perfused with calcium-free perfusion buffer oxygenated and prewarmed to 37°C. The perfusion is carried out for about 15 min at the flow rate of 5–6 mL/min by inserting at multiple sites and to variable depths a 27-gauge needle connected to the perfusion circuit.
4. The blanched tissue is sliced with a sterile scalpel blade and the resulting fragments are incubated for 45 min with 10 mL of collagenase buffer (*see* **Subheading 2.1.1.**) prewarmed in a water bath to 37°C. The suspension is oxygenated every 10 min and stirred occasionally.
5. The tissue digest is gently pressed through a 50-mesh sieve using the pestle of a 10-mL plastic syringe. The separated cells are collected in a Petri dish, transferred to a 15-mL conical tube with screw cap, and centrifuged at 50*g* for 5 min at ambient temperature. The cell pellet is washed two or three times, each time with 10 mL of HBSS, by a low-speed centrifugation under the same conditions as above until essentially a pure preparation (>97%) of hepatocytes is obtained. The purity of preparation and the number of viable hepatocytes are determined by trypan blue exclusion.

3.2. Primary Hepatocyte Cultures

1. Approximately 1×10^6 live hepatocytes are placed in a gelatin-coated 25-cm^2 culture flask (Corning, Corning, NY; cat. no. 430 168) containing 5 mL of conditioned hepatocyte culture medium (*see* **Subheading 2.2.1.**). The cells are allowed to attach for 3–4 h in a humidified CO_2 tissue culture incubator.
2. The medium with nonadhered cells is removed and 5 mL of fresh conditioned hepatocyte culture medium is added. The cells are allowed to grow for 24 h at 37°C in a humidified CO_2 atmosphere. At this stage, hepatocytes derived from livers of healthy animals can be inoculated with WHV, as described in **Subheading 3.5.**, and those isolated from WHV-infected livers tested for WHV genome and antigen expression.
3. At this stage, it would be advisable to seed as many primary hepatocytes in 25-cm^2 flasks as reasonably possible (following the procedure described above), cultivate them until confluence, collect, and preserve (*see* **Subheading 3.5.**).

3.3. Long-term Hepatocyte Cultures

1. Hepatocytes seeded under conditions described in **Subheading 3.2.** are allowed to grow until confluent, usually for 6–7 d after seeding. If lower numbers of cells are seeded, more time might be required before they reach confluence.

2. When the cell monolayer becomes confluent, culture medium is removed and hepatocytes washed by gentle swirling with 15 mL of HBSS prewarmed to 37°C.
3. The cells are harvested after treatment with 1 mL of trypsin–EDTA solution (Gibco-BRL; cat. no. 25200-056) in a humidified CO_2 atmosphere for 15 min or until dissociated from the flask. Then, 5 mL of HBSS is added to the flask and the cell suspension is transferred to a 15-mL conical tube with screw cap.
4. Hepatocytes are washed with 10 mL of HBSS by centrifugation under conditions described in **Subheading 3.1.1., step 11**.
5. The pellet is resuspended in 1 mL of conditioned hepatocyte culture medium and cells counted.
6. Hepatocytes predestined for long-term culture are seeded at 3×10^5 cells per gelatin-coated 25-cm^2 culture flask containing 5 mL of conditioned hepatocyte culture medium, whereas those used for a large-scale expansion are plated at 1×10^6 cells per a 75-cm^2 gelatin-coated flask (Corning; cat. no. 439 720) containing 10 mL of the medium.
7. Hepatocytes are harvested by trypsinization when they reach confluence and counted. If their long-term culture is intended, they are seeded again at 3×10^5 cells per a gelatin-coated 25-cm^2 culture flask. Woodchuck hepatocytes can be maintained in culture for a long period of time (months or even years) when passaged at weekly intervals following the procedure outlined above (*see* **Note 2**).

3.4. Generation and Maintenance of Woodchuck Hepatocyte Lines

1. Hepatocytes harvested at confluence by trypsinization from a 25-cm^2 flask are washed with 10 mL of HBSS by a low-speed centrifugation. The cell pellet is suspended in 1 mL of conditioned hepatocyte culture medium and hepatocytes counted.
2. Cells are diluted to an estimated 0.5 cell/mL in conditioned hepatocyte culture medium and seeded at 200 μL per well in two gelatin-coated, 96-well flat bottom plates with cover (Linbro; ICN; cat. no. 7600305). Typically, no more than a few wells show cell proliferation. It takes 3–4 wk before a confluent monolayer is formed. During this time, cell growth is monitored daily and, if required, fresh conditioned hepatocyte culture medium is added after careful collection of the aged medium with help of a sterile Pasteur pipet.
3. When the monolayer becomes confluent, cells from each well are separately harvested by trypsinization, suspended in 2 mL of HBSS in a 15-mL conical tube with screw cap. Cells are washed by centrifugation at 500 rpm for 5 min and seeded into gelatin-coated wells of a 24-well flat bottom plate with lid (ICN; cat. no. 7603305) containing 1-mL aliquots of conditioned hepatocyte culture medium. It takes between 7 and 10 d before the cells reach confluence.
4. Cells are collected after trypsinization, transferred into a 15-mL conical tube with screw cap, and washed with 5 mL of HBSS by a low-speed centrifugation. Then, they are seeded in 2 mL of conditioned hepatocyte culture medium in a gelatin-coated well of a six-well cell culture dish (ICN; cat. no. 7605805). Cells become confluent in 6–7 d.
5. Cells are released by trypsinization, washed in 10 mL of HBSS, and transferred into a 25-cm^2 culture flask containing 5 mL of conditioned hepatocyte culture medium for further expansion. Subsequently, they can be cultured for prolonged time periods (*see* **Subheading 3.3.**), cryopreserved (*see* **Subheading 3.5.**) or used in WHV infection experiments (*see* **Subheading 3.6.**).
6. To ascertain hepatocyte origin of the cell lines generated, cells are examined for transcriptional activity of genes and display of proteins specifically expressed by differentiated hepa-

tocytes (*see* **Note 2**). Typically, we periodically analyze transcription of asialoglycoprotein receptor (ASGPR) genes and presence of the ASGPR protein subunits, and test the display and secretion of woodchuck albumin *(6,10)*.

3.5. Cryopreservation and Reviving of Hepatocytes

1. Hepatocytes destined for cryopreservation are collected at confluence, as described in **Subheading 3.3.**, and suspended at 1×10^6 cells/mL in heat-inactivated FCS with 10% DMSO. One-milliliter aliquots are poured into 1.5-mL cryogenic vials. The vials are wrapped in several layers of paper towels and placed in a Styrofoam box. Hepatocytes are frozen overnight at –70°C and then transferred to a liquid nitrogen freezer for long-term storage.
2. To revitalize cells, the vial is retrieved from liquid nitrogen and placed in a water bath set at 37°C. After the content is thawed, the vial is wiped with 70% ethanol, opened, and cells transferred to a sterile 15-mL conical tube with screw cap. Ten milliliters of HBSS is added and hepatocytes are centrifuged at ambient temperature as outlined in **Subheading 3.1.1.**
3. The hepatocyte pellet is suspended in 5 mL of conditioned hepatocyte culture medium, poured into a gelatin-coated 25-cm^2 culture flask, and cultured as described in **Subheading 3.2.** Usually, more than 90% of woodchuck hepatocytes are viable after revitalization using this approach.

3.6. Infection of Hepatocytes with WHV

Primary woodchuck hepatocytes, hepatocytes from long-term cultures, and hepatocyte lines derived from WHV-naive animals are susceptible to WHV when either infected sera or culture supernatants from WHV-infected woodchuck lymphoid cells or hepatocyte cultures are used as inocula *(7)*. Hepatocytes infected with these various inocula show intracellular expression of WHV DNA, covalently closed circular DNA (cccDNA) and virus RNA transcripts, display virus specific core and envelope antigens, and are able to synthesize virus that is infectious to naive woodchucks *(7)*.

1. Under our standard conditions, 3×10^5 hepatocytes are seeded onto gelatin-coated 25-cm^2 tissue culture flask in 5 mL of conditioned hepatocyte culture medium and allowed to attach for 3–4 h in a humidified CO_2 atmosphere, as described in **Subheading 3.2.** Nonadhered cells are removed and 5 mL of fresh culture medium is added. The cells are cultured for 24 h.
2. The culture medium is poured out and WHV inoculum (*see* **Note 3**) is added at a volume of 200 μL per cm^2 of vessel surface in 5 mL of fresh conditioned hepatocyte culture medium. Inoculum is incubated with hepatocytes for 24 h at 37°C in a humidified CO_2 atmosphere.
3. The culture medium with inoculum is removed, hepatocytes washed in two 10-mL changes of HBSS and 5 mL of conditioned hepatocyte culture medium is added.
4. The cells are allowed to grow for 3 more days (i.e., 4 d after exposure to inoculum) and they are harvested by trypsinization and washed in HBSS. The recovered cells can be examined for expression of WHV genomes (*see* **Subheading 3.8.**) and virus antigens by immunohistochemistry and flow cytometry *(7)*.

3.7. Preparation of Infected Hepatocytes for WHV DNA Detection

To eliminate potential carryover of extracellular viral sequences possibly associated with the cell surface and, therefore, to ensure that only intracellular virus genome material is analyzed, hepatocytes are subjected to limited enzymatic digestion and extensive washing prior to DNA extraction *(1,2,7)*.

1. Approximately 5×10^6 hepatocytes from cultures infected with WHV are suspended in 2 mL of HBSS and supplemented with 200 μL of DNase digestion buffer and 20 μL of DNase (*see* **Subheading 2.3.1.**). The suspension is incubated at 37°C for 1 h in a CO_2 culture incubator.
2. In the next step, the cells are treated with 10 μL of trypsin in the presence of 20 μL of 0.1 *M* $CaCl_2$ for 30 min on ice. The reaction is terminated by adding 20 μL of trypsin inhibitor (*see* **Subheading 2.3.1.**). The DNase digestion step is repeated using the same conditions as outlined above (*see* **Note 4**).
3. The cells are washed twice with a total of 20 mL of PBS with 1 m*M* EDTA by centrifugation at 50g for 5 min. The final wash and the treated cells are saved for detection of WHV DNA.

3.8. Detection of Intracellular WHV DNA

3.8.1. Dot-Blot Hybridization

1. Hepatocytes (approx 1×10^6 cells/sample) recovered after DNase/trypsin/DNase treatment (*see* **Subheading 3.7.**) are suspended in 200 μL of sterile PBS in a microcentrifuge 1.5-mL tube and disrupted by three freeze–thaw cycles. The tube content is briefly centrifuged to collect condensation and loaded using a dot-blot microfiltration apparatus onto nylon membrane prewet in 6X SSC (*see* **Subheading 2.3.2.**). The spotted sample is washed twice with 200 μL of sterile PBS.
2. The membrane is removed from the apparatus, placed on filter paper soaked with denaturation solution (*see* **Subheading 2.3.2.**) for 10 min, and then transferred on filter paper prewet with neutralizing solution and kept for 10 min at room temperature.
3. After baking at 80°C for 2 h in a vacuum oven, the membrane is prehybridized in hybridization solution for 90 min at 65°C.
4. Then, the blot is hybridized for 16 h at 65°C in an aliquot of the hybridization solution supplemented with 1×10^6 cpm/mL of ^{32}P-labeled, full-length, linearized, cloned WHV DNA ***(14)*** and washed twice for 10 min at room temperature with 2X SSC, 0.1% SDS and twice for 10 min at 65°C with 0.1X SSC, 0.05% SDS.
5. The intensity of the hybridization signals is determined by densitometric quantitation using twofold serial dilutions of full-length, cloned WHV DNA as the reference. The sensitivity of this assay is 10^6–10^7 virus genome equivalents (vge)/mL.

3.8.2. PCR for Detection of WHV Subgenomic Sequences

Total DNA is extracted from hepatocytes and the final washes collected after the DNase/trypsin/DNase treatment (*see* **Subheading 3.7.**) by a standard proteinase K digestion and phenol–chloroform extraction protocol ***(15)***.

1. One microgram of total cellular DNA or DNA extracted from 100 μL of cell wash is amplified with direct polymerase chain reaction (PCR) primer pair specific for WHV core, surface (envelope), or X gene in a 100-μL reaction volume (*see* **Subheading 2.3.3.**). Amplification of WHV core subgenomic sequence is carried out by initial denaturation at 92°C for 5 min, annealing at 52°C for 2 min, and elongation at 70°C for 3 min followed by 30 cycles at 92°C, 52°C, and 70°C for 30 s at each step and at 70°C for 5 min for a final extension in a TwinBlock thermal cycler (Ericomp, San Diego, CA). Amplifications of WHV envelope and X gene sequences are done using one cycle of 5 min at 92°C, 2 min at 56°C, and 3 min for 70°C followed by 30 cycles, in which each denaturation (92°C), annealing (56°C), and elongation (70°C) was 30 s, followed by a 5-min elongation step at 70°C.

2. Following direct PCR, 20 μL of the product is analyzed by electrophoresis on a 0.9% agarose gel in the presence of 0.5 μg/mL of ethidium bromide. DNA bands are visualized by ultraviolet fluorescence.
3. If the product band is not detectable on agarose gel, 10 μL of the mixture from the direct PCR round is examined by nested PCR using appropriate primer pairs and conditions described for the direct round of amplification.
4. To ensure authenticity of WHV DNA detection, extensive precautions are taken during sample collection, DNA isolation, and PCR amplification to eliminate any potential viral and DNA contamination. Reaction controls include mock samples containing TE buffer extracted and assayed in parallel with test samples, PCR-positive and -negative controls that consist of DNA derived from livers of healthy and WHV-positive animals, and PCR contamination controls that consist of water added to the PCR mixture instead of DNA. For nested PCR, aliquots of the contamination controls from direct amplifications and water added to the nested PCR mixture instead of amplicons from direct PCR are used as controls. Southern blot analysis ***(1,16)*** of the final PCR products is routinely performed to verify detection of virus-specific amplicons and validity of controls. The sensitivity of the direct and nested PCR amplifications employing different WHV primer pairs is 10^3 and approx 10 vge/mL, respectively. Southern blot analysis of the PCR products increases sensitivity of WHV DNA detection by approx 10-fold.

3.8.3. PCR for Detection of the Full-Length WHV DNA

One microgram of hepatocellular DNA is amplified in a 50-μL volume. The reaction is run with a hot start that was followed by one cycle of 5-min denaturation at 94°C, 2-min annealing at 60°C, 3-min elongation at 72°C, 30 cycles with the denaturation time 40 s, annealing for 90 s, and elongation for 3 min with an increment of 2 min after each 10 cycles, and a final 15-min elongation step at 72°C. Reaction controls are the same as described in **Subheading 3.7.1.** We use a water heated TwinBlock thermal cycler (Ericomp) to perform this amplification.

4. Notes

1. We have tested a number of matrices to support growth of woodchuck hepatocytes but we did not find any advantage to using complex commercially available or in-house designed culture supports. In our system, the thin film of 0.1% gelatin is sufficient to settle hepatocytes and establish culture even from a single-cell seeding.
2. Although woodchuck hepatocyte lines and long-term primary cultures can be established from a single cell, seeding at the density greater than 1×10^4 hepatocytes/cm^2 of surface gives superior results and a confluent monolayer is usually formed in less than a week after seeding. Cell morphology and transcriptional activity of genes and display of proteins specific for the mature hepatocyte phenotype are routinely evaluated in newly established cultures and they are tested periodically in long-term cultures and hepatocyte lines. We observe that the continued transcription of ASGPR genes and display of the receptor protein subunits ***(6,17)***, together with the evidence of albumin secretion, are good indicators of differentiated woodchuck hepatocyte phenotype.
3. We have found that WHV content is an important determinant of the inoculum's ability to establish active infection in cultured hepatocytes. The inoculum WHV levels below 10^3 DNase-protected vge/mL are usually not sufficient to initiate infection, that is, the lack of WHV DNA detectable by PCR–Southern blot analysis (*see* **Subheading 3.6.**). In contrast,

the amounts of the intracellular WHV DNA, as well as virus covalently closed circular DNA (cccDNA) *(7)*, progressively increase when the inoculum content rises from 10^3 to 10^7 vge/mL. We also noted that the inocula with WHV levels greater than 10^7 vge/mL did not further enhance the intensity of the intrahepatocellular virus DNA signals detected. Therefore, the inocula containing approx 10^7 vge/mL produce the highest frequency of successful WHV infection in our hepatocyte culture system.

4. The conditions for the removal of extracellular WHV virions and DNA fragments using DNase/trypsin/DNase treatment must to be determined empirically. Cultured hepatocytes derived from healthy animals exposed to cloned WHV DNA suspended either in conditioned hepatocyte culture medium or in normal woodchuck serum provide a convenient system in which this enzymatic treatment can be tested.

Acknowledgments

This work was supported by operating grants MA-9256, MT-11262, and MPO-14818 from the Canadian Institutes of Health Research (formerly the Medical Research Council of Canada). T. I. Michalak is the Senior (Tier 1) Canada Research Chair in Viral Hepatitis/Immunology supported by the Canada Research Chair Program and funds from the Canada Foundation for Innovation.

References

1. Michalak, T. I., Pardoe, I. U., Coffin, C. S., et. al. (1999) Occult lifelong persistence of infectious hepadnavirus and residual liver inflammation in woodchucks convalescent from acute viral hepatitis. *Hepatology* **29,** 928–938.
2. Coffin, C. S. and Michalak, T. I. (1999) Persistence of infectious hepadnavirus in the offspring of woodchuck mothers recovered from viral hepatitis. *J. Clin. Invest.* **104,** 203–212.
3. Michalak, T. I. (2000) Occult persistence and lymphotropism of hepadnaviral infection: insights from the woodchuck viral hepatitis model. *Immunol. Rev.* **174,** 98–111.
4. Tennant, B. C. and Gerin, J. L. (1994) The woodchuck model of hepatitis B virus infection, in *The liver: Biology and Pathobiology* (Arias, I. M., Boyer, J. L., Fausto, N., Jakoby, W. B., Schachter, D. A., and Shafritz, D. A., eds.), Raven Press, New York, pp. 1455–1466.
5. Michalak, T. I. (1998) The woodchuck animal model of hepatitis B. *Viral Hepat. Rev.* **4,** 139–165.
6. Diao, J. and Michalak, T. I. (1998) Complement-mediated cytotoxicity and inhibition of ligand binding to hepatocytes by woodchuck hepatitis virus-induced autoantibodies to asialoglycoprotein receptor. *Hepatology* **27,** 1623–1631.
7. Lew, Y.-Y. and Michalak, T. I. (2001) In vitro and in vivo infectivity and pathogenicity of the lymphoid cell-derived woodchuck hepatitis virus. *J. Virol.* **75,** 1770–1782.
8. Seglen, P. O. (1976) Preparation of isolated rat liver cells. *Methods Cell Biol.* **13,** 29–83.
9. Michalak, T. I. and Churchill, N. D. (1988) Interaction of woodchuck hepatitis virus surface antigen with hepatocyte plasma membrane in woodchuck chronic hepatitis. *Hepatology* **8,** 499–506.
10. Michalak, T. I. and Bolger, G. T. (1989) Characterization of the binding sites for glutaraldehyde-polymerized albumin on purified woodchuck hepatocyte plasma membranes. *Gastroenterology* **96,** 153–166.
11. Michalak, T. I., Snyder R. L., and Churchill, N. D. (1989) Characterization of the incorporation of woodchuck hepatitis virus surface antigen into hepatocyte plasma membrane in woodchuck hepatitis and in the virus-induced hepatocelluar carcinoma. *Hepatology* **10,** 44–55.

12. Michalak, T. I. and Lin, B. (1994) Molecular species of hepadnavirus core and envelope polypeptides in hepatocyte plasma membrane of woodchucks with acute and chronic viral hepatitis. *Hepatology* **20,** 275–286.
13. Berry, M. N., Edwards, A. M., and Barritt, G. J. (1991) *Isolated Hepatocytes Preparation: Properties and Applications*. Elsevier, New York.
14. Pardoe, I. U and Michalak T. I. (1995) Detection of hepatitis B and woodchuck hepatitis viral DNA in plasma and mononuclear cells from heparinized blood by the polymerase chain reaction. *J. Virol. Methods* **51,** 277–288.
15. Moore, D. (1998) Manipulation of DNA, in *Current Protocols in Molecular Biology* (Ausubel, F. M., Brent, R., Kingstron, R. E., et al., eds.), John Wiley & Sons, New York, pp. 2.1.1–2.1.10.
16. Brown, T. (1993) Analysis of DNA sequences by blotting and hybridization, in *Current Protocols in Molecular Biology* (Ausubel, F. M., Brent, R., Kingstron, R. E., et al., eds.), John Wiley & Sons, New York, pp. 2.9.1–2.9.15.
17. Diao, J. and Michalak, T. I. (1996) Composition, antigenic properties and hepatocyte surface expression of the woodchuck asialoglycoprotein receptor. *J. Recept. Sig. Transduct. Res.*, **16,** 243–271.

16

Duck Hepatitis B Virus Primary Hepatocyte Culture Model

Olivier Hantz and Fabien Zoulim

1. Introduction

Hepadnaviruses *(1)* are essentially hepatotrophic, and hepatocytes are the main site of viral replication. Other cells of the same embryonic origin such as the biliary epithelial cells are able to efficiently replicate the virus but represent only a very minor proportion of total liver. The virus can also be found in several nonhepatic tissues, including lymphocytes, kidney, and spleen. Peripheral blood mononuclear cells (PBMCs), in particular, could represent a nonhepatic reservoir of virus *(2)*, a finding consistent with the recent demonstration that hepatocytes may originate from CD34 bone marrow cells *(3,4)*. However, primary hepatocyte cultures remain the most efficient culture system for in vitro studies of viral infection.

Owing to the lack of cellular functions that may be required for early events of the infection process, hepatoma cell lines are usually refractory to viral infection but are widely used in transfection experiments. Only primary cultures of hepatocytes can be efficiently infected and support high levels of viral replication. As a main consequence, the duck hepatitis B virus (DHBV) model became an essential and impossible to circumvent tool *(5)* for many in vitro studies: indeed, obvious difficulties in obtaining human liver cells have limited the studies of the human virus, HBV. Far more expensive and less practical, the two other models, the woodchuck and the ground squirrel, and their respective viruses, woodchuck hepatitis virus (WHV) and GSHV, have rarely been used *(6)*.

Much effort has been devoted to better defining the isolation procedure for obtaining a purified hepatocyte population *(7–9)* and to increase the survival and functional stability of these cells *(10,11)*. *In situ* perfusion of the liver is the most used technique to obtain hepatocytes *(12,13)*. Following isolation, hepatocytes can be cultivated in various conditions, on different substrates, and in well-defined media supplemented with hormones, growth factors, or chemical agents known to induce hepatocyte differentiation *(14)*. This chapter describes the main techniques for duck hepatocyte isolation, infection by DHBV *(15,16)* and the evaluation of antiviral activities of new drugs *(17–21)*.

From: *Methods in Molecular Medicine, vol. 96: Hepatitis B and D Protocols, volume 2*
Edited by: R. K. Hamatake and J. Y. N. Lau © Humana Press Inc., Totowa, NJ

In the presence of 1.5–1.8% dimethyl sulfoxide (DMSO), duck hepatocyte cultures can be maintained for at least 15 d. After in vitro inoculation, viral replication can be easily monitored by the level of virion-associated DNA secreted in culture supernatants. Typical results are shown in **Fig. 1A**: the level of extracellular viral DNA produced by untreated cells increases continously during the time of culture. Addition of antiviral compound such as 9-(2-phosphonylmethoxyethyl)adenine (PMEA) at 0.1 μ*M* 2 d after infection during 8 d of culture clearly decreases DHBV DNA levels in culture supernatants. Removal of inhibitors is followed by a rebound of viral replication. Within 3–4 d this rebound can reach a level similar or even higher than that of control culture, depending of the nature and the concentration of antiviral compounds. High doses of inhibitors generally delay the increase of viral replication by several days *(22)*.

At d 8 of treatment, the level of DHBV DNA in supernatant is represented as a function of the drug concentration (**Fig. 1B**). The IC_{50} is defined as the drug concentration that induces a 50% decrease in the level of DHBV DNA in culture supernatants and is calculated by linear regression analysis. Assays are usually made in triplicate and data from at least two independent experiments are combined.

Analysis of intracellular viral DNA allows a determination of the mode of action of the tested compound (inhibition of priming, reverse transcription, or second strand DNA synthesis) and its action on the recalcitrant viral covalently closed circular (cccDNA) (*see* **Fig. 2**). Single-strand (SS) DNA is usually the viral DNA form that is the most affected by antiviral treatment. Relaxed circular (RC) and linear (L) DNA decrease in parallel. cccDNA levels are less affected but can also be strongly diminished and even undetectable by conventional hybridization methods (not by the polymerase chain reaction [PCR]) with very potent compounds such as 2', 3'-dideoxy-2', 3'-didehydro-β-L-5-fluorocytidine (β-L-Fd4C) *(22)*. In that case, the rebound of viral replication several days after cessation of treatment indicates that complete eradication of cccDNA cannot be achieved in these experimental conditions even with highly potent anti-HBV compounds.

2. Materials

2.1. Solutions

1. 4-(2-Hydroxyethylpiperazine)-1-ethanesulfonic acid (HEPES) buffer: 160.8 m*M* NaCl, 15 m*M* KCl, 0.7 m*M* $NaHPO_4 \cdot 12H_2O$, and 33 m*M* HEPES adjusted to pH 7.65 at 37°C in distilled water (purity of water is critical). Sterilize by filtration through a 0.22 μm filter unit, dispense into 500-mL autoclaved sterile glass bottles, and store at 4°C.
2. Collagenase for perfusion (*see* **Note 1**): Dissolve collagenase (Collagenase D Roche–Boehringer Manheim) at 15–25 mg/100 mL in HEPES buffer containing 0.075% $CaCl_2$ and 0.05 mg/mL of DNase I (Roche–Boehringer Manheim). Use immediately.
3. Collagenase for dissociation of fetal liver: 0.2% Collagenase (Type V Sigma, 230 U/mg) in HEPES buffer containing 0.6 m*M* $CaCl_2$ and 0.1 mg/mL of DNase I. Sterilize by filtration through a 0.22 μm filter unit, dispense into 5-mL sterile polypropylene tubes, and store at –20°C.
4. Hepatocyte washing medium: Leibovitch L15 medium supplemented with penicillin–streptomycin and 1% normal chicken serum.
5. Isotonic Percoll solution: 45 mL of Percoll (Amersham–Pharmacia) is mixed with 5 mL of a 10-fold concentrated stock salt solution (80 g of NaCl, 4 g of KCl, 2 g of Mg $SO_4 \cdot 7H_2O$ for 1 L of H_2O) and 1 mL of phosphate buffer (12 g of Na_2HPO_4 and 2 g of KH_2PO_4 in 1 L of H_2O).

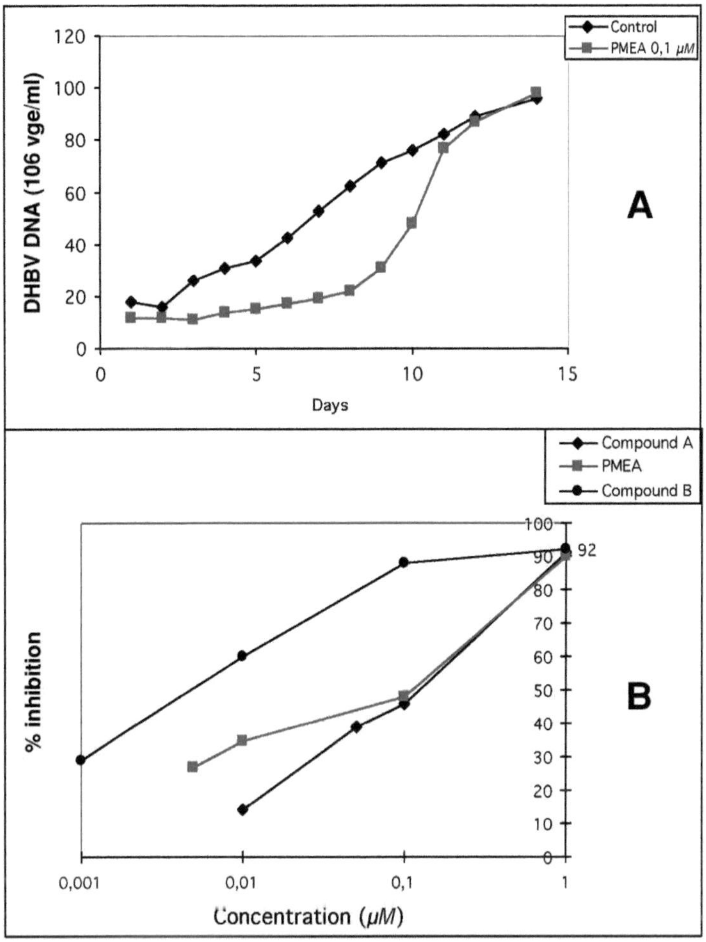

Fig. 1. (**A**) Time course of DHBV replication in duck hepatocyte primary culture untreated (♦) or treated with 0.1 μM PMEA (■). Drug is added 2 d post-plating. Extracellular DHBV DNA was quantified by dot–blot hybridization as described. Each experiment was performed in duplicate. (**B**) IC_{50} determination of antiviral compound A (♦), compound B (●), and PMEA (■). Infected duck hepatocyte primary culture are treated for 8 d with different concentrations of tested compounds. Extracellular DHBV DNA levels are determined at the end of treatment.

6. L15 or Williams medium: Standard L15 Leibovitch or Williams E medium supplemented with 50 U/mL of kanamycin (Gibco-Invitrogen), 50 U/mL of penicillin–streptomycin (Gibco-Invitrogen), 5 μg/mL of bovine insulin, and 7×10^{-5} M hydrocortisone hemisuccinate (Boehringer-Mannheim, France). For plating, add 5% fetal calf serum (FCS). For long-term culture, add 1.5% DMSO instead of FCS.
7. Neutral red: 0.4% Stock solution is made in distilled water. Dilute 1:80 in L15 medium, incubate for at least 1 h at 37°C, and filter through a 0.22-μm filter unit.

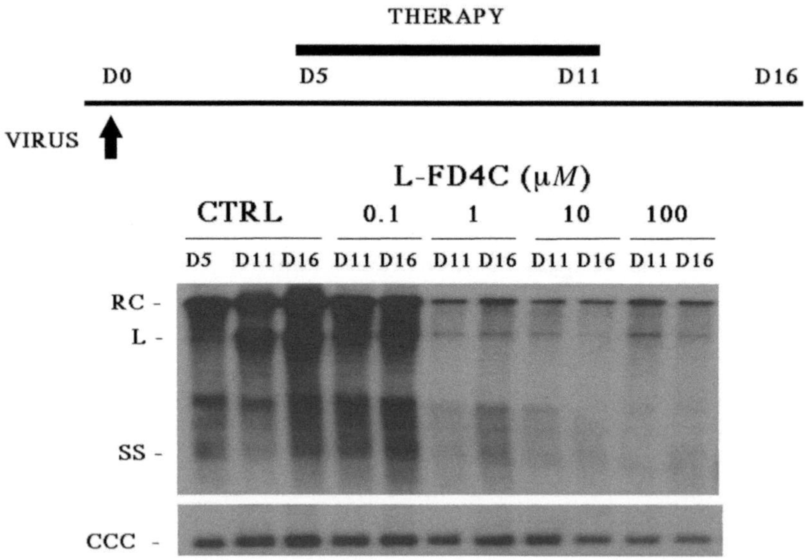

Fig. 2. β-L-Fd4C inhibits viral DNA synthesis in primary duck hepatocyte cultures. **(Top)** Primary duck hepatocyte cultures were inoculated with an infectious serum on d 1 post-seeding and intracellular viral DNA was analyzed after Southern blotting at the indicated time points during cell culture. β-L-Fd4C and 3TC were added 6 d post-inoculation (d 7), at the indicated concentrations, for 6 consecutive days with a daily medium change in the curative protocol. In this experiment viral DNA was analyzed at the end of treatment (d 13) and 4 d post-treatment (d 17). **(Bottom)** In the preventive treatment, inoculation with an infectious serum was performed 2 d post-plating. Drugs (β-L-Fd4C, 3TC) were added 1 d prior to the inoculation and maintained for 4 d post-inoculation, at the indicated concentrations. In this experiment, viral DNA was analyzed at the end of treatment (d 6), and 3 and 8 d post-treatment (d 9 and 14, respectively). The viral replicative intermediates are indicated: RC, relaxed circular; L, linear; SS, single-stranded DNAs; CCC, cccDNA.

8. Formol–calcium solution: Mix 1 mL of 40% formaldehyde with 10 mL of 10% $CaCl_2$ and 89 mL of distilled water.
9. Acetic acid–ethanol solution: One volume of acetic acid with 99 volumes of 50% ethanol in distilled water.

2.2. Equipment

1. Peristaltic pump able to give adjustable flow rate from 10 to 30 mL/min with silicon tubing and Tygon connecting tubing.
2. Thermostated water bath equilibrated at 42°C so that perfusion media are at 37°C before it enters the liver.
3. Bubble trap can be constructed with a 10 to 20-mL glass tube with a rubber stopper that has been pierced with stainless-steel tubing in two lengths, one short (inflow) and one longer (outflow) immersed in perfusion medium (one third of the tube).
4. Portal vein canulas.

5. Standard surgical equipment for dissection of small animals (scalpel, scissors, forceps, clamp, trocar, and cannulas).

2.3. Animals and Tissues for Study

Usually, 3-wk-old ducklings or 1- to 3-yr-old woodchucks are used for the preparation of fresh hepatocytes. Animals are not fed within 16 h before perfusion. Fetal liver tissue was obtained from Pekin duck embryos (3 wk post-laying) laid by DHBV-negative (or DHBV-positive if needed) ducks.

3. Methods

3.1. Primary Hepatocyte Cultures

3.1.1. In Situ *Two-Step Liver Perfusion*

1. Animals are injected with heparin as anticoagulant and then killed under anesthesia with intravenous pentobarbital (100 mg/kg body wt).
2. Place the animal abdomen upward and open the abdominal cavity from the pubis to the tips of the sternum. Uncover the portal vein in the upper intestinal loop and expose the liver.
3. Cannulate the portal vein using a trocar and a cannula. Cut the cava vein and connect the inflow tubing to the cannula. Begin the perfusion with HEPES at 37°C at a low rate (10 mL/min) for a few minutes. Rapid decoloration of the liver indicates a correct perfusion. HEPES perfusion is continued for 10 min at 30 mL/min. Avoid air bubbles.
4. The second step is made with the same HEPES buffer containing collagenase and $CaCl_2$ at 37°C for 10 min at a flow rate of 15 mL/min (*see* **Note 2**). DNase is added to decrease high viscosity of the cell preparation.
5. At the end of the perfusion, the softened liver (very careful manipulation is necessary as spontaneous disintegration of the organ can occur during this step) is transferred from the abdominal cavity to a sterile glass Petri dish.
6. Cells are dispersed by cutting the dissociated liver with a scalpel in preheated (37°C) L15 medium supplemented with bovine serum albumin (BSA). The suspension is filtered through gauze into a sterile 250 mL bottle.
7. Cells in 100–200 mL of medium are left to sediment by gravity for 10 min. Hepatocytes form a clear layer at the bottom of the bottle. The supernatant is carefully removed by aspiration.
8. The hepatocyte suspension is transferred to a 50-mL tube and washed twice with HEPES solution by centrifugation at 50*g* for 2 min. The final pellet is resuspended in 50 mL of HEPES solution.
9. Add an equal volume of isotonic Percoll solution, mix gently, and centrifuge at 4°C for 10 min at 50*g* in 50-mL tubes. Damaged hepatocytes, debris, and nonparenchymal cells float in the upper region of the tube and are removed by careful aspiration.
10. Pelleted cells are washed twice as above and diluted in L15 medium with 5% FCS. The final suspension usually contains $500–1000 \times 10^6$ viable cells for a duckling liver. The viability of the hepatocyte preparation must be more than 90% (*see* **Note 3**) as estimated by trypan blue staining.

3.1.2. Preparation of Embryonic Hepatocytes

1. Liver tissues are obtained from Pekin duck embryos, 3 wk post-laying, laid by DHBV-negative (or positive if needed) ducks. The embryos are killed by decapitation a week before they hatch.

2. After dissection, livers from 6–12 embryos are pooled and washed with HEPES solution. Tissues are then dispersed by mechanical disruption using a scalpel blade in 2.5–5 mL of freshly prepared 0.2% collagenase in HEPES buffer.
3. After 10–15 min incubation at 37°C, cell aggregates are removed by filtration through a nylon mesh (60 μm pore size) and diluted to 15 mL with Williams medium containing 2% chicken serum.
4. To remove damaged cells, the hepatocyte suspension is carefully layered on 15 mL of 20% Percoll in Williams medium and centrifuged at 20°C for 10 min at 50*g*.
5. Pelleted cells are washed twice as described above and resuspended in Williams medium containing 2% chicken serum.

3.1.3. Long-Term Hepatocyte Culture

1. Dispense 2 mL/well of cell suspension at 5–8 × 10^5 cells/mL in L15 medium containing 5% fetal calf serum into Collagen I coated six-well plates.
2. Incubate for 6 h or overnight in a 5% CO_2 atmosphere at 37°C.
3. Wash the plated cells twice with HEPES buffer and then add 2 mL/well of L15 medium with 1.5% DMSO. Renew the medium daily.

3.1.4. Embryonic Hepatocyte Culture

1. Dispense 2 mL/well of cells suspension at a density of 0.2–0.3 × 10^6 cells/mL in Williams medium with 2% chicken serum into Collagen I coated six-well plates.
2. After 4 h, wash twice, then add Williams medium without serum. Medium is renewed daily.

3.2. Antiviral Testing

3.2.1. In Vitro Infection

Viral infection is performed before or after plating by incubation of the cells with DHBV-positive duck serum at a final titer of approx 30 viral genome equivalents (vge) per cell (*see* **Note 4**) diluted in Williams medium without serum. Sterilize by filtration through a 0.22-μm filter unit (Millipore).

3.2.1.1. Infection Before Plating

1. Incubate cells (10 × 10^6 cells/mL) in suspension with virus for 2 h at room temperature with gentle agitation.
2. Dilute in medium containing 2% of chicken serum then dispense 0.4–0.6 × 10^6 cells/well in Collagen I coated six-well plate.
3. Incubate overnight in a 5% CO_2 atmosphere at 37°C.
4. Wash the cells five times with 2 mL of HEPES buffer per well and incubate with 2 mL of medium.

3.2.1.2. Infection After Plating

1. Plate 0.4–0.6 × 10^6 cells/well in a six-well plate.
2. Incubate for 3–4 h at 37°C.
3. Dispense 0.5 mL of inoculum diluted in Williams medium (usually 50–100 μL of duck serum/mL) and incubate overnight at 37°C.
4. Wash the cells five times with 2 mL of HEPES buffer per well and incubate in 2 mL of medium.

3.2.2. Antiviral Screening

1. Tested compounds are aliquoted as concentrated (usually 100 m*M*) stock solutions in DMSO.
2. Dilute at desired concentration in fresh medium just before use to avoid degradation of the compounds.
3. Renew daily for 8 d.
4. Each assay is made in triplicate and medium collected for analysis of secreted virus.
5. At the end of treatment, cells from one well are collected for intracellular viral DNA analysis. The two other wells are maintained in culture without drugs for 3–5 additional days to study the eventual rebound of viral replication.

3.2.3. Analysis of extracellular viral DNA *(23)*

1. Aliquots (800 µL out of 2 mL) of the clarified cell supernatants removed daily are pipetted onto a nitrocellulose membrane and denatured with 0.2 *N* NaOH, 1 *M* NaCl.
2. The membrane is neutralized with 0.5 *M* Tris-HCl, pH 7.4; 1 *M* NaCl, followed by a wash with 2X SSC and fixed by baking for 2 h at 80°C.
3. Hybridizations are done with a ^{32}P-labeled genomic DHBV probe. Quantitative analysis is done using a PhosphorImager System with ImageQuant®oftware (Molecular Dynamics).

3.2.4. Analysis of Intracellular Viral DNA: Isolation of Covalently Closed Circular DNA or Total Nucleic Acids Followed by Southern Blot Analysis

At the indicated times, cultures in six-well plates are rinsed twice with phosphate-buffered saline (PBS). To isolate cccDNA-enriched fractions, we used the previously described procedure *(24)*.

1. In brief, cells are lysed with buffer (20 m*M* Tris-HCl, pH 7.5, 20 m*M* EDTA) containing 0.5% sodium dodecyl sulfate (SDS).
2. Protein-bound replicative forms are precipitated as a protein–detergent complex by addition of KCl to a final concentration of 0.5 *M*.
3. After centrifugation, cccDNA, along with genomic DNA, is recovered from the soluble fraction by phenol extraction and ethanol precipitation.
4. Replicative forms (RC and SS DNA) are dissolved by digestion of the pellet with 0.83 mg/mL of proteinase K for 4 h at 55°C and purified by phenol extraction and ethanol precipitation.
5. Alternatively, for the isolation of total DNA, hepatocytes are lysed in a solution containing 0.8 mg/mL of proteinase K; 0.1% SDS, 150 m*M* NaCl; 20 m*M* Tris-HCl, pH 7.5; and 20 m*M* EDTA and incubated at 55°C for 4 h. This lysate is extracted twice with phenol–chloroform, and nucleic acids are collected by ethanol precipitation.
6. Ten micrograms of total DNA or aliquots of cccDNA extracts containing 10 µg of copurifying genomic DNA are analyzed by 1.5% agarose gel electrophoresis and transferred to an amphoteric nylon membrane (Biodyne A-Pall filtron). For RC DNA extracts, which contain only contaminating cellular genomic DNA, aliquots equivalent to the corresponding cccDNA extracts are analyzed.
7. Hybridizations are performed with a ^{32}P-labeled full-length genomic DHBV probe *(23)*. The membranes are analyzed by autoradiography and are read with the PhosphorImager System. Fifty nanograms of linear DHBV DNA obtained by *Eco*R1 digestion of plasmid is used as a standard.

3.2.5. Cytotoxicity

Cytotoxicity measurements are based on the estimation of hepatocyte viability after drug treatment using uptake of neutral red dye *(25)*.

1. For determination of CC_{50} (50% cytotoxic concentration), primary duck hepatocytes are seeded at a density of 5×10^4 cells/well in 24-well tissue culture plates.
2. After plating, cells are cultivated in 1 mL of medium containing various concentrations of the test compound with daily changes. Four wells per assay are used.
3. After 8 d of treatment, cell viability is estimated by a neutral red uptake method. In brief, cells are incubated overnight in medium containing 0.005% neutral red.
4. Remove medium by aspiration and add 0.5 mL of formol–calcium solution in each well for 1 min.
5. Discard and add 0.5 ml of acetic acid–ethanol.
6. After 15 min, mix and read the optical density at 540 nm. The minimum cytotoxic concentration or CC_{50} is defined as the concentration required to reduce cell viability by 50%.

4. Notes

1. Collagenase is the main factor affecting both the viability of the cells and their capacity to be efficiently infected. We use Collagenase D (Roche-Boeringher Manheim) at 0.28 U/mg (1.69 U/mg of Clostripain, 27.2 Einh/mg of protease, and 0.062 U/mg of trypsin).
2. Perfusion for longer times may result in higher yield of hepatocytes but cells may lose their ability to be infected. A good compromise is 10–15 min.
3. Discard the hepatocyte preparation if viability of cells is 80%.
4. From 1 to 10 vge/cell is enough to obtain a detectable infection.

References

1. Seeger, C. and Mason, W. S. (2000) Hepatitis B virus biology. *Microbiol. Mol. Biol. Rev.* **64**, 51–68.
2. Lamelin, J. P., Zoulim, F., and Trepo, C. (1995) Lymphotropism of hepatitis B and C viruses: an update and a newcomer. *Int. J. Clin. Lab. Res.* **25**, 1–6.
3. Theise, N. D., Nimmakayalu, M., Gardner, R., et al. (2000) Liver from bone marrow in humans. *Hepatology* **32**, 11–16.
4. McDonnell, W. M. (2000) Liver stem cells from bone marrow. *Hepatology* **32**, 1181.
5. Tuttleman, J. S., Pugh, J. C., and Summers, J. W. (1986) In vitro experimental infection of primary duck hepatocyte cultures with duck hepatitis B virus. *J. Virol.* **58**, 17–25.
6. Moraleda, G., Saputelli, J., Adrich, C. E., Averett, D., Condreay, L., and Mason, W. S. (1997) Lack of effect of antiviral therapy in nondividing hepatocyte cultures on the closed circular DNA of woodchuck hepatitis virus. *J. Virol.* **71**, 9392–9399.
7. Berry, M. N. and Phillips, J. W. (2000) The isolated hepatocyte preparation: 30 years on. *Biochem. Soc. Trans.* **28**, 131–135.
8. Berry, M. N., Grivell, A. R., Grivell, M. B., and Phillips, J. W. (1997) Isolated hepatocytes—past, present and future. *Cell. Biol. Toxicol.* **13**, 223–233.
9. Berry, M. N., Halls, H. J., and Grivell, M. B. (1992) Techniques for pharmacological and toxicological studies with isolated hepatocyte suspensions. *Life. Sci.* **51**, 1–16.
10. Mitaka, T. (1998) The current status of primary hepatocyte culture. *Int. J. Exp. Pathol.* **79**, 393–409.

11. Runge, D., Michalopoulos, G. K., Strom, S. C., and Runge, D. M. (2000) Recent advances in human hepatocyte culture systems. *Biochem. Biophys. Res. Commun.* **274**, 1–3.
12. Berry, M. N., Edwards, A. M., and Bariit, G. (1991) *Isolated Hepatocytes: Preparation, Properties and Applications. Laboratory Techniques in Biochemistry and Molecular Biology*, vol. 21 (Burden, R. & Knippenberg, P., eds.), Elsevier, Amsterdam/New York/Oxford.
13. Guguen-Guillouzo, C. (1992) Isolation and culture of animal and human hepatocytes, in *Culture of Epithelial Cells*, Wiley-Liss, New York, pp. 197–223.
14. LeCluyse, E. L., Bullock, P. L., and Parkinson, A. (1996) Strategies for restoration and maintenance of normal hepatic structure and function in long-term cultures of rat hepatocytes. *Adv. Drug. Deliv. Rev.* **22**, 133–186.
15. Turin, F., Borel, C., Benchaib, M., et al. (1996) *n*-Butyrate, a cell cycle blocker, inhibits early amplification of duck hepatitis B virus covalently closed circular DNA after in vitro infection of duck hepatocytes. *J. Virol.* **70**, 2691–2696.
16. Borel, C., Schorr, O., Durand, I., et al. (2001) Initial amplification of duck hepatitis B virus covalently closed circular DNA after in vitro infection of embryonic duck hepatocytes is increased by cell cycle progression. *Hepatology* **34**, 168–179.
17. Fourel, I., Gripon, P., Hantz, O., et. al. (1989) Prolonged duck hepatitis B virus replication in duck hepatocytes cocultivated with rat epithelial cells: a useful system for antiviral testing. *Hepatology* **10**, 186–191.
18. Charvet, A. S., Turin, F., Faury, P., et. al. (1994) Synthesis and antiviral activity of new carbonylphosphonate 2',3'-dideoxy-3'-thiacytidine conjugates. *Antivir. Res.* **25**, 161–168.
19. Zoulim, F., Dannaoui, E., Borel, C., et. al. (1996) 2',3'-dideoxy-beta-L-5-fluorocytidine inhibits duck hepatitis B virus reverse transcription and suppresses viral DNA synthesis in hepatocytes, both in vitro and in vivo. *Antimicrob. Agents Chemother.* **40**, 448–453.
20. Hantz, O., Borel, C., Trabaud, C., et. al. (1997) Selective inhibition of the duck hepatitis B virus by a new class of tetraazamacrocycles. *Antimicrob. Agents Chemother.* **41**, 2579–2581.
21. Delmas, J., Schorr, O., Jamard, C., et. al. (2002) Inhibitory effect of Adefovir on viral DNA synthesis and covalently closed circular DNA formation in duck hepatitis B virus-infected hepatocytes in vivo and in vitro. *Antimicrob. Agents Chemother.* **46**, 425–433.
22. LeGuerhier, F., Pichoud, C., Guerret, S., et. al. (2000) Characterization of the antiviral effect of 2',3'-dideoxy-2', 3'-didehydro-beta-L-5-fluorocytidine in the duck hepatitis B virus infection model. *Antimicrob. Agents Chemother.* **44**, 111–122.
23. Lambert, V., Fernholz, D., Sprengel, R., et. al. (1990) Virus-neutralizing monoclonal antibody to a conserved epitope on the duck hepatitis B virus pre-S protein. *J. Virol.* **64**, 1290–1297.
24. Summers, J., Smith, P. M., and Horwich, A. L. (1990) Hepadnavirus envelope proteins regulate covalently closed circular DNA amplification. *J. Virol.* **64**, 2819–2824.
25. Fautz, R., Hussein, B., and Hechenberger, C. (1991) Application of the neutral red assay (NR assay) to monolayer cultures of primary hepatocytes: rapid colorimetric viability determination for the unscheduled DNA synthesis test (UDS). *Mutat. Res.* **253**, 173–179.

17

Enhancement of Infection of HepG2 Cells in Culture by Predigestion of Hepadnavirus with V8 Protease

Xuanyong Lu and Timothy M. Block

1. Introduction

In this chapter, a method for infecting HepG2 cells with human hepatitis B virus (HBV) and woodchuck hepatitis virus (WHV) is reviewed. This chapter provides a stepwise, experimentally sensitive description of how to perform the protease infectivity assay. The assay is highly technical and sensitive to certain cell culture and virological steps. Therefore, essential technical points are emphasized, to assist the experimentalist as much as possible.

1.1. Background

Although HBV is considered to be highly efficient in establishing infection in people following parenteral exposure, tissue culture cells are generally refractory. For example, inoculation of tissue cultures of hepatocyte-like cells, such as the hepatoblastoma line HepG2, with serum-derived HBV does not usually result in an efficient production of progeny virus ***(1–3)***. This is true despite the fact that HepG2 cells transfected with appropriate vectors are capable of replicating the viral genome and producing progeny virus that is infectious in chimpanzees ***(4)***. In addition, manipulation of the cultures with chemicals such as dimethyl sulfoxide (DMSO) or polyethylene glycol (PEG) has been reported to enhance HBV infection of tissue cultures ***(5,6)***. The reason(s) that these manipulations enhance viral infectivity are unclear. Human hepatocyte primary cultures derived from liver explants have been shown to be susceptible to HBV infection, but only for a limited amount of time following explant ***(7–9)***. Therefore, although cultures of cells can be shown to support HBV replication, there is yet no easily reproducible tissue culture system of HBV infectivity, frustrating the study of the HBV life cycle as well as the pursuit of antiviral agents. Because it is clear that hepatocyte cells in culture can support replication of HBV, the data taken together suggest that the major block to tissue culture infection is at a very early step in the virus life cycle: attachment, fusion, and penetration or entry.

From: *Methods in Molecular Medicine, vol. 96: Hepatitis B and D Protocols, volume 2*
Edited by: R. K. Hamatake and J. Y. N. Lau © Humana Press Inc., Totowa, NJ

Recently, an exopeptidase, carboxypeptidase D, was reported as a putative receptor for duck hepatitis B virus (DHBV) ***(10,11)***. Significantly, the putative carboxypeptidase D receptor could apparently mediate the internalization of DHBV after attachment ***(3,12)***.

We have reported that following limited digestion with the staphylococcal protease V8, the human and woodchuck hepatitis viruses can be rendered "infectious" for tissue cultures of HepG2 cells ***(1,2)***. The viruses pretreated with V8 protease were shown to infect tissue cultures of HepG2 cells and produce progeny. In contrast, in the absence of this protease pretreatment, there is little, if any, detectable productive infection as has been observed by others. The protease enhanced the infectivity of these viruses for tissue culture by more than 100-fold.

The reason that V8 protease treatment induces viral infectivity is not clear. It is interesting that a V8 protease cleavage site is in a specific region between the C-terminus of preS2 and N-terminus of S domain of surface protein. This region contains a proteolytic sensitive motif called a "PEST region" as well as a hydrophobic motif associated with membrane fusion: FLG-LL-AG ***(1,2,13)***. This fusion motif occurs in the domains of other viral envelope polypeptides associated with fusion, including human immunodeficiency virus (HIV) and influenza virus ***(1,2,13)***. We reason that V8 cleavage of HBV and WHV results in exposure of this fusion motif, present within the virus envelope polypeptide. This in turn facilitates virus fusing with host cell and allowing entry. Because V8 protease is of bacterial origin, we further speculate that a mammalian protease exists that, during natural infection, performs a function similar to V8 protease in our experimental system.

It was recently hypothesized that a domain immediately upstream of the PEST region in pre-S2 serves as a "permeability" region for HBV internalization ***(14)***. This is consistent with the hypothesis that, during natural infection, after virus pre-S region mediated receptor binding followed by internalization via a permeability motif, a V8-like protease(s) present in susceptible hepatocytes (but lacking or not functional in HepG2 cells) would act as a post-attachment step. The action of this/these putative protease(s) would expose the fusion domain of envelope polypeptide resulting in virus–cell membrane fusion, permitting viral genome entry into the cytosol. The further details of this theory, are the subject of other publications and work.

2. Materials

2.1. Source and Abundance of Hepadnaviruses

Serum from infected persons or woodchucks containing more than 10^9 HBV genomes/mL was used as a source of virus. We have used 0.5–17 mL of infectious serum depending on the virus titer.

2.2. Cells and Reagents

1. HepG2 cells purchased from American Type Culture Collection (Rockville, MD, USA).
2. RPMI-1640 with sodium bicarbonate and L-glutamine (BioWittaker, Walkersville, MD, USA).
3. RPMI-1640 powder for 1 L without sodium bicarbonate and with L-glutamine (Gibco, Gaithersburg, MD, USA).

4. Fetal bovine serum (FBS, BioWittaker, Walkersville, MD, USA).
5. Trypsin–versine solution (BioWittaker, Walkersville, MD, USA).
6. Staphylococcal protease V8 (Beohringer, Germany).
7. 2-*N*-Morpholinoethanesulfonic acid (MES, Sigma, St. Louis, MO, USA).
8. Sucrose (Sigma, St. Louis, MO, USA).
9. 0.45-μm 500-mL bottle top filter (Nalge Nunc International, Rochester, NY, USA).
10. Ultrafree-15 centrifugal filter device (Millipore, Bedford, MA, USA).
11. Ultrafree-MC 100K NMWL (Millipore, Bedford, MA, USA).
12. Polyvinylidene fluoride (PVDF) membranes (Millipore, Bedford, MA, USA).
13. 0.45-μm Syringe driven filter (Millipore, Bedford, MA, USA).
14. 96-Well polystyrene plates (Nunc, Naperville, IL, USA).
15. Anti-preS2 antibody for HBV or WHV.
16. Anti-core protein antibody for HBV or WHV.
17. Bovine serum albumin (BSA, Bio-Whittaker, MA, USA).
18. Primers "158" (3'-AGACCACCAAATGCCCCTATC) and "159" (5'-TTCCCAAGAATAT GGTGACCC).
19. Primers XYL3 (3'-AGACCTCCTAATGCACCCATT) and XYL4 (5'-TTCCCAAGAATA TGGTTTACC).
20. Nylon membrane (Bio-Rad, Hercules, CA).
21. Ultrafree-DA (Millipore, MA, USA).
22. Random priming kit (Gibco-BRL, USA).
23. [^{32}P]dCTP (DuPont NEN, Boston, MA, USA).
24. Rapid-hyb buffer (Amersham, Piscataway, NJ, USA).
25. Proteinase K (FisherBiotech, Fair Lawn, NJ).
26. Fluorescein isothiocyanate (FITC)-conjugated goat anti-mouse antibody (Jackson ImmunoResearch West Grove, PA, USA).
27. Gelatin (Sigma, St Louis, MO, USA).
28. Mowiol 488 (Hoechst, Frankfurt/Main, Germany).

2.3. Solutions

1. 0.01 *M* Potassium phosphate buffer, pH 7.6.
2. Phosphate-buffered saline (PBS), pH 7.4.
3. TNE buffer: 0.01 *M* Tris-HCl, pH 7.4, 0.15 *M* NaCl, 0.05% EDTA.
4. Solution for sucrose gradient ultracentrifugation:
   15% (w/v) sucrose: 15 g of sucrose is solved in 85 mL of TNE buffer.
   25% (w/v) sucrose: 25 g of sucrose is solved in 75 mL of TNE buffer.
   35% (w/v) sucrose: 35 g of sucrose is solved in 65 mL of TNE buffer.
   45% (w/v) sucrose: 45 g of sucrose is solved in 55 mL of TNE buffer.
   60% (w/v) sucrose: 60 g of sucrose is solved in 40 mL of TNE buffer.
5. 0.01 *M* $NaHCO_3$–Na_2CO_3, pH 9.6.
6. Washing buffer: 1X PBS with 0.05% Tween-20, pH 7.4.
7. 0.2 *M* NaOH.
8. 0.2 *M* Tris-HCl buffer, pH 7.5.
9. 2 *M* NaOH.
10. Neutralization buffer: 1.0 M Tris-HCl, pH 8.0, 1.5 *M* NaCl.
11. Lysis buffer: 0.01 *M* Tris-HCl, pH 7.4, 0.5% Nonidet P-40 (NP-40), 0.01 *M* NaCl; and 0.003 *M* $MgCl_2$.
12. 1% Agarose gel in TAE buffer.

13. 0.01 *M* HAc–NaAc buffer, pH 2.5.
14. Cell fixer: 50% methanol and 50% acetone.
15. Block solution: 0.8% bovine serum albumin (BSA), 0.1% gelatin, 5% goat serum in PBS.
16. Washing buffer: 0.8% BSA, 0.1% gelatin in PBS.
17. Mounting solution: 1 *M* Mowiol 488 (Hoechst, Frankfurt/Main, Germany) plus 10% 1,4-diazobicyclo-[2,2,2]-octane.

2.4. Culture Media

1. Normal growth medium for culture of HepG2 cells: RPMI-1640 (with sodium bicarbonate and L-glutamine) containing 10% FBS.
2. pH 5.5 medium for viral infection: RPMI-1640 medium powders for 1 L (without sodium bicarbonate and with L-glutamine) was dissolved in 500 mL of sterilized distilled water. The pH was adjusted to 5.5 with MES. Medium was filtered with a 500 mL bottletop filter, then diluted to 1 L with sterilized distilled water. Ten percent FBS was added before use. (*See* **Note 1.**)

2.5. Equipment

1. Sanitary laminar flow safety hood.
2. CO_2 incubator.
3. Ultracentrifuge and rotors: SW41 and SW55 (Beckman).
4. High-performance liquid chromatography (HPLC).
5. Bio-Silect SEC 250 column (Bio-Rad, CA, USA).
6. Digital MultiImage system (Alpha Innotech, USA).
7. Dot-blot apparatus (Schleicher and Schuell, Keene, NH, USA).
8. "Cross linker" (Stratagene, La Jolla, CA, USA).
9. PhosphorImager (Bio-Rad, Hercules, CA, USA).
10. Polymerase chain reaction (PCR) thermocycler.
11. Fluorescence microscope.

3. Methods

3.1. Isolation of Virus

1. Prepare sucrose gradients by layering sucrose solutions from the bottom to the top. For an SW41 rotor (Beckman), use 1 mL of 60% sucrose, 2 mL of of 45% sucrose, 2 mL of 35% sucrose, 2 mL of 25% sucrose, and 2 mL of 15% sucrose. For an SW55 rotor (Beckman), use 0.5 mL of 60% sucrose, 1 mL of 45% sucrose, 1 mL of 35% sucrose, 1 mL of 25% sucrose, and 1 mL of 15% sucrose.
2. Serum containing hepadnavirus is layered on top of the 15–60% sucrose gradient cushion. If the volume to be centrifuged is larger than 1 mL, an SW41 rotor is used. The tube should be filled with TNE buffer if the sample does not reach the top of the tube. The sample is centrifuged at 38,000 rpm for 16 h at 10°C. Alternatively, smaller volumes ($<$ 1 mL) are centrifuged using an SW55 rotor at 50,000 rpm for 16 h at 10°C.
3. Fractions of either 500 μL with large samples or 200 μL with small samples are collected. The fractions between 40% and 48% sucrose should contain intact enveloped virions which can be determined by detection of HBV DNA either using dot blot hybridization or immunoabsorbance-PCR (IA-PCR, a quick test, see below).
4. Virus-containing fractions are pooled and dialyzed against 0.01 *M* potassium phosphate buffer, pH 7.6, and concentrated by the Ultrafree-15 centrifugal filter device to 500 μL.

3.2. V8 Protease Digestion of Virus

1. Half of the volume of the concentrated virion (250 μL) from the above procedure is digested with 0.8–1.0 mg/mL of V8 protease in potassium phosphate buffer for 8–12 h at 37°C. The other half of the volume is incubated with the same amount of potassium phosphate buffer for mock digestion.
2. V8 protease is removed from the sample using HPLC with a Bio-Silect SEC 250 column. PBS is used as elution buffer. Viruses are further purified during this process. The virion peak (the first peak, the second peak is V8 protease) at void volume is collected (total approx 1 mL) and concentrated to approx 300 μL for infection using Ultrafree-MC 100K NMWL (*see* **Note 2**).
3. The mock sample is treated similarly. These viruses were used as negative control in the infection assay.
4. The successful elimination of pre-S epitopes by V8 digestion is monitored by SDS electrophoresis (*see* **Subheading 3.3.**) or by enzyme-linked immunosorbent assay (ELISA) with the plate coated by anti-preS2 antibody.
5. If HPLC is not available, V8 protease can be removed from digested samples by sedimentation of virions through a cushion of 2 mL of 20% sucrose (w/v) with an SW55 rotor at 50,000 rpm overnight at 10°C. The pellet containing virions are resuspended in 300 μL of PBS (*see* **Note 3**).
6. After removal of V8 protease, the material should be filtered before using as "inocula" for tissue culture infection. Before filtration, precipitates in the inocula are removed by centrifugation at 12,800*g* in a tabletop centrifuge for 3 min. The clarified inocula supernatant is subjected to filtration with a syringe-driven filter. Viruses are diluted to approx. 10^7 viral genomes/mL with pH 5.5 medium. For infecting a T25 flask cells, 0.8 mL of inoculum is used.

3.3. SDS Polyacrylamide Gel Electrophoresis (SDS-PAGE) and Western Blotting

1. The removal of pre-S region from the virus particle by V8 protease can be examined by SDS-PAGE. One microgram of purified virus either treated with V8 or left untreated is resolved by SDS-PAGE through 12.5% gels.
2. Proteins are stained with silver or transferred to PVDF membranes.
3. The membranes are analyzed by Western blots using antibody as described elsewhere (**2**).

3.4. Infection of HepG2 Cells (see Note 4)

1. HepG2 cells (*see* **Note 5**) cultured in the normal growth RPMI 1640 medium with 10% FBS are seeded in a 25-cm^2 flask at approx 5×10^6.
2. Wash with 5 mL of pH 5.5 medium once, then incubate with virus inoculum containing 10^7 viral genomes/mL overnight (16 h) in an incubator with 5% CO_2 at 37°C.
3. Infected cells are then carefully washed, first with 10 mL of pH 5.5 medium two times, then with 10 mL of PBS two times, followed by two washes with 10 mL of normal growth medium.
4. After washing, cells are maintained in 2 mL of normal growth medium.
5. The medium is collected every day or every 2 d until cells are harvested. Days post-infection (pi) are counted from the first day of medium collection.

3.5. Detection of Progeny Produced by Infected Cells

A challenge to the success of the protease infectivity assay is distinguishing input from progeny virus. We have used several different assays for this purpose, some are protein based, and others are nucleic acid based.

Typically, progeny viral DNA can be detected in the culture medium and inside of the cell as early as the third day pi by sensitive methods such as IA-PCR, acid treatment-PCR, and dot-blot (*see* below). Progeny signal should increase as a function of time. We have found that the signal reaches a maximum between 5 and 8 d pi and decreases thereafter. Progeny can still be detected, however, after more than 20 d. The amount of gene product (polypeptide and/or genome) generated is related to the amount of virus in the inoculum as well as the success of the infection. Our data show that approx 1.5×10^8 virus genomes are secreted into the medium at the eighth day after a successful infection with 1.86×10^7 viral genome (vs 5×10^6 cells). In addition, a minimum of 222 viral genomes per cell have been synthesized in infected cells 8 d pi ***(2)***.

3.5.1. IA-PCR Detection of Progeny Virus DNA in Medium

IA-PCR is a powerful method that combines the specificity of antibody binding with the sensitivity of PCR ***(15)***. Because V8 protease digestion of the virus quantitatively removes pre-S epitopes, the anti-preS2 antibody can be used as a means of selectively precipitating progeny virus and monitoring virus gene product synthesis as a function of time after infection. However, other envelope antibodies may also be used, but may not distinguish input from progeny virions.

1. 96-Well plates are coated with anti-preS2 antibody (40 µg/mL in 0.01 *M* $NaHCO_3$–Na_2CO_3 buffer, pH 9.6) using 100 µL/well at 4°C overnight.
2. The plate is washed with washing buffer (1X PBS with 0.05% Tween-20, pH 7.4) four times.
3. The nonspecific binding is blocked by incubation of wells with 2% BSA in PBS (120 µL/well) at 37°C for 1 h.
4. The plate is washed with washing buffer two times and stored at –20°C until used.
5. To determine the amount of absorbed virus, 50 µL/well of test sample or standard serum with a series of dilution is added, and the plates are incubated at 37°C for 2 h with gentle shaking.
6. After washing four times with wash buffer, the plates are incubated with 25 µL/well 0.2 *M* NaOH at 37°C for 1 h with gentle shaking to release viral DNA. Under these conditions, proteins including both antibody and viral proteins are quantitatively hydrolyzed.
7. The samples are neutralized and mixed well with 40 µL/well 0.2 *M* Tris-HCl buffer, pH 7.5, at room temperature for 5 min.
8. An aliquot of each sample (10 µL) is used to perform PCR with primers 158 and 159 for HBV or XYL3 and XYL4 for WHV.
9. The image of PCR bands that was observed on an ethidium bromide stained gel is quantified by the Digit MultiImage system.
10. The amount of HBV DNA in the sample is determined by comparing the intensity of sample band to the standard bands.

3.5.2. Dot-Blot Detection of Viral DNA in Medium

1. Five hundred microliters of medium from infected cell cultures is incubated with 100 µL of 2 *M* sodium hydroxide at room temperature for 1 h.
2. DNA is transferred to the nylon membrane with a dot-blot apparatus according to the instructions supplied by the manufacturer.

3. The membrane is incubated with a neutralization buffer of 1.0 *M* Tris-HCl, 1.5 *M* NaCl, pH 8.0 for 5 min, followed by exposure to an ultraviolet light "crosslinker."
4. Viral DNA immobilized on the membrane is detected by incubation with a radiolabeled HBV specific probe.
5. The probe is made from a viral DNA fragment produced from PCR amplification with respective primers, which has been extracted from an agarose gel with Ultrafree-DA, and labeled with [^{32}P]dCTP using a random priming kit (Gibco-BRL, USA).
6. Hybridization is performed in Rapid-hyb buffer at 68°C.
7. Radioactivity is detected using a PhosphoriMager (Bio-Rad, CA, USA).

3.5.3. Acid Treatment (of Infected Cells)-PCR Detection of Cellular Viral DNA

1. An easy and sensitive method to detect viral DNA in infected cells was developed in our laboratory.
2. HepG2 infected by V8-digested HBV are harvested by trypsin digestion at 8 d pi.
3. From 500 to 1000 cells are incubated in 1 mL of 0.01 *M* HAc–NaAc buffer, pH 2.4, for 10 min at room temperature.
4. The same amount of infected cells are treated with PBS as control.
5. Cells are sedimented at 3200*g* for 5 min with a table top centrifuge, then washed with 1 mL of PBS.
6. Low pH treated cells are resuspended in 50–100 μL of PBS, depending on the amount of cells used.
7. A 5- to 10-μL cell suspension containing about 100–200 cells are used for performing PCR amplification with respective primers.
8. PCR cycles utilize 95°C for 3 min, then 95°C for 1 min, 55°C for 1 min and 72°C for 2 min for 30 cycles and a final one at 72°C for 5 min.

3.5.4. Southern Blot Detection of Cellular Viral DNA

1. Monolayers of HepG2 cells (10^6 cells) from the cells infected with either V8-digested or mock-digested viruses are harvested by trypsin digestion after d 8 pi.
2. After two washes by sedimentation in PBS, cells are lysed with 0.01 *M* Tris-HCl buffer, pH 7.4, 0.5% NP-40; 0.01 *M* NaCl; and 0.003 *M* $MgCl_2$ and kept on ice for 5 min.
3. Nuclei are removed by centrifugation for 5 min at 500*g* at 4°C.
4. Nuclei depleted supernatants are incubated with 0.5 μg/mL of Proteinase K at 37°C overnight.
5. DNA is extracted with phenol–chloroform and precipitated with ethanol.
6. Twenty micrograms of DNA is resolved through a 1% agarose gel, then transferred to a nylon membrane as described above.
7. The membrane is hybridized with a [^{32}P]dCTP-labeled probe made from a viral DNA fragment as above.
8. The radioactivity signal is recorded on a PhosphoriMager.

3.6. Immunofluorescent Staining of *De Novo* Viral Proteins

1. At d 8 pi, 10^3 HepG2 cells are harvested by trypsin digestion and reseeded onto eight-well glass slides by incubating for an additional 24 h.
2. The cells on the slide are then briefly washed twice with PBS and fixed with 50% methanol and 50% acetone at −20°C for 10 min.

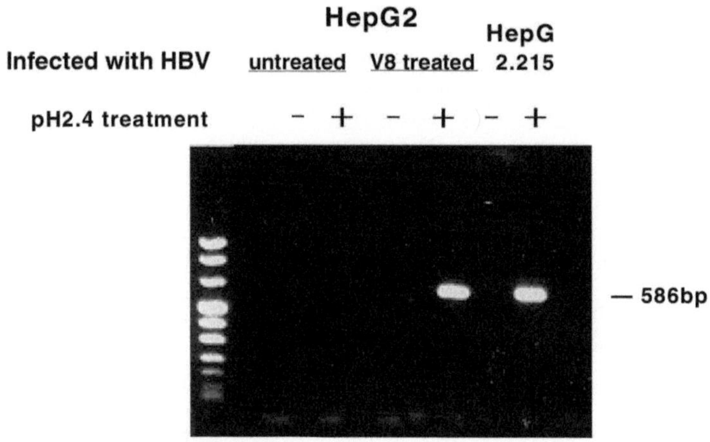

Fig. 1. Acid treatment-PCR detects the cellular HBV DNA. 10^3 cells infected with V8 digested or undigested HBV were treated with HAc–NaAc buffer, pH 2.5 for 10 min. After the cells were washed with PBS, they were suspended in 100µL PBS and 5µL of cells were taken for PCR using HBV primer 158 and 159. HepG2.215 cells were used as control. A PCR product band at 586 bp was indicated.

3. The fixed cells are incubated with 0.8% BSA, 0.1% gelatin, 5% goat serum in PBS at room temperature for 20 min to reduce nonspecific staining.
4. Cells are incubated either with mouse anti-surface protein (anti-SHBs or anti-SWHs) or anti-core protein antibody (anti-HBc or anti-WHc) at 37°C for 1 h.
5. Following five washes with 0.8% BSA, 0.1% gelatin in PBS, cells were incubated with fluorescein-conjugated rabbit anti-mouse antibody at 37°C for 1 h.
6. Cells are washed with the same buffer five times and covered with 1 *M* Mowiol 488 plus 10% 1,4-diazobicyclo-[2,2,2]-octane and viewed under a fluorescence microscope.

3.7. Results

Infection of HepG2 cell cultures with V8-treated HBV and WHV was described in detail in our two papers, which includes use of IA-PCR and dot blotting to detect the progeny viral DNA in the culture medium as well as Southern blotting to detect intracellular viral DNA and immunostaining to detect viral proteins ***(1,2)***. Thus, we limit the data here to show detection of the *de novo* cellular HBV DNA, using acid treatment-PCR. From 500 to 1000 infected cells were first treated with HAc–NaAc buffer, pH 2.5, for 10 min. pH 2.5 buffer is intended to remove residual virus from the inocula remaining attached to the cell membrane. This is important to enrich for detection of intracellular viral DNA as well as rendering the cells permeable for PCR. **Figure 1** shows that at d 8 pi, HBV DNA is detectable in HepG2 cells infected with V8 treated HBV, but not in the cells infected with untreated HBV (**Fig. 1**, *lanes 2* and *4*). However, this HBV DNA can be detected only by treatment of infected cells with pH 2.5 buffer (**Fig.1**, *lanes 3* and *4*). The same result is obtained with HepG2 2.2.15 cells, which has integrated HBV genome (**Fig. 1**, *lanes 5* and *6*). This result suggests that the cellular HBV

DNA can be released for PCR detection only after low pH treatment. It also suggests that the DNA detected in the cells infected by V8-treated HBV is progeny DNA generated by HBV infection.

4. Notes

1. It is important to use medium without sodium bicarbonate to make pH 5.5 medium. The buffer capability of sodium bicarbonate not only makes it difficult to adjust the pH with MES but also results in a high ion concentration that is harmful to cell viability.
2. A final check of the concentration of virus with either IA-PCR or dot blot is recommended. More than 10^7 viral genomes/mL is needed for infection. Fewer than 10^6 viral genomes/mL would not give determined results.
3. A final determination of the virus abundance in the sample is necessary because significant losses may occur.
4. Infection should be performed in a safety hood.
5. Before use, the cells should be reseeded a couple of times (about 4–5 d each time) to keep them healthy and growing. The optimal cells for infection are 90–95% confluent after 4–5 d growth. Complete confluence is not suggested because cells may detach from the monolayer after pH 5.5 medium treatment. For a T25 flask, cells at approx 5×10^6 is enough for infection assay. If the cells are in good condition (based on inspection under a microscope), overnight incubation in pH 5.5 medium will not generally result in major cell distress. However, some arrest of cell growth is usually observed. Nevertheless, after changing to normal growth medium, within 24 h the cells should appear to have recovered and look as refractive and morphologically intact by examination under the light microscope as they did before infection.

Acknowledgments

This work has been supported by The Hepatitis B Foundation of America and an appropriation from The Commonwealth of Pennsylvania.

References

1. Lu, X., Block, T., and Gerlich, W. H. (1996) Protease-induced infectivity of hepatitis B virus for a human hepatoma cell line. *J. Virol.* **70,** 2277–2285.
2. Lu, X., Hazboun, T. and Block, T. M. (2001) Limited proteolysis induces woodchuck hepatitis virus infectivity for human HepG2 cells. *Virus* Res. **73**, 27–40.
3. Qiao, M., MacNaughton, T. B., and Gowans, E. J. (1994) Adsorption and penetration of hepatitis B virus in a nonpermissive cell line. *Virology* **201,** 356–363.
4. Sells, M. A., Chen, M. L., and Acs, G. (1987) Production of hepatitis B virus particles in HepG2 cells transfected with cloned hepatitis B virus DNA. *Proc. Natl. Acad. Sci. USA* **84,** 1005–1009.
5. Gripon, P., Diot, C., Theze, N., et al. (1988) Hepatitis B virus infection of adult human hepatocytes cultured in the presence of dimethyl sulfoxide. *J. Virol.* **62,** 4136–4143.
6. Gripon, P., Diot, C., and Guguen-Guillouzo, C. (1993) Reproducible high level infection of cultured adult human hepatocytes by hepatitis B virus: effect of polyethylene glycol on adsorption and penetration. *Virology* **192,** 534–540.
7. Ochiya, T., Tsurimoto, T., Ueda, K., Okubo, K., Shiozawa, M., and Matsubara, K. (1989) An in vitro system for infection with hepatitis B virus that uses primary human fetal hepatocytes. *Proc Natl. Acad. Sci. USA* **86,** 1875–1879.

8. Galle, P. R., Haglestein, J., and Kommerell, B. (1994) In vitro experimental infection of primary human heptocytes with hepatitis B virus. *Gastroenterology* **106,** 664–673.
9. Paran, N., Geiger, B., and Shaul, Y. (2001) HBV infection of cell culture: evidence for multivalent and cooperative attachment. *EMBO J.* **20,** 4443–4453.
10. Li, J. S., Tong, S. P., and Wands, J. R. (1996) Characterization of a 120-kilodalton pre-S-binding protein as a candidate duck hepatitis B virus receptor. *J. Viro.* **70,** 6029–6035.
11. Eng, F. J., Novikova, E. G., Kuroki, K., Ganem, D., and Fricker, L. D. (1998) gp180, a protein that binds duck hepatitis B virus particles, has metallocarboxypeptidase D-like enzymatic activity. *J. Biol. Chem.* **273**, 8382–8388.
12. Qiao, M., Scougall, C. A., Duszynski, A., and Burrell1, C. J. (1999) Kinetics of early molecular events in duck hepatitis B virus replication in primary duck hepatocytes. *J. Gen. Virol.* **80,** 2127–2135.
13. Gerlich, W. H., Lu, X., and Heermann, K. H. (1993) Studies on the attachment and penetration of hepatitis B virus. *J. Hepatol.* **17 (Suppl. 3),** S10–S14.
14. Oess, S. and Hildt, E. (2000) Novel cell permeable motif derived from the PreS2-domain of hepatitis-B virus surface antigens. *Gene Ther.* **7**, 750–758.
15. Simsek, E., Ouzounov, S., Hazboum, T., Block, T. M. and Lu, X. A specific and sensitive method for quantification of HBV DNA. In preparation.

18

Construction of Recombinant Adenoviruses that Produce Infectious Hepatitis B Virus

Martin Sprinzl, Jérôme Dumortier, and Ulrike Protzer

1. Introduction

Hepatitis B viruses (HBVs) are characterized by their high species and tissue specificity. Because of the large number of patients chronically infected with HBV, the development of new treatment strategies remains a major goal but is hindered by the lack of infection systems that would allow testing. Only primary human or humanoid hepatocytes are fully permissive for HBV infection. Consequently, no permissive cell line and no convenient small animal model are available to study HBV infection. However, highly differentiated liver cell lines support virus replication following transfection of replication competent HBV constructs. Stable cell lines with integrated HBV genomes, for example, HepG 2.2.15 cells *(1)*, are commonly used for assessing the action of drugs on HBV replication. HBV-transgenic mice *(2)* and have been generated and were proven to be very useful for immunological studies. However, stable cell lines as well as transgenic mice, unlike in natural infection, replicate HBV from an integrated genome that cannot be eliminated. In addition, they cannot mimic an acute infection and the level of virus replication cannot be varied or adjusted.

We describe a system that allows the initiation of HBV replication across the species barrier in a broad range of liver cells and in the livers of animals by circumventing receptor-mediated uptake. This system employs adenoviral vectors that transfer 1.3-fold overlength HBV genomes from which infectious HBV is produced at high titers and with high liver specificity. These HBV constructs have proven to be superior over other replication-competent HBV constructs in transgenic mice *(2)* and were used for a baculovirus-mediated HBV genome transfer *(3)*.

The adenovirus-mediated genome transfer described here efficiently initiates hepadnavirus replication from an extrachromosomal template in established cell lines, in primary hepatocytes from various species, and in the livers of mice *(4,5)*. Following the genome transfer, HBV proteins, genomic RNA, and all replicative DNA intermediates

From: *Methods in Molecular Medicine, vol. 96: Hepatitis B and D Protocols, volume 2*
Edited by: R. K. Hamatake and J. Y. N. Lau © Humana Press Inc., Totowa, NJ

were detected. Detection of covalently closed circular DNA (cccDNA) in hepatoma cell lines and in primary hepatocytes indicated that an intracellular replication cycle independent from the transferred linear viral genome was established ***(4,5)***. High titer hepatitis B virions were released into the culture medium of hepatoma cells and the various primary hepatocytes following AdHBV transduction. In addition, using the duck hepatitis B virus, we showed that infectious virions were secreted into the serum of mice ***(4)***.

Adenoviral vectors became our first choice to transfer HBV genomes to establish a HBV replication system, as a broad range of resting or dividing cells of various species are transduced. In addition, adenoviral vectors allow the transfer of defined quantities of foreign DNA into cells. Finally, adenoviral vectors efficiently target the liver following in vivo gene transfer and transduced DNA is not integrated into the cellular chromosome. Extrachromosomal transduction of HBV genomes appears to be essential to mimic natural HBV infection, because integration of HBV genomes into cellular chromosomes is a rare event during HBV infection. It usually marks the switch from a highly replicative phase to a low replication state occurring late during chronic HBV infection. Replication of HBV from an extrachromosomal template might therefore be an attractive target for antiviral strategies, which this system allows to be tested in cell culture and in living animals. In addition, a HBV genome transfer is so far the only way to study the immune response against HBV during acute infection in mice ***(10)***.

Commonly used adenoviral vectors are derived from a modified human adenovirus serotype 5. The vector genome includes the entire adenoviral DNA sequence except the genes responsible for the initiation and propagation of an adenoviral replication. This region is named E1 in respect to their early expression during the adenoviral replication cycle and was replaced by the HBV genome construct. Additional deletions in region E3 reduce adenoviral genome size and facilitate integration of transgenes without exceeding the adenoviral encapsidation capacity ***(6)***.

Unfortunately, conventional generation of recombinant adenoviruses by ligation of transgenes into the adenoviral genome backbone or by recombination in mammalian cell cultures proved to be technically challenging and time consuming. To generate AdHBV, we therefore employed a method first published by T-C. He et. al. ***(7)*** that allows the generation of recombinant adenoviral genomes by homologous recombination in *E. coli.* On transfection of the defined recombinant adenoviral genome into mammalian 293 or 911 cells, the adenoviral vectors grow.

The so-called AdEasy system employs a large adenoviral backbone plasmid and an easy-to-manipulate shuttle plasmid that contains overlapping adenoviral sequences and allows insertion of a gene of interest. If desired, a shuttle plasmid containing a green fluorescent protein (GFP) reporter cassette is available that facilitates monitoring of vector growth and titration of vector stocks and allows monitoring of transduction ***(7)***. Following linearization of the shuttle plasmid, adenoviral sequences are exposed to the DNA ends and can participate in homologous recombination with the supercoiled adenoviral backbone in recombination competent *E. coli* BJ5183. On recombination, the shuttle plasmid confers a kanamycin resistance gene that allows for the efficient selection of recombinants. Restriction analysis of recombinant DNA isolated from the *E. coli* reveals characteristic restriction patterns (**Fig. 1**). Recently, *E. coli* (BJ5183) already containing the adenoviral backbone plasmid pAdEasy1 became available that eliminates the rate-limiting step of transforming the large plasmid. Once a proper recombinant has been identified, further amplification of plasmid DNA is recommended in standard *E. coli* to avoid further DNA sequence alterations and to increase the yield of DNA. The recombinant adenoviral genome is excised from the plasmid backbone via artificial *Pac*I sites to expose the adenoviral inverted terminal repeats (ITRs) and is transfected into suitable cell lines (e.g., 293 or 911 cells). These cell lines must provide the missing E1 gene products by transcomplementation to allow growth of the adenoviral vectors *(7)*. Cell lysates and culture medium contain the adenoviral vectors and can be used for further propagation. Once a suitable titer is reached, vector stocks are either used directly for experimental infections or processed further for applications in vivo.

Using AdHBV vectors produced as described, we could not only initiate efficient hepatitis B virus replication in cultured liver cells *(4,5)*, but could also transduce HBV genomes into the livers of mice which then start to replicate the virus from an extrachromosomal template (**Fig. 2**). This will allow development of small animal models of HBV infection and will help to study pathogenicity of wild-type and mutant viruses as well as virus–host interaction and new therapeutic and prophylactic approaches.

2. Materials

2.1. Plasmids

The system employs an adenoviral backbone plasmid (pAdEasy) and adenoviral shuttle plasmid (pShuttle/pAdTrack) containing overlapping adenoviral sequences that allow homologous recombination. All adenoviral plasmid constructs used were generously provided by Tong-Chuan He and Bert Vogelstein, Howard Hughes Medical Institute, Baltimore, MD, USA. The constructs are commercially available from Stratagene, La Jolla, CA, USA and from Qbiogen, Illkirch, France. (*See* **Note 1.**)

1. pAdEasy: Adenoviral backbone plasmid pAdEasy1 contains all Ad5 sequences except those encompassing the E1 region, the left ITR, and the E3 region, and is used for generation of E1/E3 deleted Ad5 vectors. The pAdEasy2 is identical to pAdEasy1 except that it contains an additional deletion encompassing the E4 region. It is used for generation of E1/E3/E4 deleted Ad5 vectors. Both adenoviral plasmids contain an ampicillin resistance gene and are used in a supercoiled form *(7)*.
2. pShuttle/pAdTrack: Adenoviral shuttle plasmid pShuttle contains a multiple cloning site to allow convenient insertion of the "gene of interest"—in our case the replication competent HVB 1.3 genome—into the E1 deletion. This site is surrounded by Ad5 sequences that allow homologous recombination with pAdEasy and confer the left ITR and packaging signal sequences (nucleotides 1–480 of Ad5). Artificial *Pac*I restriction sites flank the Ad5 genome *(7)*. pAdTrack is identical to pShuttle except that it contains a CMV promoter driven enhanced GFP expression cassette downstream of the multiple cloning site. A unique *Pme*I restriction site between the adenoviral sequences is used for linearization of the shuttle plasmids which forces homologous recombination with the adenoviral backbone. On recombi-

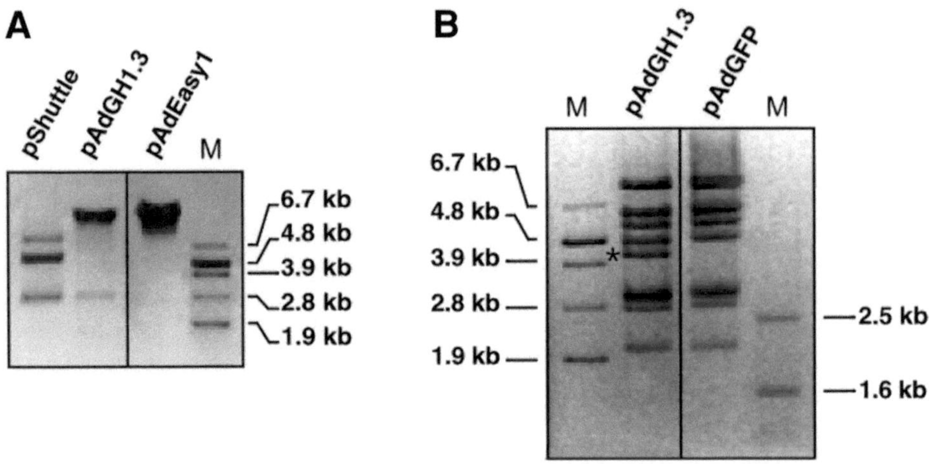

Fig. 1. Restriction analysis of adenoviral recombinants. **(A)** The first analysis of candidate recombinants is performed with *PacI* resulting in excision of a 3-kb or a 4.5-kb fragment containing sequences derived from the integrated shuttle plasmids. To confirm that a large plasmid was grown, pAdEasy was analyzed in parallel. **(B)** Restriction digestion with *Hin*dIII results in a typical restriction pattern of Ad5-based genomes as demonstrated for a recombinant containing a GFP gene (pAdGFP). The HBV 1.3 genome integrated into the adenoviral recombinant (pAdGH1.3) is excised by flanking *Hin*dIII sites and migrates as a 4.3-kb band (marked by an *asterisk*). M, DNA marker.

nation, the shuttle plasmids provide a kanamycin resistance gene that allows antibiotic selection of *E. coli* containing recombinant adenoviral vector genomes.

3. pHBV1.3: The parental plasmid for HBV was pHBV1.3 (kindly provided by Heinz Schaller, ZMBH, University of Heidelberg). It contains an 1.3-fold overlength genome of HBV, subtype ayw, with a 5' terminal redundancy encompassing enhancers I and II, the origin of replication (direct repeats DR1 and DR2), the X- and pregenomic/core promoter regions, the transcription initiation site of the pregenomic RNA, the unique polyadenylation site, and the entire X open reading frame that serves as a template for transcription of HBV pregenomic and subgenomic RNAs **(2,4)**. This construct has been proven to initiate replication of HBV efficiently and with high liver specificity in transfection experiments in cell culture and in transgenic mice *(2)*. The 1.3-fold HBV genome was excised via flanking *Pst*I/*Nhe*I restriction sites and cloned into the multiple cloning site of pAdTrack using adapters that included *Hind* III sites flanking the HBV construct.

2.2. Bacterial Strains

E. coli BJ 5183, which are not *recA* but are deficient in other enzymes mediating bacterial recombination, were employed for recombination. BJAdEasy cells already contain a pAdEasy1 plasmid and thus avoid the limiting step of transforming a large plasmid. They show resistance against ampicillin and streptomycin. Standard *recA*-deficient *E. coli* strains (e.g., DH5α, DH10B, XL1) are used for growth of plasmids to increase DNA yields without further unwanted recombinations.

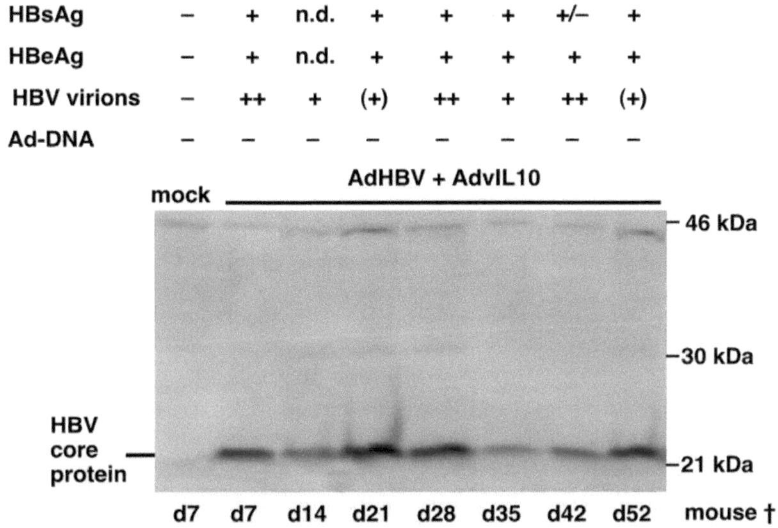

Fig. 2. AdHBV infection of mice results in productive HBV replication. Mice were injected into the tail vein with 10^9 IU AdHBV and 10^8 IU of an adenoviral vector expressing a viral analog of the immunosuppressive cytokine IL-10 (kindly provided by Thomas Ritter, Freie Universität Berlin, Germany). A control mouse was injected with PBS (mock). Secretory HBV antigens (HBsAg and HBeAg) were determined in mouse sera (1:20 diluted in PBS) using commercial assays. HBV virions were immunoprecipitated from mouse sera using an anti-HBs antibody and HBV DNA in the virions was assayed by PCR. Adenoviral DNA was amplified by PCR from DNA extracted from mouse sera. HBV core protein in mouse livers was analyzed by Western blot analysis of liver lysates using a polyclonal rabbit antiserum and a peroxidase-coupled secondary antibody and chemiluminescence. Animals were killed at consecutive time points (7–52). Secretion of HBsAg, HBeAg, and HBV virions into the mouse sera as well as expression of HBV core protein in mouse livers shows replication of HBV following adenoviral genome transfer.

2.3. Cell Culture

For propagation of pAdEasy1-based vectors, we routinely use E1 transformed human embryonic kidney cells (293 cells) ***(4)***. Alternatively, E1 transformed embryonic retinal cells (911 cells) are available ***(7,8)***. Cells were maintained in minimum essential medium Eagle supplemented with 10% fetal calf serum, 2 m*M* L-glutamine, 50 IU/mL of penicillin, and 50 μg/mL of streptomycin at 37°C in 5% CO_2.

2.4. Solutions

1. Phosphate-buffered saline (PBS) buffer: 140 m*M* NaCl, 10 m*M* Na_2HPO_4, pH 7.4.
2. TE buffer: 10 m*M* Tris-HCl, pH 8; 0.1 m*M* EDTA.
3. 2X HBS buffer: 137 m*M* NaCl; 0.5 m*M* KCl, 0.7 m*M* $Na_2HPO_4{\cdot}2H_2O$; 6 m*M* dextrose, 21 m*M* *N*-(2-Hydroxyethylpiperazine)-l-ethanesulfonic acid (HEPES), adjust final pH to 7.05 with NaOH. For an HBS-buffer stock (2X) dissolve 1.6 g of NaCl, 0.074 g of KCl, 0.027 g of Na_2HPO_4, 0.2 g of dextrose, 1 g of HEPES; add H_2O to 100 mL

4. Virus storage buffer: 137 m*M* NaCl, 5 m*M* KCl, 10 m*M* Tris-HCl, pH 7.5, 1 m*M* $MgCl_2$, 10% glycerol.
5. 2X Storage buffer: 10 m*M* Tris-HCl, pH 8.0, 100 m*M* NaCl, 0.1% bovine serum albumin (BSA), and 50% glycerol.

3. Methods

3.1. Homologous Recombination in E. coli (BJAdEasy)

1. Shuttle plasmids (0.1–0.5 μg) pAdTrack or pAdShuttle containing an HBV 1.3-fold genome are linearized with restriction nuclease (*Pme*I). We usually add 1 U of *Pme*I to cleave a total amount of 0.1 μg DNA. As *Pme*I is meta-stable at 37°C, we add one half of total *Pme*I for 2 h at 37°C and then digest further after adding the second half of total *Pme*I for 2 h to overnight at room temperature. To ensure complete linearization, the restriction digest is monitored by gel electrophoresis of an aliquot in a 0.8% agarose gel. Following digestion, DNAs are ethanol precipitated and resuspended in 10 μL of distilled H_2O. Complete linearization is critical for reducing the background. Therefore, plasmid purification by preparative gel electrophoresis may be used.
2. Cotransform *E. coli* BJ5183 with 0.1–0.5 μg of linearized pShuttle/pAdTrack and 1 μg (45 fmol) of pAdEasy. *E. coli* BJAdEasy are only transformed with 0.05–0.1 μg linearized shuttle plasmid. As *E. coli* BJ5183 tends to show a low competency, it is essential to prepare these cells carefully for transformation. Standard protocols for preparation of electrocompetent *E. coli* and standard transformation procedures are sufficient to obtain a yield of $>10^4$ cfu/fmol plasmid DNA. Competency of *E. coli* is tested with 0.1 fmol of plasmid DNA, for example, pUC13. Preincubation of the transformation mixture at 37°C without antibiotic selection should not exceed 15 min. Subsequently, the transformed bacteria are plated onto L-Broth agar plates containing 50 μg/mL of kanamycin. (*See* **Note 2**.)
3. Following 12–16 h of incubation at 37°C, choose the smallest colonies for further growth in liquid L-Broth medium containing 50 μg/mL of kanamycin. Perform plasmid DNA mini-preparations by standard alkaline lysis. Correct recombinants are identified by restriction analysis with *Pac*I or *Hind*III. Following *Pac*I digestion, recombinant clones will yield a large fragment (>30 kb) representing the adenoviral DNA and a small fragment (3 or 4.5 kb), which is derived from the integrated pShuttle or pAdTrack and contains the plasmid backbone. *Hind*III restriction digestion will result in a characteristic restriction pattern **(Fig. 1).**
4. Once confirmed, supercoiled DNA of correct recombinants are transformed into your standard *recA E. coli* (e.g., DH5α or DH10B) for further propagation. Finally, purify plasmid DNA from midi- or maxi-cultures by CsCl-banding or by ion-exchange columns that allow binding of large DNAs (e.g., Nucleobond®).

3.2. Amplification of Adenoviral Vectors in Cell Culture

1. At 24 h prior to transfection, 293 cells or 911 cells are seeded onto 25-cm² cell culture flasks. Confluence of cells should be around 50% at the time of transfection. (*See* **Note 3**.)
2. Before transfection, digest the recombinant adenoviral plasmids with *Pac*I to liberate the ends of the respective adenoviral genome to allow replication. Usually 4–7 mg of DNA are sufficient to transfect one culture dish. Precipitate digested DNA with ethanol, centrifuge the precipitate, and dry the pellet under sterile conditions. Dissolve DNA in 450 μL of distilled water and add 50 μL of 2.5 *M* $CaCl_2$ solution. During thorough mixing, add 500 μL of HBS buffer (2X) to the solution drop by drop. DNA precipitates will form during 10–15 min incubation at room temperature and subsequently are added to the cell culture medium. Alterna-

tive transfection protocols may be used. After 12–16 h incubation, cells are washed and maintained as described.

3. If pAdTrack has been employed during recombination, transfection of cells can be monitored by expression of green fluorescent protein using fluorescence microscopy. At 12–24 hours after transfection, the first GFP-expressing cells can be observed. After 2–3 d, single cells replicating the adenovirus round off and give rise to virus-producing cell-foci or plaques *(7)*. Plaques can be observed after 7–10 d as groups of rounded cells by phase-contrast microscopy and represent the typical cytopathic effect elicited by adenoviruses. However, GFP expression largely facilitates the identification of plaques for an inexperienced person. When the majority of cells start to detach from the cell culture plastic, it is time to mobilize them completely with a rubber policeman or a pipet. Do not use trypsin!
4. Transfer the cell suspension into a conical 50-mL tube and recover cells by centrifugation (10 min at 500*g*). Resuspend the cell pellet in 2 mL of sterile PBS and subject cells to three or four freeze–thaw cycles with vigorous vortex-mixing to free all virus from the cells. Cellular debris is removed by brief centrifugation and the adenovirus containing supernatant is stored at –70°C after addition of 10% glycerol for stabilization. (*See* **Note 4.**) The procedure will yield about 10^6–10^7 infectious particles/mL at this point. Avoid freezing on dry ice because adenoviruses are sensitive to low pH. (*See* **Note 5.**)
5. For further amplification of adenoviral vectors, use 30–40% of your primary cell lysate to infect a 75-cm² flask of 80–90% confluent 293 or 911 cells. To increase infection efficacy, remove cell culture medium, apply virus stocks in a low volume (1–2 mL), and allow viruses to bind to the cells for 15–20 min at room temperature before cell culture medium is added. Cells are maintained as described and when the majority of cells start to detach from the cell culture dish (usually after 2–5 d), follow the protocol listed above. Repeated amplification may be necessary. Each infection cycle will lead to a 10- to 100-fold increase of viral titers. When adenoviral titers increase, the cell culture medium containing approx 1% of the total virus may also be preserved or the cells may be lysed in the culture medium. To ensure that a clonal adenovirus is grown, plaque purification may be desired which can be performed following standard protocols.
6. Because rare recombination events with the adenoviral DNA integrated in 293 cells may lead to unwanted contamination with wild-type adenovirus, it is recommended that continuous passaging of adenoviral vector stocks be avoided. Rather, a low passage vector stock should be kept for growing new vector stocks, or the virus should be plaque purified in between.

3.3. Assays to Quantify Adenoviral Vectors

If the construct contains GFP, titration of the viral stock can be done by dilution assays on permissive cells (typically 293, 911, or HeLa cells). Expression units can be determined by counting GFP expressing cells, for example, by FACS analysis 18–24 h post-infection (i.e., before the first round of replication is finished!). Triplicate dilutions are recommended. If the adenoviral vector contains no GFP marker, the cytopathic effect observed at the end of the first round of replication (i.e., after 36 h) and after 8–10 d using at least triplicate limiting dilutions may be used to determine infectious units. Because the cytopathic effect is hard to quantify, we prefer an immunofluorescence staining of adenoviral proteins in 293 or 911 producer cells for precise titration of vector stocks.

To determine the amount of adenoviral particles contained in a vector stock, the amount of DNA may be quantified and used as a surrogate marker. Because the protein content alters the optical density at 260 nm, only serum-free virus stocks can be quantified by this method. To determine the amount of viral particles, add 15 µL of virus to 15 µL of blank solution. As a blank solution use 1.35 g/mL of CsCl mixed with an equal volume of 2X storage buffer. Add 100 µL of TE/0.1% Sodium dodecy/sulfate (SDS), vortex-mix for 30 s, and centrifuge for 5 min. From the supernatant, determine the OD_{260}. One A_{260} unit contains approx 10^{12} viral particles. Depending on the quality of the vector preparation, the ratio of total adenovirus particles to infectious particles ranges between 20:1 and 100:1. (*See* **Note 6.**)

3.4. Preparation of High-Titer Vector Stocks

1. To produce high titer vector stocks, usually 8–16 cell culture flasks (150-cm^2) containing 293 or 911 cells at a confluence of 80–90% (approx 2×10^7 cells/flask) are required. These cells are infected with the respective adenovirus stock at a multiplicity of infection of 5 IU per cell. After 2–3 d post-infection, when 80% of the cells are rounded and detached from the flask, cells are harvested as described above. The cell suspensions are collected in sterile 50-mL tubes.
2. Cells are sedimented at 500*g* for 10 min, resuspended in 2.5–3 mL of 0.1 *M* Tris-HCl, pH 8.0, buffer per 150-cm^2 flask, and lysed by four freeze–thaw–vortex cycles as described above. Cell debris is carefully removed by centrifugation at 5000–7000*g* for 5–10 min at 4°C.
3. Virus is purified in a CsCl density gradient. To prepare the gradient, add 4.4 g of CsCl into a 50-mL tube and mix it with 8 mL of cleared cell lysate by vortex-mixing. Transfer the solution with an approximate density of 1.35 g/mL to a 12-mL SW41 rotor tube. Overlay the solution with 2 mL of mineral oil to prevent formation of infectious aerosol during centrifugation. Ultracentrifuge for 18–24 h at 10°C (32,000 rpm using an SW40 rotor in a Beckman ultracentrifuge).
4. The fraction containing virus equilibrates at a density of 1.35 g/mL and can be visualized as a dull milky band. In a typical gradient, the band containing virus will be clearly separated from a band containing mainly defective particles that sediment at a lower density and should be collected in a total volume of 0.5–1 mL. Alternatively, the first gradient can be run as a discontinuous gradient using equal amounts of CsCl at 1.4 g/mL and 1.2 g/mL for 2 h. To obtain a high grade of purification, a second continuous gradient using CsCl at 1.35 g/mL is recommended following dilution of the banded virus in an equal volume of TE. The virus is stable in CsCl at 4°C for several weeks. If longer storage is required, mix the collected virus with an equal volume of filter sterilized 2X storage buffer and store it at –70°C.
5. To avoid toxicity, CsCl has to be completely removed before virus stocks are used in vivo. For dialysis under sterile conditions, 1–2 L of storage buffer and a pot containing a magnet stirrer must be autoclaved for each vector stock. UV-irradiated, sealed dialysis chambers are recommended (Slyde-A-Lyzer, 0.5–3 mL, Perstorp Life Science). To avoid contamination and to fulfill biosafety conditions, dialysis should be performed at room temperature in a laminar flow hood. Following injection of the vector stock into the dialysis chamber, it is dialyzed against the 200-fold volume of virus storage buffer for 2–3 h. After exchanging the buffer, dialysis is repeated. Dialyzed virus is removed from the chamber, titered and stored at –80°C until further use. (*See* **Note 7.**)

4. Notes

1. Excellent and detailed protocols to generate adenoviral vectors with the help of the AdEasy system, plasmid maps, and sequence information are in the meantime available at the following Internet sites:
   http://www.coloncancer.org/adeasy.htm

http://www.qbiogene.com/products/gene-expression/adeasy.html
http://www.stratagene.com/vectors/expression/adeasy.htm

2. In our hands, electrocompetent and chemically competent *E. coli* worked comparably. However, it proved crucial that cells were highly competent. They have to form at least 10^4 colonies on transformation with 1 fmol of pUC plasmid.
3. For efficient production of adenoviral vectors, 293 cells have to be in a good condition. It proved advantageous to keep them constantly growing. It is critical not to use high passages (>30) of the cells.
4. Repeated thawing of adenoviral vector stocks lead to decreased infectivity and should be avoided. Once thawed, stocks can be stored at 4°C for several days.
5. Adenoviruses are sensitive to pH changes; for example, freezing or transport on dry ice should therefore be done with care.
6. Quantification of adenoviral particles by determining the OD_{260} as described above is recommended before dialysis or further processing because high particle concentrations may cause insoluble aggregation dependent on the pH.
7. Because the adenoviral vectors contain replication-competent HBV genomes they are able to initiate HBV replication and produce infectious HBV. Therefore, only persons with an appropriate vaccination status (anti-HBs >100 IU/mL) should be allowed to participate in the experiments. Vector stocks have to be handled under appropriate biosafety conditions. However, the infectious potential of the adeno-HBV vectors described does not exceed that of naturally occurring HBV because the adenoviral vector is replication deficient and thus solely serves as a transfer vehicle of HBV DNA. The 1.3-fold overlength HBV construct used does not employ any foreign promoter and thus shows the same liver cell restriction as HBV. HBV DNA causes an HBV infection only if it is directly delivered into hepatocytes, which is usually done by the virion. It has been shown that the injection of even large amounts of HBV DNA into the bloodstream of chimpanzees is not sufficient to cause HBV infection *(9)*. Because of size restrictions of the adenoviral genome, replication competent HBV genomes cannot accidentally be integrated into wild-type adenoviruses which would allow replication of HBV DNA outside the liver.

References

1. Acs, G., Sells, M. A., Purcell, R. H., et al. (1987) Hepatitis B virus produced by transfected Hep G2 cells causes hepatitis in chimpanzees. *Proc. Natl. Acad. Sci. USA* **84**, 4641–4644.
2. Guidotti, L. G., Matzke, B., Schaller, H., and Chisari, F. V. (1995) High-level hepatitis B virus replication in transgenic mice. *J. Virol.* **69**, 6158–6159.
3. Delaney IV, W. E. and Isom, H. C. (1998) Hepatitis B virus replication in human HepG2 cells mediated by hepatitis B virus recombinant baculovirus. *Hepatology* **28**, 1134–1146.
4. Sprinzl, M. F., Oberwinkler, H., Schaller, H., and Protzer, U. (2001) Transfer of hepatitis B virus genome by adenovirus vectors into cultured cells and mice: crossing the species barrier. *J. Virol.* **75**, 5108–5118.
5. Ren, S. and Nassal, M. (2001) Hepatitis B virus (HBV) virion and covalently closed circular DNA formation in primary tupaia hepatocytes and human hepatoma cell lines upon HBV genome transduction with replication-defective adenovirus vectors. *J. Virol.* **75**, 1104–1116.
6. Graham, F. L., Smiley, J., Russel, W. C., and Nairn, R. (1977) Characteristics of a human cell line transformed by DNA from human adenovirus type 5. *J. Gen. Virol.* **36**, 59–72.
7. He, T. C., Zhou, S., da Costa, L. T., Yu, J., Kinzler, K. W. and Vogelstein, B. (1998) A simplified system for generating recombinant adenoviruses. *Proc. Natl. Acad. Sci. USA* **95**, 2509–2514.

8. Fallaux, F. J., Bout, A., van der Velde, I., et al. (1998) New helper cells and matched early region 1-deleted adenovirus vectors prevent generation of replication-competent adenoviruses. *Hum. Gene Ther.* **9**, 1909–1917.
9. Will, H., Cattaneo, R., Darai, G., Deinhardt, F., Schellekens, H., and Schaller, H. (1985) Infectious hepatitis B virus from cloned DNA of known nucleotide sequence. *Proc. Natl. Acad. Sci. USA* **82**, 891–895.
10. Yang, P. L., Althage, A., Chung, J., and Chisari, F. V. (2002) Hydrodynamic infection of viral DNA: a mouse model of acute hepatitis B virus infection. *Proc. Natl. Acad. Sci. USA* **21**, 13825–13830.

19

Baculovirus-Mediated Gene Transfer for the Study of Hepatitis B Virus

Harriet C. Isom, Ayman M. Abdelhamed, John P. Bilello, and Thomas G. Miller

1. Introduction

Establishing novel in vitro model systems for studying hepatitis B virus (HBV) pathogenesis and the effects of antivirals on HBV replication is necessary because of the limitations encountered studying HBV in vivo. However, there are many challenges to in vitro studies as well.

The first challenge is selection of the appropriate exogenous sequences including regulatory sequences to be introduced into a hepatic cell in culture. HBV replication starts with the formation of pregenomic RNA (pgRNA) from the HBV template, HBV covalently closed circular (ccc) DNA. pgRNA is 3.5 kilobases (kb), while the full-length HBV genome itself is 3.2 kb. To obtain a productive viral replication, more than a one-genome-length DNA construct must be used. The HBV construct ideally should be controlled by its authentic regulatory elements or by foreign regulatory elements that are active in the mammalian milieu. These foreign regulatory elements could be either weaker or stronger than the authentic HBV regulatory elements, and hence the level of expression would not be identical to the natural infection. A good candidate system is one that has authentic HBV regulatory elements and permits rapid detection of HBV replication cycle including all HBV viral proteins, RNAs, and DNAs.

The second challenge is to select a method for gene delivery. Available methods for gene delivery can be characterized as chemical (calcium phosphate precipitation), physical (electroporation), or viral (adenovirus, baculovirus, vaccinia, and retrovirus). A good candidate method should have high transfection efficiency without cellular toxicity, expression of vector virus genes, or generation of recombinant human pathogens.

The third challenge is to avoid integration of HBV genetic information into the host genome. Some in vitro systems use cell lines that contain integrated HBV DNA *(1)*. However, in natural infection, HBV DNA is present in the cells as nuclear extrachro-

From: *Methods in Molecular Medicine, vol. 96: Hepatitis B and D Protocols, volume 2*
Edited by: R. K. Hamatake and J. Y. N. Lau © Humana Press Inc., Totowa, NJ

mosomal DNA called minichromosomes *(2)*. Therefore, the ideal in vitro culture system is the one that would mimic the natural extrachromosomal HBV DNA.

The fourth challenge is the ability to manipulate experimentally the timing of initiation of HBV replication and the level of HBV expression. This enables treatment of cells with antivirals or other agents either at specified times prior to or after initiation of replication. Many established stably transfected HBV expressing cell lines lack this attribute.

The fifth challenge is to provide sufficiently high levels of DNA expression and replication that they can be easily detected by simple and direct methods. In addition, replication needs to persist for sufficient time to permit antiviral studies.

The sixth challenge is to be able to quantify reproducibly HBV DNA expression. This will facilitate the judgment of the efficacy of antiviral compounds.

Baculoviruses constitute one of the largest and most diverse groups of insect pathogenic viruses *(3)*. They have a double-stranded DNA genome of 88–153 kb. The family Baculoviridae has a single genus, *Baculovirus*, that is divided into three subgroups. Baculoviruses have been isolated only from arthropods. Subgroup A contains the nuclear polyhedrosis viruses (NPVs), which have many virions (enveloped nucleocapsids) that are occluded within intranuclear protein crystals known as polyhedra or occlusion bodies. These polyhedra are usually 1–10 μm in size, and up to 30 or more may be produced in each infected cell. The polyhedra have a crystalline protein lattice, comprised primarily of a single viral-encoded protein, named polyhedrin, with a molecular weight of 29 kDa. The virions are present within the polyhedra as singly enveloped nucleocapsids (SNPVs) or bundles of multiply enveloped nucleocapsids (MNPV). The NPVs replicate in the nucleus of infected cells. *Autographa californica* multiple nuclear polyhedrosis virus (AcMNPV) has a host range of more than 30 insect species and can grow in several permissive insect cell lines. It has been used widely for high-level expression of recombinant proteins in insect cells *(4,5)*. Subgroup B contains the granulosis viruses (GVs) that exist as singly enveloped nucleocapsids and are individually occluded with small (0.1–1.0 μm) capsule-shaped polyhedra termed granules. GVs undergo replication in both the nuclear and cytoplasmic compartments of an infected cell. Subgroup C represents a small group of baculoviruses that have one nucleocapsid per envelope and are not occluded at any stage in their life cycle.

It has been shown that AcMNPV can effectively transfer genes into mammalian cells of hepatic origin *(6–9)*. Baculovirus promoters do not drive transcription in mammalian cells. Primary rat hepatocytes *(9)*, HepG2 cells *(8)*, and other mammalian cell types including nonhepatic cells *(10)* have been efficiently transfected using recombinant baculovirus vectors having a promoter normally active in mammalian cells. Baculoviruses have several features that make them attractive as a vector for gene transfer including: (1) baculoviruses on their own do not replicate or express viral genes in mammalian cells, but through the addition of a mammalian promoter it is feasible to achieve transcription of an exogenous gene in mammalian cells; (2) generation of recombinant baculoviruses is relatively simple; (3) baculoviruses can accommodate large DNA inserts; (4) transfection efficiencies of $>$ 70% are possible; and (5) large quantities of recombinant baculoviruses can be easily produced and purified from cultured insect cells.

Delaney and Isom ***(11)*** demonstrated that HBV replicated in human HepG2 cells after infection with a recombinant HBV baculovirus. A 1.3-genome-length HBV construct previously shown to drive high-level liver-specific HBV replication in transgenic mice was used to generate a recombinant HBV baculovirus. In HepG2 cells infected with this recombinant HBV baculovirus, HBV transcripts, and secreted HBV antigens, HB surface antigen (HBsAg) and HB e antigen (HBeAg), were produced. HBV replication occurred as evidenced by the presence of high levels of intracellular replicative intermediates (RI) and secreted HBV DNA in the medium. HBV cccDNA was also present in the infected HepG2 cells, indicating that HBV core particles are capable of delivering newly synthesized HBV genomes back into the nucleus of infected HepG2 cells. HB core antigen (HBcAg) was detected in the infected cells as shown by immunohistochemical staining. Density gradient analysis of extracellular HBV DNA indicated that DNA was contained predominantly in enveloped HBV virions. The major differences in natural HBV infection and HBV recombinant baculovirus-mediated gene transfer are the following (follow the green arrow in **Fig. 1**). In a natural infection, the HBV Dane particle enters the host cell. The envelope is removed. The HBV particle travels to the nucleus by a currently unknown mechanism. Core disassembly occurs and the HBV genome is deposited in the nucleus. Once in the nucleus, viral DNA is repaired to the cccDNA form and transcription of the four HBV transcripts occurs from the cccDNA. In HBV recombinant baculovirus-mediated gene transfer, the enveloped baculovirus enters the cell through a receptor-mediated process (follow the red arrows in **Fig. 1**). The baculovirus loses its envelope in transit to the nucleus. Once in the nucleus, the baculovirus DNA serves as the template for the four HBV transcripts. To our knowledge, once the HBV RNAs, including the pregenome, are synthesized, replication proceeds in the same fashion for natural infection and baculovirus-initiated infection. It is important to note that, in both systems, recycling of HBV DNA to the nucleus occurs.

The recombinant HBV baculovirus system, initially reported by Delaney and Isom ***(11)***, has many advantages. (1) HBV expression can be initiated any time relative to seeding of HepG2 cells. (2) Levels of HBV replication can be regulated over a wide range simply by changing the baculovirus multiplicity of infection. (3) HBV replication is readily detectable by 1 d post-infection (pi) with HBV baculovirus and persists at least through d 11 pi. (4) The transient nature of the infection can be extended and/or enhanced by superinfection of the cultures. (5) The system is transient and gene expression is driven in the absence of integration of HBV genome into the host genome. (6) Levels of HBV gene expression and replication achieved in HBV baculovirus-infected HepG2 cells far exceed the levels found in HepG2 2.2.15 cells. (7) cccDNA is expressed at sufficiently high levels that it can be readily detected by Southern blot analysis (**Fig. 2**). (8) HBV baculovirus infection, even at high multiplicities, is not toxic to HepG2 cells. (9) Endogenous HBV enhancers and promoters are sufficient for high levels of HBV expression and replication in HepG2 cells. (10) The system is highly

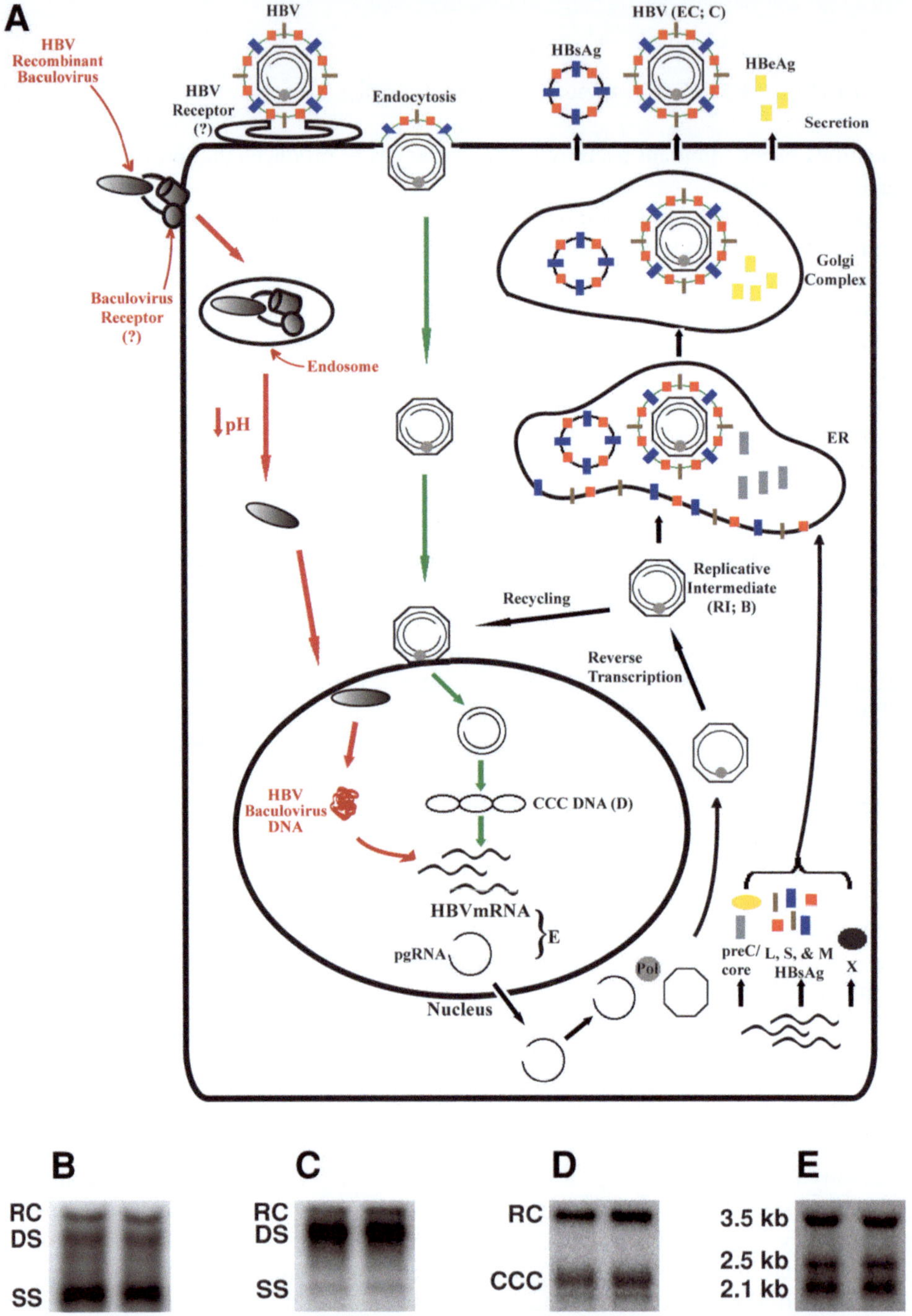

Fig. 1. Natural HBV and recombinant HBV baculovirus-mediated infection of mammalian cells. **(A)** Schematic of natural HBV and recombinant HBV baculovirus-mediated gene transfer. HBV DNA **(B–D)** and RNA **(E)** species were detected in HepG2 cells infected with the recombinant HBV baculovirus. HepG2 cells were infected with HBV recombinant baculovirus at 100 pfu/cell. Infected cells were harvested at d 7 pi for **(B)** replicative intermediate DNA (RI), **(C)** extracellular DNA (EC), **(D)** cccDNA (CCC), and **(E)** HBV RNA. The HBV bands from Southern and Northern blot analyses were visualized with a PhosphorImager and the digital images are shown. The HBV bands are relaxed circular, RC; double stranded, DS; single stranded, SS; and covalently closed circular, CCC.

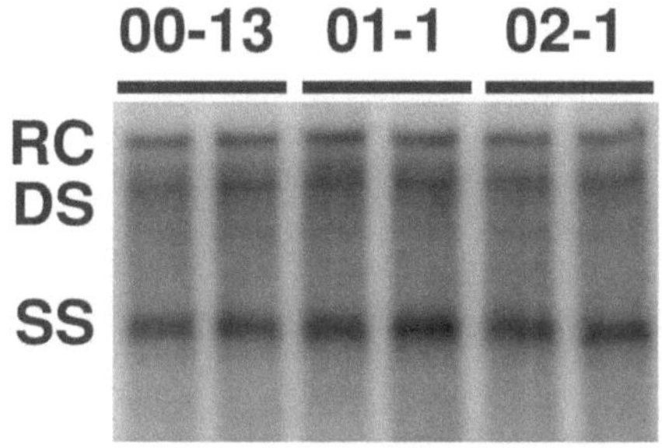

Fig. 2. Comparative study among three different viral stocks. Three different HBV recombinant baculovirus stocks, 00-13, 01-1, and 02-1, made and titrated at different time points, were used to infect HepG2 cells at 100 pfu/cell. The infected cells were harvested at d 4 pi for RI. The HBV bands from Southern blot analysis were visualized with a PhosphorImager and the digital image is shown. The HBV bands are relaxed circular, RC; double stranded, DS; and single stranded, SS. This result shows that the titer determined in insect cells can be equated with transfection efficiency in HepG2 cells. Hence reproducible studies can be carried out using different stocks of HBV recombinant baculovirus.

reproducible; titration of HBV recombinant baculovirus in insect cells can be equated with gene transfer efficiency to HepG2 cells (**Fig. 3**).

The HBV recombinant baculovirus system has been used for antiviral drug studies such as lamivudine ***(12)*** and clevudine ***(13)***. In addition, HBV recombinant baculoviruses which encode drug-resistant strains of HBV have been generated and used for drug studies ***(14)*** (Miller et al., *in preparation*). Recently, HBV recombinant baculovirus has been used in HepG2 cells to study the rebound phenomenon seen in patients after discontinuation of the nucleoside analog lamivudine ***(13)***. The system has also been used to determine the EC_{50} and EC_{90} of antiviral nucleoside analogs for HBV DNA species ***(15)***. The HBV recombinant baculovirus/HepG2 system has unique advantages over existing transient transfection systems and stably transfected cell lines for studying HBV replication and the effects of specific drugs on this process.

2. Materials

2.1. Solutions and Chemicals

1. Agarose: Ultrapure agarose (Invitrogen, Carlsbad, CA) and Seaplaque agarose (low-melting-temperature agarose) (Biowhittaker Molecular Applications, Walkersville, MD).
2. 0.5 *M* EDTA: Dissolve 186.1 g of disodium ethylenediaminetetraacetate·$2H_2O$ in 600 mL of H_2O. Adjust the pH to 8.0 with 10 *N* solution of NaOH (or approx 20 g of NaOH pellets). Adjust the volume to 1 L with H_2O. The disodium salt of EDTA will not dissolve until the pH of the solution is adjusted to approx 8.0 by the addition of NaOH.
3. 1 *M* $MgCl_2$: Dissolve 203.3 g of $MgCl_3 \cdot 6H_2O$ in 800 mL of H_2O. Adjust the volume to 1 L with H_2O.
4. 1 *M* Tris-HCl: Dissolve 121.1 g of Tris base in 800 of H_2O. Adjust the pH to 7.4 with concentrated HCl (approx 70 mL). Adjust the volume to 1 L with H_2O.

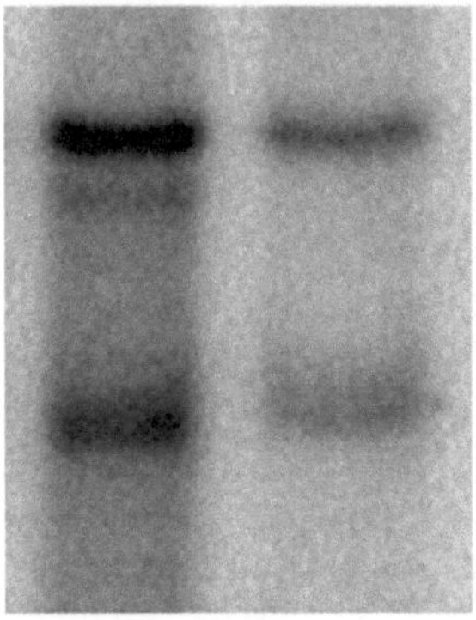

Fig. 3. Comparative study of two methods of non-protein bound cccDNA extraction. HepG2 cells were infected with recombinant HBV baculovirus at a multiplicity of 100 pfu/cell and harvested at 6 d pi. The figure shows Southern blot analysis of non-protein bound cccDNA extracted from the nuclei of the infected HepG2 cells. During the process of extraction, plasmid-safe DNase (PSD) was included *(lane 2)* or not *(lane 1)*. PSD has the benefit of decreasing the background and degrading any nicked linear DNA or circular DNA. It is crucial to note that the ratio of RC to cccDNA is not changed.

5. 10% Nonidet P-40 (NP40) (or 10% IGEPAL CA-630).
6. 2.5 *M* KCl: Dissolve 186.4 g of KCl to 1 L.
7. 20% SDS: Dissolve 200 g of sodium dodecyl sulfate (SDS, also called sodium lauryl sulfate) in 800 mL of H_2O. Heat to 68°C until dissolved. Adjust the volume to 1 L with H_2O.
8. 3 *M* Sodium acetate: Dissolve 246 g of sodium acetate anhydrous in 800 mL of H_2O. Adjust the pH to 5.2 with glacial acetic acid. Adjust the volume to 1 L with H_2O.
9. 4% SDS: Dissolve 40 g of SDS in 800 mL of H_2O. Adjust the volume to 1 L with H_2O.
10. 5 *M* NaCl: Dissolve 292.2 g of NaCl in 800 mL of H_2O. Adjust the volume to 1 L with H_2O.
11. 50% PEG 8000: Dissolve 500 g of polyethylene glycol (PEG) in 800 mL of H_2O. Adjust the volume to 1 L with H_2O.
12. 5X Digestion buffer for extracellular HBV DNA extraction: 0.25% SDS–0.25 *M* Tris–0.25 *M* EDTA: Dissolve 2.5 g of SDS, 30.27 g of Tris and 93.05 g of EDTA in 800 mL of H_2O. Adjust the volume to 1 L with H_2O.
13. [^{32}P]dCTP.
14. 25 m*M* ATP solution.
15. Bac-N-Blue transfection kit (Invitrogen).
16. Chloroform ($CHCl_3$): HPLC grade.
17. DNase I, RNase-free: 10 U/L.
18. GTC buffer: Dissolve 94.53 g of guanidine isothiocyanate (GTC) in 150 mL of H_2O. Add 1.47 g sodium citrate and 0.27 g n-lauroyl sacrosine. Adjust the pH to 7. Adjust the volume to 200 mL with H_2O.

19. Isopropanol anhydrous.
20. Neutral red dye.
21. Phosphate-buffered saline (PBS), pH 7.4: Dissolve 8 g of NaCl, 0.2 g of KCl, 1.44 g of Na_2HPO_4, and 0.24 g of KH_2PO_4 in 800 mL of distilled H_2O. Adjust the pH to 7.4 with HCl. Add H_2O to 1 L, aliquot, and sterilize by autoclaving. Store at 4°C.
22. Plasmid safe ATP-dependent DNase 10 U/μL.
23. Proteinase K: 15.3 mg/mL in 10 m*M* Tris-HCl, pH 7.5.
24. Random prime labeling kit (Roche, Indianapolis, IN).
25. RNase, DNase-free : 500 μg/mL.
26. Sephadex-G50.
27. Sodium hydroxide.
28. Sucrose cushion: 27% Sucrose (w/w) PBS.
29. Sucrose gradient solutions: 20% and 60% (w/w) in PBS.
30. TE (10:1), pH 8.0: 10 m*M* Tris-HCl, pH 8.0, and 1 m*M* EDTA, pH 8.0.
31. TE (50:1), pH 8.0: 50 m*M* Tris-HCl, pH 8.0, and 1 m*M* EDTA, pH 8.0.
32. TNM-FH medium: Grace's Insect Medium with supplements (lactalbumin hydrolysate, L-glutamine, TC-yeastolate, and 10% fetal bovine serum [FBS]).
33. Tris-saturated phenol: Thaw fresh phenol (total 25 mL) in a 65°C water bath, and add one equal volume of 1 *M* Tris-HCl, pH 8.0, into one volume of phenol. Add 0.025*g* 8-hyroxyquinoline. Mix well. Centrifuge at 3,000*g* for 10 min and transfer aqueous phase to a fresh tube and add 100 m*M* Tris-HCl, pH 8.0; shake, and centrifuge at 3,000*g* for 10 min. Remove the aqueous phase. Store at 4°C for approx 1 mo.
34. tRNA: 10 μg/μL.
35. Trypan blue dye.
36. X-gal (20 mg/ml of dimethyl formamide).

2.2. Equipment

1. 1.5-mL and 2-mL microcentrifuge tubes.
2. 15- and 50-mL conical tubes.
3. −20°C and −80°C freezers.
4. 4°C Storage space.
5. High-speed ultracentrifuge and Beckman SW 28 rotor.
6. Magnetic stirrer.
7. pH meter.
8. Refractometer.
9. Rocking platform.
10. Several temperature adjustable water baths: 37, 56, 65°C.
11. Slow-speed magnetic stirrer.
12. Snap-cap, polypropylene tube.
13. Sonicator.
14. Spectrophotometer, UV and visible range.
15. Spinner flasks.
16. Tabletop microcentrifuge.
17. Ultracentrifuge tubes (e.g., for Beckman SW28 rotor, cat. no. 344058).
18. Variable micropipets, P10, P20, P200, and P1000.
19. Water purification equipment. Use of triple-distilled deionized water, milliQ water, or water of equivalent quality.

3. Methods

3.1. Generation of Baculovirus Transfer Plasmid.

The baculovirus transfer plasmid can be generated by the standard laboratory subcloning method. The detailed method of subcloning is present in other cloning manuals, such as those by Sambrook et al. ***(16)*** and Ausubel et al. ***(17)***.

In brief:

1. Subclone the *Pst*I/*Sac*I fragment containing the 1.3 ***(11)*** unit length HBV construct from pTHBV1.3 into the multiple cloning region of pBlueBac4.5 (Invitrogen).
2. Analyze the recombinant transfer plasmid, pBB4.5HBV1.3, by restriction mapping to demonstrate the presence of only one copy of the HBV 1.3 construct.

3.1.1. Summary of Generation of Recombinant Baculoviruses Containing the 1.3 HBV Construct

1. Cotransfect both the purified pBB4.5HBV1.3 ***(11)*** and linear AcMNPV baculovirus DNA into Sf21 cells using the Bac-N-Blue transfection kit (Invitrogen). (*See* **Subheading 3.2.**)
2. Isolate recombinant viruses by plaque assay. (*See* **Subheading 3.3.**)
3. Amplify the isolated recombinant virus plaques by infecting 100-mm dishes of Sf21 cells. (*See* **Subheading 3.4.**)
4. Extract viral DNA from the amplified viruses. (*See* **Subheading 3.4.**)
5. Digest purified viral DNA with restriction enzymes and then fractionate by electrophoresis in a 1.0 % agarose gel. (*See* **Subheading 3.4.**)
6. Perform Southern blotting to determine which virus isolates contained the intact 1.3 HBV construct. (*See* **Subheading 3.4.**)
7. Amplify virus clone with correct HBV 1.3 insert to a high titer stock. (*See* **Subheadings 3.5.** and **3.6.**)

3.2. Generation of HBV Recombinant Baculovirus (Homologous Recombination) (See Note 1)

1. Seed 2 × 10^6 Sf21 cells in complete TNM-FH medium (Grace's Insect Medium with supplements) in a 60-mm dish. Four 100-mm plates are enough to seed ten 60-mm plates. Shake gently side to side to distribute the cells evenly.
2. Allow the cells to fully attach and form a monolayer of cells for 2 h. In addition to the number of dishes needed for transfection, perform one experimental control (Bac-N-Blue DNA) and one negative control (without any DNA). Examine the cells under inverted microscope to verify their attachment.

Tube	pBB4.5HBV1.3	Bac-N-Blue	Grace's	Insectin
pBB4.5HBV1.3	+	+	+	+
Experimental control		–	+	+ +
Negative control	–	–	+	–

3. To a 1.5 mL microcentrifuge tube add the following reagents:
   a. 10 μL (0.5 μg) of the Bac-N-Blue DNA.
   b. 4 μL (4 μg) recombinant transfer plasmid containing 1.3 HBV DNA (pBB4.5HBV1.3).
   c. 1 mL of Grace's Insect Medium (without supplements or FBS).
   d. 20 μL Insectin-Plus Liposomes (vortex before use and always add last).

4. Vortex the transfection mixture vigorously for 10 s.
5. Incubate the transfection mixture at room temperature for 15 min.
6. Carefully remove the medium from the cells without disrupting the monolayer and wash the cells with 2 mL of fresh Grace's Insect Medium without supplements or FBS.
7. Carefully remove the medium from the monolayer and add the entire transfection mix dropwise into the 60-mm dish. Distribute the drops over the monolayer.
8. Incubate the dishes at room temperature for 4 h on a side-to-side rocking platform. Adjust speed to approx 2 side-to-side motions per minute. This can also be done manually by side-to-side rocking of the plate every 15 min.
9. After the 4-h incubation period, add 1 mL of complete Grace's Medium to each 60-mm dish, seal the dish with parafilm, and incubate at 27°C for 72 h.
10. After 72–96 h, check cells under inverted microscope for signs of infection (*see* **step 12**). If infection is confirmed, collect the conditioned medium and transfer to a sterile 15-mL, snap-cap, polypropylene tube, and centrifuge cell debris at 3,000*g* for 10 min, then store at 4°C (first collection). This conditioned medium will be used to identify the HBV recombinant baculovirus by plaque assay (*see* **Subheading 3.3.**).
11. Add 4 mL of fresh complete Grace's Medium to the transfected cells and incubate at 27°C for an additional 48 h (second collection). Centrifuge cell debris at 3,000*g* for 10 min. This conditioned medium will be used as a backup for the first collection.
12. Using an inverted microscope at × 250–400 magnification, check the cells for visual signs of successful transfection including:

    a. Early signs:
    Cell diameter increased by about 25–50%.
    Increased size of cell nuclei, nuclei fill the cells.
    b. Late signs:
    Cessation of cell growth compared to nontransfected control.
    Granular appearance, signs of viral burst.
    Viral occlusions which appear as refractive crystals in the nuclei of a few cells containing wild-type virus.
    Detachment of the cells from the dish.
    c. Very late signs:
    A few cells may fill with occluded virus, die, and burst, leaving signs of clearing in the monolayer.

13. Once confirmation of transfection is confirmed, purify HBV recombinant baculovirus by plaque assay (*see* **Subheading 3.3.**).

3.3. Plaque Purification Assay (Following Homologous Recombination)

1. Set the water bath to 42–43°C with two beakers containing water (used as a portable water path).
2. Combine confluent 100-mm plates of Sf21 cells into a 50-mL conical tube.
3. Do a cell count of the combined cells.
4. Seed Sf21 cells in complete Grace's Insect Medium at 7×10^6 cells per 100-mm dish. It is recommended to prepare two plates per viral dilution, but, if purifying more than one virus, one plate per dilution is acceptable. Allow cells to attach for about 30 min. Proceed to the next step while cells are attaching. Confirm that the cells look about 75% confluent before using.
5. Use first collection of the conditioned medium from cotransfection (from **Subheading 3.2., step 10**) to set up viral dilutions. Use large 15-mL snap-cap tubes and vortex the virus after each dilution. Set up viral dilutions in complete Grace's Medium:

10^{-2} : 20 μL of conditioned medium in 1980 μL of medium
10^{-3} : 200 μL of previous dilution in 1800 μL of medium
10^{-4} : 200 μL of previous dilution in 1800 μL of medium
10^{-5} : 200 μL of previous dilution in 1800 μL of medium

6. Use 10^{-3}, 10^{-4}, and 10^{-5} dilutions to infect Sf21 cells. Aspirate medium from newly seeded Sf21 cells and add the viral dilutions, 1 mL/plate. Feed one plate with just medium as a negative control. Allow the infection to proceed for 1 h, rock every 15 min. While the infection is proceeding, prepare the agarose and set up the flow hood for the agarose overlays.
7. Prepare agarose: The final concentration is 1%. Calculate the volume needed using 12.5 mL/100-mm plate plus one extra plate. Equilibrate a bottle of complete Grace's Insect Medium to 42°C in the water bath. Prepare the agarose by making up 25% of the total volume as 4% agarose in sterile water. Microwave until there are no clumps, try not to let too much evaporation occur and keep it sterile. Allow 4% agarose to cool slightly and then place in 42°C water bath. After the agarose has equilibrated, add 75% of the total volume of prewarmed Grace's Insect Medium to the agarose and swirl quickly to mix the solution. Place agarose in the water bath. Allow a few minutes for all the reagents to equilibrate. Add X-gal to achieve a final concentration of 150 μg/mL of agarose.
8. Prewarm a 25-mL pipet in a 37°C incubator. Aspirate plates (no more than three at a time). Tilt plates and let them sit for about 30 s, and aspirate again. It is imperative that the plates are dry before adding the agarose, as excess liquid underneath the agarose will lead to smeared plaques. However, be careful not to let the monolayer dry out. Quickly move the 42°C beaker and agarose into the hood. Draw 25 mL into the pipet and overlay two plates with 12.5 mL each. To avoid disturbing the cell monolayer, pour the agarose gently down the side of the plate at a moderate pace (if too slow, the agarose will harden). After the overlays are poured, place the lid over the top of the plate but allow room for steam to escape. Carefully move the plates to the back of the hood and repeat for all dilutions. Allow 15–30 min for the agarose to harden and the condensation to escape. Then tightly wrap each plate in parafilm and place the plates in the 27°C insect incubator. Check for *lacZ*-positive plaques every day. Plaques take 5–7 d to become well formed and visible.
9. Once plaques are visible, mark them and examine under inverted microscope to rule out any wild-type plaques. This step is very important, not only for selection of recombinant plaques but also to make sure that you will pick only one recombinant per plaque pick. Wild-type plaques are *lacZ* negative and the cells have black occlusion bodies. Recombinant plaques are *lacZ* positive and the cells do not have occlusion bodies.
10. Using a Pasteur pipet and bulb, remove a plug of agarose over the plaques that were selected.
11. Discharge the agarose plugs into individual cryovials containing 1 mL of insect cell medium. This allows the virus to diffuse out of the plug.
12. Label cryovials by number and place tubes at 4°C overnight.

3.4. HBV Recombinant Baculovirus Isolation (Following Homologous Recombination and Plaque Assay)

1. Seed one 100-mm plate of cells per cryovial at light density (split insect cells 1:8 or 1:10) and allow to attach for more than 30 min at room temperature.
2. Add 0.5 mL of the medium from each cryovial containing low-melting-point agarose plug to a correspondingly numbered plate. Seed one plate without medium containing virus as a control.
3. Parafilm and incubate at 27°C.

4. Incubate for 4–5 d and observe for infection (occlusion$^+$ or occlusion$^-$).
5. Discard any plates that contain wild-type baculovirus (occlusion$^+$).
6. Once full infection is confirmed, collect the plate supernatant in a 15-mL conical tube and centrifuge cell debris at 3,000*g* for 10 min in a tabletop centrifuge. This is the P1 viral stock.
7. In a 2-mL microcentrifuge tube, place 1 mL of P1 viral stock and 1 mL of cold (4°C) 20% PEG in 1 *M* NaCl. Invert to mix and incubate at room temperature for 30 min.
8. Keep the remainder of the supernatant at 4°C; it will be used for initiation of infection of spinner flasks (*see* **Subheading 3.5.**).
9. Centrifuge precipitated virus at 20,000*g* for 10 min at room temperature. Discard the supernatant.
10. Resolubilize pellet with 100 μL of sterile dH_2O.
11. Add 10 μL of Proteinase K (5–10 mg/mL) and incubate at 50ºC for 1 h.
12. Extract with 110 μL of 1:1 phenol–chloroform. Centrifuge at 20,000*g* for 5 min.
13. Transfer aqueous top phase to a new microcentrifuge tube and precipitate the DNA with 1/10 volume of 3 *M* NaAc, 3 μL of glycogen (3.5 μg/μL stock), and two volumes of 100% ethanol. Incubate at –20°C for > 1 h.
14. Centrifuge at 20,000*g* for 15 min at 4°C.
15. Resuspend pellet in 13 μL of sterile dH_2O. Quantitate DNA by measuring the absorbance at 260 nm of 1 μL at a 1:50 dilution. Store at 4°C.
16. Digest the purified DNA with restriction enzymes (*Pst*I/*Sac*I, *Fsp*I) and then fractionate by electrophoresis in a 1.0% agarose gel.
17. Restriction digest:
    Set up the following restriction enzyme digestions using 1 μg of DNA.

Condition	Uncut DNA	*Pst*I/*Sac*I digestion	*Fsp*I digestion
DNA	1 μg	1 μg	1 μg
Restriction enzyme	—	2 μL each	2 μL
10X buffer	2.5 μL	2.5 μL	2.5 μL
Water	Up to 25 μL	Up to 25 μL	Up to 25 μL
Expected bands	One high mol wt	4.1-kb represent 1.3 HBV construct	3.2-kb represent unit length HBV monomer

18. Incubate at 37°C for 1.5–2 hours.
19. Add 3 μL of 10X loading buffer to each sample.
20. Load 20 μL sample into each well of an agarose gel, including standard lanes for each enzyme used.
21. Run gel at 65–80 V for approx 3 h.
22. Once done, take a picture of the gel on a UV transilluminator, with ruler beside the standard for reference.
23. Perform a Southern blot to determine which virus isolates contain the intact 1.3 HBV construct using a ^{32}P-radiolabeled probe generated from a full-length, double-stranded HBV genome as a template (*see* **Subheading 3.12.**).

3.5. Initiation and Infection of Spinner Flask Culture (Amplification of Viral Recombinants)

This procedure follows confirmation of recombinant identification by Southern blot. Carry out all procedures in the flow hood. All spinner flasks are carefully sterilized (*see* **Note 2**).

1. Initiate spinner flask: Pour water out of flask and add 200 mL of medium.
2. Seed flask with four confluent plates. Place in a 27°C incubator on a stirrer plate. Adjust plate speed for 70–80 rpm.
3. On the third day post-seeding, remove cap on one arm of the flask and take up 5 mL with a pipet. Count the number of cells. From this count, calculate how many days it will take to reach 2×10^6 cells/mL, taking into account that insect cells double every day. While culturing, aerate the flask daily to allow for oxygenation. This is accomplished by placing the flask in a flow hood and carefully removing the caps on both arms of the flask. Gently swirl the flask to force the stale air out of it and allow fresh air in. Place the caps back on the arms and return the flask to the incubator. Care should be taken to be as sterile as possible during this procedure as it is performed daily, therefore increasing the chances of contamination being introduced into the spinner flask (*see* **Note 3**).
4. When the proper cell density is achieved, add 200 mL of medium to the flask (this acts as a 1:2 split).
5. The next day pipet out 200 mL and add to a fresh flask (after pouring its water out). Put 200 mL of fresh medium into each flask. This is now another 1:2 split forming two flasks with 400 mL each. If you are amplifying only one recombinant virus (the first time after homologous recombination), proceed to next step; otherwise repeat this procedure until the required number of flasks is obtained (four flasks for every recombinant being amplified).
6. Following the final split, infect each flask with 1 mL of viral supernatant, one recombinant per flask. (The 1 mL of supernatant is from the 8–9 mL of P1 stock that was stored at 4°C prior to recombinant identification; **Subheading 3.4., step 8.**)
7. If the flask is being infected from a viral stock that has already been titered, do a cell count and infect at a multiplicity of infection (MOI) of 0.2 plaque-forming units (pfu)/mL. Infecting at such a low MOI is necessary to allow the virus to proliferate for a few days, allowing a larger yield before the cells begin to lyse. Also, in the event that a mutated construct exists in the stock, the low MOI will allow the recombinant of choice to amplify at a much faster pace, therefore diluting out the unwanted virus. To infect at an MOI of 0.2, gently shake the flask then remove 10 mL of cell suspension and place it into a 50-mL conical tube. From this, do a cell count to calculate how many cells are in the flask. Use this count plus the virus titer to calculate what volume of virus is needed to attain the MOI. Add the virus to the cells in the conical tube, swirl, and pipet back into the flask. Incubate as before.
8. Feed the infected flask as follows:
   D 1 pi: Add 50 mL of fresh medium to each flask.
   D 2 and 3 pi: Add 25 mL of fresh medium to each flask.
   D 5–7 pi: For each flask, remove 3 mL, add to 7 mL of medium to a plate. Once cells attach (it takes about 15 min), observe for active infection (the cell membrane is not well defined). If infection is not evident, carry flask cultures for another day or two and repeat until observed. Five to six days are regularly required to produce full-blown infection. It has been shown that waiting an extra day will slightly increase the yield of virus as well.

9. Once infection is confirmed, pour the medium into several 50-mL conical tubes and centrifuge in a tabletop centrifuge, 3,000*g* for 10 min.
10. Collect all supernatants of each recombinant into 0.45-μm bottletop filter mounted on a 2-L bottle.
11. Apply vacuum pressure to filter the supernatant, store in 4°C.
12. Virus stocks must be concentrated prior to infection of hepatocytes.

3.6. Virus Concentration and Purification

3.6.1. D 1: Virus Concentration

Starting point: Medium that has been collected from infected cells, centrifuged, and filtered through 0.45-μm bottletop filter.

1. Fill six SW28 tubes with the medium containing virus, 33 mL per tube (use a plastic 25-mL pipet).
2. Underlay the medium of each tube with 3 mL of 27% sucrose in PBS. Take 6 mL into a 5-mL plastic pipet and use it to underlay two tubes. Do not go back into the 27% sucrose with a dirty (infected) pipet. Sucrose concentration should be confirmed using refractometer. If the amount of virus stock is not enough to fill the tube, add PBS until there is at least 35 mL/tube.
3. Balance tubes on the scale (add PBS to equalize weights). Load the SW28 rotor and spin in the ultracentrifuge at 25,000 rpm for 90 min at room temperature.
4. When the run is completed, remove the tubes and examine the contents; a small yellowish-white and opaque pellet should be visible at the bottom of the tube. Aspirate off the supernatant.
5. Add 0.33 mL of PBS to each tube and allow them to stand for about 30 min. Pipet up and down with 1-mL pipetteman to resuspend all pellets. Parafilm and allow pellets to resuspend overnight at 4°C.
6. Repeat **steps 1–5** until all infected medium containing virus is concentrated.
7. Carefully and thoroughly clean all rotors exposed to virus with a detergent (soap) to eliminate the possibility of cross-contaminating the next viral preparation (*see* **Note 4**).

3.6.2. D 2: Viral Purification

Starting point: Multiple aliquots of concentrated virus resuspended in 0.33 mL (**Subheading 3.6.1., step 5**).

1. Prepare sucrose gradients. For each SW28 tube add 18 mL of 60% sucrose, overlay 60% sucrose with 18 mL of 20% sucrose, tightly wrap each tube with parafilm, place in a tight-fitting rack, gently lower all the gradients sideways, and allow gradient to form by diffusion for 3 h at room temperature. Again, the sucrose concentration should be confirmed with a refractometer.
2. Combine all aliquots of virus into one 15-mL polystyrene tube. Rinse all SW28 tubes with one or two 0.5-mL aliquots of PBS to minimize loss of virus.
3. Tune a sonicator before using. Make sure that the cup horn is dry and tune the sonicator at 50%, then at 100% amplitude.
4. Add ice and water to the sonicator cup and sonicate the virus between settings 28 and 31 amplitude (up to 50% pulse) for about 2 min total time. Make sure the sonicator is visibly mixing the concentrated virus.
5. Carefully layer the virus onto the gradients, 2–3 mL per gradient. Balance the gradients by adding PBS or redistributing the virus among tubes. Centrifuge at 27,000 rpm for 3 h at 4°C.

6. The virus should band at 47% sucrose (about halfway down the tube). Collect the band by puncturing the tube wall with a 10-cc syringe and 18-gauge needle. Do this approx 1 cm below the band and collect as much virus as possible.
7. Deposit the virus into a fresh SW28 tube for each gradient and fill the tube with PBS to decrease the concentration of residual sucrose that was collected with the virus.
8. Balance with PBS, and centrifuge again at 27,000 rpm at 4°C for 1 hr.
9. Aspirate the supernatant and resuspend pelleted virus in 1 mL of PBS/tube for 30 min in the flow hood. Pipet up and down a few times with a pipetteman, wrap with parafilm, and store overnight at 4°C.
10. The next day, pipet up and down four or five times, then combine aliquots into a 15-mL conical tube. Rinse all empty SW28 tubes with one 0.5 mL of PBS to collect leftover virus and add this to the conical tube as well.
11. Sonicate virus once more as described above.
12. Sterilize the virus: Prewet a 0.45-µm filter with PBS then filter the virus and collect filtrate into a 15-mL conical tube. Store at 4°C.

3.7. Titration of Purified Virus "Plaque Assay"

Perform the titration and plaque assay as described in **Subheading 3.3., steps 1–8** with the following modifications.

1. The X-gal may be omitted as plaques will be visualized by staining with neutral red.
2. Set up viral dilutions in complete Grace's Medium:

   10^{-2}: 20 µL of virus stock in 1980 µL of medium **(Subheading 3.6.2., step 12)**
   10^{-4}: 20 µL of previous dilution in 1980 µL of medium
   10^{-6}: 20 µL of previous dilution in 1980 µL of medium
   10^{-8}: 40 µL of previous dilution in 3960 µL of medium → use to infect three plates, 1 mL each.
   10^{-9}: 400 µL of previous dilution in 3600 µL of medium → use to infect three plates, 1 mL each.

3. After 6–7 d, overlay with neutral red stain:

   a. Prepare neutral red solution by dissolving 0.01 g of neutral red in 10 mL of PBS.
   b. Prepare 0.75% agarose by dissolving 0.75 g of agar in 20 mL of sterile water, adding 70 mL of Grace's Medium at 45°C, and then adding 10 mL of neutral red solution (the final concentration is 100 µg/mL). Cool the agarose to 40–42°C before adding to the plates.
   c. Overlay each plate with 6 mL. Let harden and incubate at 27°C overnight.

4. Plaques will appear as clear, circular areas approx 0.5–3 mm in diameter against a red background.
5. Calculate the titer of the virus stock by counting the number of plaques per plate. Take the average from replicate plates. The most reliable count is between 10 and 100 plaques/plate. Multiply the plaque number by the dilution factor. For example, if an average of 25 plaques are counted on the plates infected with a 10^{-8} dilution, the titer of the stock is $25 \times 10^8 = 2.5 \times 10^9$ pfu/mL.

3.8. Baculovirus Infection (See *Note 1*)

1. Seed the desired number of 60-mm dishes with HepG2 cells plus three additional dishes that will be used to determine the number of cells per dish prior to infection. Allow the cells to grow for 16–24 h before the infection is started.

2. After 16–24 h, count the three extra dishes of cells to determine the exact number of cells per dish and average these values to determine the average number of cells per dish. The desired cell density range for infection is $1.0–1.5 \times 10^6$ cells per dish.
3. Based on the desired MOI, calculate the amount of virus that is needed to infect one dish of HepG2 cells. This is done by multiplying the cell number by the desired MOI to yield total pfu needed per cell. This number is then divided by the virus titer and multiplied by 1000 to convert the milliliter value into a microliter value.
4. To infect multiple dishes, multiply the amount of virus needed to infect one dish by the number of dishes to be infected plus two additional dishes to make sure that there is enough of virus available to infect all of the dishes.
5. To infect a 60-mm dish, a volume of 0.5 mL is needed. To determine the total number of milliliters needed, multiply 0.5 mL by the total number of dishes to be infected plus two additional dishes to make sure that there is enough virus available to infect all of the dishes.
6. To a conical tube add the total number of milliliters of medium needed to do the infection. Remove the virus from the refrigerator and vortex the tube to resuspend the virus and then add the total number of microliters needed to do the infection. Vortex the medium and virus mixture.
7. Add 0.5 mL of the virus and medium suspension to each of the dishes in a dropwise circular fashion. Gently rock the dishes to distribute the virus evenly over the entire surface area of the dish.
8. Incubate the cells at 37°C for 1 h. Rock the dishes every 15 min to keep the virus mixture evenly distributed over the cells.
9. After 1 h, rinse the cells two times with PBS and refeed the cells with 4 mL of medium.
10. The cells are fed as required for each experiment but must be refed 24 h prior to harvesting and the medium collected at the time of harvest. The medium is then analyzed for HBV extracellular (EC) DNA as well as for HBV proteins.
11. The cells are harvested at the desired time point and analyzed for HBV replicative intermediates (RI) and covalently closed circular DNA (cccDNA).

3.9. Extraction of HBV RIs

1. Collect medium from the dish and place it into a centrifuge tube. Centrifuge the medium at 3,000*g* for 10 min to pellet cellular debris and then transfer medium to a new tube. Store at –20°C until needed. The medium can be analyzed later for HBV extracellular (EC) DNA, HBsAg, or HBeAg.
2. Scrape the cells in 1 mL of PBS and pipet into a 1.5-mL centrifuge tube. Rinse the dish with 0.5 mL of PBS and add to the centrifuge tube to optimize cell recovery.
3. Centrifuge the cells at 3,000*g* for 5 min. Remove the PBS and resuspend the pellet in 750 μL of PBS and then add 37.5 μL of 10% IGEPAL CA-630 (replaces NP-40). Allow the cells to lyse for 20 min on ice.
4. Pellet nuclei by centrifugation at 20,000*g* (maximum speed) for 10 min at 4°C. Pipet the supernatant into a fresh tube. Store the nuclei at –20°C until needed.
5. To the supernatant, add 4.5 μL of 1 *M* $MgCl_2$ and 1 μL of DNase I. Incubate at 37°C for 1 h.
6. After 1 h, add the following in order:

EDTA to 10 m*M*	15.7 μL of 0.5 *M* stock
SDS to 1%	39.3 μL of 20% stock
NaCl to 100 m*M*	15.7 μL of 5 *M* stock
Proteinase K	To 500 μg/mL

Incubate at 37°C for 2 h.

7. Extract once with an equal volume of phenol saturated with 0.1 *M* Tris-HCl, pH 8.0, and transfer the aqueous phase to a fresh tube.
8. Extract once with an equal volume of chloroform and transfer the aqueous phase to a fresh tube.
9. Precipitate the nucleic acids by adding 0.05 volume of 3 *M* sodium acetate and one volume of isopropanol. Place at –20°C overnight.
10. Pellet the nucleic acid by centrifugation at 20,000*g* (maximum speed) for 15 min at 4°C. Aspirate off the isopropanol and allow the pellets to dry.
11. Resuspend the pellet in 50 μL of TE. Add 2 μL of DNase-free RNase and incubate at 37°C for 1 h.
12. Add loading dye to samples and load onto an agarose gel for Southern analysis (*see* **Note 5**).

3.10. Extraction of HBV cccDNA

1. Thaw the nuclei pellet that was placed in the –20°C freezer during the isolation of replicative intermediates (from **Subheading 3.9., step 4**).
2. Resuspend the pellet in 400 μL of 50:1 TE and transfer to a 2.0-mL centrifuge tube. Add 400 μL of 4% SDS and allow the nuclei to lyse for 20 min.
3. Add 200 μL of 2.5 *M* KCl. Mix gently by inversion and centrifuge at 20,000*g* (maximum speed) for 20 min at 4°C.
4. Transfer the supernatant to a new tube and extract once with an equal volume of phenol saturated with 0.1 *M* Tris-HCl, pH 8.0, and transfer the aqueous phase to a fresh tube.
5. Extract once with an equal volume of chloroform and transfer the aqueous phase to a fresh tube.
6. Precipitate the DNA by adding 2.0 μL of 10 μg/μL of tRNA, 0.05 volume of 3 *M* sodium acetate, and one volume of isopropanol. Place at –20°C overnight.
7. Pellet the DNA by centrifugation at 20,000*g* (maximum speed) for 15 min at 4°C. Aspirate off the isopropanol and allow the pellets to dry.
8. Resuspend the pellet in 20 μL of sterile water.
9. Add 2.0 μL of Plasmid-Safe 10X reaction buffer, 1.0 μL of 25 m*M* ATP, 1.0 μL of DNase-free RNase, and 1.0 μL of Plasmid-Safe DNase. Incubate at 37°C for 15 min followed immediately by an incubation at 65°C for 30 min to inactivate the DNase.
10. Add loading dye to samples and load onto an agarose gel for Southern analysis (*see* **Note 5**).

3.11. Extraction of HBV EC DNA

1. Aliquot 1.5 mL of medium into a 2.0-mL centrifuge tube (from **Subheading 3.9., step 1**).
2. Add 0.5 mL of 50% PEG 8000. Mix thoroughly by inversion and place the tubes at 4°C for 1 h.
3. Pellet the virions by centrifugation at 20,000*g* (maximum speed) for 20 min at 4°C.
4. Aspirate off the supernatant and resuspend the virion pellet in 0.5 mL of PBS.
5. Add 125 μL of 5X digestion buffer (0.25% SDS, 0.25 *M* Tris, 0.25 *M* EDTA) and add proteinase K to 500 μg/mL. Incubate for 2 h at 37°C.
6. Extract once with an equal volume of phenol saturated with 0.1 *M* Tris-HCl, pH 8.0, and transfer the aqueous phase to a fresh tube.
7. Extract once with an equal volume of chloroform and transfer the aqueous phase to a fresh tube.
8. Precipitate the viral DNA by adding 2.0 μL of 10 μg/μL of tRNA, 0.05 volume of 3 *M* sodium acetate, and one volume of isopropanol. Place at –20°C overnight.

9. Pellet the viral DNA by centrifugation at 20,000*g* (maximum speed) for 15 min at 4°C. Aspirate off the isopropanol and allow the pellets to dry.
10. Resuspend the pellet in 30 μL of TE. Add 2 μL of DNase-free RNase and incubate at 37°C for 1 h.
11. Add loading dye to samples and load onto an agarose gel for Southern analysis (*see* **Note 5**).

3.12. Generation of HBV Radioactive Probe (See Note 6)

1. Digest pTHBV1.3 with *Pst*I and *Sac*I restriction enzymes to excise a fragment containing the 1.3-unit-length HBV construct.
2. Separate the 1.3-unit-length fragment by gel electrophoresis.
3. Cut HBV band and extract HBV DNA from the gel.
4. Run 1 μL of the DNA eluate along with *Hin*dIII marker.
5. Determine DNA concentration by comparing HBV DNA band density to a band density of *Hin*dIII marker. Store at –20°C; this is the DNA probe template.
6. Dilute DNA probe template so that there are 50–100 ng of DNA in 9 μL of dH_2O.
7. Boil the DNA probe template for 5 min, then cool on ice and centrifuge the condensation.
8. Make core reaction mixture using Random Prime DNA Labeling Kit (Roche): 2 μL of oligonucleotides/buffer, 3 μL of AGT mixture 1:1:1, and 1 μL of Klenow DNA polymerase.
9. Add 9 μL of denatured DNA probe to the core reaction mixture.
10. Add 50 μCi of [^{32}P]dCTP.
11. Incubate in a water bath at 37°C for 30–45 min.
12. Set up a Sephadex-G50 elution column.
13. Pipet the reaction onto the column and elute with 150 μL of TE (10:1).
14. Add 3 μL of eluate to 5 mL of scintillation fluid, shake to mix, and count on a scintillation counter.
15. Calculate the amount of probe that gives final concentration in the range of $2–4 \times 10^6$ cpm/mL of hybridization buffer.

4. Notes

1. The HBV recombinant baculovirus, although replication deficient in human cells, contains a 1.3-fold overlength HBV genome and should be handled with the same precautions used for HBV. Infection of HepG2 and other cell lines with the HBV recombinant baculovirus results in the production of infectious HBV particles. Therefore, all work with the HBV recombinant baculovirus (generation of viral stocks, infection of cells, etc.) should be done using BSL-2 guidelines and only with personnel showing appropriate anti-HBs status after being immunized.
2. Cleanup of the spinner flasks:

   a. Care must be taken to ensure that the used spinner flasks are cleaned and sterilized properly to avoid contamination during the next use. It is extremely important that soaps or detergents are NOT used to clean the flasks. These products could leave a residue in the flask and prevent the growth of cells in future cultures.

   b. Rinse flask out several times with water and then allow to sit with arms open and one arm under running water for about 30 min. It is not necessary to remove the top cap that has the propeller attached, but be sure to invert several times while washing and rinse out arm caps extremely well.

   c. Add 2000 mL of 10% acetic acid to the flask and tighten caps. Spin on a stirrer plate overnight. Be sure to invert the flask every couple of hours to wash the caps.

d. Rinse the flask with water again as described above except that you now disassemble the cap and stirring rods to rinse them thoroughly. Be sure to rinse thoroughly as any residual acetic acid in the flask would be detrimental to growing cells in the future. Once done, rinse once with distilled water. Place the flask on the tabletop with caps off to dry overnight.

e. The next day, add approx 500 mL of sterile distilled water to the flask, loosely screw caps back on arms, and autoclave. Two autoclave runs will be necessary, as baculovirus can survive one run.

f. Pour water out, fill with 500 mL sterile distilled water again, and loosely screw caps onto arms. Cover the arms with foil and autoclave tape. Autoclave again and store in the cabinet without removing foil or water.

3. Every day the flasks are aerated and before splitting, check for signs of contamination. Let the cells in the flasks settle down for about 5 min and look at the upper surface of the cell culture (meniscus); it should be clear. If it is turbid, this most probably indicates contamination and this flask should be discarded.
4. Do not purify two different viruses in the same rotor at the same time.
5. HBV RNA extraction, prehybridization and hybridization, and Southern blot analysis can be performed using standard laboratory methods.
6. The method we described can be used for generation of the HBV probe; other methods can be used as well.

References

1. Sells, M. A., Chen, M. L., and Acs, G. (1987) Production of hepatitis B virus particles in Hep G2 cells transfected with cloned hepatitis B virus DNA. *Proc. Natl. Acad. Sci. USA* **84**, 1005–1009.
2. Newbold, J. E., Xin, H., Tencza, M., et al. (1995) The covalently closed duplex form of the hepadnavirus genome exists in situ as a heterogeneous population of viral minichromosomes. *J. Virol.* **69**, 3350–3357.
3. Wood, H. A. and Granados, R. R. (1991) Genetically engineered baculoviruses as agents for pest control. *Annu. Rev. Microbiol.* **45**, 69–87.
4. Smith, G. E., Summers, M. D., and Fraser, M. J. (1983) Production of human beta interferon in insect cells infected with a baculovirus expression vector. *Mol. Cell. Biol.* **3**, 2156–2165.
5. Pennock, G. D., Shoemaker, C., and Miller, L. K. (1984) Strong and regulated expression of *Escherichia coli* beta galactosidase in insect cells with a baculovirus vector. *Mol. Cell. Biol.* **4**, 399–406.
6. Hofmann, C., Sandig, V., Jennings, G., Rudolph, M., Schlag, P., and Strauss, M. (1995) Efficient gene transfer into human hepatocytes by baculovirus vectors. Proc. *Natl. Acad. Sci. USA* **92**, 10099–10103.
7. Sandig, V., Hofmann, C., Steinert, S., Jennings, G., Schlag, P., and Strauss, M. (1996) Gene transfer into hepatocytes and human liver tissue by baculovirus vectors. *Hum. Gene Ther.* **7**, 1937–1945.
8. Boyce, F. M. and Bucher, N. L. (1996) Baculovirus-mediated gene transfer into mammalian cells. *Proc. Natl. Acad. Sci. USA* **93**, 2348–2352.
9. Bilello, J. P., Delaney, W. E. IV, Boyce, F. M., and Isom, H. C. (2001) Transient disruption of intracellular junctions enables baculovirus entry into nondividing hepatocytes. *J. Virol.* **75**, 9857–9871.
10. Shoji, I., Aizaki, H., Tani, H., et al. (1997) Efficient gene transfer into various mammalian cells, including non-hepatic cells, by baculovirus vectors. *J. Gen. Virol.* **78**, 2657–2664.

11. Delaney, W. E. IV and Isom, H. C. (1998) Hepatitis B replication in human HepG2 cells mediated by hepatitis B virus recombinant baculovirus. *Hepatology* **28**, 1134–1146.
12. Delaney, W. E. IV, Miller, T. G., and Isom, H. C. (1999) Use of the hepatitis B virus recombinant baculovirus-HepG2 system to study the effects of (–)-β-2',3'-dideoxy-3'-thiacytidine on replication of hepatitis B virus and accumulation of covalently closed circular DNA. *Antimicrob. Agents Chemother.* **43**, 2017–2026.
13. Abdelhamed, A. M., Kelley, C. M., Miller, T. G., Furman, P. A., and Isom, H. C. (2002) Rebound of hepatitis B virus replication in HepG2 cells after cessation of antiviral treatment. *J. Virol.* **76**, 8148–8160.
14. Delaney, W. E. IV, Edwards, R., Colledge, D., et al. (2001) Cross-resistance testing of antihepadnaviral compounds using novel recombinant baculoviruses which encode drug-resistant strains of hepatitis B virus. *Antimicrob. Agents Chemother.* **45**, 1705–1713.
15. Abdelhamed, A. M., Kelley, C. M., Miller, T. G., Cable, E. E., Furman, P. A., and Isom, H. C. (2003) Comparison of the anti-hepatitis B virus activity of lamivudine and clevudine using a quantitative assay. *Antimicrob. Agents Chemother.* **47**, 324–336.
16. Sambrook, J., Fritsch, E. F., and Maniatis, T. (1989) Analysis and cloning of eukaryotic genomic DNA, In *Molecular Cloning: A Laboratory Manual* 2nd edit. Cold Spring Harbor Laboratory Press, Cold Spring Harbor, NY, pp. 9.1–9.62.
17. Ausubel, F. M., Brent, R., Kingston, R. E., et al. (2002) In *Current Protocols in Molecular Biology*. John Wiley & Sons, New York.

20

Transgenic Hepatitis B Virus Mouse Model in the Study of Chemotherapy

John D. Morrey

1. Introduction

Much of the knowledge about hepatitis B virus (HBV) has been obtained from the infection of natural hosts with nonhuman hepatitis viruses that possess similar characteristics to HBV, such as in the duck and woodchuck. Transgenic mouse models have also been valuable in recent years for studying the biology of the virus ***(1–7)*** and for evaluating antiviral compounds ***(3,8–11)***. The development of the transgenic mouse model carrying the infectious HBV genome has been motivated in part by the expense and minimal availability of the HBV chimpanzee model, and the absence of more convenient, small non-primate animal models that can be infected with HBV.

Transgenic lines (1.3.32 and 1.3.46) were reported in 1995 ***(1)*** to replicate virus in the liver and produce quantifiable levels of HBV in the serum. HBV DNA replicative intermediates (relaxed circular, double-stranded linear, and single-stranded) and virus particles with infectious Dane particle-like morphology were identified in liver. RNA species (3.5 kb, 2.4 kb, and 2.1 kb) were also identified in comparable proportions as found in chronically infected human liver. HBV antigens found in infected human subjects were also identified in these mice, namely, hepatitis B surface antigen (HBsAg) and hepatitis B envelope antigen (HBeAg) in both the serum and liver, and hepatitis B core antigen (HBcAg) in the liver ***(1)***. These HBV transgenic mice are the ones described in this chapter. HBV transgenic mice generated previously ***(12–14)*** did not yield high levels of virus replication, presumably because of suboptimal tandem repeated copies of the viral genome. Subsequently, other HBV transgenic mice that express quantifiable levels of HBV have also been produced (P. Marion, Stanford University, Stanford, CA, personal communications).

Interest in using HBV transgenic mice for antiviral studies has increased since the development of mice that replicate quantifiable levels of virus ***(1,15)***. Studies have reported the efficacy of cytokines and nucleotides to reduce viral parameters in viral hep-

From: *Methods in Molecular Medicine, vol. 96: Hepatitis B and D Protocols, volume 2*
Edited by: R. K. Hamatake and J. Y. N. Lau © Humana Press Inc., Totowa, NJ

atitis mouse models *(3,16–22)*. This chapter describes the use of this HBV transgenic animal model for antiviral experiments, which includes details on the use of the mice, and the assays for serum HBV DNA, serum antigens, liver HBV DNA, RNA, and HBcAg.

2. Materials

2.1. Transgenic Mice

2.1.1. Source

Hepatitis B transgenic mice were obtained from Dr. Francis V. Chisari (Scripps Research Institute, La Jolla, CA), which were derived from founder 1.3.32 *(1)*. The transgenic line had been backcrossed to obtain a C57BL/6 genetic background. (*See* **Note 1**.)

2.1.2. Transgenic Animal Experiments

1. Oral gavage needle, ball diameter 1.25 mm, 20-gauge, 1-inch length (Fisher Scientific cat. no. 01-290-3A).
2. Disposable 27-gauge needle and syringe.
3. BL3-N animal facility with standard animal care supplies.
4. Refrigerator/freezer with stored compounds.

2.2. Necropsy

1. Avertin anesthesia: 2.5% Solution of 1 g of tribromoethanol/mL of tertiary amyl alcohol in water, 0.3 mL/20 g mouse, 3 mg.
2. 27-Gauge needle and disposable syringes.
3. Necropsy instruments: Scissors, forceps, pins, cork board.
4. 3% Hydrogen peroxide and 10% bleach for dipping instruments after each mouse.
5. Pasteur pipets for collecting blood.
6. Petri dishes for liver samples.
7. Incinerator (USU Veterinary Diagnostics Laboratory) for infected mice.

2.3. Sample Processing

1. Microcentrifuge tubes and microcentrifuge.
2. Liquid nitrogen and Dewer flasks.
3. 4-mm diameter biopsy punches (Uni-punch, Disposable Biospy Punch, Premier Medical Products, cat. no. 9033504, King of Prussia, PA).
4. Proteinase K digestion solution (freshly prepared) for DNA extraction: 0.2 mg/mL of proteinase K, 10 m*M* Tris-HCl, pH 8.0, 1 m*M* EDTA, 10 mM NaCl, 0.5% sodium dodecylsulfate (SDS) *(23)*.
5. Grinder to fit microcentrifuge tubes dedicated to DNA extraction.
6. Forceps for handling liver samples.
7. Grinder to fit microcentrifuge tubes dedicated to RNA extraction.
8. Trizol reagent (Gibco/BRL, Gaithersburg, MD) for RNA extraction.
9. Sealable containers for formalin.

2.4. Liver HBV DNA Assay

Standard alkaline transfer method of the Southern blot hybridization was done *(24)*. The supplies listed in the following are only the unique items, with the common items left out of the list.

1. *Hind*III restriction enzyme and buffer.
2. Imager (Alphaimager2000TM, Alpha Innotech, out of business).
3. Biodyne B positive-charged nylon membrane (PALL).
4. UV Stratalinker 1800 (Stratagene).
5. BioMax film (cat. no. 8294985, Kodak).

2.5. Liver HBV RNA Assay

A standard salt-transfer procedure for Northern blot analysis was preformed *(26)*. The same membrane (Biodyne B) and film (BioMax) as for the Southern blot analysis were used.

2.6. ELISA for Detection of HBeAg in Serum

1. Black opaque 96-well plates (Greiner).
2. Capture anti-HBeAg antibody (cat. no. 10-H10, clone no. M2110147, Fitzgerald).
3. Horseradish peroxidase (HRP) conjugated tracer anti-HBeAg antibody (cat. no.10-H10, clone no. M2110146, Fitzgerald Industries). The antibody was conjugated per instructions using a commercial kit (Pierce, cat. no. 31485, EZ-Link maleimide-activated HRP).
4. HBe protein (BioDesign International, Massachusetts) to make a standard curve.
5. Normal mouse serum (Sigma) for diluent and blanks.
6. Sensitization buffer: 0.05 *M* Tris-HCl, 0.3 *M* KCl, 0.002 *M* EDTA, pH 8.0.
7. Blocking buffer: 0.3% Tween-20, 0.25% bovine serum albumin (BSA) in phosphate-buffered saline (PBS).
8. Quanta Blu™ fluorogenic peroxidase substrate kit which includes fluorogenic substrate and stop solution (cat, no. 15169, Pierce Biochemical).
9. Molecular Devices fMax fluorimeter with 320/405 filter pair.
10. Rocker, 37°C incubator.

2.7. ELISA for Detection of HBsAg in Serum

1. Sensitization, blocking buffers, Quanta Blu™ fluorogenic peroxidase substrate kit, fluorimeter, rocker, and normal mouse sera as in **Subheading 2.6.**
2. Capture anti-HBsAg (East Coast Biologics, cat. no. B04-95-33M-P).
3. Biotinylated goat anti-HBsAg (Accurate, cat. no. YV51807).
4. Streptavidin HRP conjugate (Pierce).
5. Molecular Devices fMax fluorimeter.
6. HBs protein (BioDesign International, Massachusetts) to make a standard curve.

2.8. Liver HBcAg Assay (Immunocytochemistry)

1. Charged glass slides.
2. Histoclear (National Diagnostics, cat. no. HS200).
3. Humidified slide chamber.
4. Modified Harris stain (contains no alcohol).
5. DAKO Biotin Blocking system cat. no. X0590 (blocking reaction for avidin and biotin reagents).
6. DAKO LSAB peroxidase kit no. K0684 (3% hydrogen peroxide, blocking agent, linked antibody to core, streptavidin, chromagen substrate, with buffers).
7. DAKO no. B0586 rabbit anti-HBcAg antigen.
8. 0.05 *M* Tris-HCl, pH 7.7, with 0.1 % Tween-20.

9. 0.05 *M* Tris-HCl, pH 7.7, without 0.1 % Tween-20 (last washes).
10. 10% Buffered neutral formalin (BNF) for hematoxylin and eosin (H & E) and immunocytochemistry.
11. DAKO Glycergel mounting media (cat. no. CO563, DAKO) (Carpinteria, CA).
12. Graded series of ethanol from absolute down to 70%.
13. Concentrated ammonia.

2.9. Serum HBV DNA Assay (15)

The interpretation of this parameter has been problematic because of variability and a trauma/placebo effect (*see* **Note 2**); therefore, the use of this parameter is optional. Liver HBV DNA parameter is by far the more dependable of the two parameters.

1. Reference serum HBV standard (Eurohep study group, Dr. K.-H. Heerman, Universitatskliniken Gottingen, Kreuzbergring, Germany).
2. 96-Well polymerase chain reaction (PCR) plate (MBP no. 3416).
3. 0.2 mL, eight tube strip caps (MBP no. 3418C).
4. 0.2 mL, eight tube strips (MBP no. 3418).
5. Gene releaser (Bioventures).
6. Thermoseal tape, Genemate (ISC Bioexpress, cat. no. T-2417-5).
7. TE buffer, pH 8; obtain from separate lab to control for contamination.
8. dNTPs, stock, 2 m*M* concentration each (Amersham Pharmacia Biotech).
9. Blue dextran dye (diluted 1:2 in 1.5X TBE).
10. Forward primer, 20 μ*M*, sequence GATTGAGACCTTCGTCTGCGAG.
11. Reverse primer, 20 μ*M*, sequence CATTGTTCACCTCACCATACTGCAC.
12. Internal control plasmid-target sequence with extraneous insert to make larger than wild-type signal.
13. Cloned PFU DNA polymerase (Stratagene).
14. 10X Cloned PFU buffer (Stratagene).
15. 96-Well thermocycler (heated lid so does not require oil overlay).
16. 10X TBE to make 1X and 1.5X solutions for polyacrylamide gel electrophoresis (PAGE).
17. 40% Acrylamide (PAGE-PLUS, Amresco, E562).
18. Tetraethylmethyldiamine (TEMED). Store at 4°C.
19. Ammonium persulfate (APS). Store at 4°C.
20. Ethidium bromide: 0.5 μL of 10 mg/mL EtBr into 150 mL of 1.5X TBE.
21. 800-W microwave oven.

3. Methods

3.1. Use of Transgenic Mice

3.1.1. Selection of Mice for Experiments

1. Male mice are preferred (*see* **Note 3**).
2. Screen mice for serum HBeAg titers, remove 15% of the mice having the lowest titers, and block randomize the mice according to serum HBeAg titers across treatment groups (*see* **Note 4**).
3. Age-match transgenic mice for experiments whenever possible.

3.1.2. Mouse Breeding

1. Establish some male homozygous transgenic mice by breeding two heterozygote mice. Identify transgenic mice by serum HBV DNA or HBeAg (*see* **Note 5**).

2. Test male mice for homozygosity by breeding the resulting progeny in **step 1** with female nontransgenic C57BL/6 mice. If homozygote, all littermates will be transgenic.
3. Breed verified male homozygous mice with nontransgenic female C57BL/6 mice to obtain 100% heterozygous mice, which are the animals used for experiments. Five to eight heterozygote pups are typically obtained per litter.

3.1.3 Gender

Male transgenic mice are preferentially used but female mice might be used if numbers are limited and caging of single mice is problematic (*see* **Note 3**).

3.1.4. Safety Issues

1. Use BL2-N, or preferably, BL3-N animal containment facility (*see* **Note 6**).
2. Vaccinate all personnel with clinically approved hepatitis B vaccine (Engerix-B, SmithKline Beecham Pharmaceuticals, Philadelphia, PA).
3. Confirm seroconversion of all personnel to vaccine by testing for antibodies. We use the local health clinic for this.
4. The personnel receive laboratory safety training and special training on blood-borne pathogen handling by our institution's Environmental Health and Safety Office.

3.2. Experimental Design, Treatment Schedules, and Routes

The design of a typical experiment for evaluating a compound such as a nucleoside analog would be as follows:

- Two treatment groups containing a high and a low dosage of drug based on pharmacokinetic studies.
- Placebo control group.
- Untreated group.
- Number of mice per group—10 each.
- Route of administration—usually oral gavage or intraperitoneal administration once or twice per day.
- Duration of treatment—10 d has been sufficient for previous evaluation of nucleoside analogs, but this can extended to 14 d or longer depending on the nature of the compound.

3.3. Necropsy and Sample Collection

This will depend in part on the specific Institutional Animal Care and Use Committee.

1. Periodical bleeding from individual mice is performed by ocular bleeding technique *(25)*.
2. For necrospy, mice are anesthetized with Avertin (2.5% solution of 1 g of tribromoethanol/mL tertiary amyl alcohol in water), and blood is collected by exsanguination from the subclavian artery, while being careful to avoid virus or DNA contamination from hair or instruments (*see* **Note 7**).
3. Uniform liver biospies are obtained by using 4.0-mm punches:
   a. Two punches in cryotube snap-frozen in liquid nitrogen.
   b. One punch grounded in 0.5 mL of proteinase K solution using a grinder fitted to a microcentrifuge tube. Incubate for 5–10 min (min) at room temperature (RT), then snap-freeze in liquid nitrogen.
   c. One punch grounded in 1 mL of Trizol reagent. Incubate for 5 min at RT and snap-freeze in liquid nitrogen.

4. Serum processing: Coagulate for 30 min in a refrigerator, centrifuge at 3000–3500*g*, collect serum while leaving a substantial volume of serum near the interface to avoid aspirating cells (*see* **Note 7**), and freeze at –80°C until use for PCR or antigen assays.

3.4. Southern Blot Hybridization for Detection of Liver HBV DNA

1. Remove liver homogenized in proteinase K solution (*see* **Subheading 3.3., step 3**) from the freezer and incubate at 52°C for 2 h.
2. Purify the DNA with phenol–chloroform and ethanol precipitation using standard protocols.
3. Restriction digest liver DNA by adding 31 μL of liver DNA solution to 5 μL of *Hin*dIII and 4 μL of R+ buffer (MBI Fermentas, Hanover, MD). *Hin*dIII is used because it does not cut the DNA within the transgene.
4. The reaction is incubated at 37°C for >3 h, after which 8 μL of 6X running dye is added to each sample.
5. A 1% agarose gel is then loaded with the *Hin*dIII-digested liver DNA and run at 60 V for 20 min, after which the voltage is raised to 90 V for 2 h.
6. After the electrophoresis, the DNA is stained with ethidium bromide and photographed.
7. DNA is then transferred for 2–3 h to BioDyne™ B positive-charged nylon membrane by the alkaline transfer method ***(24)***.
8. The membrane is baked for >30 min at 80°C and UV-fixed using the UV Stratalinker™ 1800 (Stratagene, La Jolla, CA).
9. Prior to hybridization, the filter is rinsed twice for 30 min in a neutralizing solution of 0.1X SSC and 0.1% SDS.
10. Hybridization using a [^{32}P]CTP-labeled, HBV genomic probe (digested with *Hae*III; *see* **Note 8**) cloned into the pBluescript plasmid (gift of Dr. Luca Guidotti, The Scripps Institute, La Jolla, CA) occurs overnight at 60°C in a solution of 10% PEG-8000, 0.05 *M* $NaPO_4$, 0.21 mg/mL of salmon sperm DNA, and 7% SDS.
11. The membrane is washed to remove background radiation and exposed on Biomax film (Kodak, Rochester, NY) at –80°C. The transgene and viral DNA bands on the X-ray film are measured using densitometric analysis (AlphaImager2000TM, Alpha Innotech).
12. Quantification. The ratio of the viral DNA bands to the transgene band is used to determine the concentration of viral DNA per host DNA. This calculation is based on the knowledge that there are 1.3 copies of the transgene present per host cell with this line of transgenic mice (F. Chisari, The Scripps Research Insitute, personal communication). The transgene is used as an internal indicator to calculate the picograms of HBV DNA per microgram of cellular host DNA.

3.5. Northern Blot Analysis for Detection of Liver HBV RNA

1. Thaw samples homogenized in Trizol reagent (*see* **Subheading 3.3., step 3**) and incubate for 5 min at RT.
2. The Trizol procedure is followed using the manufacturer's instructions.
3. After ethanol precipitation, RNA pellets are dried and stored until use. Before electrophoresis, they are suspended in diethyl pyrocarbonate (DEPC)-treated water.
4. An agarose–formaldehyde gel is prepared by dissolving 1.5 g of agarose in 108 mL of DEPC-treated water and cooling the gel to 60°C in a water bath.
5. A volume of 15 mL of 10X 3-(*N*-morpholino)propanesulfonic acid (MOPS) running buffer and 27 mL of 12.3 *M* formaldehyde is mixed well with the dissolved agarose and the gel is poured immediately and allowed to solidify. An electrophoresis unit is filled with sufficient 1X MOPS buffer to cover the gel ***(26)***.

6. Samples are prepared by combining 6 μL of dissolved RNA with 2.5 μL of 10X MOPS running buffer, 4.5 μL of 12.3 *M* formaldehyde, and 12.5 μL of formamide in a microcentrifuge tube.
7. After brief mixing by vortexing, samples are centrifuged for 5–10 s in a microcentrifuge and incubated for 15 min at 55°C.
8. A volume of 5 μL of formaldehyde loading buffer is added and the samples are loaded onto the gel and run at 5 V/cm until the loading dye migrates between one half and two thirds of the length of the gel.
9. The gels are rinsed four times with DEPC-treated water and allowed to soak in 10 gel volumes of 20X saline sodium citrate (SSC) for 45 min.
10. RNA is transferred to BioDyne™ B positive-charged nylon membrane by salt transfer method of Northern blot analysis ***(26)***.
11. After transfer, the membrane is rinsed in 2X SSC and allowed to dry. The membranes are baked and crosslinked as outlined in the HBV DNA procedure.
12. To prepare for hybridization, the membranes are wetted in 6X SSC. Hybridization, exposure of the probed membrane onto film, and analysis of the exposure are carried out as described for DNA membranes except that they are probed for both GAPDH and HBV in separate reactions, with the GAPDH serving as an internal control.
13. The relative RNA concentration is calculated by dividing the density of the HBV autoradiographic signal with the density of the housekeeping gene RNA (GAPDH) or the total RNA.
14. This parameter may or may not respond to antiviral therapy because it depends on the mode of action of the compounds (*see* **Note 9**).

3.6. ELISA for Quantification of HBeAg in Serum

1. Coat wells of black opaque 96-well plates with 100 μL of capture anti-HBeAg antibody at a concentration of 2.4 μL/mL diluted in sensitization buffer at 37°C for 2 h.
2. Remove the capture antibody with a multichannel pipettor, wash wells three times with water, and add 200 μL of blocking buffer. Incubate at RT for 30 min.
3. Wash wells three times with 300 μL of pure water.
4. Add 100 μL of serum samples diluted 1:20 in blocking buffer to wells. Also include two negative controls (normal mouse serum diluted 1:20 in blocking buffer) and four to eight serially diluted HBeAg protein controls to make a standard curve (each diluted 1:20 in blocking buffer). Incubate at 4°C for 2 h.
5. Remove solution and wash three times with water. Add 200 μL of blocking buffer and incubate for 10 min at RT and wash as described in **step 3**.
6. Add 100 μL of horseradish peroxidase conjugated tracer anti-HBeAg antibody (Fitzgerald Industries) at a concentration of approx 0.6 μg/mL into blocking buffer. Incubate at 4°C for 2 h.
7. Block and wash as described in **step 5**.
8. Add 100 μL of working solution of fluorogenic substrate Quanta-Blue (Pierce Biochemical). Incubate for 10 min at RT.
9. Read using filter pairs 320/405.
10. Construct a standard curve with an equation for the line and determine the concentration of HBeAg in the serum samples.

3.7. ELISA for Quantification of HBsAg in Serum

1. Coat wells of black opaque 96-well plates with 100 μL capture anti-HBsAg antibody at a concentration of 5.6 μg/mL diluted in sensitization buffer at 37°C for 2 h.

2. Remove the capture antibody with a multichannel pipettor, wash wells three times with water, and add 200 μL of blocking buffer. Incubate at RT for 30 min.
3. Wash wells three times with 300 μL of pure water.
4. Add 100 μL serum samples diluted 1:20 in blocking buffer to wells. Also include two negative controls (normal mouse serum diluted 1:20 in blocking buffer) and four to eight serially diluted HBsAg protein controls to make a standard curve (each diluted 1:20 in blocking buffer). Incubate at RT for 2 h.
5. Remove solution and wash three times with water. Add 200 μL of blocking buffer and incubate for 10 min at RT and wash as in **step 3**.
6. Add 100 μL of HRP-conjugated tracer anti-HBsAg antibody diluted at 1:1000 (concentration from manufacturer not known) in blocking buffer. Incubate at RT on a rocker for 1 h.
7. Block and wash as described in **step 5**.
8. Add 100 μL of streptavidin–horseradish peroxidase conjugate diluted to 1 μg/mL in blocking buffer. Incubate at RT on a rocker for 1 h. Block and wash as described in **step 5**.
9. Add 100 μL of working solution of fluorogenic substrate Quanta-Blue (Pierce Biochemical). Incubate for 20 min at RT, at which point 100 μL of stop solution is added. Block and wash as described in **step 5**.
10. Read using filter pairs 320/405.
11. Construct a standard curve with an equation for the line and determine concentration of HBsAg in serum samples.

3.8. Immunocytochemical Staining for HBcAg of Liver Sections

3.8.1. Staining

1. Cut paraffin-embedded sections on gelatin-free deionized (DI) water. Use charged slides.
2. Deparaffinize with Histoclear using three changes at 5 min each. Dehydrate in graded series of alcohols (absolute ethanol down to 70% ethanol) and then running tap water. Rinse well in distilled water before beginning the procedure.
3. Perform all incubations in a humid chamber.
4. Add avidin reagent and incubate for 10 min.
5. Rinse (*see* **Subheading 3.8.2.**).
6. Add biotin reagent and incubate for 10 min.
7. Rinse (*see* **Subheading 3.8.2.**).
8. Add 3% hydrogen peroxide and incubate for 5 min.
9. Rinse in DI water, followed by Tris-HCl without Tween-20.
10. Add blocking reagent and incubate for 5 min.
11. Tap off excess reagent, **Do not rinse.**
12. Add antibody and incubate 10 min (for greater sensitivity, incubate for 30 min).
13. Rinse (*see* **Subheading 3.8.2.**).
14. Add the link reagent and incubate 10 min (for greater sensitivity, incubate for 30 min).
15. Rinse (*see* **Subheading 3.8.2.**).
16. Add streptavidin peroxidase and incubate for 10 min (for greater sensitivity, incubate for 30 min).
17. Rinse (*see* **Subheading 3.8.2.**).
18. Add substrate–chromogen solution and incubate for 10 min.
19. Rinse (*see* **Subheading 3.8.2.**).
20. Counterstain with modified Harris stain (contains no alcohol) for 3 min.
21. Rinse with DI water to remove excess stain.

22. Add 10 drops of diluted ammonia (two drops of concentrated ammonia in 100 mL).
23. Rinse with DI water.
24. Mount in glycergel (glycerin jelly).
25. Score staining 1–4. Viral staining is red in cytoplasm and nuclei. (*see* **Note 10** for alternative scoring of HBcAg staining.)

3.8.2. Rinsing Technique (Used in Procedures Described in Subheading 3.8.1.)

1. Squirt Tris-HCl Tween-20 solution over the slide while holding the slide over a sink.
2. Shake the slide three times to remove excess solution.
3. Add 10 quick dips of slide in a Coplin jar of Tris-HCl Tween-20. **Important: Change this bath for each reaction**.
4. Squirt the slide with Tris-HCl (without Tween-20).
5. Hold the slide in a Tris-HCl bath.
6. Shake Tris-HCl from each slide and blot semidry before adding the next reagent.

3.9. Quantitative PCR for Serum HBV DNA

The interpretation of this parameter has been problematic because of variability and a trauma/placebo effect (*see* **Note 2**); therefore, the use of this parameter is optional. Liver HBV DNA parameter is by far the more dependable of the two parameters.

3.9.1. Sample Preparation—Single-Step Purification (See ***Notes 7*** *and* ***11****)*

1. Thaw serum samples and mix thoroughly.
2. Make 1:8 dilutions of the serum in TE buffer, pH 8.0, using a 96-well plate. Seven microliters of serum and 49 μL of TE for a final volume of 56 μL is convenient. (*See* **Note 12**.)
3. Cover the plate with Thermoseal tape and vortex-mix the plate moderately for approx 15 s to ensure a homogeneous mixture. Dilutions can be frozen and reused for subsequent PCR reactions *(27)*.
4. Add 2.3 μL of diluted serum to 6 μL of Gene Releaser, while being careful to not create a contaminating aerosol by covering both ends of the plate with lids that have been cleaned with Chlorox.
5. After serum has been added to each well, overlay plate with thermoseal tape. Vortex-mix the reaction plate to mix evenly with Gene Releaser (approx 15 s).
6. Microwave the plates containing Gene Releaser and serum samples at 800 W for 6 min. Also, add a 1-L beaker of water to act as a heat sink for the microwave energy.
7. Cool the plate by placing the well tips in cool water to minimize condensation.
8. The PCR reaction mixture can be prepared directly in the wells with Gene Releaser depending on the PCR protocol being used. (*See* **Note 13**.)
9. Set up and perform the PCR reaction.
10. If Gene Releaser is still present, store the PCR at RT, that is, do not store the plates at 4°C because the PCR products will associate with the resin.
11. Heat the plates to 65°C to release the PCR products from the Gene Releaser resin, centrifuge the warm resin to the bottom of the tubes, remove the supernatant, and process for electrophoresis to detect PCR products.

3.9.2. PCR Setup

1. Place reaction plate from previous step on ice until needed.
2. The components in a total 40 μL of PCR reaction were: 0.02 U of cloned Pfu DNA polymerase, 1X Pfu buffer, 200 n*M* of each deoxynucleotide triphosphate, and 0.2 μ*M* of each of

the forward and reverse primers. The internal control DNA is added between 10 and 450 genome equivalents (ge) per reaction (*see* **Notes 14** and **15**).

3. Chill the tubes. Mix master mix gently by lightly vortexing with caps on tubes.
4. Add master mix to each well, keeping the other wells covered to avoid contamination.
5. Cap wells with 0.2 mL-eight tube strip caps, and transfer the plate (still on ice) to the amplification lab area.
6. Vortex-mix the samples moderately for approx 15–30 s or until GeneReleaser is mixed into solution.
7. Place the plate in a preheated thermocycler, 94°C, for hot start. Heat at 94°C for 2 min and then run 40 cycles of 1 min at 94°C, 1 min at 55°C, and 1 min at 72°C. End with 5 min at 72°C and then hold at RT. (Do not chill.)

3.9.3. PCR Analysis

1. Add 10 µL of a 1:2 dilution of blue dextran dye (Perkin Elmer, Foster City, CA) in 1.5X TBE to each 40 µL PCR reaction.
2. Vortex-mix, heated to 60°C for 10 min and vortex-mix again before pelleting the Gene Releaser™ resin at 500 rpm for 30 s. (*See* **Note 16**.)
3. After a prerun for 30 min at 300 V in 1X TBE in which the lower reservoir contained 0.02 mg/mL of ethidium bromide, samples were loaded and electrophoresed for 12 min at 360 V in a 4.5% nondenaturing polyacrylamide gel. A NucleoScan 2000 system was used, however, the instrument has been discontinued so a sequencing instrument may be used.
4. Determine the area under the curve for each band.
5. The gel is reloaded with more samples for up to five times, which resulted in relatively high throughput.
6. The titers of the serum samples are determined by running multiple PCR reactions with each serum sample using different amounts of internal control. The objective is that at least two different ratios (lower/upper bands) are to be obtained, with one greater and one less than a ratio of 1. The point at which each band is equal to the other (ratio = 1) is called the "crossover" point. This crossover point is calculated by linear regression of the logarithm of the ratio vs logarithm of the concentration of the internal control added ***(15***). (*See* **Note 17**.)

4. Notes

1. Dr. Pat Marion, Stanford University, also has mice suitable for these types of studies. We have also generated HBV transgenic mice with a Balb/C background. They appear to have better breeding vigor and perhaps higher serum titers than the transgenic mice with a C57BL/6 background. We have not yet used these Balb/C background mice, however, in antiviral experiments.
2. We have determined that treatment of these transgenic mice using per os, intraperitoneal, or orbital sinus bleeding, and different drug vehicles will result in reduction of serum HBV DNA in control animals, which is referred to as "trauma/placebo effect" ***(15)***. This undesirable trauma/placebo effect and the inherent variability of the serum HBV DNA causes difficult and sometimes ambiguous analysis of serum HBV DNA. Consequently, we depend on the liver HBV DNA parameter for consistent results.
3. Male mice have slightly higher viral titers and titers may be less variable presumably because female transgenic mice can sporadically generate antibodies to HBsAg over time (Frank Chisari, The Scripps Research Institute, La Jolla, CA, *personal communication*). We have found that female mice can be used to obtain statistically valid data; however, caution should be used because the differences between male and female mice are not well defined.

In short, male mice are preferred, but female mice can be used if available numbers are low and single mouse caging is problematic.

4. Approximately 3% of male and 11% of female transgenic mice express < 0.2 pg viral DNA/μg of cellular DNA as determined by liver HBV DNA Southern blot hybridization, that is, the transgene signal can be readily detected, but viral DNA products are not readily detected. Serum HBeAg is a useful marker for this anomaly; therefore, pretreatment screening of serum HBeAg should be used to block-randomize mice across groups. We know that by excluding the lowest 15% of the transgenic mice having the lowest serum HBeAg titers, one can eliminate the transgenic mice that produce undetectable liver HBV DNA, and the numbers of potential "outliers" can be reduced from the experiment, which decreases the variability.
5. Female homozygous transgenic mice do not have good breeding vigor, whereas the male homozygous mice breed adequately. Male homozygous mice are used as breeders with non-transgenic mice to produce 100% heterozygous transgenic mice. The breeding strategy described in **Subheading 3.** is for obtaining large numbers of transgenic mice efficiently.
6. The safety classification of the human hepatitis B virus is biosafety level 2 or 3 (BSL-2 or -3), depending on the potential for droplet or aerosol production ***(28,29)***. We use HBV transgenic mice (lines 1.3.32) ***(1)*** under BL-3N containment. All personnel who handle the animals are required to receive the commercially available hepatitis B vaccination (Engerix-B, SmithKline Beecham Pharmaceuticals, Philadelphia, PA). Individuals must seroconvert to the vaccination (anti-HBV positive) before working with the animals. The personnel receive laboratory safety training and special training on blood-borne pathogen handling by our institution's Environmental Health and Safety Office. Vigilant efforts are made to ensure safety of those working with the mice.
7. As with any PCR, contamination with extraneous DNA, particularly products from previous PCRs, should be avoided. We process tissues, set up PCRs, and do analysis all in different buildings. Gowns and gloves are worn in the PCR setup building, which does not have any HBV research activity in the building. When collecting blood during necropsy, the instruments are soaked in 3% hydrogen peroxide, dipped in 10% Chlorox™, and wiped with a fresh tissue. The skin is peeled from the incision site to avoid contamination from hair. Serum is collected to avoid aspiration of cells, that is, substantial volume of serum is left near the interface of the cells and tubes are handled very gently.
8. We have experienced that the HBV probe length has an influence on the hybridization ***(30)***. The probe should not be longer than 1000 bp, because this increases the chance of heterologous duplexes, which remain stable during stringent washes. Consequently, we cut our probe with a four-basepair (bp) cutting enzyme.
9. Since the HBV infectious life cycle is incomplete in the transgenic mice, probably only those parameters "downstream" from the antiviral target will be affected by the therapeutic substance. This incomplete life cycle is a disadvantage, but it is also an advantage in that it helps to identify modes of action. For example, adefovir dipivoxil (Gilead Sciences, Foster City, CA), a known inhibitor of polymerase, predictably affected the HBV DNA parameters, but not the HBV RNA ***(15)***.
10. Three different HBcAg parameters can be obtained from each tissue section. The first two measurements are based on the observation that cells surrounding the central veins of the liver are more strongly stained than in other areas of the liver ***(1)***, and that drug administered intravenously should have ready access to the luminal cells of the veins. The first two parameters are obtained from counting cells surrounding central veins as follows. The total number of cells, the number of cells with stained nuclei, and the number of cells with stained cyto-

plasms are counted around central veins. The stained nuclei counts or the stained cytoplasm counts are divided by the total cells. Five central vein areas are counted with each slide sample. For the third parameter, a field, not in a central vein area, is counted for the total number of stained nuclei. One quarter of the field is counted. Five such fields are counted per liver section.

11. The use of Gene Releaser resin has been very convenient with the transgenic mice because of one-step extraction, use of small volume of serum (7 μL), and the ability to set up the PCR reaction directly in the Gene Releaser resin. The extraction of the DNA from the virus and the PCR reaction is all done in the same tube. There is no phenol–chloroform extraction or other multistep extraction on very small volumes of mouse serum. Because our quantitative PCR reaction is unique to our laboratory, we will cite only the protocol ***(15)*** or refer the reader to commercially available kits. Our quantification method using GeneReleaser does not use fluorescence-labeled primers, because when we tried to develop our PCR assay using such primers, we did not obtain acceptable results. One possible explanation is that the Gene Releaser may have removed or interfered with fluorescence primers, but the answer is not know for certain.
12. Mouse serum possesses inhibitory substances for the PCR reaction and must be diluted at least eightfold to reduce the concentration of the inhibitory substances.
13. If Gene Releaser resin is not suitable for the PCR being used, such as real-time PCR in which the resin would interfere with spectrophotometric detection, the DNA must be removed from the resin solution. This is done by heating the plate to 65°C, centrifuging the resin to the bottom of the plate, and then removing the supernatant to be used for the PCR reaction. Because of the nature of the in-house quantitative PCR reaction used in our laboratory, we perform the PCR reaction directly in the tubes containing the Gene Releaser resin.
14. The internal control consisted of a 42-bp fragment inserted into a plasmid clone of the HBV target sequence. The sizes of the internal control and the virion PCR products were 412 bp and 370-bp, respectively. A 370 bp region was chosen within the core gene sequence of the HBV genome to amplify using PCR. The oligonucleotide primers utilized for these analyses were complementary to the HBV sequence (accession no. V01460). The forward primer sequence was GATTGAGACCTTCGTCTGCGAG (position 776–797) and the reverse primer sequence was CATTGTTCACCTCACCATACTGCAC (position 1146–1122).
15. The total PCR reaction volumes varied between 30 μL and 220 μL using different concentration of internal control and serum virus to determine the exact amount of viral DNA.
16. Heating the PCR reaction mixture containing GeneReleaser resin will dissociate the PCR products from the resin. Chilling the samples will cause unwanted association so that PCR products will not be contained in the supernatant.
17. Serum titers in units of genome equivalents per milliliter of serum are reported on a log scale. The means are calculated from the log scale and statistics performed. Liver HBV DNA in units of pg viral DNA/μg cellular DNA is not reported on a log scale. All other parameters are not reported or analyzed on a log scale.

References

1. Guidotti, L. G., Matzke, B., Schaller, H., and Chisari, F. V. (1995) High-level hepatitis B virus replication in transgenic mice. *J. Virol.* **69**, 6158–6169.
2. Wirth, S., Guidotti, L. G., Ando, K., Schlicht, H.-J., and Chisari, F. V. (1995) Breaking tolerance leads to autoantibody production but not autoimmune liver disease in hepatitis B virus envelope transgenic mice. *J. Immunol.* **154**, 2504–2515.

3. Cavanaugh, V. J., Guidotti, L. G., and Chisari, F. V. (1997) Interleukin-12 inhibits hepatitis B virus replication in transgenic mice. *J. Virol.* **71**, 3236–3243.
4. Guidotti, L. G., Matzke, B., and Chisari, F. V. (1997) Hepatitis B virus replication is cell cycle independent during liver regeneration in transgenic mice. *J. Virol.* **71**, 4804–4808.
5. Larkin, J., Clayton, M., Sun, B., et al. (1999) Hepatitis B virus transgenic mouse model of chronic liver disease. *Nat. Med.* **5**, 907–912.
6. Raney, A. K., Eggers, C. M., Kline, E. F., et al. (2001) Nuclear covalently closed circular viral genomic DNA in the liver of hepatocyte nuclear factor 1 alpha-null hepatitis B virus transgenic mice. *J. Virol.* **75**, 2900–2911.
7. Sette, A. D., Oseroff, C., Sidney, J., (2001) Overcoming T cell tolerance to the hepaititis B virus surface antigen in hepatitis B virus-transgenic mice. *J. Immunol.* **166**, 1389–1397.
8. Kajino, K., Kamiya, N., Yayasa, S., Takahara, T., Sakurai, J., Yamamura, K.-I., and Hino, O. (1997) Evaluation of anti-hepatitis B virus (HBV) drugs using the HBV transgenic mouse: application of the semiquantitative polymerase chain reaction (PCR) for serum HBV DNA to monitor the drug efficacy. *Biochem. Biophys. Res. Commun.* **241**, 43–48.
9. Marion, P. L., Salazar, F. H., Liittschwager, K., and Bordier, B. B. (1998) Transgenic mouse lineages with potential for testing antivirals targeting hepatitis B virus. *ICAAC* **Session 201-H**, H-150.
10. Morrey, J. D., Korba, B. E., and Sidwell, R. W. (1999) Transgenic mice as a chemotherapeutic model for hepatitis B virus infection. *Antiviral Ther.* **3 (Suppl 3)**, 59–68.
11. Morrey, J. D., Bailey, K. W., Korba, B. E., and Sidwell, R. W. (1999) Utilization of transgenic mice replicating high levels of hepatitis B virus for antiviral evaluation of lamivudine. *Antiviral Res.* **42**, 97–108.
12. Perfumo, S., Amicone, I., Colloca, S., Giorgio, M., Pozzi, I., and Tripodi, M. (1992) Recognition efficiency of the hepatitis B virus polyadenylation signals is tissue specific in transgenic mice. *J. Virol.* **66**, 6819–6823.
13. Araki, K., Miyazaki, J., Hino, O., et al. (1989) Expression and replication of hepatitis B virus genome in transgenic mice. *Proc. Natl. Acad. Sci. USA* **86**, 207–211.
14. Gilles, P. N., Fey, G., and Chisari, F. V. (1992) Tumor necrosis factor alpha negatively regulates hepatitis B virus gene expression in transgenic mice. *J. Virol.* **66**, 3955–3960.
15. Julander, J. G., Sidwell, R. W., and Morrey, J. D. (2002). Characterizing antiviral activity of adefovir dipivoxil in transgenic mice expressing hepatitis B virus. *Antiviral Res.* **55**, 27–40.
16. Guidotti, L. G., Guilhot, S., and Chisari, F. V. (1994) Interleukin-2 and alpha/beta interferon down-regulate hepatitis B virus gene expression in vivo by tumor necrosis factor-dependent and-independent pathways. *J. Virol.* **68**, 1265–1270.
17. Guilhot, S., Guidotti, L. G., and Chisari, F. V. (1993) Interleukin-2 downregulates hepatitis B virus gene expression in transgenic mice by a posttranscriptional mechanism. *J. Virol.* **67**, 7444–7449.
18. Nagahata, T., Araki, K., Yamamura, K.-I., and Matsubara, K. (1992) Inhibition of intrahepatic hepatitis B virus replication by antiviral drugs in a novel transgenic mouse model. *Antimicrob. Agents Chemother.* **36**, 2042–2045.
19. Petersen, J., Dandri, M., Gupta, S., and Rogler, C. E. (1998) Liver repopulation with xenogenic hepatocytes in B and T cell-deficient mice leads to chronic hepadnavirus infection and clonal growth of hepatocellular carcinoma. *Proc. Natl. Acad. Sci. USA* **95**, 310–315.
20. Elmore, L. W., Hancock, A. R., Chang, S.-F., et al. (1997) Hepatitis B virus X protein and p53 tumor suppressor interactions in the modulation of apoptosis. *Proc. Natl. Acad. Sci. USA* **94**, 14707–14712.

21. Kawashima, T. (1964) The lymph system in mice. *Jpn. J. Vet. Res.* **12**, 69–81.
22. Mehta, A., Lu, X., Block, T. M., Blumberg, B. S., and Dwek, R. A. (1997) Hepatitis B virus (HBV) envelope glycoproteins vary drastically in their sensitivity to glycan processing: evidence that alteration of a single N-linked glycosylation site can regulate HBV secretion. *Proc. Natl. Acad. Sci. USA* **94**, 1822–1827.
23. Baginski, I., Ferrie, A., Watson, R., and Mack, D. (1990) Detection of hepatitis B virus, in *PCR Protocols: A Guide to Methods and Applications* (Innis, M. A., Gelfand, D. H., Sninsky, J. J., and White, T. J., eds.), Hartcourt Brace-Jovanovich Publishers, San Diego.
24. Budelier, K. and Schorr, J. (1995) Preparation and analysis of DNA, in *Current Protocols in Molecular Biology*, Vol. 1 (Ausubel, F. M., Brent, R., Kingston, R. E., et al., eds.), John Wiley & Sons, New York, pp. 2.9.7–2.9.8.
25. Cate, C. (1969) A successful method for exsanguinating unanesthetized mice. *Lab. Anim. Care* **19**, 256–258.
26. Greenberg, M. E. (1995) Preparation and analysis of RNA, in *Current Protocols in Molecular Biology*, Vol. 1 (Ausubel, F., Brent, R., Kingston, R. E., et al. eds.), John Wiley & Sons, New York, pp. 4.9.1–4.9.8.
27. Krajden, M., Minor, J. M., Rifkin, O., and Comanor, L. (1999) Effect of multiple freeze-thaw cycles on hepatitis B virus DNA and hepatitis C virus RNA quantification as measured with branched-DNA technology. *J. Clin. Microbiol.* **37**, 1683–1686.
28. NIH (1994) Appendix B-II-D. Class 2 viral, rickettsial, and chlamydial agents, in *Guidelines for Research Involving Recombinant DNA Molecules (NIH Guidelines).* U.S. Government Printing Office, Washington, D.C.
29. Richmond, J. Y. and McKenney, R. W., eds. (1993) *Biosafety in Microbiological and Biomedical Laboratories* U.S. Government Printing Office, Washington, D.C.
30. Brown, T. (1994) Analysis of DNA sequences by blotting and hybridization, in *Current Protocols in Molecular Biology* (Ausubel, F. M., Brent, R., Kingston, R., et al., eds.), John Wiley & Sons, New York, pp. 2.9.1–2.10.16.

21

Transplantation of Human Hepatocytes in Immunodeficient UPA Mice

A Model for the Study of Hepatitis B Virus

Jörg Petersen, Martin R. Burda, Maura Dandri, and Charles E. Rogler

1. Introduction

Persistent infection with hepatitis B virus (HBV) is a major worldwide health problem, and chronically infected individuals are at high risk for developing liver cirrhosis and hepatocellular carcinoma ***(1,2)***. Despite the availability of an HBV vaccine, there are still more than 350 million chronically infected people worldwide, and the few antiviral treatments currently available have a limited rate of efficacy. As for other infectious diseases in humans, advances in the study of viral hepatitis have been critically dependent on the development of suitable experimental systems. Replication of HBV can be successfully achieved by transfecting hepatoma cell lines with cloned HBV DNA genomes. However, the lack of culture systems permissive for hepadnavirus infection and the narrow host range of HBV have hampered the understanding of some crucial events of the hepadnavirus life cycle, as well as the development of more effective antiviral drugs aimed at eradicating the virus from chronic carriers. Although HBV has been grown successfully in cultures of human hepatocytes, primary human hepatocytes are difficult to maintain in culture and become nonpermissive for HBV very soon after plating. In addition, they normally differ in function and gene expression from hepatocytes integrated in the liver architecture. Therefore, any technique that would allow keeping human hepatocytes in an environment that supports both cell growth and liver-specific differentiation would offer unique opportunities to study human hepatotropic viral infections and to evaluate the efficacy of novel antiviral drugs in a system closely mimicking the in vivo situation.

Previous studies demonstrated that transplanted hepatocytes have the capacity to engraft, survive, and function in the host liver parenchyma ***(3–5)***; however, transplanted hepatocytes show very limited proliferative activity in a healthy normal liver ***(6)***. Stud-

From: *Methods in Molecular Medicine, vol. 96: Hepatitis B and D Protocols, volume 2*
Edited by: R. K. Hamatake and J. Y. N. Lau © Humana Press Inc., Totowa, NJ

ies in transgenic mice have shown that the liver can be repopulated by rodent hepatocytes harboring a selective growth advantage over resident hepatocytes ***(7–10)***. In the past years, a novel liver repopulation model, the urokinase-type plasminogen activator (uPA) transgenic mouse model, was developed. In this system, the expression of the albumin-uPA transgene is toxic to the hepatocytes and, as a consequence, livers undergo continued necrosis of hepatocytes carrying the transgene, which results in a strong stimulus for liver regeneration. During the regenerative process, transgene deletion takes place in some endogenous mouse hepatocytes, which then compete with transplanted hepatocytes ***(7,8)***. The hepatocyte proliferative stimulus lasts approx 8 wk after birth until the transplanted hepatocyte mass becomes comparable to the hepatocyte mass in the liver of nontransgenic normal mice ***(7,11)***. Recently, it was shown by our group ***(12)*** and by others ***(13)*** that human hepatocytes isolated from the adult normal liver are able to engraft and partially repopulate the liver of immunodeficient uPA transgenic mice.

To develop a novel hepatitis B mouse model that allows transplantation of xenogenic hepatocytes, we crossed *Alb-uPA* transgenic mice with *RAG-2* mice, which lack mature T and B lymphocytes because of a deletion in the recombination activation gene 2 (*RAG-2*) ***(14)***. From our experience, it appears that one of the most critical and limiting factors for successful transplantation of normal human hepatocytes is the scarce availability of liver tissues that underwent a very short ischemia time before perfusion. To isolate primary human hepatocytes, we used both donor liver specimens that were not utilized for human liver transplantation and surgical liver tissues from partial hepatectomies (PHs). Immediately after cell isolation, 500,000 viable human hepatocytes were transplanted into multiple uPA/RAG-2 mice by intrasplenic injection (*see* below). By screening of the mice for the production of human serum albumin (HSA), we estimated that engraftment of human hepatocytes was successful (HSA ⩾1%) in 70% of the transplanted mice. Levels of human albumin ranged between approx 1% and 15% (mean of 5%) in the sera of mice transplanted with hepatocytes (viability ⩾80%) obtained by perfusing donor liver specimens ***(12)***. Previous studies indicated that only approx 20% of splenically injected cells reach the liver and survive (which corresponds in our experiments to about 1×10^5 cells), while a mouse liver contains about 1×10^8 hepatocytes ***(15,16)***. In this case, engraftment without repopulation could result in only 0.1–0.5% human hepatocytes in transplanted mice. The presence of 1–15% human hepatocytes in mouse livers, as indicated by the levels of human albumin in the serum, and human genomic DNA in the liver (*see* below), strongly suggests that transplanted human hepatocytes have undergone several cell doublings. Recently, we also successfully transplanted hepatocytes that were isolated from PH livers that underwent a considerable time (up to 4 h) of warm ischemia (*unpublished data*). However, in those cases, engraftment without repopulation was mainly observed. Hepatocytes that had been liberated from cirrhotic livers or from healthy donors in other liver centers, and were sent to us as cell solutions, were not successfully transplanted. Therefore, the limited degree of cell growth achieved so far by transplanting human liver cells appears to be mainly due to differences in the quality of hepatocytes recovered from human livers compared to those routinely obtained by *in situ* perfusion of animals. In the latter case, transplantation of hepatocytes isolated from rodents ***(11,17)*** constantly led to high levels of hepatocyte repopulation (up to 90%) in these mice. The work of Mercer et al. ***(13)*** showed that homozygosity of *SCID/Alb-uPA* mice was critical to achieve higher levels of liver repopulation with transplanted human hepatocytes. This suggests that less growth by the competing endogenous mouse hepatocytes facilitates sustained engraftment and expansion of those fragile human hepatocytes. Moreover, it is possible that evolutionary differences between human and rodent hepatocyte-specific proteins involved in cell–cell interactions or in other functions are responsible for the limited repopulation efficacy using human hepatocytes. Further efforts to improve both the recipient animal model and the human hepatocyte isolation technique would help to overcome these difficulties. Here, we describe the criteria and the methods we have been using to liberate primary hepatocytes from human livers, as well as the transplantation and screening procedures we have been performing to repopulate mouse livers partially with HBV-permissive human hepatocytes.

2. Materials

2.1. Solutions

1. Leffert's stock buffer (10X): 23.83 g of 4-(2-hydroxyethyl)-l-piperazineethanesulfonic acid (HEPES), 2.24 g of KCl, 75.87 g of NaCl, 1.38 g of $NaH_2PO_4 \cdot 4H_2O$, and 18.02 g of D-glucose dissolved in 800 mL of H_2O, adjusted with 10 *N* NaOH to pH 7.4 and brought to a volume of 1 L.
2. EGTA solution (10X): 1.9 g was added to 100 mL of 10X Leffert's buffer and 800 mL H_2O. Thirteen drops of 10 *N* NaOH were then added and the solution was stirred until it cleared and then brought up to 1 L with H_2O.
3. $CaCl_2$ solution (100X): A 2.79% solution of $CaCl_2$ is made by adding 14 g of $CaCl_2$ to 500 mL of H_2O.
4. After preparation, all stock solutions are filter sterilized.
5. University of Wisconsin (UW) solution (Du Pont, Wilmington, DE, USA).
6. Preperfusion EGTA solution (1X): To 54 mL of 10X Leffert's buffer add 60 mL of EGTA solution and bring volume to 500 mL with H_2O. Adjust the pH to 7.4 and then the volume to 600 mL.
7. Leffert's buffer (1X): To 50 mL 10X Leffert's buffer add 400 mL H_2O. Adjust the pH to 7.4 and then the volume to 500 mL.
8. Digestion solution: To 150 mL of 10X Leffert's buffer add 1200 mL of H_2O and 15 mL of $CaCl_2$. Adjust the pH to 7.4, and add collagenase D (Worthington Biochemical). Adjust the volume to 1.5 L (*see* **Note 1**).
9. Rompun/Ketamin solution: 2% Rompun is diluted 1:100 and 100 mg/mL of Ketamin is diluted 1:10 into an isotonic salt solution.
10. Mouse monoclonal antibody against human serum albumin (HSA-11, Sigma, St. Louis, Mo, USA).

2.2. Polymerase Chain Reaction PCR-Reagents

1. For PCR analysis, DNA sequences were amplified by using the Robocycler (Stratagene, La Jolla, CA, USA).
2. *Taq* polymerase, nucleotide mix, and buffer were provided by Roche.

2.3. Equipment

1. Individually ventilated cages: To ensure that the immunodeficient mice are kept in a pathogen-free environment, they should be held in racks with individually ventilated cages (Tecniplast, Buguggiate, Italy).
2. Heating plate: To prevent hypothermia of mice during surgery, the anesthetized mice are placed on a heating plate at 37°C.
3. Tools for surgery: 1-mL Luer lock syringes, 1-cm 27-gauge Luer lock cannulas, 14-cm blunt tipped forceps, a 12-cm pin-tipped forceps, a pair of straight 12-cm scissors, an autoclip applier (Becton Dickinson) for 9-mm wound clips, a 100 μL gas-tight Hamilton syringe, 12.7 mm RN cannulas (Hamilton) with gauge 26 and a 45° taper, 2/0 surgical silk suture cut into pieces of 8 cm length.
4. A pump with variably adjustable speed (Millipore, cat. no. xx82002200), a pump head (Millipore, cat. no. xx8000003), 3-mm diameter silicon tubing (cat. no. xx8000023), a bubble trap (Dahlhausen, Cologne, Germany), a perfusor tubing, an intravenous cannula, a water bath that allows the equilibration of three 1-L bottles at 42°C, and a water bath that allows the equilibration of a 20-cm diameter glass dish for perfusion of liver tissue at 37°C.
5. A centrifuge with a rotor for swingout buckets for separating hepatocytes from nonparenchymal cells (Beckman, Allegra 6 R).
6. An 80-μm nylon filter for separation of tissue debris and cells, rubber spatula for mechanical disruption of perfused liver tissue, and scalpels (shape 22) for cutting of liver tissue.

2.4. Liver Specimens

Either nontumorigenic pieces of human tumor resections (PH) or whole or split livers that were refused for transplantation in humans were utilized for the perfusion experiments.

2.5. Animals

uPA transgenic mice and *RAG-2* knockout mice were purchased from Jackson Laboratories (Bar Harbor, ME, USA) and Taconic Farms (Germantown, NY, USA), respectively. uPA transgenic mice were crossed with RAG-2 knockout mice and chimeric mice were characterized by PCR (*see* below).

3. Methods

3.1. Genotyping of Mice

For analysis of genomic DNA, nucleic acids were extracted from mouse tail tips using the Qiagen DNeasy Tissue Kit (Qiagen, Germany) according to the instructions for rodent tails.

3.1.1. Detection of the *RAG-2* KO Gene by PCR

1. Use the following three primers: rag1 (5'-CGG CCG GAG AAC CTG CGT GCA A-3'), rag 2 (5'-GGG AGG ACA CTC ACT TGC CAG TA-3'), and rag 3 (5'-AGT CAG GAG TCT CCA TCT CAC TGA-3').
2. Per reaction setup: 39 μL of H_2O, 5 μL of 10X Roche PCR Buffer, 1 μL of Roche dNTP Mix, 1 μL of rag1 (20 pmol/μL), 1 μL of rag2 (20 pmol/μL), 1 μL of rag3 (20 pmol/μL), 1 μL of Taq Roche (2.5 U/μL), and 1 μL of DNA preparation. Cover the sample with mineral oil.
3. The program for PCR amplification is (40 cycles): 94°C, 3 min, 62°C, 45 s; 72°C, 1 min 30 s.

4. A *RAG-2* double knockout results in a single band at 350 basepairs (bp), a *RAG-2* hemizygous results in a band at 350 bp and a band at 250 bp, and a wild-type mouse in a band at 250 bp.

3.1.2. *Detection of the* Alb/uPA *Transgene*

1. For analysis of the genomic DNA use the following primers: upa⁺ (5'-CAT CCC TGT GAC CCC TCC-3') and upa⁻ (5'-CTC CAA ACC ACC CCC CTC-3).
2. Per reaction setup: 40 µL of H_2O, 5 µL 10X Roche PCR Buffer, 1 µL of Roche dNTP Mix, 1 µL of upa⁺ of (20 pmol/µL), 1 µL of upa⁻ (20 pmol/µL), 1 µL of Taq Roche (2.5 U/µL), and 1 µL of DNA preparation. Cover the sample with mineral oil.
3. The program for PCR amplification is (30 cycles): 94°C, 3 min; 57°C, 45 s; 72°C, 1 min 30 s. A uPA-positive mouse results in a 180-bp band.

3.2. Isolation of Human Hepatocytes

Donor human livers that were reduced in size for transplantation into children or were rejected for transplantation because of traumatic lesions, as well as liver tissues obtained from patients undergoing PHs because of metastasis of colorectal carcinoma, were used for cell isolation. Cell isolation and transplantation procedures were performed in accordance with institutional guidelines. In all cases, patients were negative for HBV, hepatitis C virus (HCV), and human immunodeficiency virus (HIV) serological markers, liver biopsies were negative for HBV markers, and isolated hepatocytes were checked for the absence of specific HBV-DNA sequences by PCR ***(12)***.

1. The donor livers were perfused *in situ* with cold UW solution before explantation and kept on ice until use. In the case of tumor resections, a wedge from the resected liver lobe was cut at a distance of at least 3 cm from the metastasis. Warm ischemia time, defined as the time after clamping of the branches of the hepatic artery and portal vein until excision of the piece of tissue, varied from 90 min to 4 h.
2. Immediately after excision, the liver tissue was placed on ice and immediately perfused with ice cold UW solution by means of multiple catheters inserted into the vessels on the cut surface of the resected fragment. Afterwards, human hepatocytes were isolated using the two-step collagenase perfusion method.
3. A branch of the portal vein was cannulated, the liver or liver segment was placed on a sterile glass plate, in a 37°C water bath, half submersed in prewarmed isotonic solution, and perfused for 5 min with the preperfusion solution. All solutions were prewarmed at 42°C and the flow rate of the perfusate was 100 mL/min. For small liver specimens (< 200 g) use a lower flow rate (60 mL/min) (*see* **Note 2**).
4. Leffert's buffer not containing EGTA was allowed to run through the liver for 3–5 min, and then the tissue was perfused with the collagenase buffer. Perfusion time with collagenase varied between 10 and 30 min according to the size of the tissue (*see* **Note 3**).
5. Subsequently, the digested liver tissue was placed in cold RPMI, the liver capsule was cut, and cells were dissociated and then filtered through 80-µm nylon filters.
6. Cell suspensions were centrifuged three times (50*g*, 5 min) to separate hepatocytes from nonparenchymal cells.
7. Hepatocyte viability was assessed by trypan blue exclusion.
8. Immediately after isolation, 5×10^5 viable human hepatocytes were resuspended in a volume of 50 µL of phosphate-buffered saline (PBS) and transplanted into 13- to 21-d old recipient *uPA/RAG-2* mice by intrasplenic injection.

3.3. Transplantation of Human Hepatocytes

1. Mice were anesthetized with 10 μL/g of Rompun/Ketamin solution.
2. Their left sides were disinfected with 70% (v/v) ethanol and a 1.5-cm cut was applied 5 mm below the lower rim of the ribs without injuring the peritoneum.
3. The spleen was localized and the covering peritoneum cut (5 mm).
4. The spleen was protracted slightly with the blunt-ended forceps and the lower pole smoothly ligated with a suture.
5. The injection needle of the Hamilton syringe was inserted through the ligation into the spleen and 50 μL of cell suspension injected slowly into the spleen.
6. The needle was retracted and the ligation pulled tight.
7. The spleen was pushed back into the body cavity and the skin and peritoneum closed with two or three autoclips.

3.4. Analysis of Cell Engraftment

3.4.1. Detection of Human Serum Albumin in Mice

1. Samples of mouse and human sera were subjected to sodium dodecyl sulfate-polyacrylamide gel electrophoresis (SDS-PAGE) and blotted onto polyvinylidene fluoride (PVDF) membranes.
2. The blots were probed with a commercially available mouse monoclonal antibody (MAB) against HSA (1:10,000 dilution) that does not cross-react with the mouse proteins. Specific binding was detected by using peroxidase coupled anti-mouse IgG antibodies and an enhanced chemiluminescence system (Pierce, Rockford, IL, USA).
3. For semiquantitative determination of the relative amount of HSA in transplanted mouse sera, the mouse serum samples to be quantified plus a set of artificial mixtures composed of known ratios of human and mouse sera were used to prepare Western blots ***(12)***.

3.4.2. Detection of Human Genomic DNA in the Livers of Transplanted Mice

1. Genomic DNA is extracted from frozen liver tissues by proteinase K digestion (Roche), phenol extraction, and ethanol precipitation.
2. The following primers specific for the human *Alu* sequences were chosen for PCR amplification, as they produce a specific band of 440 bp that is not detectable using mouse tissue as a template: Primer 1, 5'-GCT TCC TGA GTA ACT GGA CAA CAG C-3', and Primer 2, 5'-TGC GAT GGC ATG TTT CCA AG-3'.
3. To estimate the percentage of human versus mouse genomic DNA in transplanted mice, 2 μg of DNA extracted from liver tissues may be also dot-blotted onto a nylon membrane ***(18)*** and hybridized under high stringency conditions overnight with a 440-bp *Alu* DNA ^{32}P-labeled probe, which is obtained by PCR using the aforementioned *Alu* primers and human genomic DNA as template. Test mixtures of known amounts of human and mouse genomic DNAs are loaded in parallel on the blots to serve as a standard. Hybridization signals are quantitated by scanning densitometry using the TINA program from Raytest and a FujiX/2000 laser densitometer (Fuji).

3.5. HBV Infection

For infection studies, human serum containing high-titer HBV DNA ($>1 \times 10^8$ virus genome equivalents/mL serum) is used. Samples may be aliquotted and kept at –70°C until use. At 5 d after transplantation, mice are injected subcutaneously with 20 μL of HBV-infectious serum (1×10^8 HBV DNA genome equivalent / mL).

3.6. Detection of Hepatitis B Surface Antigen (HBsAg) in Sera of Inoculated Mice

Human HBsAg was measured using the HBsAg Axsym Test (Abbott, Wiesbaden, Germany) using a 1:100 dilution of the mouse sera. Approximately 4–6 wk after virus inoculation, HBsAg is detectable in sera of successfully transplanted mice.

3.7. Detection of HBV DNA in Sera of Inoculated Mice

1. Viral DNA is extracted from mouse and human sera using the QIAamp Blood Kit (Qiagen, Hilden, Germany).
2. The following primers are used for PCR amplification:
   Primer 1: 1823 (+): 5'-TTTTTCACCTCTGCCTAATCATC-3'
   Primer 2: 2121 (–): 5'-ACCCACCCAGGTAGCTAGAGTCAT-3'.
3. The program for PCR amplification is (30 cycles): 94°C, 50 s; 57°C, 50 s; 72°C, 50 s.
4. An HBV DNA positive signal results in a 350-bp band.

4. Notes

1. The digestion solution may be prepared without collagenase the day before the perfusion and stored overnight at 4°C. Collagenase must be added to the buffer shortly before the perfusion, the pH checked, and then the solution sterile filtered.
2. For efficient perfusion of very large liver specimens or whole human livers higher speed flow-through (>120 mL/min) of the perfusate is recommended, which involves the use of different equipment. Highly viable hepatocytes can also be obtained by cutting a small (< 200 g) piece of liver and then performing the cell isolation as described above.
3. It is essential to keep the collagenase temperature throughout the whole procedure at 37°C. This includes the temperature of the liver tissue during digestive perfusion. Deviations to lower temperatures will especially reduce quality and viability of isolated hepatocytes. However, temperatures that are too high will damage the tissue and inactivate the collagenase.

Acknowledgment

We thank David Zuckerman for critical reading of the manuscript.

References

1. Blumberg, B. S. (1997) Hepatitis B virus, the vaccine, and the control of primary cancer of the liver. *Proc. Natl. Acad. Sci. USA* **94**, 7121–7125.
2. Rogler, C. E. (1991) Cellular and molecular mechanisms of hepatocarcinogenesis associated with hepadnavirus infection. *Curr. Top. Microbiol. Immunol.* **168**, 103–140.
3. Gupta, S., Rajvanshi, P., Bhargava, K. K., and Kerr, A. (1996) Hepatocyte transplantation: progress toward liver repopulation. *Prog. Liver. Dis.* **14**, 199–222.
4. Gunsalus, J. R., Brady, D. A., Coulter, S. M., Gray, B. M., and Edge, A. S. (1997) Reduction of serum cholesterol in Watanabe rabbits by xenogeneic hepatocellular transplantation (see comments). *Nat. Med.* **3**, 48–53.
5. Brown, J. J., Parashar, B., Moshage, H., et al. (2000) A long-term hepatitis B viremia model generated by transplanting nontumorigenic immortalized human hepatocytes in Rag-2-deficient mice. *Hepatology* **31**, 173–81.
6. Gupta, S., Rajvanshi, P., Aragona, E., Lee, C. D., Yerneni, P. R., and Burk, R. D. (1999) Transplanted hepatocytes proliferate differently after CCl4 treatment and hepatocyte growth factor infusion. *Am. J. Physiol.* **276**, G629–638.

7. Sandgren, E. P., Palmiter, R. D., Heckel, J. L., Daugherty, C. C., Brinster, R. L., and Degen, J. L. (1991) Complete hepatic regeneration after somatic deletion of an albumin-plasminogen activator transgene. *Cell* **66**, 245–256.
8. Rhim, J. A., Sandgren, E. P., Palmiter, R. D., and Brinster, R. L. (1995) Complete reconstitution of mouse liver with xenogeneic hepatocytes. *Proc. Natl. Acad. Sci. USA* **92**, 4942–4946.
9. Overturf, K., Al-Dhalimy, M., Tanguay, R., et al. (1996) Hepatocytes corrected by gene therapy are selected in vivo in a murine model of hereditary tyrosinaemia type I (see comments) (published erratum appears in *Nat. Genet.* 1996 Apr; **12** 458). *Nat. Genet.* **12**, 266–273.
10. Mignon, A., Guidotti, J. E., Mitchell, C., et al. (1998) Selective repopulation of normal mouse liver by Fas/CD95-resistant hepatocytes. *Nat. Med.* **4**, 1185–1188.
11. Petersen, J., Dandri, M., Gupta, S., and Rogler, C. E. (1998) Liver repopulation with xenogenic hepatocytes in B and T cell-deficient mice leads to chronic hepadnavirus infection and clonal growth of hepatocellular carcinoma. *Proc. Natl. Acad. Sci. USA* **95**, 310–315.
12. Dandri, M., Burda, M. R., Torok, E., et al. (2001) Repopulation of mouse liver with human hepatocytes and in vivo infection with hepatitis B virus. *Hepatology* **33**, 981–988.
13. Mercer, D. F., Schiller, D. E., Elliott, J. F., et al. (2001) Hepatitis C virus replication in mice with chimeric human livers. *Nat. Med.* **7**, 927–933.
14. Shinkai, Y., Rathbun, G., Lam, K. P., et al. (1992) RAG-2-deficient mice lack mature lymphocytes owing to inability to initiate V(D)J rearrangement. *Cell* **68**, 855–867.
15. Gupta, S., Rajvanshi, P., Sokhi, R., et al. (1999) Entry and integration of transplanted hepatocytes in rat liver plates occur by disruption of hepatic sinusoidal endothelium. *Hepatology* **29**, 509–519.
16. Jamal, H. Z., Weglarz, T. C., and Sandgren, E. P. (2000) Cryopreserved mouse hepatocytes retain regenerative capacity in vivo (see comments). *Gastroenterology* **118**, 390–394.
17. Dandri, M., Burda, M. R., Gocht, A., et al. (2001) Woodchuck hepatocytes remain permissive for hepadnavirus infection and mouse liver repopulation after cryopreservation. *Hepatology* **34**, 824–833.
18. Scotto, J., Hadchouel, M., Hery, C., Yvart, J., Tiollais, P., and Brechot, C. (1983) Detection of hepatitis B virus DNA in serum by a simple spot hybridization technique: comparison with results for other viral markers. *Hepatology*, **3**, 279–284.

22

Duck Hepatitis B Virus Model in the Study of Hepatitis B Virus

Lucyna Cova and Fabien Zoulim

1. Introduction

Because of the narrow host range of hepatitis B virus (HBV) that infects only humans and chimpanzees, the closely related duck HBV (DHBV) provides a particularly useful model, which plays a pivotal role in study of hepadnavirus life cycle, virus–host interactions, and antiviral strategies ***(1–3)***. This chapter describes the use of DHBV-infected Pekin duck as an in vivo model and Chapter 16 describes the DHBV primary hepatocyte culture for in vitro studies.

One of the major advantages of the DHBV model is that its natural host, domestic Pekin duck (*Anas domesticus*), is inexpensive, easy to handle, and available from commercial breeders. Naturally occurring DHBV infections seem to be endemic in most parts of the world, as they have been reported among ducks from the United States, Australia, China, Germany, and France ***(1,2,4)***. The DHBV isolates originating from different geographic areas have been cloned and the sequence data are available from the GenBank database.

To use the DHBV model as an in vivo experimental system, it is essential to have an efficient and reproductive duck infection method leading to the development of persistent infection in all animals. Because the experimental inoculation of DHBV to adult ducks results only rarely (5–10%) in chronic infection, different modes of DHBV transmission to neonatal ducklings have been investigated ***(1)***. The congenital virus transmission from infected breeding ducks to their progeny, via the egg yolk, leads to the development of chronic infection in all animals. However, this transmission mode is only rarely used because it does not allow the generation of a large number of infected animals of the same age that is frequently required for experimental studies. Another approach consists of intrahepatic transfection of ducklings with cloned DHBV DNA ***(5)***. Although this approach is very useful for DHBV mutant infectivity testing, it cannot be used for early stages of viral infection and host–cell interaction studies.

From: *Methods in Molecular Medicine, vol. 96: Hepatitis B and D Protocols, volume 2*
Edited by: R. K. Hamatake and J. Y. N. Lau © Humana Press Inc., Totowa, NJ

Finally, ducklings can be experimentally infected with a pool of DHBV-positive serum. In this chapter we focus on this last method of DHBV transmission, which is currently used by ourselves and others, as it allows a rapid generation of a large flock of chronically infected ducklings of the same age *(6,7)*. Pekin ducklings are susceptible to DHBV during their first few weeks, although the highest rates of infection and viremia were observed following inoculation of newly hatched ducklings. Therefore, we have chosen in our protocol to inoculate ducklings that are < 5 d old.

The inoculum is usually a pool of DHBV-positive duck sera that has been quantified in virus genome equivalents (vge) assuming that one DHBV genome contains 3×10^{-6} pg of DNA *(8)*. The DHBV DNA content of the sera pool is estimated by quantitative hybridization using successive dilutions (10 ng to 0.1 pg) of cloned DHBV DNA that has been excised from the plasmid. To this end, the pooled duck serum and dilutions of cloned DHBV DNA are spotted on a membrane and hybridized with a radiolabeled DHBV probe as described previously *(9)* and detailed in **Subheadings 2.** and **3.** The quantified inoculum is diluted in phosphate-buffered saline (PBS) and inoculated into neonatal ducklings by the intraperitoneal or intravenous route. We use the intravenous route for duckling inoculation via the occipital sinus, which gives more reproducible results and works better in our hands. Blood samples are taken daily during the first week post-inoculation and twice a week thereafter during the following weeks. Viremia is quantified by serum dot-blot hybridization as detailed in **Subheadings 2.** and **3.** The DHBV content of serum can also be quantified by the infectivity titer (ID_{50}) determination method which is performed by inoculating ducklings with successive serum dilutions. The ID/mL titer has been found to be similar to the titer in vge/mL for infectious serum. However, a lower infectivity than the number of genomes of the same serum sample may reflect the presence of defective DHBV mutants *(8)*.

An important factor that determines the outcome of infection is the DHBV dose used for duckling inoculation. Several studies have demonstrated that the onset of viremia is inversely proportional to the inoculum dose *(6,8)*. We have chosen the protocol based on a high inoculum dose (5×10^7–5×10^8 vge/duckling), which is administered intravenously to the 3 to 4 d old ducklings. The advantage of this protocol is that it leads to a very fast and reproducible development of viremia in 100% of inoculated ducklings *(6,7,10)*. This is illustrated further in **Fig. 1**, which shows that following inoculation of four ducklings with 6×10^7 vge/duckling the viremia evolution is similar in all inoculated animals. Viremia starts to be detectable at d 4 and reaches a peak at d 5–7 post-inoculation, followed by a decrease and fluctuations (**Fig. 1**). Alternatively, the use of a lower inoculum dose will lead to the delay in the appearance of the viremia peak *(data not shown)*.

Figure 2 illustrates the use of the duck infection model for the in vivo testing of the antiviral efficacy of two different nucleoside analogs (β-L-Fd4C and 3TC), which inhibit in vitro DHBV reverse transcription *(10)*. Four weeks of oral administration of these antiviral drugs leads to a significant decrease in viremia peak during drug administration (**Fig. 2A**). This effect is not sustained, as a rebound in viremia is observed after drug withdrawal, although the peak of viremia is delayed as compared with the untreated controls. This delay in the onset of viremia is similar to that observed when ducklings are

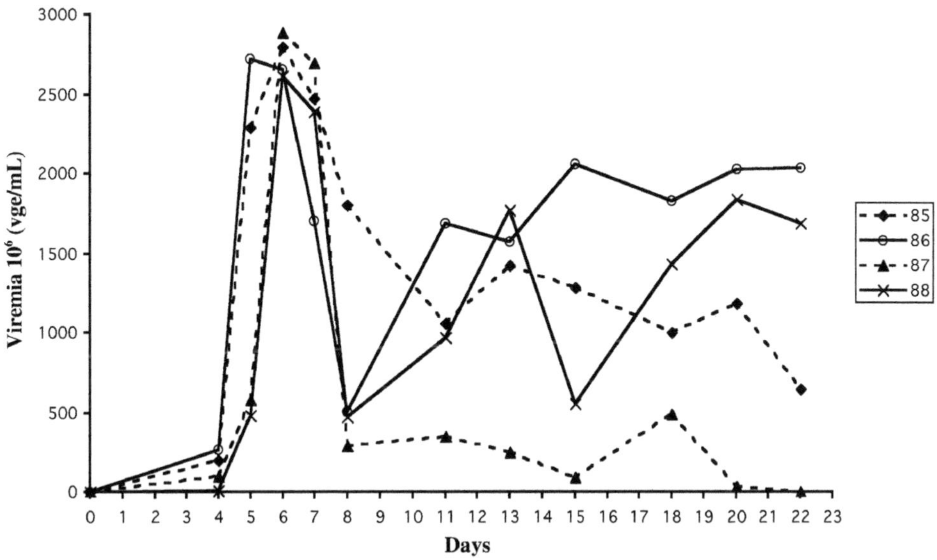

Fig. 1. Viremia follow-up in ducklings following experimental DHBV infection. Four 3-d-old ducklings were inoculated intravenously with the DHBV-positive serum pool (6×10^7 vge/animal). Ducklings were bled daily during the first week post-inoculation and thereafter every 2–3 d. The individual serum DHBV DNA titer in vge/mL is represented for each animal. Note the viremia peak at d 5–7 post-inoculation.

inoculated with a lower inoculum dose. Tolerance of antiviral administration is assessed by daily monitoring of animal weight **(Fig. 2B)**. In addition, cellular toxicity is determined by monitoring lactic acid levels in the duck serum using Lactate PAP (bioMerieux, Marcy L'Etoile, France) **(Fig. 2C)**. The results show an absence of toxicity, as neither weight loss nor an increase in the serum lactic acid levels was observed in the treated duck groups as compared with the untreated controls **(Fig. 2B, C)**.

To assess the impact of the treatment on intrahepatic viral replication, ducks are killed and their livers are removed. Part of the liver is snap frozen for DHBV DNA analysis as detailed in **Subheading 3.** and part is formalin fixed for immunochemical visualization of viral proteins. For viral DNA analysis, the liver tissue is first crushed in liquid nitrogen to a fine powder and divided into two parts. One is used for isolation of total viral DNA (protein bound) analysis (detailed in **Subheading 3.3.**) and another for isolation of covalently closed circular (ccc) DNA (non-protein bound) as described in the accompanying chapter on DHBV primary hepatocyte infections.

Figure 3 shows a typical Southern blot analysis of liver DNA from untreated ducks, which reveals the presence of different DHBV DNA replicative forms, that is, 3-kb viral DNA in relaxed circular (RC) and linear (L) form as wells as single-stranded (SS) viral DNA and cccDNA. By contrast, the analysis of liver biopsies at the end of β-L-Fd4C treatment shows a marked decrease in DHBV DNA to levels unde-

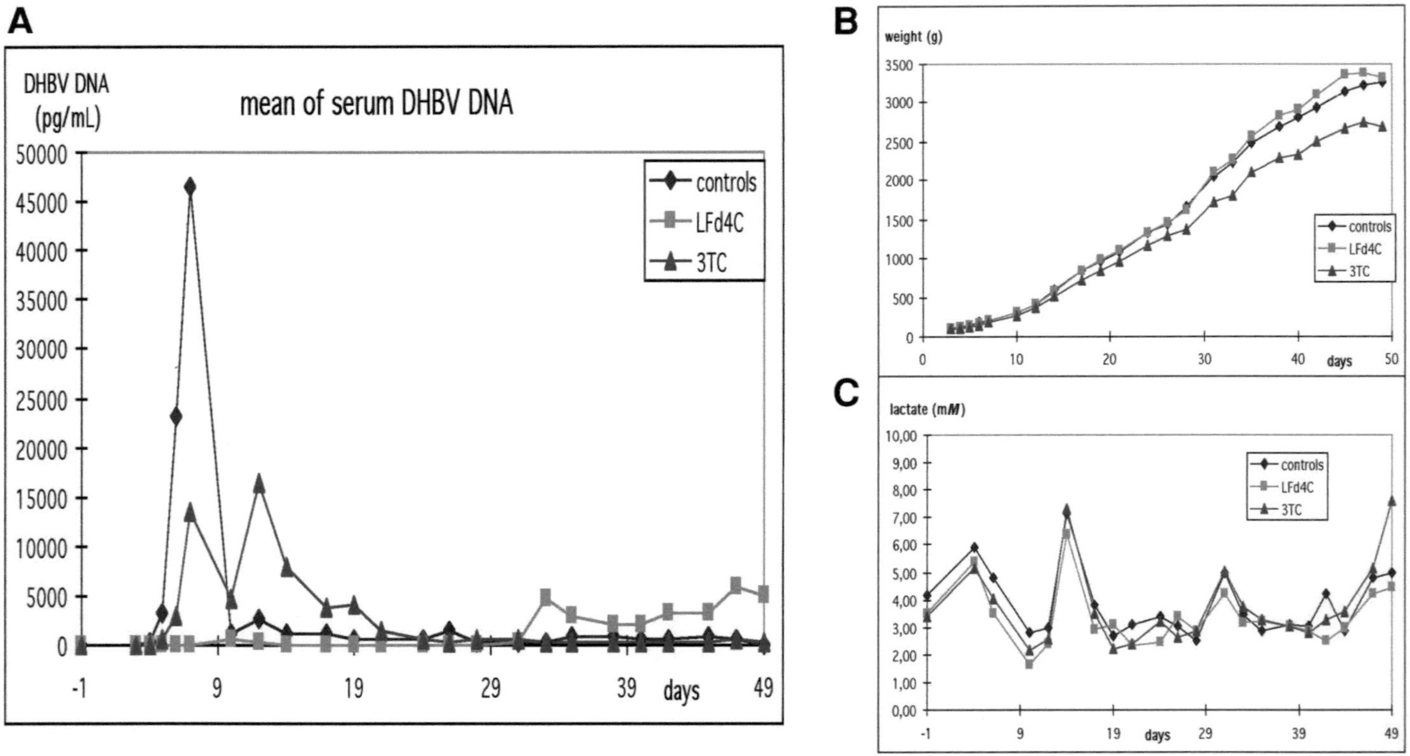

Fig. 2. Course of viremia in the DHBV-infected duck groups during antiviral drug treatment. Ducklings were inoculated with a DHBV-positive serum at 3 d of age and antiviral treatment was started 3 d post-inoculation. Animals received intraperitoneal injections with either β-L-Fd4C or 3TC at a dose of 25 mg/kg/d for 5 d, followed by a maintenance therapy at 25 mg/kg thrice weekly for 3 more weeks. Viremia was quantitatively analyzed by dot-blot hybridization as detailed in **Subheading 3.3.** **(A)** Mean DHBV DNA titers of nine animals, which have been included in each of the treatment group (β-L-Fd4C, 3TC) as wells as in the untreated control group are represented. **(B)** Mean duck weight values for each treatment and control group. **(C)** Serum lactic acid levels for each duck group.

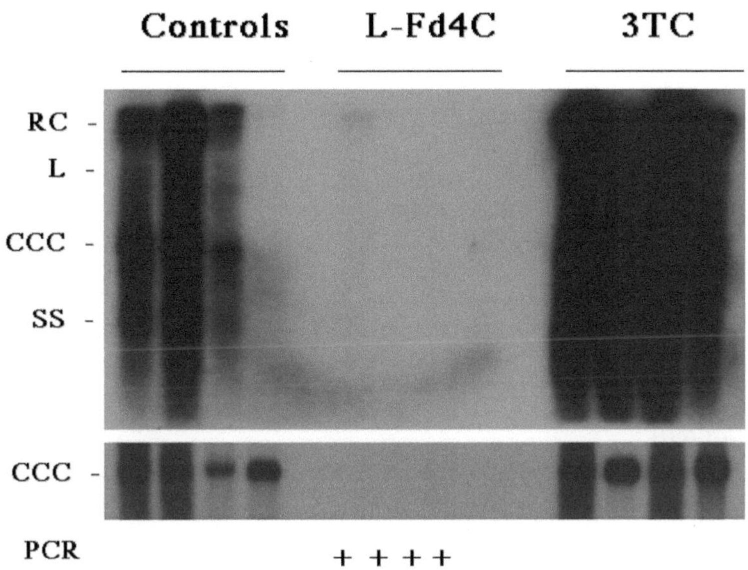

Fig. 3. Analysis of DHBV DNA in the duck livers at the end of antiviral drug treatment. Total viral DNA including the replicative intermediates (RC, relaxed circular; L, linear; SS, single-stranded viral DNAs) as well as viral cccDNA were extracted from the β-L-Fd4C, 3TC-treated and control groups. Southern blot analysis of liver biopsies at the end of antiviral drug treatment was followed by specific hybridization with the radiolabeled full-length DHBV DNA probe. Note that β-L-Fd4C therapy suppresses viral DNA synthesis in the livers of infected animals, but is not sufficient to eradicate viral infection, as a low level of DHBV DNA was detectable by a specific PCR test (indicated by *crosses*).

tectable by Southern blot analysis. However, after drug withdrawal a rebound of intrahepatic DHBV DNA is observed in duck livers *(data not shown)*. The rebound of viral replication is essentially due to the pool of intranuclear DHBV cccDNA, a transcriptional template for viral RNA synthesis, which was detectable by PCR in the duck liver biopsies at the end of antiviral treatment **(Fig. 3)**. This cccDNA plays an essential role in the persistence of infection and in the long-term resistance to the antiviral drug treatment.

This example illustrates the usefulness of the DHBV infection model for the in vivo evaluation of new anti-HBV strategies, which is essential before their use in clinical trials.

2. Materials

2.1. Animals

1. Purchase 1-d old Pekin ducklings (*Anas domesticus*) from a commercial breeder.
2. Maintain ducklings indoors, in suspended cage floors, under heating lamps during the first 2 wk of age and thereafter without lamps. Feed the animals with a commercially prepared diet,

with free access to food and water, and handle them in accordance with the guidelines for animal care under veterinary control.

3. Keep DHBV-positive and -negative ducks separately.

2.2. Solutions

1. Dolethal (sodium pentobarbitol) (Vetoquinol, Lure, France).
2. 20X Saline sodium citrate (SSC): Dissolve 175.3 g of NaCl and 88.2 g of sodium citrate in 800 mL of H_2O. Adjust the pH to 7.4 with 10 *N* NaOH, and adjust the volume to 1 L.
3. 20X SSPE: Dissolve 174 g of NaCl and 27.6 g of $NaH_2PO_4 \cdot H_2O$ and 7.4 g of EDTA in 800 mL of H_2O. Adjust the pH to 7.4 with 10 *N* NaOH, and adjust the volume to 1 L.
4. Prehybridization and hybridization solution: Mix 125 mL of 10X SSPE, 25 mL of Denhardt's solution, 250 mL of formamide, 12.5 mL of 20% sodium dodecyl sulfate (SDS). Complete with 50 mL of H_2O to 500 mL.
5. TE buffer: 10 m*M* Tris-HCl, pH 8.0, 1 m*M* EDTA, pH 8.0.

2.3. Equipment

1. Duck animal facility should be heated (20°C) and divided in boxes with suspended grating floors and constant water supply. For newly hatched ducklings, additional heating with lamps is required.
2. HybriDot manifold apparatus (BRL) for serum and DNA dot-blot analysis.
3. Water bath.
4. Microcentrifuge.
5. Sterile mortars and pestles.
6. Hybridization oven (e.g., Appligene Minihybridization oven).

3. Methods

3.1. Preparation of the Viremic Serum Pool

1. Inoculate 3-d-old Pekin ducklings with DHBV-positive serum (5×10^7–5×10^8 vge/duckling) diluted in phosphate-buffered saline (PBS) (final volume 200 µL/duckling) using a 1-mL syringe by intravenous injection, either via an occipital sinus (located at the back of duck head) puncture or via the foot sinus.
2. At d 5–7 post-inoculation anesthetize ducklings by intravenous injection of Dolethal (1 mL/200 g body wt) and bleed them by a cardiac puncture using a 1-mL syringe.
3. Sterilize serum by filtration and store all serum samples at –20°C. Save a 50-µL aliquot of each duck serum for DHBV DNA quantification.
4. Quantify DHBV DNA in 50 µL of each duck serum by dot-blot hybridization as detailed in **Subheading 3.3.**
5. Pool together sera samples that have similar DHBV DNA concentrations in vge/mL. Check the DHBV DNA concentration of the pooled sera by quantitatitive dot-blot hybridization as detailed in **Subheading 3.3.**
6. Filter the serum pool and aliquot in 0.5- and 1-mL samples and store them at –20°C. Thaw the aliquots of pooled sera immediately prior to duck inoculation.

3.2. Establishment of DHBV Chronic Carrier Duck Flock

1. Inoculate 3-d old ducklings by intravenous injection with 200 µL of DHBV-positive serum pool diluted in PBS as detailed in **Subheading 3.1.**
2. Bleed ducklings by the intravenous route each day post-infection during the first week and twice a week during the following weeks.

3. Confirm the chronic carrier state of inoculated ducks by DHBV DNA detection in duck serum samples by spot hybridization as detailed in **Subheading 3.3.**

3.3. Detection and Quantification of DHBV DNA in Duck Serum by Dot-Blot Hybridization

1. Apply 50 μL of each duck serum sample under vacuum directly onto a 0.45-nm Biodyne® (PALL, Gelman Laboratory, AnnArbor, MI, USA) membrane using a HybriDot manifold apparatus (BRL) that allows analysis of 96 samples. Cut off the vacuum and lay the membrane on a sheet of Whatman 3MM paper.
2. Denature the DNA by floating the membrane for 20 min on 0.2 *M* NaOH, 1 *M* NaCl solution. Carefully remove the membranes from this bath and soak them for 5 min in another bath containing 1 *M* Tris-HCl, pH 7.4, 1 *M* NaCl for neutralization, and finally rinse it for 5 min in a 2X SSC bath.
3. Prepare tubes with successive dilutions of cloned DHBV DNA (ranging from 10 ng to 0.1 pg) in a final volume of 100 μL of water. Denature DNA by boiling tubes for 5 min and rapid cooling in ice. Add 100 μL of 20X SSC to each tube and apply the total (200 μL) of each DHBV DNA dilution on a separate membrane using the HybriDot manifold.
4. Air-dry the membranes and bake them for 30 min at 80°C between two glass plates followed by UV fixation at 0.44 J/cm^2.
5. Prehybridize the membranes by inserting them in a hybridization tube containing 10–20 mL of hybridization solution. Incubate the filters at 42°C in a hybridization oven for at least 30 min.
6. Hybridize together the serum and DHBV DNA dilutions containing membranes by overnight incubation at 42°C with the genome-length DHBV DNA probe labeled with α-^{32}P (Ready-to-go™ DNA labeling kit, Amersham). Wash the membranes at 68°C twice (20 min each wash) in 2X SSC, 0.2% SDS, then twice in 1X SSC, 0.1% SDS and once in 0.5X SSC, 0.1% SDS. Air-dry the membranes and autoradiograph them using intensifying screens followed by PhosphorImager scanning.
7. Quantitate the relative amounts of DHBV DNA in each serum sample by the Image Quant software using the values obtained for successive dilutions of cloned DHBV DNA. Express the viremia in (vge/mL) assuming that one DHBV genome contains 3×10^{-6} pg of DNA.

3.4. DHBV DNA Extraction from Duck Liver

1. Cut duck liver biopsy or autopsy tissue samples into small pieces. Quickly freeze liver tissue by immersion in liquid nitrogen and store at –80°C for DNA analysis. Fix a part of the tissue in formalin for liver histology
2. Quickly weigh about 0.2 g of frozen liver sample without defrosting and rapidly crush the liver tissue into a fine powder using a mortar containing liquid nitrogen.
3. For protein bound DNA extraction, transfer the powdered liver tissue to a tube containing 3 mL of ice-cold TE buffer. Do this step quickly before the mortar warms up. Add 30 μL of proteinase K (300 μg/mL final) and 150 μL of 20% SDS (1% final concentration), mix well, and incubate at 37°C for 3 h.
4. Perform two phenol–chloroform extractions and one chloroform extraction (to be done in the hood) followed by ethanol precipitation. The total nucleic acids recovered after ethanol precipitation can be treated with RNase followed by phenol–chloroform extractions to eliminate RNAs.
5. Analyze liver DNA by Southern blotting followed by hybridization with radiolabeled DHBV DNA probe as described above for viremia quantification.

References

1. Schödel, F., Weimer, T., Fernholz, D., et al. (1991) The biology of avian hepatitis B viruses, in *Molecular Biology of the Hepatitis B Viruses* (McLachlan, A., ed.) CRC Press, Boca Raton, FL, pp. 53–80.
2. Cova, L., Fourel, I., Vitvitski, L., et al. (1993) Animal models for the understanding and control of HBV and HDV infections. *J. Hepatol.* **17,** S143–S148.
3. Zoulim, F. (2000) Design and evaluation of hepatitis B virus inhibitors. *Curr. Pharmaceut. Design* **6**, 503–523.
4. Triyatni, M., Ey, P. L, Tran, T., et al. (2001) Sequence comparison of an Autralian DHBV strain with other avian hepadnaviruses. *J. Gen. Virol.* **82**, 373–378.
5. Sprengel, R., Kuhn, C., Manso, C., and Will, H. (1984) Cloned DHBV DNA is infectious in Pekin ducks. *J. Virol.* **52**, 932.
6. Sunyach, C., Chassot, S., Jamard, C., Kay, A., Trepo, C., and Cova, L. (1997) In vivo selection of duck hepatitis B virus pre-S variants which escape from neutralization. *Virology* **234,** 291–299.
7. Robaczewska, M., Guerret, S., Remy, J. S., et al. (2001) In vivo inhibition of duck hepatitis B virus replication by polyethylenimine-delivered antisense phosphodiester oligodeoxynucleotides. *Gene Ther.* **8**, 874–881.
8. Jilbert, A. R., Miller, D. S., Scougal, C. A., Turnbull, H., and Burrel, C. J. (1996) Kinetics of duck hepatitis B virus infection following low dose virus inoculation: one virus DNA genome is infectious in neonatal ducks. *Virology* **226**, 338–345.
9. Cova, L., Wild, C. P., Mehrotra, R., et al. (1990) Contribution of Aflatoxin B1 and Hepatitis B virus infection in the induction of liver tumours in ducks. *Cancer Res.* **50**, 2156–2163.
10. Le Guerhier, F., Pichoud, C., Chevallier, M., et al. (2000) Characterization of the antiviral activity of 2', 3'-dideoxy-2', 3'-didehydro-β-L-5-fluorocytidine in the duck hepatitis B virus infection model. *Antimicrob. Agents Chemother.* **44**, 111–122.

23

Hepatitis B Virus Transgenic Severe Combined Immunodeficient Mouse Model of Acute and Chronic Liver Disease

Mark A. Feitelson, Jonathan D. Larkin, and Raymond F. Schinazi

1. Introduction

With the advent of blood tests capable of identifying hepatitis B virus (HBV), and the development of an effective vaccine *(1)*, one of the major challenges that remains is what to do with people who are chronic carriers of HBV. This is important because there are an estimated 350 million chronic carriers of HBV worldwide *(2)* who are at high risk for the development of hepatitis, cirrhosis, and hepatocellular carcinoma (HCC) *(3)*. There are up to a million newly diagnosed cases of HCC each year, making this one of the most common tumor types worldwide. In addition, the risk of carriers developing HCC is in excess of 100, which makes it one of the strongest associations between a cancer and an infectious agent ever reported *(4)*. While the survival rate for HCC is < 3% over 5 y, the development of hepatitis is often associated with considerable morbidity, and its progression to cirrhosis is a leading cause of death worldwide. Treatment options for carriers with chronic liver disease are few, with interferon-α (IFN-α), lamivudine, and adefovir dipivoxil the only licensed drugs for clinical use *(5)*. Interferon produces a sustained virus response in only about 20% of patients following the end of therapy *(5,6)*. Lamivudine is highly effective against both virus and liver disease, although a high rate of virus resistance has been reported *(7,8)*. Adefovir is effective against lamivudine-resistant virus.

Although many other drugs are under development, part of the problem in targeting chronic hepatitis B is the lack of knowledge concerning the virus and host elements that contribute to the pathogenesis of chronic liver disease (CLD). Although it is generally agreed that the pathogenesis of chronic infection is immune mediated *(9)*, there is considerable debate as to which virus encoded proteins trigger the accumulation of inflammatory cells in the liver, and the nature of the immune responses that contribute importantly to the clearance of virus and pathogenesis of CLD. The problem in address-

From: *Methods in Molecular Medicine, vol. 96: Hepatitis B and D Protocols, volume 2*
Edited by: R. K. Hamatake and J. Y. N. Lau © Humana Press Inc., Totowa, NJ

ing these types of questions is the lack of suitable small animal model(s) that develop CLD. HBV-like viruses, for example, naturally infect woodchucks and ground squirrels ***(10)***, and may result in the development of CLD and HCC ***(11,12)***, but the immune mediated pathogenesis in these naturally occurring animal models cannot be studied easily. This is because the immune system of these animals is poorly characterized, they are expensive to maintain and breed, and none of these animals have inbred strains upon which to dissect the immune reactions relevant to pathogenesis on an otherwise constant genetic background. Chimpanzees are one of a small number of primates susceptible to HBV ***(13)***, and do develop a mild CLD, but their cost, endangered species status, and difficulty in working with these animals have limited their use. Hence, the amount of information that could be obtained from such model systems has been limited.

The host range for HBV is quite narrow, and attempts to establish easily manipulated laboratory animal models of HBV infection have not been successful. As a consequence, a number of labs have created transgenic mice that express one or more virus gene products or support viral replication ***(14–18)***. The success of these attempts suggest that mouse hepatocytes are fully capable of supporting HBV replication, and suggests that the inability to infect such animals with virus may be due to the lack of appropriate host encoded cell surface receptor(s). A major limitation with this approach is the fact that the transgenic mice are immunologically tolerant to the virus gene products, so that transgenic mice demonstrating virus gene expression and/or replication do not develop hepatitis. While this situation appears to be analogous to the asymptomatic carrier state in people ***(19)***, this does not provide an opportunity to study the pathogenesis of CLD or to evaluate experimental therapeutics against disease. Adoptive transfer of T-cell lines with reactivity to individual HBV antigens has resulted in the appearance of acute or fulminant hepatitis ***(20,21)***, but not CLD. In the models of acute and fulminant hepatitis, cytokines (such as tumor necrosis factor-α, interleukin-2, and IFN-γ) in addition to inflammatory cells appear to be very important to pathogenesis, to the down regulation of virus gene expression, and to the clearance of replicating virus ***(9,22)***. When HBV envelope antigen expressing transgenic mice were irradiated, thymectomized, reconstituted with bone marrow from severe combined immunodeficient (SCID) mice, and then adoptively transferred with envelope-antigen-specific T-cell clones, CLD was observed ***(23)***. The importance of envelope-antigen-specific T cells to the pathogenesis of chronic HBV infection in humans, however, is not clear. In part, this is because HBV carriers have detectable envelope antigen in blood whether or not they have underlying CLD ***(24)***. In addition, there does not seem to be a correlation between envelope antigen staining in the liver and the distribution of intrahepatic inflammatory cells in patients with CLD ***(25)***. Hence, the introduction of previously primed T cells may give rise to CLD, but its relevance to the pathogenesis of natural infection in human remains to be established.

Immune-mediated liver disease has also been experimentally generated in several other laboratory animal models. For example, when a competent clone of HBV DNA was introduced by liposomes into the liver of normal rats, HBV DNA appeared in serum within a few days, followed by clearance of virus, a transient elevation of alanine aminotransaminase in blood, and histopathological evidence of acute hepatitis in the liver. When the same experiment was conducted in T-cell-deficient nude rats, no clearance of virus or development of liver disease was observed, suggesting that T lymphocytes play a central role in liver cell injury and the clearance of HBV *(25)*. These findings independently confirm the immune-mediated nature of fulminant and acute hepatitis and provide information regarding the putative mechanisms of disease. Likewise, when normal rats were injected with a liposome formulation containing an expression plasmid encoding the HBV envelope polypeptides, the rats seroconverted to envelope antibodies and developed transient, acute hepatitis *(26)*.

Chronic liver disease is a major target for therapeutics. As outlined above, there has been no easily manipulated small animal model for HBV. In a recent report *(27)*, transgenic mice supporting HBV replication were constructed using SCID mice hosts that lacked mature T and B cells *(28)*. Because the T and B cell compartments account for the bulk of specific antiviral immunity, these transgenic mice were not tolerant to HBV. A single adoptive transfer of 10 million unprimed, syngeneic splenocytes resulted in the development of chronic hepatitis, whereas a similar transfer of 50 million cells resulted in a bout of acute, resolving hepatitis. Hepatitis was accompanied by mononuclear infiltrates resembling acute and chronic hepatitis in humans and with the clearance of virus gene expression and replicative forms from the liver as well as clearance of virus DNA from the blood. Although this model confirms the immune-mediated nature of HBV associated acute and chronic liver disease, it will permit dissection of the immune components and virus antigen targets that contribute to pathogenesis. Importantly, this model will permit the evaluation of experimental therapeutics against CLD.

The following sections outline and reference protocols that were used in the construction of the transgenic mice, in the measurement of viral nucleic acids and proteins in the mice, and in the development of liver disease following adoptive transfer of naive, syngeneic splenocytes into these transgenic mice. They also list key materials and equipment needed for the conduct of each procedure.

2. Materials

2.1. Animals and Accessories

1. Swiss Webster mice (Taconic Farms, Germantown, NY).
2. B6C3F1 mice (Taconic Farms).
3. C.B.-17 SCID mice (Taconic Farms).
4. C3H/SCID mice (C3H SMN.C SCID, Jackson Laboratory, Bar Harbor, ME).
5. Fluoromethane spray (Gebauer Company, Cleveland, OH).
6. Cauterizer (cat. no. 106205 from NLS Animal Health, Pittsburgh, PA).
7. Ketamine (Ft. Dodge Animal Health).
8. Xylazine (Phoenix).
9. Betadine (Fisher, Pittsburgh, PA).
10. Alcohol pads (Fisher).
11. Hemoclips (Weck, Research Triangle Park, NC).
12. Specimen bag (Bitran, Fisher).
13. Braided suture (Ethicon, Somerville, NJ).
14. Tail vein injection apparatus (wedge-type) (LJ Shore Acrylic Designs, Philadelphia, PA).

2.2. Equipment

1. Microfuge (Eppendorf Model 5415D; Eppendorf, Westbury, NY).
2. Turboblotter (Schleicher & Schuell, Keane, NH).
3. Microtome (Leitz, model 1512).
4. Fluorescent microscope (B×60 Universal Fluorescent Microscope, Olympus, Melville, NY).
5. Light microscope (Olympus BH-2).
6. Camera (DKC 5000 Sony 3 CCD, Sony, NY).
7. Thermocycler (Hybaid Touchdown; Hybaid, Franklin, MA); Perkin Elmer 9600 (Perkin Elmer, Norwalk, CT).
8. UV/VIS spectrophotometer (Spectronic Genesys 5; Spectronic, Garforth, Leeds, UK).
9. Enzyme-linked immunosorbent assay ELISA) plate reader (Dynatech MR5000, Dynatech, Germantown, MD).
10. Water bath (Fisher Tissue Prep Flotation Bath 135).
11. Heating block (Thermolyne DB16525, Barnstead International, Dubuque, IA)
12. Hybridization incubator (Hybridizer 600, Stratagene, La Jolla, CA).
13. Transilluminator (FotoPrep I, Fotodyne, Hartland, WI).

2.3. Buffers and Solutions

1. TE: 10 m*M* Tris-HCl, 1 m*M* EDTA, pH 8 (Sigma Chemical, St. Louis, MO).
2. TAE: 0.04 *M* Tris-acetate, 0.001 *M* EDTA, pH 8.0 (Sigma).
3. TBE running buffer: 90 m*M* Tris base, 90 m*M* boric acid, and 2 m*M* EDTA.
4. Homogenization buffer: 10 m*M* Tris-HCl, 25 m*M* EDTA, pH 8, 100 m*M* NaCl, 0.5% sodium dodecyl sulfate (SDS).
5. Formaldehyde loading buffer: 1 m*M* EDTA, pH 8, 0.25% (w/v) bromophenol blue, 50% (w/v) glycerol, and 0.5 μg/mL of ethidium bromide.
6. 1X MOPS: 40 m*M* MOPS [3-(*N*-morpholino)-propanesulfonic acid], pH 7, 10 m*M* sodium acetate, 1 m*M* EDTA.
7. Phosphate-buffered saline (PBS) (Ca^{2+}- and Mg^{2+}-free) (Invitrogen, Carlsbad, CA).
8. AL buffer (QIAGEN, Chatsworth, CA).
9. Hybridization buffer: 50% formamide, 12.5% dextran sulfate; 2X saline sodium citrate (SSC), 50 m*M* sodium phosphate, pH 7.5, 1X Denhardt's solution, 10 m*M* dithiothreitol (DTT), 1m*M* EDTA, 25 μg of yeast tRNA per milliliter.

2.4. Molecular Biology Reagents

1. Restriction enzyme *Eco*RI (Promega, Madison, WI).
2. Low-melting-temperature agarose (Seaplaque, FMC, Philadelphia, PA).
3. Ethidium bromide (Sigma).
4. Phenol–chloroform–isoamyl alcohol: 25:24:1 (by vol) (Invitrogen).
5. Phenol–chloroform: 1:1 (v/v) (Invitrogen).
6. 10 *M* ammonium acetate (Fisher).
7. Ethanol (Pharmco, Brookfield, CT).
8. QIAamp Tissue Kit (QIAGEN).
9. HBV core specific primer MF03 (ATGGACATCGACCCTTATAAAGAATTTG, spanning HBV residues 1903–1929).
10. HBV core specific primer MF04 (CTAAGATTGAGATCTTCTGCG ACGCGG, spanning HBV residues 2436–2412).
11. *Taq* polymerase (Perkin Elmer, Norwalk, CT).
12. DNA size marker: 100-bp DNA ladder (Promega, Madison, WI).

13. RQ1 DNase 1 (Promega).
14. Qiamp DNeasy column (QIAGEN).
15. AmpliTaq Gold (Applied Biosystems, Foster City, CA).
16. DNAzol® (Molecular Research Center, St. Louis, MO).
17. TriReagent® (Molecular Research Center).
18. RNase Protection Assay Kit: RPAII (Ambion, Austin, TX) or RiboQuant® (Pharmingen, San Diego, CA).
19. Competent cells: Max-efficiency DH5-α (Invitrogen).
20. QIAprep Spin Miniprep Kit (QIAGEN).
21. RNA Transcription Kit: MEGAscript™ kit (Ambion) or the RiboQuant® System (Pharmingen).
22. pGEM plasmid (Promega, Madison, WI).

2.5. Reagents for Tissue Staining

1. Xylene (Fisher).
2. Gill's Hematoxylin (GHS-2-16, Sigma).
3. Ammonium hydroxide (A6899 from Sigma).
4. Eosin-phloxine B (HT110-3-6, Sigma).
5. Permount (cat. no. 8310-4 from Stephens Scientific).
6. Trypsin (T-8003, Sigma).
7. Glycine (BP381-1, Sigma).
8. Acetic anhydride (A-6404, Sigma).
9. Triethanolamine (T1377, Sigma).
10. Hydrogen peroxide (H325-500, Fisher).
11. 50% formamide–2X SSC (T-7503, Sigma).
12. DIG-Nick Translation Kit (cat. no. 1745816, Roche, Indianapolis, IN).
13. Anti-digoxygenin antibody conjugated to horseradish peroxidase (HRP) (cat. no. 1207733, Roche).
14. Diaminobenzidine (DAB, cat. no. K4011, DAKO, Carpinteria, CA).
15. Probe-on Plus (Fisher).
16. 10% neutral buffered formalin (Fisher).
17. Paraffin (Fisher).
18. Normal pig blocking solution (Sigma).
19. Fetal bovine serum (FBS, Sigma).
20. Primary antibodies:
    Anti-HBs (DAKO)
    Anti-HBc (DAKO)
    Anti-CD3, clone 17A2 (BD Pharmingen, San Diego, CA)
    Anti-CD4, clone GK1.5 (BD Pharmingen)
    Anti-CD8, clone 53-6.7 (BD Pharmingen)
    Anti-CD45R/B220, clone RA3-6B2 (BD Pharmingen)
    Anti-Mac1, clone M18/2.a.12.7 hybridoma supernatant (ATCC, Manassas, VA)
21. Secondary antibodies:
    Affinity-purified fluorescein isothiocyanate (FITC)-conjugated goat anti-rabbit Ig (Sigma)
    FITC-labeled anti-rat Ig κ light chain, clone MRK-1 (BD Pharmingen)
    HRP-conjugated anti-mouse Ig (Accurate Chemical & Scientific, Westbury, NY)
22. Biotin-free Fc receptor blocker (Accurate).
23. 2% paraformaldehyde (Sigma).

24. Colorimetric substrate: 20 mL of 0.05 *M* phosphate citrate buffer containing 0.014% hydrogen peroxide, pH 5 (Sigma, cat. no. P-9305) mixed with one 15-mg tablet of *o*-phenylenediamine dihydrochloride (OPD) (Sigma, cat. no. P-4664).

2.6. Other Materials

1. 100-mm cell culture dishes (Falcon, Fisher).
2. Ground-glass slides (Fisher).
3. ALT/GPT assay (ALT/GPT 50, Sigma).
4. Removawell Strip Holders (Fisher, cat. no. 6604).
5. Removawell strips (Immunolon 4, Fisher, cat. no. 6404).
6. Microtome blades (Accuedge, cat. no. 4689).

3. Methods

3.1. Construction of Transgenic Mice

3.1.1. Isolation of HBV Dimer DNA

The plasmid, pTKHH2, which contains a head-to-tail *Eco*R1 dimer of HBV DNA, and is infectious in chimpanzees ***(29)***, was used for making transgenic mice.

1. pTKHH2 was partially digested with *Eco*R1 using increasing amounts of enzyme in separate tubes. For this work, 30 μg of pTKHH2 plasmid DNA was added to 360 μL of TE buffer along with 40 μL of 10X restriction enzyme buffer "H" provided by the manufacturer. The assay was set up by transferring 60 μL of the DNA solution to each of nine Eppendorf tubes in ice, adding 2 U of *Eco*R1 to tube 1, and after thorough mixing, transferring 30 μL of the mixture to the next tube. This process was repeated serially through and including tube 8, from which 30 μL is discarded. Tube 9 serves as an enzyme negative control. The digestions were incubated for 1 h at 37°C, and then the enzyme was heat inactivated at 70°C for 15 min.
2. The HBV dimer was resolved by gel electrophoresis using low temperature melting agarose (1% gels) in 1X TAE buffer at 2.5 V/cm.
3. The HBV DNA dimer (6.4 kb) was then visualized by ethidium bromide staining (0.5 μg/mL of ethidium bromide for 15 min), cut out, added to five volumes of TE buffer, and melted at 65°C for 5 min. The released nucleic acid was recovered by adding an equal volume of phenol–chloroform–isoamyl alcohol, vortex-mixing, recovering the aqueous phase, then reextracting the aqueous phase with an equal volume of phenol–chloroform, and finally with chloroform alone. In these extractions, it is important not to collect the interface, if possible.
4. The aqueous phase was then transferred to a fresh tube containing 0.2 volume of 10 *M* ammonium acetate, vortex-mixed, and then two volumes of ethanol added. Ethanol precipitation was carried out at –20°C for 30 min, and recovered by microcentrifugation at full speed. The pellet was rinsed with 70% ethanol, dried, and resuspended in the proper amount (10–50 μL) of TE buffer.

3.1.2. Microinjections

The pTKHH2 insert was microinjected into eggs from two strains of mice at concentrations of 1 ng/μL and 5 ng/μL. Detailed protocols for the construction of these transgenic mice have previously been published ***(30,31)***. All microinjected embryos were implanted into pseudopregnant Swiss Webster females.

1. B6C3F1 and C.B.-17 SCID females were superovulated as described *(30)* and mated to males of the same strains.
2. Twenty plugged B6C3F1 females released 674 eggs, 394 of which were fertilized and microinjected; 264 fertilized eggs survived microinjection. Following overnight culture, 238 embryos were implanted, and 13 of 64 liveborn offspring carried the transgene.
3. In contrast, C.B.-17 SCID females were poor superovulators, with 118 plugged C.B.-17 SCID females releasing 1875 eggs, 690 of which were fertilized. C.B.-17 SCID fertilized eggs were fragile; of the 637 microinjected, only 256 survived. Half of the embryos were cultured overnight prior to implantation and half were implanted directly after microinjection. Of the 219 embryos implanted, only one of 15 liveborn offspring carried the transgene. This single C.B.-17 SCID transgenic founder was the progenitor of all mice in the colony.
4. Founder mice (F0) were screened for the transgene by extracting whole cell DNA from tail snips and performing Southern blot hybridization of undigested and *Eco*R1 digested samples or by polymerase chain reaction (PCR) amplification (*see* **Subheading 3.2.**).
5. Mice scoring positive for the HBV transgene were tested for virus in blood (*see* **Subheading 3.3.**). Virus-positive animals were mated to C3H/SCID mice.
6. Virus-positive littermates were mated to each other to establish a transgenic colony. In addition, littermates that did not carry the viral transgene were also mated together to establish a line of mice for use as virus-negative controls, hereafter referred to as nontransgenic littermates.

3.2. Detection of the Transgene

1. Shortly after weaning (21 d after birth), mice were topically anesthetized with fluoromethane spray at the ends of their tails, tail tips (0.25–0.5 cm) were then clipped and placed into 1.5-mL microfuge tubes for further analysis. The cut tails on the mice were then cauterized.
2. Mouse tail tissue was minced, Dounce homogenized, treated with proteinase K, and then extracted with phenol, phenol–chloroform, and chloroform in successive steps using the QIAamp Tissue Kit *(32)*. Additional details were supplied by the instructions provided by the manufacturer.
3. DNA was recovered by ethanol precipitation in the presence of carrier tRNA, washed, and redissolved in PCR reaction buffer. One microgram of extracted DNA was analyzed by PCR (32 cycles at 95°C for 30 s; 52°C for 30 s; and finally 72°C for 1 min) utilizing HBV core region specific primers MF03 and MF04 and 1.25 U of *Taq* polymerase, as previously described *(33,34)* using a Hybaid Touchdown Thermocycler.
4. Ten-microliter samples of amplified products were analyzed by agarose gel electrophoresis (1.0% gels containing 0.5 μg of ethidium bromide/mL) and run in 1X TAE buffer. Size markers consisted of a 100-bp DNA ladder. The products were visually inspected under ultraviolet light on a transilluminator and photographed using a Polaroid camera and w/667 film.

3.3. Detection of HBV DNA in Serum by PCR

1. Viral DNA in blood was detected by semiquantitative PCR. One hundred microliters of blood, drawn from the retroorbital plexus of mice under isoflurane anesthesia, was collected in a sterile 1.5-mL microfuge tube. When bleeding was performed more than once a month, the alternate eye was chosen for each session. In each case, blood was allowed to clot, and serum collected after centrifugation at 6610*g* for 10 min with a refrigerated microcentrifuge set at 4°C.

2. Twenty-five microliters of serum from each animal was RQ1 DNase 1 digested at 37°C for 30 min. The DNase was heat-inactivated (95°C for 10 min) and the samples digested with proteinase K (0.1 mg/mL) at 37°C for 60 min in lysis buffer (AL buffer). Each sample was processed through a Qiamp DNeasy column according to the manufacturer's instructions and eluted in 200 μL of nuclease-free water.
3. Semiquantitative PCR was conducted with 6-μL aliquots of isolated DNA template containing 10-fold dilutions of spike in competitive PCR reactions. The spike consisted of the same sequence as in the virus PCR amplicon, except that it had an internal deletion of 120 bp, which allowed the spike to be distinguished from the virus amplicon by gel electrophoresis. For PCR amplification, 1.25 U of AmpliTaq Gold was added to each reaction mixture (5 μL of 10X AmpliTaq Gold reaction buffer), 1 μL of MF03 primer (10 μ*M*), 1 μL of MF04 primer (10 μ*M*), 1 μL of dNTP mix (10 m*M* each NTP), 1 μL of spike (ranging from 10^1 to 10^7 HBV copies), 6 μL of mouse DNA sample, and 32.75 μL of PCR-grade water). The tubes were heated at 95°C for 10 min in a Perkin Elmer 9600, and amplified for 40 cycles under the following conditions: 95°C for 30 s, 52°C for 30 s, 72°C for 1 min. At the end of the last cycle, the samples were incubated at 72°C for 8 min.
4. PCR products were separated by agarose gel electrophoresis (**Fig. 1**). Quantitation was accomplished by conducting densitometry scans of a photographic negative image from an ethidium bromide stained gel of lanes having equal amounts of amplified samples and spike or by conducting Southern blot hybridization and scanning the appropriate bands. Negative controls included conducting PCR in the presence of extracted nucleic acids from normal mouse serum, in the absence of template, with an irrelevant template, or with irrelevant primers. Sera from tail blot [+], virus [–] mice were used as additional negative controls to exclude detection of the transgene within cells. A positive control consisted of amplifying 100 copies of the HBV DNA spike in a separate reaction tube.

3.4. Detection of Viral Replication in the Liver

1. Hepatic genomic DNA was extracted by mincing snap-frozen liver (250–500 mg) in 5 mL of homogenization buffer, Dounce homogenizing the pieces (5–10 strokes), treating the homogenate with proteinase K (0.1 mg/mL), and then extracting the DNA by addition of phenol, as previously described ***(35–37)***. Alternatively, genomic DNA was also isolated using DNAzol® according to the manufacturer's directions.
2. Total RNA was isolated from liver tissue using TriReagent® according to enclosed instructions.
3. Twenty micrograms of purified DNA was resolved by agarose gel electrophoresis (1.5% agarose gel containing 0.5 μg of ethidium bromide/mL) in 1X TAE buffer. In addition, 20 μg of purified total liver RNA dissolved in formaldehyde loading buffer was heated to 60°C for 10 min, loaded onto a denaturing agarose gel (1.5% agarose gel containing 2.2 *M* formaldehyde), and separated under electrophoresis in 1X MOPS.
4. Following electrophoresis, nucleic acids were transferred to positively charged nylon membranes via pressure blotting (Turboblotter) and HBV replicative forms were probed with a full-length HBV DNA probe (3.2-kb product of *Eco*RI digested pTKHH2 plasmid) radioactively labeled with [^{32}P]dNTP by random priming ***(38)***. DNA extracted from HepG2.2.15 cells, which support HBV replication ***(39)***, was used as a positive control for the presence of HBV DNA replicative forms as well as viral transcripts, while DNA extracted from the parental HepG2 cells ***(40)*** serves as a negative control. An example of intrahepatic HBV DNA replicative forms, as detected by Southern blotting, is presented in **Fig. 2A,** while an example of the major viral mRNAs, as detected by Northern blotting, is shown in **Fig. 2B**.

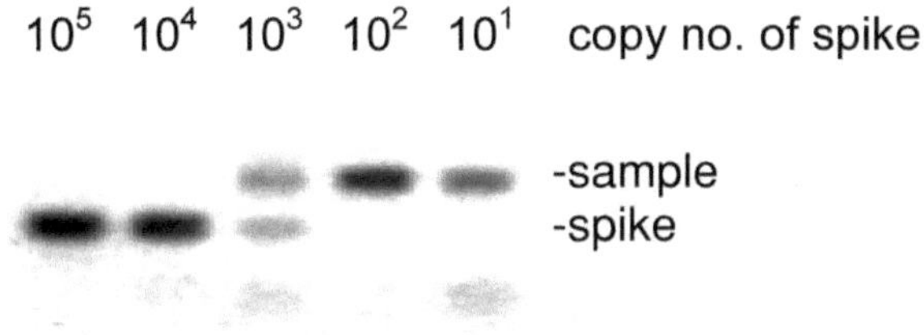

Fig. 1. Example of quantitative PCR using a single serum sample. Extracted samples were submitted to PCR amplification using core region primers in the presence of decreasing amounts of a spiked DNA, which was amplified by the same primers, but migrated faster (i.e., the lower band) during agarose gel electrophoresis. Quantitation was based on gel scanning of Southern blots.

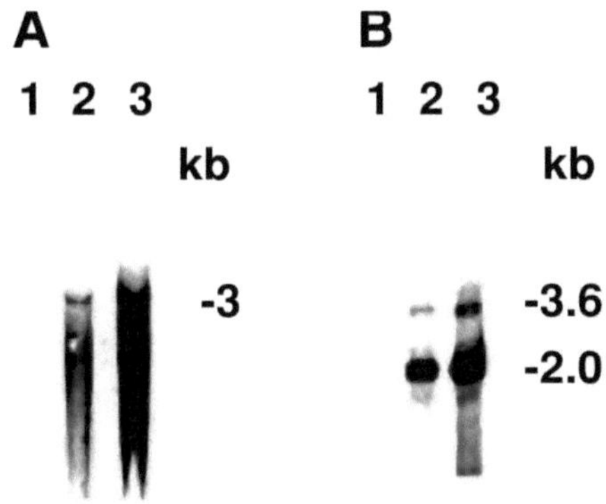

Fig. 2. Evidence for virus replication in the livers of HBV transgenic SCID mice. (**A**) Southern blot hybridization of whole cell DNA isolated from the liver of a nontransgenic mouse (*lane 1*), and from two transgenic littermates (*lanes 2* and *3*). The results show intrahepatic virus replicative forms ≤ 3 kb among the livers of mice with detectable HBV in serum. (**B**) Northern blot analysis of virus RNAs from a nontransgenic SCID mouse (*lane 1*), and from two different HBV transgenic SCID mice (*lanes 2* and *3*). The pregenomic RNA at 3.6 kb is characteristic of virus replication. The other RNA at 2 kb encodes the HBsAg polypeptides.

3.5. Immunofluorescence

1. Liver tissues were fixed in 10% buffered formalin for at least 24 h, embedded in paraffin, and sectioned using a microtome, and 5 μm thick sections were mounted on poly-L-lysine coated slides (Probe-on Plus).
2. Slides were deparaffinized and incubated with (normal pig) blocking serum diluted 1:100 in PBS for 20 min at room temperature.
3. Slides were washed twice for 5 min in PBS containing 0.5% fetal bovine serum, and incubated with primary antibody (ranging from 1:50 to 1:2000 dilutions) for 1 h at room temperature in a humidified hybridization chamber (plastic container with lid and wet paper towels). The primary antibodies, anti-HBs or anti-HBc, were used according to enclosed instructions. Anti-HBx was used according to published procedures ***(34)***. In brief, rabbit

antisera was raised to three HBx synthetic peptides (LPAMSTTDLEAYFKDC, spanning residues 99–115; VFKDWEELGEEIRLKVC, spanning residues 116–131; and DPSRDVL-CLRPVGAESRGRP; spanning residues 10–29) ***(41)***. Previous results showed that anti-100–115 worked well for the detection of HBxAg in tissue sections ***(42)***.

4. For secondary antibody, affinity-purified FITC-conjugated goat anti-rabbit Ig was added and each slide was then incubated for 30 min at room temperature in the dark. Following three washes, the slides were mounted, visualized using an epifluorescent microscope equipped with a dual FITC/rhodamine or HiQ FITC filter and a digital camera. (*See* **Note 1.**)

3.6. Partial Hepatectomy

1. Transgenic mice and nontransgenic littermates were prebled and subjected to a 30–40% partial hepatectomy (PH) ***(43,44)***. For PH, mice were anesthetized using ketamine (200 mg/kg) and xylazine (10 mg/kg) delivered intraperitoneally.
2. The abdomen was shaved, thoroughly swabbed with betadine and an alcohol pad, and small incisions (approx 2 cm) made through the skin and peritoneum.
3. Holding the mouse upright and applying gentle pressure to the abdomen with both thumbs then exposes the right lateral lobe of the liver, which was held using sterile gauze. Hemoclips were used for isolation and ligation of the liver lobe. The lobe was excised with sterile scissors, taking care to leave liver tissue distal to the clip.
4. Following lobe removal it was cut in half using a scalpel and half placed in 10% neutral buffered formalin. The remaining piece was placed in a specimen bag, snap frozen in liquid nitrogen, and stored at –70°C.
5. Each incision (peritoneum and skin) was then closed with braided suture, and mice were placed on paper towels on a heating pad set to low and allowed to wake up, at which time they were returned to a cage. The recovery time was 1 wk to allow for complete regeneration of the liver mass.

3.7. Splenocyte Preparation

1. After the donor mice were killed by cervical dislocation, whole spleens were aseptically isolated by spraying the abdomen with 70% ethanol, making a left abdominal incision, and peeling back the skin to expose the peritoneal cavity.
2. The spleen, visible through the peritoneum as a dark red organ on the upper left abdomen just below the rib cage, was isolated through another incision made directly above the organ. The spleen was removed with sterile scissors and forceps, taking care to remove any connected fat, and immediately placed in 5 mL of sterile PBS in a 100-mm cell culture dish.
3. A single-cell suspension of splenocytes was generated by grinding the spleen between the ends of sterile ground-glass slides and passing the remaining clumps, containing connective tissue and splenocytes, through a 1-cc syringe held against the bottom of the dish.
4. The remaining clumps (connective tissue only) were removed with sterile forceps, leaving a splenocyte suspension that was counted and assessed for viability using trypan blue exclusion. (*See* **Note 2.**)

3.8. Adoptive Transfer

1. Transgenic mice (>6 wk old) were adoptively transferred with normal splenocytes from syngeneic donors (C3H/C.B.-17 F1) by a single tail vein injection. For adoptive transfer, recipient mice were placed under an infrared heat lamp set at intensity level 5 for 30 s to dilate the tail vein.

2. Mice were then immobilized in the barrel of a 50-mL centrifuge tube or a tail vein injection apparatus (wedge-type) and immediately injected intravenously in the tail vein with 0.5 mL of splenocyte cell suspension using a 1-cc syringe fitted to a 27-gauge needle. The entire injection volume should be delivered in approx 20 s. The dose of splenocytes administered was dependent on the desired disease state, with 1×10^7 generating chronic hepatitis and 5×10^7 generating an acute disease.
3. Another group of transgenic mice was injected with an equal volume of saline (negative control).
4. Groups consisting of nontransgenic littermates adoptively transferred with normal splenocytes were analyzed in parallel (negative control).
5. Serial serum samples were collected weekly and assayed for HBV by quantitative PCR **(Fig. 1)**.
6. Mice were killed at 35 wk following adoptive transfer and livers removed for further analysis. Immunofluorescent staining of liver samples obtained at the time of PH and at 35 wk post-adoptive transfer showed that adoptive transfer resulted in a partial clearance of viral antigens from the liver **(Fig. 3)**. Adoptive transfer also resulted in the clearance of HBsAg and viral DNA from serum, as well as the appearance of viral antibodies **(Fig. 4)**, suggesting the priming and appearance of antiviral immune responses following adoptive transfer.

3.9. Measurement of Alanine Aminotransferase (ALT)

1. ALT levels were determined in fresh serum samples by measuring enzyme activity in a commercial kit (ALT/GPT 50) with a protocol adapted for analysis of smaller volumes. In brief, freshly isolated serum (10 μL) (*see* **Subheading 3.3.**) was mixed with ALT reagent (100 μL) and incubated in a 30°C water bath for 1 min.
2. The change in absorbance [ΔA] was measured every 30 s for 90 s at 340 nm in a spectrophotometer.
3. ALT activity was determined as follows.

$$\text{ALT (U/L)=} \frac{\Delta\text{A per minute} \times \text{Total volume (0.11 mL)} \times 1000}{6.22 \times \text{Light path (1 cm)} \times \text{Sample volume (0.01 mL)}}$$

3.10. Assessment of Immune Reconstitution

1. After the adoptively transferred transgenic and nontransgenic littermates and saline injected transgenic SCID mice were killed, spleens were removed under sterile conditions (*see* **Subheading 3.7.**) and splenocytes resuspended in sterile PBS supplemented with 5% FBS at 1×10^7 splenocytes/mL.
2. Aliquots of 100 μL (containing 1×10^6 cells) were processed for quantitation of immune cell reconstitution by flow cytometry using antibodies to cell surface markers (*see* below). To eliminate potential nonspecific binding of detection (fluorochrome-labeled) antibodies to Fc receptors on B cells, natural killer cells, macrophages, and so forth, splenocytes were treated with biotin-free Fc receptor blocker using 0.3 mL/10^6 cells for 10 min at room temperature. Splenocytes were then washed twice in PBS wash (*see* **Subheading 2.5.**).
3. Individual cell subsets were identified using rat primary monoclonal antibodies specific for mouse cell surface molecules (CD3, CD4, CD8, CD45R/B220, and Mac1) and FITC-labeled anti-rat Ig κ light chain. Purified primary antibodies were diluted (1:100) in PBS wash and hybridoma supernatant was used neat to label splenocytes (0.3 mL/10^6 cells) at room temperature for 30 min.
4. The cells were then washed twice in PBS wash and incubated with FITC-labeled secondary antibody (diluted 1:100, 0.3 mL/10^6 cells) in the dark for 30 min at 4°C.

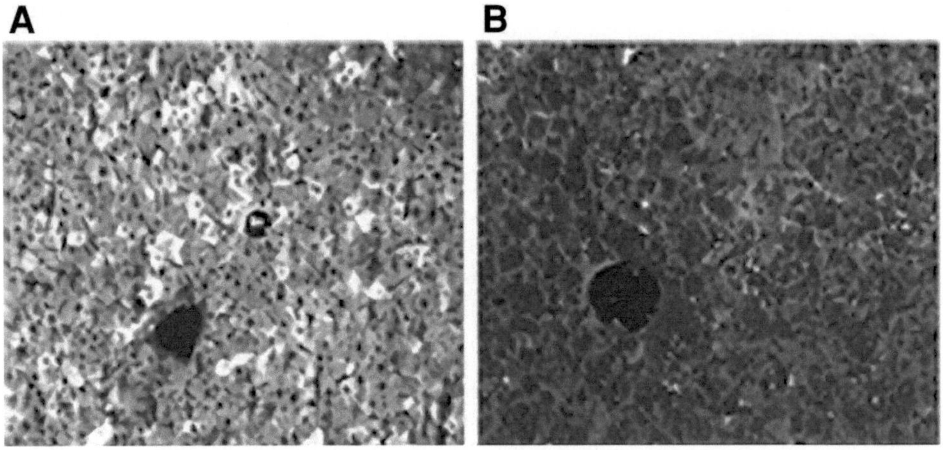

Fig. 3. Patterns of HBsAg gene expression in the liver of a transgenic mouse prior to (**A**) and 35 wk after (**B**) adoptive transfer of 1×10^7 unprimed, syngeneic splenocytes. Prior to adoptive transfer, liver material was obtained by PH. Similar decreases in the expression of HBcAg and HBxAg were also noted in the same mice (*data not shown*). The results suggest that adoptive transfer results in in vivo priming of cell-mediated immune responses against virus antigens.

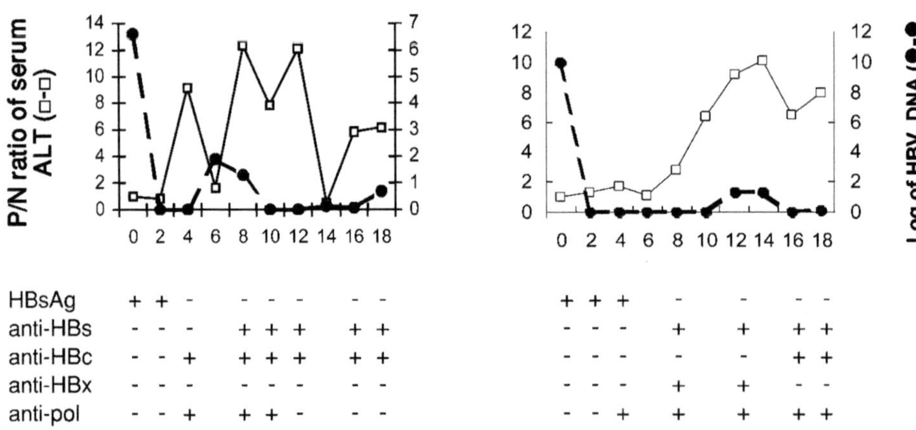

Fig. 4. Development of the host–virus relationship following adoptive transfer. The panels show virus serology and the course of liver disease in two transgenic mice injected with 1×10^7 normal, syngeneic splenocytes at wk 0. ALT was measured by a commercial kit (Sigma) and HBV DNA by quantitative PCR. HBsAg, anti-HBs, and anti-HBc were measured by adaptations of commercially available assays (Abbott) while anti-HBx and anti-pol were measured by ELISAs developed in the laboratory (*see* **Subheading 3.11.**). The results show the development of virus antibodies, spikes of liver enzymes, and intermittent appearance of HBV DNA, as in chronic human infections.

5. Following antibody treatments, splenocytes were stabilized by fixation in 0.5 mL of 2% paraformaldehyde in PBS–5% BSA and stored in the dark at 4°C until processing. Flow cytometry was performed in the cytometric analysis core facility of the Kimmel Cancer Center at Thomas Jefferson University.

3.11. Detection of Circulating Viral Antigens and Antibodies

ELISA was utilized to detect serum HBV antigen and antibody levels. Ninety-six-well plates, consisting of Removawell Strip Holders and Immunolon 4 Removawell strips, were used for this work.

1. To detect virus-specific antibodies, each well was coated with virus-specific peptides made by solid phase peptide synthesis. For coating, each well received 1 μg of one or more synthetic peptides dissolved in 50 μL of PBS, pH 7.4, containing 10% FBS. Plates were wrapped with parafilm to prevent evaporation and stored at 4°C overnight.
2. Alternatively, to detect virus specific antigens, commercially available anti-HBs was diluted in PBS–FBS, and used to coat wells, as outlined above.
3. Control plates were also processed in parallel by coating with PBS–FBS in place of the viral antigens or antibodies to control for nonspecific binding.
4. Following overnight incubation, all wells were washed seven times with PBS at room temperature using a Nunc 12-port Well Washer to remove unbound proteins.
5. Serum samples (5 μL) from experimental transgenic and nontransgenic mice were diluted 1:10 in PBS–FBS, applied in triplicate to the coated and control plates, and then incubated at 4°C for 30 min.
6. Following incubation, wells were washed seven times with PBS and then incubated with secondary antibody for 60 min at 37°C. For HBsAg detection in serum, the secondary antibody was HRP-conjugated anti-HBs diluted 1:2500 in PBS–FBS, while for virus antibody detection, HRP-conjugated anti-mouse-Ig was used.
7. Wells were again washed seven times with PBS to remove unbound antibody. Fifty microliters of freshly prepared colorimetric substrate was then added to each well and allowed to develop for 5–15 min.
8. Plates were read spectrophotometrically at 450 nm on a Dynatech ELISA Plate Reader at 5-, 10-, and 15-min time points. A sample was considered positive if the OD was greater than the mean plus two standard deviations above the negative controls, which were serum samples from nontransgenic mice. Positive serum samples were derived from human HBV carriers. These assays were used to characterize the host–virus relationship that developed following adoptive transfer (**Fig. 4**).

3.12. Liver Pathology

Hematoxylin and eosin staining was utilized to analyze liver pathology following immune reconstitution as previously described ***(46)***.

1. Tissues were processed by fixation in 10% phosphate-buffered formalin, embedded in paraffin, and 5 μm sections prepared on the microtome using low-profile disposable blades.
2. Tissue sections were then floated on a lighted water bath at 45°C, the sections captured on poly-L-lysine coated slides (Probe-on Plus), and allowed to air-dry.
3. Sections were deparaffinized in xylene by immersing the slides in xylene for 5 min. This step was then repeated with fresh xylene.

4. Rehydration was carried out by immersing the slides in 100% ethanol for 5 min, and the step then repeated with fresh ethanol. Rehydration was continued in 95% ethanol (once for 5 min). then in 85% ethanol (once for 5 min), and finally in running tap water for 5 min.
5. Staining was carried out with Gill's hematoxylin for 1–2 min, and the slides then washed in tap water for 5 min. Slides were then incubated in 0.25% ammonium hydroxide for 10 s, washed in running tap water for 5 min, and counterstained by immersion into eosin–phloxine B solution for 45 s ***(46)***.
6. Sections were dehydrated sequentially through alcohol to xylene (85% ethanol for 5 min, 95% ethanol for 5 min, twice in fresh batches of 100% ethanol for 5 min each, and finally by two incubations in fresh xylene for 5 min each).
7. Sections were then mounted with Permount and then protected by a cover glass before viewing by standard light microscopy.

3.13. RNase Protection Assay (RPA) for HBV RNA

Total liver RNA was isolated using TriReagent (*see* **Subheading 2.4.**). The RPA ***(47–50)*** was conducted using commercially available kits according to enclosed instructions.

1. In brief, antisense probes were produced by directionally cloning fragments of the HBV genome, spanning the HBx, HBpol, HBc, or HBs region, into pGEM plasmids between the Sp6 and T7 phage polymerase transcription initiation sites. These recombinant plasmids were then used to transform competent bacteria in accordance with the manufacturer's protocol.
2. Following transformation, competent cells were used to seed 10-mL sterile LB media containing ampicillin (100 μg/mL), and cultured overnight at 37°C in a bacterial shaker. Plasmids were isolated and purified from the cultured cells using the QIAprep Spin Miniprep Kit. Other antisense probe template sets specific for mouse cell surface molecules and cytokines were custom designed and obtained from commercial sources (PharMingen).
3. The ^{32}P-labeled sense or antisense RNA probes were produced by transcription from one or the other polymerase start sites with [^{32}P]UTP at 30°C for 16 h using an RNA transcription kit according to enclosed instructions ***(51–54)***.
4. The labeled antisense probe was mixed with 20–25 μg of total liver RNA and precipitated by the addition of five volumes of ethanol and pelleted by microcentrifugation (16,000*g* at 4°C).
5. Pellets were resuspended in hybridization buffer supplied in the RPA kits and denatured at 90–95°C for 5 min in a heat block. Hybridization was conducted for 16–22 h at 50°C in a cabinet-type incubator.
6. Following hybridization, the samples were supplemented with 60 μL of RNase digestion buffer (RDB; supplied in RPA kits) without RNase and incubated at 15°C for 30 min in the cabinet-type incubator. Samples were then treated with 40 μL of a mix of RNase A–T1 (supplied in RPA kits) diluted in RDB (1 μL of RNase A/T1: 39 μL of RDB per sample) and incubated at room temperature for 60 min. to digest unprotected RNA.
7. RNase was inactivated and protected RNA fragments were precipitated in one step by the addition of RNase inactivation/precipitation buffer. Pellets were resuspended in gel loading buffer and subjected to 5% polyacrylamide gel electrophoresis in 1X TBE running buffer.
8. Gels were applied to TBE prewetted Whatman filter, desiccated with a gel dryer system equipped with a liquid trap, wrapped in plastic wrap, and exposed to X-ray films for 5–48 h at –80°C using autoradiographic cassettes without intensifying screens. X-ray films were developed using an automated developer system.

9. The RPA was also carried out with RNA isolated from HepG2.2.15 cells ***(39)*** (positive control) and from parental HepG2 cells (negative control). For quantitation, the RPA kit provided a probe for β-actin, which was in the same reaction mixtures as the HBV probes. Accordingly, quantitation was carried out by scanning of the autoradiographic images (Canon Scanner linked to a Hewlett–Packard desktop computer), where the intensity of the viral RNA band was compared to the intensity of the β-actin RPA product on the same gel using densitometry software (Scion Corporation, www.scioncorp.com). An example of an RPA conducted prior to and 35 wk after adoptive transfer is shown (**Fig. 5**).

3.14. In Situ *Hybridization (ISH)*

1. Liver tissues were fixed in 4% paraformaldehyde solution, embedded in paraffin, and 5 μm thick sections mounted on poly-L-lysine coated slides.
2. Slides were deparaffinized by immersing in xylene and hydrated through a graded alcohol series (100, 90, and 75% ethanol) for 10 min each followed by three washes in PBS for 10 min each.
3. Sections were treated with 0.2 *N* HCl for 20 min to denature protein, and then permeabilized with 0.1% trypsin for 10 min at room temperature. Protein digestion was stopped by addition of 2 mg/mL of glycine for 30 s.
4. Slides were treated again with 4% paraformaldehyde solution for 5 min and washed with PBS. Background was reduced by acetylating samples with 0.25% acetic anhydride in 0.1 *M* triethanolamine for 10 min, and then washing with 2X SSC.
5. Slides were then dehydrated through 50, 75, 90, and 100% ethanol baths for 10 min each and finally air-dried.
6. Endogenous peroxidase was inactivated by treatment with 3% hydrogen peroxide for 10 min followed by air-drying.
7. Slides were rinsed in water and prehybridized with 50% formamide–2X SSC for 1 h.
8. Hybridization was carried out in hybridization buffer containing 1 μg/mL of HBV genomic DNA probe labeled with digoxygenin in the DIG-Nick Translation Kit. The mixture was heated to 95°C for 10 min, placed on ice for 5 min, and 20 μL added to each section.
9. The samples were covered with a plastic coverslip and incubated overnight at 42°C in a humidified chamber (covered glass jar with water at bottom).
10. The slides were then washed as follows: 2X SSC for 20 min at 22°C , 1X SSC for 20 min at 42°C , and finally 0.5X SSC for 10 min at 50°C.
11. An HRP-conjugated anti-digoxigenin antibody, was diluted 1:40 in 0.05 *M* Tris-HCl, pH 7.6, containing 0.15 *M* NaCl, and then applied to the liver sections for 60 min.
12. HBV DNA/RNA nucleic acids in the section were then detected by incubating the section for 1–10 min in 1 m*M* DAB. Sections were then counterstained lightly in hematoxylin, mounted with Permount under a coverslip, and viewed through a light microscope (with ×10, ×20 and ×40 ocular lenses) equipped with a 35-mm camera for photo documentation.
13. Negative controls included conducting ISH with no probe or an irrelevant probe, performing ISH after the pretreatment of tissue sections with RNase, or performing ISH on liver sections from normal (nontransgenic) mice. Positive controls include performing ISH on mouse liver epithelial cells stably transfected with full-length HBV DNA or liver from human HBV carriers.

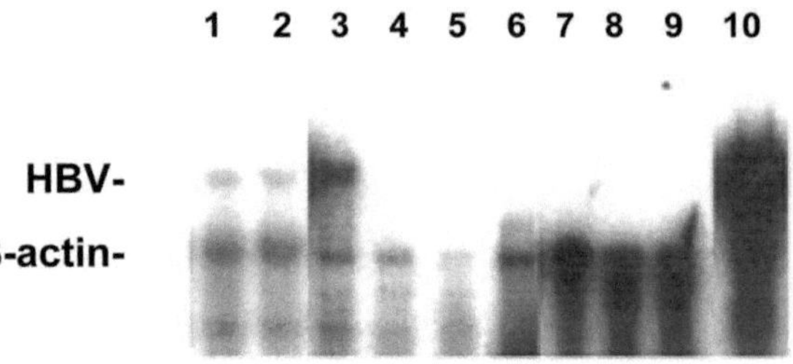

Fig. 5. HBV transcription in the liver of transgenic and nontransgenic SCID mice before and after adoptive transfer of 5×10^7 naive, syngeneic splenocytes as measured by the RNase protection assay (RPA). Hepatic HBV mRNA levels were assayed in individual transgenic mice prior to (*lanes 1–3*) and 35 wk after (*lanes 4–6*) adoptive transfer. Hepatic HBV mRNA levels were also assayed in nontransgenic littermates prior to (*lane 7*) and 35 weeks (*lanes 8* and *9*) after adoptive transfer. *Lane 10*: HBV mRNA in a mouse liver epithelial cell line transfected with an HBV DNA (positive control). The β-actin mRNA signal in each lane was used for normalization of the corresponding HBV mRNA levels.

4. Notes

1. To calibrate antibodies for immunofluorescence, staining with different dilutions of viral antibodies was carried out on liver sections from nontransgenic mice to control for nonspecific sticking. The lowest dilution for each antibody that yielded no background color on virus-negative livers was then used for staining livers from transgenic mice. The specificity of the signal obtained in livers from transgenic mice was determined further by asking whether an immunofluorescent signal in a tissue sample was blocked by preincubation of the primary antibody with an excess (25 μg) of corresponding antigen for 1 h at 37°C prior to staining. In addition, liver powder prepared from uninfected mouse liver ***(43)*** should not block the signal, while staining of transgenic mouse livers with preimmune sera at the same dilution and under the same conditions as the primary antibody should not result in any signal.
2. A typical splenocyte yield from 8- to 16-wk old mice ranged from $1.5–2 \times 10^8$ cells with a >98% viability.

Acknowledgments

This work was supported by NIH Grants CA79512 and Al-99-001.

References

1. Blumberg, B. S. (1977) Australia antigen and the biology of hepatitis B. *Science* **197**, 17–25.
2. Maddrey, W. C. (2001) Hepatitis B—an important public health issue. *Clin. Laboratorio* **47**, 51–55.
3. Arbuthnot, P. and Kew, M. (2001) Hepatitis B virus and hepatocellular carcinoma. *Int. J. Exp. Pathol.* **82,** 77–100.
4. Beasley, R. P., Hwang, L. Y., Lin, C. C., and Chien, C. S. (1981) Hepatocellular carcinoma and hepatitis B virus. A prospective study of 22 707 men in Taiwan. *Lancet* **2,** 1129–1133.
5. Lok, A. S., Heathcote, E. J., and Hoofnagle, J. H. (2001) Management of hepatitis B: 2000—summary of a workshop. *Gastroenterology* **120,** 1828–1853.

6. Hilleman, M. R. (2001) Overview of the pathogenesis, prophylaxis and therapeutics of viral hepatitis B, with focus on reduction to practical applications. *Vaccine* **19,** 1837–1848.
7. Zoulim, F. (2001) Detection of hepatitis B virus resistance to antivirals. *J Clin. Virol.* **21,** 243–253.
8. Mutimer, D. (2001) Hepatitis B virus infection: resistance to antiviral agents. *J. Clin. Virol.* **21,** 239–242.
9. Feitelson, M. A. (1996) Hepatocellular injury in hepatitis B and C infections, in *Hepatitis Viruses and Alcohol in the Pathogenesis of Chronic Liver Diseases. Clinics in Laboratory Medicine* (Feitelson, M. A. and Zern, M., eds.), W. B. Saunders, Philadelphia, pp. 307–324.
10. Summers, J. (1981) Three recently described animal virus models for human hepatitis B virus. *Hepatology* **1,** 179–183.
11. Tennant, B. C. (2001) Animal models of hepadnavirus-associated hepatocellular carcinoma. *Clin. Liver Dis.* **5,** 43–68.
12. Buendia, M. A. (1992) Mammalian hepatitis B viruses and primary liver cancer. *Semin. Cancer Biol.* **3,** 309–320.
13. Prince, A. M. and Brotman, B. (2001) Perspectives on hepatitis B studies with chimpanzees. *Ilar J.* **42,** 85–88.
14. Araki, K., Miyazaki, J., Hino, O., et al. (1989) Expression and replication of hepatitis B virus genome in transgenic mice. *Proc. Natl. Acad. Sci. USA* **86,** 207–211.
15. Babinet, C., Farza, H., Morello, D., Hadchouel, M., and Pourcel, C. (1985) Specific expression of hepatitis B surface antigen (HBsAg) in transgenic mice. *Science* **230,** 1160–1163.
16. Chisari, F. V., Pinkert, C. A., Milich, D. R., et al. (1985) A transgenic mouse model of the chronic hepatitis B surface antigen carrier state. *Science* **230,** 1157–1160.
17. Farza, H., Hadchouel, M., Scotto, J., Tiollais, P., Babinet, C., and Pourcel, C. (1988) Replication and gene expression of hepatitis B virus in a transgenic mouse that contains the complete viral genome. *J. Virol.* **62,** 4144–4152.
18. Guidotti, L. G., Matzke, B., Schaller, H., and Chisari, F. V. (1995) High level hepatitis B virus replication in transgenic mice. *J. Virol.* **69,** 6158–6169.
19. Hoofnagle, J. H., Shafritz, D. A., and Popper, H. (1987) Chronic type B hepatitis and the "Healthy" HBsAg carrier state. *Hepatology* **7,** 758–763.
20. Ando, K., Moriyama, T., Guidotti, L. G., et al. (1993) Mechanisms of class 1 restricted immunopathology. A transgenic mouse model of fulminant hepatitis. *J. Exp. Med.* **178,** 1541–1554.
21. Moriyama, T., Guilhot, S., Klopchin, K., et al. (1990) Immunobiology and pathogenesis of hepatocellular injury in hepatitis B virus transgenic mice. *Science* **248,** 361–364.
22. Chisari, F. V. (1995) Hepatitis B virus immunopathogenesis. *Annu. Rev. Immunol.* **13,** 29–60.
23. Nakamoto, Y., Guidotti, L. G., Kuhlen, C. V., Fowler, P., and Chisari, F. V. (1998) Immune pathogenesis of hepatocellular carcinoma. *J. Exp. Med.* **188,** 341–350.
24. Feitelson, M. A. (1989) Hepatitis B virus products as immunological targets in chronic infection. *Mol. Biol. Med.* **6,** 367–393.
25. Takahashi, H., Fujimoto, J., Hanada, S., and Isselbacher, K. J. (1995) Acute hepatitis in rats expressing human hepatitis B virus transgenes. *Proc. Natl. Acad. Sci. USA* **92,** 1470–1474.
26. Kato, K., Kaneda, Y., Sakurai, M., Nakanishi, M., and Okada, Y. (1991) Direct injection of hepatitis B virus DNA into liver induced hepatitis in adult rats. *J. Biol. Chem.* **268,** 22071–22074.
27. Larkin, J., Clayton, M. M., Sun, B., et al. (1999) Hepatitis B virus transgenic SCID mouse model of chronic liver disease. *Nat. Med.* **5,** 907–912.
28. Schuler, W., Weiler, I. J., Schuler, A., et al. (1986) Rearrangement of antigen receptor genes is defective in mice with severe combined immune deficiency. *Cell* **46,** 963–972.

29. Will, H., Cattaneo, R., Koch, H. G., et al. (1982) Cloned HBV DNA causes hepatitis in chimpanzees. *Nature* **299,** 740–742.
30. Hogan, B., Beddington, R., Costantini, F., and Lacy E. (1994) *Manipulating the Mouse Embryo: A Laboratory Manual*, 2nd edit. Cold Spring Harbor Laboratory Press, Cold Spring Harbor, NY.
31. Jackson, I. J. and Abbott, C. M. (2000) *Mouse Genetics and Transgenics: A Practical Approach.* Oxford University Press, Oxford, England.
32. Sambrook, J., Fritsch, E. F., and Maniatis, T. (1989) Measuring DNA, in: *Molecular Cloning: A Laboratory Manual*, 2nd edit. Cold Spring Harbor Press, Cold Spring Harbor, NY.
33. Feitelson, M. A. (1986) Products of the "X" gene in hepatitis B and related viruses. *Hepatology* **6,** 191–198.
34. Feitelson, M. A. and Clayton, M. M. (1990) X antigen/antibody markers in hepadnavirus infections. Antibodies to the X gene product(s). *Gastroenterology* **99,** 500–507.
35. Dejean, A., Bougueleret, L., Grzeschik, K. H., and Tiollais, P. (1986) Hepatitis B virus DNA integration in a sequence homologous to v-erb-A and steroid receptor genes in a hepatocellular carcinoma. *Nature* **322,** 70–72.
36. Miller, R. H., Marion, P. L., and Robinson, W. S. (1984) Hepatitis B viral DNA-RNA hybrid molecules in particles from infected liver are converted to viral DNA molecules during an endogenous DNA polymerase reaction. *Virology* **139**, 64–72.
37. Yeh, C. T., Chiu, H. T., Chu, C. M., and Liaw, Y. F. (1998) G1 phase dependent nuclear localization of relaxed-circular hepatitis B virus DNA and aphidicolin-induced accumulation of covalently closed circular DNA. *J. Med. Virol.* **55,** 42–50.
38. Feinberg, A. P. and Vogelstein, B. (1983) A technique for radiolabeling DNA restriction endonuclease fragments to high specific activity. *Analyt. Biochem.* **132,** 6–13.
39. Sells, M. A., Chen, M. L., and Acs, G. (1987) Production of hepatitis B virus particles in HepG2 cells transfected with cloned hepatitis B virus DNA. *Proc. Natl. Acad. Sci. USA* **84,** 1005–1009.
40. Knowles, B. B., Howe, C. C., and Aden D. P. (1980) Human hepatocellular carcinoma cell lines secrete the major plasma proteins and hepatitis B surface antigen. *Science* **209,** 497–499.
41. Feitelson, M. A., Clayton, M. M., and Blumberg, B. S. (1990) X antigen/antibody markers in hepadnavirus infections. Presence and significance of hepadnavirus X gene product(s) in serum. *Gastroenterology* **98,** 1071–1078.
42. Wang, W., London, W. T., Lega, L., and Feitelson, M. A. (1991) Hepatitis B x antigen in liver from carrier patients with chronic hepatitis and cirrhosis. *Hepatology* **14,** 29–37.
43. Schaeffer, D. O., Hosgood, G., Oakes, M. G., St Amant, L. G., and Koon, C. E. (1994) An alternative technique for partial hepatectomy in mice. *Lab. Anim. Sci.* **44,** 189–190.
44. Waynforth, H. B. (1992) *Experimental and Surgical Techniques in the Rat*, 2nd edit. Academic Press, London.
45. Taboas, J. O. and Ceremsak, R. J. (1967) A rapid hematoxylin and eosin stain. *Tech. Bull. Regist. Med. Technol.* **37,** 119–120.
46. Azrolan, N. and Breslow, J. L. (1990) A solution hybridization/RNase protection assay with riboprobes to determine absolute levels of apoB, A-I, and E mRNA in human hepatoma cell lines. *J. Lipid Res.* **31,** 1141–1146.
47. Belin, D. (1996) The RNase protection assay. *Methods Mol. Biol.* **58,** 131–136.
48. Ma, Y. J., Dissen, G. A., Rage, F., and Ojeda, S. R. (1996) *RNase Protect. Assay Methods* **10,** 273–278.

49. Tymms, M. J. (1995) Quantitative measurement of mRNA using the RNase protection assay. *Methods Mol. Biol.* **37,** 31–46.
50. Krieg, P. A. and Melton, D. A. (1984) Functional messenger RNAs are produced by SP6 in vitro transcription of cloned cDNAs. *Nucleic Acids Res.* **12,** 7057–7070.
51. Krieg, P. A. and Melton, D. A. (1987) *In vitro* RNA synthesis with SP6 RNA polymerase. *Methods Enzymol.* **155,** 397–415.
52. Melton, D. A., Krieg, P. A., Rebagliati, M. R., Maniatis, T., Zinn, K., and Green, M. R. (1984) Efficient *in vitro* synthesis of biologically active RNA and RNA hybridization probes from plasmids containing a bacteriophage SP6 promoter. *Nucleic Acids Res.* **12,** 7035–7056.
53. Milligan, J. F., Groebe, D. R., Witherell, G. W., and Uhlenbeck, O. C. (1987) Oligoribonucleotide synthesis using T7 RNA polymerase and synthetic DNA templates. *Nucleic Acids Res.* **15,** 8783–8798.
54. Tabor, H. (1955) Acetylation of amines with pigeon liver enzyme. *Methods Enzymol.* 608–612.

24

The Chimpanzee Model

Contributions and Considerations for Studies of Hepatitis B Virus

Pascal Gagneux and Elaine A. Muchmore

1. Introduction

Efforts to control the global pandemic of human hepatitis B virus (hHBV) infection have been hampered by incomplete understanding of viral–host interactions in this disease. This situation has been confounded by the fact that hHBV has a limited host range and cannot be propagated in simple cell culture ***(1)***. Reproducible experimental infection with determination of infectivity was demonstrated in chimpanzees (*Pan troglodytes*), but not other primates ***(2–4)***, long before other animal models such as the woodchuck were identified. After successful inoculation of chimpanzees was reported in 1972, multiple institutions, including a multigroup collaboration between the FDA, CDC, and NIH, initiated studies to evaluate them as a model for the study of HBV. For the majority of studies only chimpanzees "with no prior exposure" to virus were used because those with positive serology [either from exposure to hHBV or chimpanzee HBV (chHBV)], with an estimated prevalence of 3–6% in Africa ***(5)***, were not reproducibly susceptible to infection ***(3)***. It has been widely reported that the effects of HBV infection in chimpanzees are milder than in humans, that is, few have developed fulminant hepatitis, and inoculated chimpanzees exhibit few symptoms or signs of infection. Furthermore, the incidence of chronic infection with HBV (*see* Table 2) and horizontal and vertical transmission (from mother to offspring) in chimpanzees is lower than in humans ***(6,7)***. Chimpanzees have been the cornerstone of all research on infectivity of HBV and safety and efficacy of vaccines.

Chronic HBV infection occurs in approx 5% of experimentally infected chimpanzees, defined as persistence of hepatitis B surface antigen (HBsAg) for > 12 months (approx ⅔ clear HBsAg between 6 and 12 months of infection) ***(8)***. Liver biopsies of chimpanzees with chronic HBsAg have never been reported to have more severe abnormalities than mild persistent hepatitis ***(8–11)***, but we were unable to find published

From: *Methods in Molecular Medicine, vol. 96: Hepatitis B and D Protocols, volume 2*
Edited by: R. K. Hamatake and J. Y. N. Lau © Humana Press Inc., Totowa, NJ

reports of liver biopsies performed later than 36 mo after inoculation with HBV, and found few reports of chimpanzees with chronic infections of unknown source ***(12–14)***. Likewise, liver biopsies performed since 1972 have not been reexamined for the presence of covalently closed circular DNA (cccDNA) or integrated HBV-DNA, indicative of the chronic carrier state, in hepatocytes. In addition, other tissues that could harbor HBV ***(15)***, such as lymphocytes ***(9–11)*** and splenic tissues ***(16)***, are generally not available from these animals. Thus, it has not been possible to make histological and molecular comparisons between humans and chimpanzees with either serologically resolved or chronic infections. This information would be particularly interesting because of the demonstration by Penna ***(17)*** of the persistence of cccDNA in hepatocytes of humans with apparently "resolved" infections, which indicates that HBV can persist at low levels chronically, even in the absence of traditional serological markers. These issues raise questions about the utility of the chimpanzee model to predict the outcome of chronic infection, including cirrhosis and hepatocellular carcinoma, and the long-term efficacy of currently available treatments and vaccines. In addition, the only reported cases of hepatocellular carcinoma in chimpanzees involve two animals that had been experimentally infected with hepatitis C virus ***(18)***.

This chapter recounts the history of HBV studies in chimpanzees and explains the importance of the chimpanzee model to the study of human HBV disease and to HBV vaccine development, comparing and contrasting both host and viral factors, and revisiting the potential issues about the utility of this model for future research in the area.

2. Appreciation of Multiplicity of Infectious Agents Capable of Causing Hepatitis in Chimpanzees

Hepatitis of apparent viral origin in nonhuman primates was first described many years before HBV was identified in 1966 ***(19)***. There are reports in the 1930s and 1940s of jaundice following parenteral administration of blood products ***(19)*** or injection of a yellow-fever vaccination prepared in Rhesus monkeys ***(20)***. Between 1958 and 1960 there were multiple reports of primate-related spontaneous hepatitis (approx 26 clusters involving at least 106 veterinary personnel), associated primarily with exposure to chimpanzees rather than other primates ***(20)***, with as many as 43% in some groups infected (e.g., workers at Holloman Air Force Base ***[21]***). It was rapidly recognized that infected workers had handled chimpanzees newly arrived from Africa, indicating that the chimpanzees had only recently contracted the illness, as none of the chimpanzees quarantined for longer than 3 mo showed evidence of hepatitis. Microbiological analysis of stool, urine, and sera demonstrated that many of the infected chimpanzees had become ill with viruses such as reo-1, polio-1, ECHO-8, adenovirus 14 and 17, and an "unknown" type. This raised the question of whether chimpanzees, known to have occasionally been inoculated with pooled human sera after capture by animal dealers to protect them from development of human infections ***(21)***, had, in fact, developed significant infectious sequelae to this practice. The "unknown" infectious agent(s) remained elusive, but it was clear that there was both intercage transmission and transmission to veterinary personnel, indicating that fecal–oral transmission of what was later identified as hepatitis A virus (HAV) was most common in this period.

One chimpanzee at the Delta Regional Primate Research Center developed fulminant hepatitis 1 mo after arrival at the facility and two workers developed significant hepatitis, 4 and 7 wk after that chimpanzee became ill *(20)*. Both humans and the chimpanzee had "unusual" liver histology, consistent with "acute yellow atrophy." Although this may have been an infection with HBV, this was not confirmed. In another early study *(22)*, three of six chimpanzees inoculated with human serum from inhabitants of the Willowbrook State School (New York) developed evidence of hepatitis; although this serum may have contained more than one hepatotropic virus, HBV was later identified to be endemic in this population. The first case of documented transmission of HBV from chimpanzee to human was reported in 1970 after a cross-circulation experiment between a young girl and a chimpanzee positive for HBsAg *(23)*. The specific medical history of the infected chimpanzee was not included, so the source of HBV is unknown. In 1972, Maynard demonstrated that serologically negative chimpanzees could be infected with serum derived from humans infected with HBV *(3)*. The issue of whether apes could represent a reservoir for the human infection was briefly addressed but the prevailing attitude was that all chimpanzees serologically positive for HBV had been infected by human viruses prior to their arrival at research facilities.

One of the confounding factors to discriminate between incidence and prevalence of HBV and other forms of hepatitis in the natural habitat is that the vast majority of captive chimpanzees arrived in the United States with poor records, if any at all. Similarly, the precise geographic origin of the animals was unknown. In addition, all animals were treated as belonging to the same population. Based on recent population genetic surveys, it is now clear that some chimpanzee populations have been separated for long evolutionary periods *(24)*, and that when using these animals for biomedical studies, it may be relevant to identify the geographical origin of the animal *(25, 26)*.

The assignment of chimpanzees currently in NIH facilities (230 founder animals) into one of the four possible subspecies based on sequencing of mitochondrial DNA is still incomplete (Ely and Gagneux, *unpublished observations*). Preliminary results suggest that the vast majority originate from western Africa (West of the Niger River), but a smaller number of animals were also imported from central and East Africa, e.g., imported from Cameroon *(21)* and Rwanda *(27)*.

3. Use of Chimpanzees for HBV Research

Early studies of hepatitis involved large groups of humans (U.S. armed forces recruits) and many individuals who would today not be considered suitable candidates for human research because of ethical considerations, such as children at institutions for the mentally ill (e.g., the Willowbrook State School) *(28)*. Subsequently efforts to develop animal models were undertaken.

Although there were multiple reports of chimpanzees positive for HBV on arrival to captive facilities (**Table 1**), it was soon appreciated that serologically negative animals were susceptible to HBV infection. Maynard reported that as many as 55% of captured chimpanzees had HBV antibodies *(3)*, and two animals that did not were susceptible to infection with a 1:10 dilution of human serum containing HBsAg. Several groups expanded these observations to demonstrate that most serologically negative chimpanzees are susceptible to experimental inoculation with HBV *(3,4,29)*.

Table 1
HBV Prevalence Studies of HBV in Newly Captured Chimpanzees Housed in U.S. Facilities

	Positive/surveyed HBsAg	HBV antibodies	Site
1969 ***(117)***		3/62	Holloman AF base, LEMSIP
1971 ***(118)***	6/97	29/97	Phoenix Labs
1972 ***(119)***		46/81	Holloman AF Base
1980 ***(120)***	2/82	24/82	Southwest Foundation

All studies used serological methods for the detection of antibodies, but not all assayed for the presence of viral antigen. No retrospective analysis of these specimens has been performed to discriminate whether the infectious agent was chHBV or hHBV.

Chimpanzees selected for experimental studies were all negative by serologic assay to HBV and had no known exposure to blood, blood products, or plasma derivatives. In many cases liver enzyme assays and liver biopsies were performed to qualify the animals as noninfected. Radioimmunoassays were widely used after the mid-1970s and significantly improved detection levels. However, it is now known that none of these selection criteria rule out previous infection because infectious episomes can be detected in hepatocytes in humans serologically negative for HBV ***(17,30,31)***.

Apart from polio vaccine safety and other studies done on 300–400 chimpanzees at Lindi Camp near Stanleyville in the Belgian Congo in the 1950s, which included preliminary studies by Deinhardt and colleagues on hepatitis, HBV research was the first large-scale application of the chimpanzee in biomedical research ***(32)***.

The reaction of chimpanzees to inoculation with human serum positive for HBsAg varied between animals, but appeared to be consistently milder than in humans ***(4,8,29)***. Despite the inoculation of hundreds of animals, the first cases of confirmed fulminant HBV infection were reported in 1993 ***(33)***. Antibody production, changes in liver enzyme values, and changes in hepatic tissue architecture have been clearly documented and appear to follow a time course similar to that in humans. Transmission studies, reinfection, and combined infection (superinfection) with more than one hepatotropic virus have been carried out. In addition to their importance to the study of infectivity of HBV and in HBV vaccine safety and efficacy trials, the use of chimpanzees was instrumental in the identification of hepatitis C virus (HCV) ***(34)***.

4. Safety Testing (the "Chimpanzee Assay")

The reproducibility of infection and its temporal sequence in chimpanzees made it possible to use chimpanzees as an "assay" for the presence of HBV in human serum and serum-derived products, such as immunoglobulins and clotting factors. Between 1980 and 1993 multiple methods for decreasing infectivity of serum were reported, each of which used chimpanzees in traditional experimental format, with some animals serving as control (untreated product) and others receiving the treated product or, alternately, treated animals serving as their own controls. These studies were pivotal for reducing viral contamination of blood and serum products, and for determining the activity of serum proteins after various treatments. Specific agents tested included antibodies to HBV ***(35,36)***, ultraviolet irradiation ***(37)***, urea/formalin treatment of human sera ***(38)***, Tween-80 treatment ***(39)***, a combination of Tween-80–propiolactone and UV irradiation ***(40,41)***, chloroform ***(42)***, Tween-80–20% ether and cold (4°C) treatment ***(43)***, glutaraldehyde ***(44)***, heat treatment ***(45,46,47)***, ion exchange treatment ***(48)***, photochemical treatment ***(49)***, and disinfectants (two quaternary and one phenolic) ***(50)***. Later, when the polymerase chain reaction (PCR) became widely used, it became the preferred method for detection of HBV contamination.

Chimpanzees were also used to assay the presence of trace amounts of HBV in vaccine lots. Chimpanzees born in captivity to mothers serologically negative for HBV were the principal animals used until the U.S. moratorium on breeding in captivity came into effect in 1998. Despite improvements in the sensitivity of assays for markers of HBV, it is now recognized that an indeterminate number of animals must have escaped detection as a result of false negative assay results.

5. Experimental Inoculation of Chimpanzees with HBV

The earliest studies (**Table 2**) demonstrated that infectivity was related to both dose and serotype of HBV; inocula were diluted in fetal calf sera serologically negative for HBV. Later reports described neither the serotype nor precise source of HBV, so it is possible that the inocula for many of the experiments could have contained more than one hepatotropic virus. Infectivity of HBV inocula was calculated by the Reed–Muench method ***(8)*** and a high percentage of infected animals were achieved using an inoculum of 10^7–10^8 CID_{50} (chimpanzee infectious doses)/mL for subtypes adw, ayw, adr, and 10^0–10^3 CID_{50} for 1 yr ***(4)***. Interestingly, no such differences in infectivity were apparent in the human host. There was a roughly inverse relationship between the amount of virus inoculated and the time to appearance of HBsAg in chimpanzees, with some serotypes exhibiting more reproducible incubation times than others. The longest incubation time was 19 wk, which was comparable to infections in humans.

Animals successfully infected have typical biochemical, serological, and histological patterns of mild type B hepatitis and responses are not distinguishable based on viral subtype. Barker ***(29)*** reported that 27/29 chimpanzees developed HBsAg, which persisted in 2/29; antibodies to HBsAg were detected in 24/29 and antibodies to HBcAg in 23/29. As can be seen, and calculated from **Table 2**, the rate of infection of susceptible chimpanzees is approx 80–90%, with variation probably based on viral titer of inocula, as early studies reported complete susceptibility to infection of seronegative chimpanzees ***(3,51)***. This rate of infectivity is similar to that reported in human populations with endemic infections, such as the Willowbrook School population, where 90% of children housed at the center for 3–5 yr had detectable antibodies to HBV ***(52)***. Karasawa et al. ***(9–11)*** and others have carefully documented histologic features of mild hepatitis. Notably, there have been no reports of hepatocellular carcinoma in HBV-inoculated chimpanzees. Of the more than 150 chimpanzees reportedly infected with HBV from various sources **(Table 2)**, detection of chronic HBsAg in serum, using standard serologic assays, has occurred in < 5% of cases, or 5 of >150 reported [one addi-

Table 2
Infectivity Studies of Chimpanzees Previously Unexposed to HBV or to Human Serum Products

Date	No.	HBV type	Route	HBsAg	HBsAb	Histologic changes of hepatitis	Persistence of HBsAg	F/U
1962 (***32***)	6	WB serum (?MS-2 strain)	IP	NR	NR	3/6	NR	2 mo
1972 (***3***)	2	hHBV-plasma	IV	1/2	2/2	0/2	0/2	>1 yr
1973 (***4***)	6	hHBV-plasma (NIH) and partially purified plasma (SQ)	SQ	5/6	5/6	2/5	0/6	20–44 wk
1973 (***5***)	3	Serum from hemophiliac with chronic HBV	IV	1/3	1/3	NR	NR	6 mo
1974 (***121***)	8	hHBV (MS-2) and chimp serum from infected chimps	IV	8/8	6/8	NR	1/8	2 yr
1974 (***122***)	4	HBV	IV	3/4	3/4	3/4	0/4	6 mo
1975 (***123***)	6	HBV + cytoxan	IV	6/6 (one spontaneous infection)	4/6	6/6	2/6 treated with cystoxan during primary infection were positive at death at 11 and 42wk	13 mo
1975 (***51***)	12	NIH plasma pool, MS-2 strain	IV	9/12	12/12	8/12	2/12	NR
1975 (***124***)	2	MS-2 strain	IV	2/2	2/2	2/2	0/2	9 mo
1975 (***29***)	34	hHBV: 4 serotypes; ayw strain was MS-2	IV	27/34	29/34	23/29	1/34	7–16 mo

1977 ***(125)***	4	HBV-saliva, semen	IV	2/4	2/4	2/4	NR	6 mo
1977 ***(126)***	7	Serum with HBeAg or anti-HBeAg	IV	4/4	1/3	NR	NR	NR
1977 ***(127)***	1	hHBV+ SQ and IV ethanol	IV	1/1	1/1	0/1	0/1	6 mo
1979 ***(128)***	3	hHBV	IV	3/3	3/3	NR	0/3	22 mo
1979 ***(129)***	1	HBV human plasma	IV	1/1	1/1	0/1	0/1	1yr
1979 ***(130)***	1	hHBV (pooled serum)	IV	1/1	NR	NR	—	9 mo
1980 ***(131)***	9	hHBV, multiple sources	IV	8/9	9/9	NR	1/9	>2 yr
1980 ***(76)***	7	JHB 001 hHBV	IV	7/7	7/7	7/7	1/7	3 yr
1982 ***(132)***	1	huHBV (plasma)	corneal	1/1	NR	NR	NR	9 wks
1982 ***(133)***	1	HBV2,6,14; cloned	IV,IM,IH	1/1	1/1	0/1	0/1	1 yr
1985 ***(134)***	8	Varied sequences, routes of inoculation	IV,IP	3/6	3/6	3/6	ND	1 yr
1985 ***(8)***	6	JHB001	IV	6/6	6/6	5/6	0/6	>2 yr
1986 ***(135)***	3	hHBV variants (hu sera + anti-HBc, anti-HBe, -HBsAg)	IV	4/4	4/4	4/4	0/4	1 yr
1987 ***(136)***	2	Media from HEPG2 cells transfected with HBV	IV	2/2	1/2	2/2	1/2	NR
1988 ***(137)***	1	Media from HEPG2 cells transfected with HBV	IV	1/1	NR	1/1	NR	NR
1988 ***(138***	2	Plasma from HBsAb-negative patients	IV	2/2	2/2	1/2 (2/2 by PCR)	0/2	8 mo
1990 ***(139)***	1	Media from rat hepatoma cell line transfected with HBV	IV	1/1	1/1	NR	0/1	8 mo

Table 2
Infectivity Studies of Chimpanzees Previously Unexposed to HBV or to Human Serum Products

Date	No.	HBV type	Route	HBsAg	HBsAb	Histologic changes of hepatitis	Persistence of HBsAg	F/U
1990 ***(30)***	1	hHBV from serologically negative, PCR + individual	IV	1/1	1/1	0/1	PCR +	17 mo
1993 ***(33)***	3	hHBV mutated in pre-core region	IV	3/3	3/3	NR	0/3	1yr
1997 ***(140)***	6	hHBV, Arg-Gly at codon 145 S	IV	5/6	5/6	ND	0/6	24 wk
2001 ***(73)***	3	Serum/lymphocytes from patients HBV DNA + by PCR, HBsAg-	IV	0/3 (by PCR)	ND	ND	ND	55 wk
Total	154							

As explained in the text, the preinoculation history of most captive chimpanzees was limited. The rate of infectivity was >80%, as determined by detection of viral antigen and antiviral antibodies. Many studies did not examine liver histology, but those that did reported changes consistent with mild hepatitis. A calculation of percentage of infected animals that develop chronic infections is difficult because duration of follow-up was extremely limited, in most cases less than the 12 mo required for viral clearance in chimpanzees. NR indicates not reported.

tional case was detected using PCR in a serologically negative animal ***(30)***]. This percentage of chronically infected chimpanzees remains constant even if the calculation is restricted to animals followed for longer than 1 yr, which is the minimum follow-up required to ensure that spontaneous clearance of HBsAg has not occurred ***(8)***.

Infection with more than one hepatotropic virus has been reported to be associated with altered response to infection with HBV ***(53,54)***. Brotman et al. ***(55)*** reported that chimpanzees inoculated with "standard" doses of HBV have 100% antigenemia with HBsAg (18/18), with 15/18 having at least one abnormal alanine aminotransferase (ALT). However, simultaneous exposure to non-A, non-B, and HBV in seven animals yielded milder results: five of seven developed HBsAg, in each case with a greatly delayed onset, and three of seven had only borderline ALT abnormalities. Kos et al. ***(56)*** demonstrated decreased levels of HBV in a chronically HBV-infected chimpanzee inoculated with HDV. However, Dienes et al. ***(14)*** reported that chronic HBV carriers experimentally infected with either HAV or non-A, non-B agents developed more severe disease than infected native animals. This indicates that the number of animals that have been experimentally (knowingly) infected with more than one hepatotropic virus is too low to allow definite conclusions.

6. Reinfection of Chimpanzees with HBV

The presence of detectable antibodies to HBV was found to be associated with resistance to experimental reinfection with HBV. In 1974, Wilson and Logan ***(57)*** reported two chimpanzees with low antibody titers to HBV who did not develop detectable circulating HBsAg after injection of highly infectious serum; in fact, antibody titers increased substantially. In 1975, Maynard et al. ***(51)*** reported that chimpanzees reinfected with HBV of a different serotype did not develop hepatitis. Furthermore, Trepo et al. ***(58)*** demonstrated the presence of Arthus reactions in 7/7 animals with measurable anti-HBV that had been immunized 1 yr earlier. These observations formed the basis for vaccine development. Early studies demonstrated that immune function was directly related to outcome of infection. Wilson reported a chimpanzee treated with cyclophosphamide and prednisone around the time of challenge with HBV serum, and with prednisone for 7 wk when HBsAg levels decreased. At necropsy, abundant Dane particles were present in both serum and liver, implying that effective immune response to infection had been blunted by treatment with prednisone. In contrast, reinfection with HDV, even if associated with antibodies to HDV, has been reported ***(59)***.

7. Sequelae of Infection with HBV in Chimpanzees

Studies to determine hepatic sequelae of chronic infection with HBV in chimpanzees have been sparse because of the generally short duration of follow-up in most experimental infection studies. However, it was appreciated as early as 1982 ***(60)*** that in chronically infected animals, HBV-DNA existed in a covalently closed, supercoiled circular configuration (cccDNA) not integrated into the host genome, and was infectious. Thus, although no findings beyond minimal hepatitis have been recorded in the 1- to 3-yr follow-up of the inoculation experiments, the follow-up may have been insufficient to document chronic changes. There are several reports of biopsies performed in chronically infected chimpanzees. Krawczynski et al. ***(12)*** described liver biopsies in four chimpanzees between the ages of 6 and 15 yr who were positive for HBsAg, due to unknown exposures, for 2–8 yr; all had histopathologic features consistent with "minimal hepatitis" of humans. Similarly, Shouval et al. ***(13)*** reported liver biopsy results from five chimpanzees with chronic HBsAg (the source of the infectious inoculum was known in only two animals, infected for a minimum of 5 and 10 yr); only one of the specimens showed borderline findings for chronic aggressive, or active, hepatitis. Dienes et al. ***(14)*** described liver biopsies from seven carrier chimpanzees, with mild activation of sinusoidal cells, rare and mild fibrosis of portal tracts, and slight proliferation of bile ductules. If the pathology from these 12 chronically infected chimpanzees is representative of the course of infection in the general population, it appears unlikely that chimpanzees chronically infected with HBV would develop cirrhosis or hepatomas, as occurs with greater incidence in chronically infected humans and in chimpanzees infected with HCV ***(18)*** or chronic *Schistosoma mansoni* ***(61)***.

8. Vaccine Trials in Chimpanzees

The discovery that animals previously exposed to HBV were not susceptible to reinfection opened the way to the study of the immune modulation of infection. The first vaccines (**Table 3**) involved injection of the empty 22-nm particles purified from the plasma of chronically infected carriers. To minimize the risks of infection during immunization, multiple steps were taken to purify human plasma containing HBV, including centrifugation, fractional precipitation, chromatography, and molecular exclusion. To inactivate the HBV, various detergents, formaldehyde, heat, pH changes, and ultraviolet radiation were used. Within a few years after successful inoculation of a chimpanzee with HBV, there were multiple vaccines based on noninfectious 22-nm subviral particles (containing mostly S antigen) isolated from chronic human HBV carriers. The initial findings were somewhat confusing, perhaps because different evaluation criteria were applied to the studies, but sufficiently promising that second generation vaccines were developed. Unfortunately, all published studies used unique injection schedules regarding number of boosters and timing of injections.

The second generation of vaccines contained recombinant subviral particles produced in stably transfected eukaryotic cell lines. The sources of subviral particles for vaccine development included plasma-derived polypeptides and synthetic polypeptides expressed in *E. coli,* yeast, and murine cells. Live recombinant adenovirus vaccines were introduced in 1989 ***(62)*** but both these and synthetic polypeptides did not prove to be effective. It was recognized in the late 1980s that the M and L proteins, containing the pre-S region of HBV, in addition to the S protein, were essential for vaccine effectiveness ***(63)***. The latest generation of vaccines and treatments are intended to target the HBV carrier state.

Chimpanzees have been used successfully for all vaccine safety and efficacy trials ***(64–66)***. Cross-protection afforded by antibodies induced by different HBsAg subtypes ***(51,67)*** was also first demonstrated in chimpanzees. Antibodies to the viral envelope confer protective immunity; and 10 mIU/mL is considered sufficient to confer immunity. HBcAg is highly immunogenic but although anti-HBcAg protects chimpanzees

Table 3
HBV Immunization Studies Conducted in Chimpanzees

Date and first author	Type of vaccine	Number of chimpanzees	Failure rate	Duration of follow-up
1971 ***(118)***	Hypersensitivity test purified HBsAg	2	—	—
1974 ***(120)***	Partially purified chimpanzee HBsAg	2	—	
1974 ***(141)***	Vaccine safety HBsAg +/– CFA	28	—	—
1975 ***(58)***	Vaccine safety HBsAg purified + CFA	15		1 mo
1975 ***(64)***	HBsAg 22-nm CsCl gradient purified, formalin inactivated	7	1/4	6 mo
1976 ***(142)***	Ad and ay HBsAg from pooled serum	10	1/16	10 mo
1978 ***(143)***	HBV polypeptide vaccine efficacy	4	—	3 mo
1978 ***(144)***	Bivalent NIH vaccine HBeAg active and passive immunization	7	—	—
1978 ***(145)***	HbsAg vaccine efficacy	2		
1978 ***(146)***	Safety and efficacy NIAID subunit vaccine	16	0/4	6 mo
1981 ***(147)***	Vaccine efficacy bivalent ad/ay HBsAg (Hepagen)	46	4/46	32 mo
1982 ***(148)***	Vaccine efficacy HBeAg and HBsAg	4	—	
1983 ***(149)***	Vaccine efficacy for transfusion protection HBsAg from pooled serum	8	3/4	16 mo

Continued

Table 3
HBV Immunization Studies Conducted in Chimpanzees

Date and first author	Type of vaccine	Number of chimpanzees	Failure rate	Duration of follow-up
1983 ***(150)***	Heptavax B safety	—		6 mo
1984 ***(151)***	Vaccine efficacy HBsAg ayw MS-2 10^8 PFU (Hevac B, Pasteur)	42	—	6 mo
1984 ***(152)***	Vaccine efficacy recombinant vaccinia virus intradermal	2	0/2	8 mo
1984 ***(153)***	Treatment safety IgG anti-HBcAg and anti-HBcAg	10	—	12 mo
1985 ***(68)***	Vaccine efficacy recombinant HBcAg in *E. coli* and adjuvant	5	1/3	16 mo
1987 ***(47)***	Inactivation safety human HBsAg-plasma	4	0/4	5 mo
1987 ***(154)***	Vaccine efficacy recombinant HBsAg in yeast	7	0/4	—
1988 ***(155)***	Vaccine efficacy cloned adw 226 aa HBsAg adw & alum adjuvant (Amgen)	6	0/5	12 mo
1989 ***(62)***	Vaccine efficacy oral live recombinant adenovirus	3	1/2	11 mo
1990 ***(63)***	Vaccine efficacy recombinant pre-S and S HBsAg adr in yeasts	9	0/8	10 mo
1993 ***(50)***	Test of disinfectants	4		7 mo

1997 ***(156)***	Vaccine efficacy for offspring of chronic carriers DNA vaccine pCMV S2-S	3		16 mo
1997 ***(138)***	Vaccine efficacy recombinant HBsAg effective against surface mutant	6	0/4	8 mo
1998 ***(157)***	Vaccine efficacy Pre s1 pre-S2 and S in mouse c127i cells	5	0/3	9 mo
1998 ***(71)***	DNA vaccine safety and efficacy recombinant retrovirus (Chiron)	3 chronic carriers of chHBV	HBV DNA down	12 mo
2001 ***(70)***	Treatment efficacy/safety chronic carrier DNA prime/canary pox boost	1 chronic carrier		20 mo
	Total	>250		

Most studies did not include information about the animals used in the study, such as the previous experimental studies for which the chimpanzees had been used. The failure rate was essentially negative after 1985. The few studies that have tested vaccines in chronic chimpanzee carriers of HBV are noted. The duration of follow up, when included, after vaccine injection was universally short. (—) indicates information not included in publication.

from challenge from live HBV, high titers of maternal antibodies to HBc fail to protect the few infants of chronically infected mothers from perinatal infection ***(68)***.

In the past 25 yr, more than 250 chimpanzees have been used in vaccine safety and efficacy trials. The record in terms of safety is impressive: not a single batch of tested vaccine appeared to have contained infectious HBV. In terms of efficacy, there was a rather steep learning curve, with high efficacy for all trials since the mid-1980s. However, the number of animals involved in individual vaccine efficacy trials has been very limited, owing to the difficulty and high cost of keeping large numbers of chimpanzees. Some of the earlier trials that had used more than 40 animals reported failure rates of up to 25%. The current failure rate for HBV vaccine in humans is substantially lower (5–10%), which highlights the importance the chimpanzee has had in protecting humans at risk, or with chronic infection, with HBV.

The cost of producing the currently available vaccines has precluded generalized use in poor nations. There are recent promising reports for treatment of chronic HBV infection using DNA vaccines. This method is attractive because the response induces cytotoxic T lymphocyte (CTL) and antibody responses to the same level as the most successful subunit vaccines. All current vaccine trials have used small numbers of chimpanzees because it is so rare to have chronic chimpanzee carriers: most infected after birth spontaneously resolve infection with HBV ***(6)***. Davis et al. ***(69)*** used pre-S2 + S of ayw strain, with boost of S, adw subtype at 52 wk and demonstrated early high titers against pre-S2 domain (10-fold higher against M and S envelope proteins than those composed entirely of S), but did not subsequently challenge with HBV. The Pancholi et al. study ***(70)*** used a chimpanzee inoculated with HBV in 1985, with persistent positive serology for 12 yr, and injected first HBsAg-encoding plasmid, followed by boost with recombinant canarypox virus encoding HBsAg, preS-1, and pre-S2. There was a decline in HBV DNA coincident with increase in interferon-γ (IFN-γ)-secreting cells. The Sällberg et al. study ***(71)*** used three chimpanzees chronically infected with HBV, at least one of which almost certainly was infected with chHBV. The Sällberg group used a recombinant vector expressing HBC core antigen–neomycin phosphotransferase II fusion protein. Although two of the three animals showed no change in HBV viral load, the third animal developed antibodies to HBV core antigen and decreased HBV DNA levels. Further studies are required to develop a safe and effective vaccine with production costs that will be conducive to widespread use in the chronic carrier human population.

9. Potential Problems with the Chimpanzee Model

There are many unresolved issues raised by the review of the studies thus far performed using chimpanzees. The first is that the tests performed between 1969 and the mid-1980s to determine "susceptibility" of chimpanzees to infection with HBV were insensitive, and can safely be assumed to have produced many false-negative results, despite the fact that many included preinoculation serology, biopsy, and chemical analysis. Animals could have previously been exposed and yet been serologically negative, and there has been more than one report of transmission of HBV from serologically negative, but PCR positive, humans to chimpanzees ***(72)***. With the benefit of hindsight it would not be unrealistic to posit that infectious particles could have been recovered from serologically negative chimpanzees, had an organized effort been undertaken, or if universal archiving of biopsy and serum specimens had been applied. Another (troubling) possibility is that the animals could have been chronically infected in the wild with chHBV variants carrying mutations in the S region, as epitopes in this area mediate recognition of HBsAg in both humans and chimpanzees *(73)*. Such mutations have so far not been reported in chHBV, but we have only a minute sample of the existing chHBV diversity documented, as complete genomic sequences have been completed from only 11 chHBV sequences (**Table 4**). Such mutations are likely to be one reason for the failure, albeit small, of currently used vaccines. The existence of similar antigenic mutants in chimpanzees, because they manifest few to no clinical signs of infection, could have gone unnoticed. If a large number of chimpanzees had been previously exposed to HBV, or if the inocula contained a mixture of hepatotropic viruses, experimental reinoculation would have altered the course of infection *(14,55)*. Furthermore, rather than simply interfering, reinoculation could reactivate a latent infection as shown by Bock et al. *(74)*. Therefore, conclusions made about the course of infection with HBV in chimpanzees have been compromised by insensitive serologic studies, lack of archived serologic and pathologic specimens for reanalysis, and, most of all, generally limited duration of experimental follow-up.

A second issue regarding the value of the chimpanzee model relates to the applicability of the model data to human infection with HBV. Although infectivity of HBV is similar between chimpanzees and humans, the course of the infection in chimpanzees is milder than in humans, and vertical transmission, the major transmission in humans, in chimpanzees is rare; in addition, horizontal transmission seems clearly limited in captive chimpanzee populations *(6)*. The experimental conditions for inoculation of chimpanzees may not mirror those in which humans are infected, because humans may be infected repeatedly and with mixed hepatotropic viruses. When chimpanzees were simultaneously infected with HCV and HBV the result was a milder infection *(55)*, but also metachronous infections resulted in more significant infections *(14)*. This said, when infection with HBV occurs in a naive individual, both humans and chimpanzees exhibit a biphasic response *(75)*, and both phases are milder in chimpanzees. As can be seen in **Table 2,** substantially fewer chimpanzees (<5% in published studies) with chronic infections have been reported than in humans. This indicates that there are fundamental differences in immune response between humans and chimpanzees with regard to HBV.

A third problem is that the total number of chimpanzees infected has been too small to address the major public health risk associated with HBV, which is the number of chronic human carriers of the virus (approx 350 million) in the world. Even if one were able to identify all chronic chimpanzee carriers, the total is almost certainly too small to use for efficacy testing of all candidate therapeutic vaccines. Chimpanzees chronically infected with chHBV would probably have comparable responses as carriers for hHBV, based on the reports of vaccine efficacy in a small population of chimpanzee carriers that had almost certainly been infected with chHBV. However, it is not clear that the group of chronic carrier chimpanzees can be identified.

Table 4
Chimpanzee Hepatitis B Viruses (chHBV) for Which Complete Genome Sequence Information Exists

GenBank accession number	Chimpanzee subspecies	Facility	Authors	Virus name/ Serotype	Host alive or dead
DOOO22O	*P.t. verus*	London Zoo	Vaudin et al. ***(82)***	LSH Chimp K	Dead?
AF222322	*P.t. troglodytes*	CDC	Hu et al. ***(77)***	HBV CH109	Dead?
AF222323	*P.t. verus*	CDC	Hu et al. ***(77)***	HBV CH926	Dead?
AB032431	*P.t. verus*	Vilab Liberia	Takahashi et al. ***(78)***	HBV/E-ch195	Dead?
AB032432	*P.t. verus*	Vilab Liberia	Takahashi et al. ***(78)***	ChHBV-Ch256?	Dead
AB032433	*P.t. verus*	Vilab Liberia	Takahashi et al. ***(78)***	ChHBV-Ch258	Dead?
AF242585	*P.t. troglodytes*	Cameroun	MacDonald et al. ***(79)***	HBV Chimp 2	Alive
AF242586	*P.t. verus*	Univ of Edinburgh	MacDonald et al. ***(79)***	HBV Chimp4	Alive
AB046525	*P.t. troglodytes*	Gabon	Takahashi et al. ***(78)***	PttHBV Ch Bassi	Alive?
AF305327	*P.t. vellerosus*	Coulston Foundation	Hu et al. ***(25)***	ChHBV CB0376	Alive
AF305326	*P.t. verus*	Coulston Foundation		CB0031	Alive
AF305328	*P.t. troglodytes*	Coulston Foundation		CH116	Alive
AF305329	*P.t. verus*	Coulston Foundation		CH1435	Alive
AF305330	*P.t. verus*	Coulston Foundation		CH1436	Alive
AF498266	*P.t. schweinfurthii*	wild	Vartianan et al. ***(80)***	Chimp FG	Dead

The number of chimpanzees currently housed in U.S. facilities chronically infected with chHBV is at least eight; the number of chimpanzees chronically infected with hHBV is more difficult to determine because of the short follow-up of infected animals noted in **Table 2**.

Finally, ethical considerations have led many scientists to reconsider the use of chimpanzees for invasive biomedical research. The European Union has passed laws seriously limiting biomedical research on chimpanzees and other primates. The public acceptance for large-scale biomedical studies on chimpanzees is likely to be low in North America and Japan. In the United States several large facilities with captive chimpanzees have closed, and in 2000 Congress passed a "Chimpanzee Health Improvement, Maintenance, and Protection (CHIMP) Act," which permits "noninvasive behavioral studies of the chimpanzees, or medical studies conducted during the course of normal veterinary care that is provided for the benefit of the chimpanzees" ***(76)***. The use of the conjunction "or" indicates an acceptance that some studies that are not beneficial may be performed on chimpanzees.

10. Relevance of Distinct Chimpanzee HBV (chHBV) to the Chimpanzee as a Model for Human HBV Infection

Many investigators have explored the differences in genetic sequences of HBV to understand individual differences in viral handling. Since it had been recognized in the early 1970s that previous infections with HBV were at least potentially protective against reinfection, the presence of an endemic infection in the study population, in this case chimpanzees with chHBV, would be highly relevant to their use as a model for human disease. The discovery of chimpanzee HBV in 2000 gave a partial explanation for the large number of chimpanzees found to be serologically positive for HBV upon arrival to captivity. Two retrospective studies used banked sera from chimpanzees positive for HBsAg ***(77,78)*** and one study analyzed two wild-caught, orphaned chimpanzees ***(79)*** to document that chHBV is distinct from all forms of hHBV. Only one study looked at tissues from animals that died in the wild and found a distinct chHBV in an east African chimpanzee ***(80)***.

The first observed case of confirmed hepatitis B in captive chimpanzees was reported in 1978 when several animals of a London Zoo breeding group showed clinical symptoms ***(81)***. The virus responsible for this infection was sequenced in 1988 and its sequence was 10% divergent from that of any human HBV sequence ***(82)***. At the time it was thought to resemble African hHBV because its serotype was identical to adw1. However, based on abundant HBV sequence data, it is now apparent that serotypes do not strictly correspond to genotypes, which is why all recently described chHBV can share serotype adw, despite having divergent sequences. Two HBV with typical sequences for gibbon HBV were found in two different captive chimpanzees, both of serotype ayw, and both very likely to have been infected by gibbons in captivity ***(83,84)***. There are now 11 published sequences of the complete chHBV genome derived from chimpanzees (**Table 4**). These must represent a minimum of the HBV diversity existing in the wild chimpanzee populations.

These chHBV sequences have been used repeatedly to attempt reconstructing the phylogeny of primate HBV. Initial analysis of genomic sequences of various viral strains used only short sequences (usually parts of the S-gene), and did not take into account the frequent recombination occurring between HB viruses. A more recent analysis by Fares and Holmes ***(85)*** is based on total HBV genome sequence but excluded obviously recombinant sequences as well as all segments with overlapping reading frames for methodological reasons. While it is now clear that there are several specific chHBV strains, the precise history of direction of infection, human to nonhuman primates, or nonhuman primates to human, or complex combinations of both, cannot be clearly deduced. Thus a simple explanation for presence of hHBV in nonhuman primates by human to animal infection is not possible. The question arises whether some of the nonhuman primate species could represent reservoirs, whereas others may have been infected by another animal species (e.g., gibbons from orangutan, or vice versa). If chimpanzees are a reservoir, then this would beg the question why chHBV diversity appears so much more restricted than that of hHBV. The curious case of a very divergent HBV in woolly monkeys is puzzling and its relationship to the most divergent strain of hHBV, hHBV-F, is a total mystery. To our knowledge, 9 of 16 animals positive for wmHBV were housed in the same facility in a North American zoo ***(86)***. There are no prevalence studies in or near natural woolly monkey habitat and no neotropical primates have tested positive for HBV in any other facility. The existence of a unique strain of HBV combined with the lack of African strains in the New World is puzzling and raises questions about why "African" hHBV was not imported despite the forced movement of millions of humans during the slave trade.

Several factors may explain why we still lack a clear reconstruction of HBV evolution. The first is that HBV mutates under selection pressure, so the mutation rate is difficult to predict. This has been best demonstrated in humans who developed recurrent HBV after orthotopic liver transplantation and while receiving regular doses of anti-HBV-immunoglobulin. Ghany et al. ***(87)*** sequenced the HBV genome before and after transplantation and demonstrated a change in "a" determinant in 50% of those expressing subtype adw2 and of the "S" gene in 85% posttransplantation. Thus the mutation rate of hHBV is subject to strong fluctuations and this variable has yet to be incorporated into phylogenetic analyses. Second, there appear to be recombination hot-spots along the HBV genome. Bowyer and Sim ***(88)*** found in their analysis of 65 whole HBV genome sequences that at least 14 carry clear signs of recombination ***(89)***. They concluded that the HBV genome consists of alternating conserved and highly variable domains, with the core region apparently most involved in recombination. The persistence of HBV in the host genome long after the acute infection subsides undoubtedly provides ample opportunity for viral recombination during subsequent infections. It would be important to study the precise nature, number, and degree of variation of persistent HBV genomes in host cells of chronic carriers, as has been done for HIV ***(90)***.

We are left with several hypotheses to explain the origin of HBV, and the nature of the correct hypothesis is highly relevant to the adequacy of the use of the chimpanzee model for research on HBV. If one examines the nonoverlapping areas of genomes to minimize effects of functional constraints on sequence evolution, and assumes a constant mutation rate, it appears that HBV arose within the past 6000 yr and that, because of similarities between ape and human HBV, both groups were infected at approximately the same time. However, if one makes comparisons of complete genome sequences ***(91)*** using calculated mutation rates (based on intra-host HBV evolution), it appears that the virus may be ancient. In support of this is the observation that hHBV-F is found primarily in Polynesians and 70% of Amazon Indians ***(92)***, where different strains persist in geographically isolated populations. This indicates a more ancient divergence of human HBV (>15,000 yr) because of lack of substantial contact in intervening years. Alternatively, there could have been contact between Polynesia and the New World within the past 2000 yr. Another observation in favor of prolonged coevolution between HBV and its host is that there are geographic similarities of chHBV based on mt DNA sequence comparisons and HBV data ***(25)***; however, the generally higher genetic variability of chimpanzees as compared to humans is not reflected in the variability of their HBV. This latter point may be due to a strong bias in sample size for human viruses, leaving us with a strong underestimation of the real diversity of HBV in wild chimpanzees. The origin of HBV could be reconstructed if substitution rates were constant and recombination patterns known. To complicate matters further, the mutation rate of chHBV has not been calculated, and could differ from that of hHBV. Taken together, it is currently not possible to make a definitive statement about the origin of HBV because there are inconsistencies with both current theories. It is likely that HBV has a complex evolutionary history that may include recurrent cross-species infection between humans and apes, and periods of accelerated mutation rates in some of the host species. The consequences of the existence of chHBV for the use of the chimpanzee model for HBV infection cannot be safely determined at this point.

11. Differences in Host Genetics Between Chimpanzees and Humans

At the genomic level, humans and chimpanzees share more than 98% identity ***(93)***. Despite this high level of genetic similarity, chimpanzees have obvious phenotypic and significant functional differences, as exemplified by differing responses to HBV and other viruses. Recently, several groups have reported specific genetic differences between humans and chimpanzees. It is perhaps not surprising that several of the known genetic differences between humans and chimpanzees are connected to the immune system. It has been reported that the normal range of peripheral leukocytes in chimpanzees in captivity is 60% higher than in humans ***(94)***, but because the increase is in the number of polymorphonuclear leukocytes, this has not been considered to be the mechanism for differences in susceptibility to viral infections.

The primary host defense to viral infection is recognition of viruses by the major histocompatibility class (MHC) system. Although the functional orthologs in the MHC I genes of the human (HLA-A through G) have been described and found to be similar in chimpanzees ***(95,96)***, there are also notable differences. Chimpanzees have a much reduced repertoire of MHC I A alleles, lacking alleles falling into one of the two class I A lineages (based on exon 2 and 3 sequence data) ***(97–99)***. Furthermore, a recent study of intronic variation has demonstrated that chimpanzees must have undergone a selective sweep causing a marked reduction of gene repertoire at all three MHC Ia loci (A, B, and C) ***(100)***. Despite this loss of numerous ancient MHC I lineages and at least two MHC II lineages, chimpanzees still harbor more variation at exon 2 and 3 sequences (coding for the binding region of the molecule) of their class I B and C loci ***(101)***. Because the immediate response in both humans and chimpanzees is a strong, polyclonal CTL response to envelope, capsid, and polymerase proteins of HBV, and in humans this response has been shown to be restricted to certain HLA alleles (HLA-A2, HLA-A3, HLA-B7 supertypes), this difference may be important to the outcome of HBV infection.

Despite this observation, it has been shown that infection of two chimpanzees with HBV with a terminally redundant copy of the HBV genome transgenically expressed in mice resulted in acute but self-limited HBV infection with identical CTL responses as humans ***(100)***. In fact, one chimpanzee responded to HLA-A2 supertype-restricted CTL epitopes (Env 183–191 and 335–343) and Pol (575–583) regions. This indicates that chimpanzees can mount effective responses to HLA-A2 and HLA-B7 supertype epitopes. Studies of MHC recognition of HIV by chimpanzees and human nonprogressors have shown that MHC molecules recognizing identical HIV epitopes belonged to very different allele lineages ***(102)***. The lack of certain MHC lineages may be protective, as several viruses have been shown to exploit host MHC molecules for immune subversion (e.g., *nef* gene in HIV ***[103]***).

Perhaps more relevant to interaction of HBV, chimpanzees have a nonclassical MHC I gene *Patr-AL*, which is lacking in humans ***(104)***. The rapid evolution documented for the KIR (killing inhibitory receptors) genes of ape and human natural killer (NK) cells has generated unique sets of genes in chimpanzees and copy number polymorphisms in humans and chimpanzees ***(105)***. KIRs have lectin-like domains that may interact with carbohydrate moieties on MHC molecules of target cells. The inactivating mutation of the single copy gene for the sialic acid modifying enzyme CMP–*N*-acetylneuraminic acid hydroxylase (CMAH) uniquely in humans has caused a change in the terminal cell surface glycosylation of virtually every cell. Humans have been shown to lack a form of sialic acid (*N*-glycolylneuraminic acid) otherwise common in mammals including chimpanzees ***(106)***. The biological consequences of this loss of function mutation are still being investigated. One known consequence is a change in macrophage biology due to a dramatic change in ligand density for sialoadhesin (Siglec 1) ***(107)***. These results provide potential for differences in how the immune system deals with HBV and other infections.

Another human-specific loss of function mutation is found for the gene coding for Siglec-L1, which in humans has lost the capacity to bind to sialic acid, while it retains this capacity in chimpanzees ***(108)***. The existence of differences between chimpanzee and human immune systems must obviously be kept in mind when contemplating the further use of chimpanzees as models for human disease.

12. Viral Envelopes and Differences in Host Cell Surfaces Between Humans and Chimpanzees

HBV is an enveloped virus and thus viral particles carry large numbers of cell surface glycoconjugates: proteins or lipids decorated with carbohydrate chains (glycans). The vast majority of these glycans are capped by sialic acid molecules. Potential roles of sialic acids in natural immunity have been proposed ***(109)***. The potential role of glycosylation variants in vaccines has not been sufficiently addressed, especially with regard to the glycan structure and composition produced in different recombinant expression systems. Yeast, insect, and mammalian cells have drastically different *N*-glycans, and yeast high-mannose glycans have previously compromised vaccine design (as demonstrated by the failed vaccine attempt targeted at HIV gp120). Furthermore, it has been shown that blocking the assembly of *N*-glycans on S proteins of HBV leads to the retention of viruses inside the host cell and prevents viral replication cycles ***(110)***. Because *N*-glycolylneuraminic acid is known to be antigenic in humans but not in chimpanzees, its presence on vaccines may alter the antigenicity, and thus the effectiveness, of the vaccine in these two closely related species.

In this context, it is interesting that one inoculation attempt with woolly monkey HBV into chimpanzee produced only minimal infection ***(86)***. The enveloped HBV from the New World woolly monkey must have carried the strongly antigenic α Gal epitope. α 1–3 linked galactose (to another galactose) a structure that is completely absent in old world primates (Catarrhines). Old world primates combine the lack of this α Gal with high titers of natural antibody (IgG) against this carbohydrate epitope found in most other mammals, and it has been suggested that this forms an efficient barrier to infection by enveloped viruses from other species ***(111)***.

Unfortunately, the nature of the receptor(s) used by HBV remains elusive. Atkins et al. showed that glycosaminoglycans (proteoglycans) influence HBV liver and leukocyte interactions ***(112)***. Budkowska et al. ***(113)*** found a soluble HBV binding factor in human serum. It is a glycoprotein and binding can be decreased more than fourfold by coincubation with wheat germ agglutinin and *Helix pomatia* (*N*-acetyl-b-D-glucosamine and to *N*-acetylgalatosamine residues) but is not affected by incubation with peanut agglutinin (Galbeta1-3GalNAc) or concanavalin A (high mannose type glycans). It was purified after incubation of human serum with pre-S1 and pre-S2-specific monoclonal antibodies but demonstrates no binding to HBV S protein. The fact that this soluble protein interacts with pre-S epitopes is interesting because HBV appears to bind to cells via this region ***(114)***. However, as long as the receptor(s) used by HBV remain unknown, it is impossible to speculate on similarity of receptors in chimpanzees, or on the impact of the glycosylation differences on cell surfaces.

13. Conclusions

The chimpanzee model has been crucial for vaccine development and for improving safety of blood products. Despite the large amount of work carried out on HBV in chimpanzees and the impressive numbers of animals used for infection and vaccine work, we are left with a confusing picture of long-term effects of infection with human HBV in chimpanzees, and a nearly complete ignorance of the native chHBV infection in wild chimpanzee populations. Although chimpanzees were important in the development and testing of the currently used HBV vaccines, it is questionable whether chimpanzees will be of much help in the development of therapeutic DNA vaccines or drugs for treatment of chronic HBV infection. There is an urgent need for a concerted effort to identify the surviving chimpanzees chronically infected with hHBV or chHBV. Only a careful longitudinal study of this very small group of animals would allow determination of whether the chronic carrier state is really comparable between chimpanzees and humans. The small number of chimpanzees that develop chronic infection, in addition to ethical issues surrounding use of primates for research ***(115)***, make it likely that future studies will have to be carried out in naturally infected human populations.

Several other human viruses have been documented to have counterparts in wild chimpanzees, including HIV1/SIVcpz and HTLV1/STLV1, Ebola, TT, Spuma, Kaposi sarcoma herpes, and monkeypox viruses. Efforts are ongoing to document the epidemiology of these agents in wild ape populations in Africa. Concerted efforts to obtain good quality noninvasive samples from field research sites across Africa could provide valuable opportunities. Fecal samples, urine samples, and samples of chewed fruit ("wadges" containing saliva and many buccal cells) can easily be collected in large numbers at field sites where wild animals have been habituated to human observers (at least 10 such sites exist across Africa) and samples can be obtained even from nonhabituated populations (Gagneux, *personal experience*, ***116***). Considering the endangered status of most wild chimpanzee populations in Africa, which face human encroachment on their habitats, habitat destruction, and most of all growing hunting pressure by humans, it may very well be the last opportunity to document the epidemiology of such viruses in wild chimpanzee populations, and to relate this epidemiology to their human counterparts.

References

1. Deinhardt, F. (1976) Hepatitis in primates. *Adv. Virus Res.* **20,** 113–57.
2. Prince, A. M. (1972) Infection of chimpanzees with hepatitis B virus, in *Hepatitis and Blood Transfusion* (Vyas, G. N., Perkins, H. A., and Schmid, R. S., eds.) Grune and Stratton, New York.
3. Maynard, J. E., Berquist, K. R., and Krushak, D. H. (1972) Experimental infection of chimpanzees with the virus of hepatitis B. *Nature* **237,** 514–515.
4. Barker, L. F., Chisari, F. V., McGrath, P. P., et al. (1973) Transmission of type B viral hepatitis to chimpanzees. *J. Infect. Dis.* **127**, 648–662.
5. Desmyter, J., Liu, W. T., de Somer, P., and Mortelmans, J. (1973) Primates as model for human viral hepatitis: transmission of infection by human hepatitis B virus. *Vox Sang.* **24**, 17–26.
6. Prince, A. M., Goodall, J., Brotman, B., Dienske, H., and Schellekens, H., and Eichberg, J. W. (1989) Appropriate conditions for maintenance of chimpanzees in studies with bloodborne viruses: an epidemiologic and psychosocial perspective. *J. Med. Primatol.* **18**, 27–42.
7. Pancholi, P., Lee, D. H., Liu, Q., et al. (2001) DNA prime/canarypox boost-based immunotherapy of chronic hepatitis B virus infection in a chimpanzee. *Hepatology* **33,** 448–454.
8. Tabor, E. (1985) Chimpanzee model for the study of hepatitis B, in *Hepatitis B* (Gerety, R. J., ed.), Academic Press, Orlando, FL.
9. Karasawa, T., Shikata, T., Abe, K., Kondo, R., Noro, M., and Oda, T. (1985) Ultrastructural studies on liver cell necrosis and lymphocytes in experimental hepatitis B. *Acta Pathol. Jpn.* **35**, 1359–1374.
10. Karasawa, T., Shikata, T., Abe, K., Kanayama, S., Kondo, R., and Oda, T. (1985) Ultrastructural changes of the bile secretory apparatus and bile ductule in experimental hepatitis B with neither apparent biochemical nor light-microscopic cholestasis. *Acta Pathol. Jpn.* **35**, 1343–1358.

11. Karasawa, T., Shikata, T., Abe, K., Kanayama, S., Noro, M., and Oda, T. (1985) HBV-associated ultrastructures in the chimpanzees' livers with experimental hepatitis B. *Acta Pathol. Jpn.* **35**, 1333–1342.
12. Krawczynski, K., Prince, A. M., and Nowoslawski, A. (1979) Immunopathologic aspects of the HBsAg carrier state in chimpanzees. *J. Med. Primatol.* **8**, 222–232.
13. Shouval, D., Chakraborty, P. R., Ruiz-Opazo, N., et al. (1980) Chronic hepatitis in chimpanzee carriers of hepatitis B virus: morphologic, immunologic, and viral DNA studies. *Proc. Natl. Acad. Sci. USA* **77**, 6147–6151.
14. Dienes, H. P., Purcell, R. H., Popper, H., and Ponzetto, A. (1990) The significance of infections with two types of viral hepatitis demonstrated by histologic features in chimpanzees. *J. Hepatol.* **10**, 77–84.
15. Omata, M. (1990) Significance of extrahepatic replication of hepatitis B virus. *Hepatology* **12**, 364–366.
16. Lieberman, H. M., Tung, W. W., and Shafritz, D. A. (1987) Splenic replication of hepatitis B virus in the chimpanzee chronic carrier. *J. Med. Virol.* **21**, 347–359.
17. Penna, A., Artini, M., Cavalli, A., et al. (1996) Long-lasting memory T cell responses following self-limited acute hepatitis B. *J. Clin. Invest.* **98,** 1185–1194.
18. Tabor, E., Hsia, C. C., and Muchmore, E. (1996) Histochemical and immunohistochemical similarities between hepatic tumors in two chimpanzees and man. *J. Med. Primatol.* **23**, 271–279.
19. Millman, I., Loeb, L. A., Bayer, M. E., and Blumberg, B. S. (1970) Australia antigen (a hepatitis-associated antigen): purification and physical properties. *J. Exp. Med.* **131**, 1190–1199.
20. Smetana, H. F. and Felsenfeld, A. D. (1969) Viral hepatitis in subhuman primates and its relationship to human viral hepatitis. *Virchows Arch. A Pathol. Pathol. Anat.* **348**, 309–327.
21. Hillis, W. D. (1971) An outbreak of infectious hepatitis among chimpanzee handlers at a United States Air Force base. *Am. J. Hyg.* **73,** 316–328.
22. Deinhardt, F. (1976) Hepatitis in primates. *Adv. Virus Res.* **20,** 113–157.
23. Rivers, S. L. and Keeling, M. (1970) A study of the incidence of Australia antigen and antibody in nonhuman primates. *Vox Sang.* **19**, 270–272.
24. Morin, P. A., Moore, J. J., Chakraborty, R., Jin, L., Goodall, J., and Woodruff, D. S. (1994) Kin selection, social structure, gene flow, and the evolution of chimpanzees. *Science* **265**, 1193–1201.
25. Hu, X., Javadian, A, Gagneux, P., and Robertson, B. H. (2001) Paired chimpanzee hepatitis B virus (ChHBV) and mtDNA sequences suggest different ChHBV genetic variants are found in geographically distinct chimpanzee subspecies. *Virus Res.* **79**, 103–108.
26. Gagneux, P., Gonder, M. K., Goldberg TL, Morin PA. (2001) Gene flow in wild chimpanzee populations: what genetic data tell us about chimpanzee movement over space and time. *Philos. Trans. R. Soc. Lond. B Biol. Sci.* **356**, 889–897.
27. Rahm, U. (1967) Observations during chimpanzee captures in the Congo. In *Neue Ergebnisse der Primatologie-Progress in Primatology.* (Starck, D., Schneider, R., and Kuhn, H. J., eds.), Fischer, Stuttgart, pp. 195–207.
28. Krugman, S. (1971) Experiments at the Willowbrook State School. *Lancet* **1**, 966–967.
29. Barker, L. F., Maynard, J. E., Purcell, R. H., Hoofnagle, J. H., Berquist, K. R., and London, W. T. (1975) Viral hepatitis, type B, in experimental animals. *Am. J. Med. Sci.* **270**, 189–195.
30. Liang, T. J., Blum, H. E., and Wands, J. R. (1990) Characterization and biological properties of a hepatitis B virus isolated from a patient without hepatitis B virus serologic markers. *Hepatology* **2**, 204–212.

31. Chen, P. J., Chen, M. L., and Chen, D. S. (1994) A viral mechanism in acute exacerbations of chronic type B hepatitis: hepatitis B virus reinfection and subsequent reactivation of two viral strains. *J. Biomed. Sci.* **1**, 7–12.
32. Deinhardt, F., Courtois, G., Oberle, P., et al. (1962) Studies on liver function tests in chimpanzees after inoculation with infectious hepatitis virus. *Am. J. Hyg.* **75**, 311–321.
33. Ogata, N., Miller, R. H., Ishak, K. G., and Purcell, R. H. (1993) The complete nucleotide sequence of a pre-core mutant of hepatitis B virus implicated in fulminant hepatitis and its biological characterization in chimpanzees. *Virology* **194**, 263–276.
34. Lanford, R. E., Bigger, C., Bassett, S., and Klimpel, G. (2001) The chimpanzee model of hepatitis C virus infections. *ILAR J.* **42**, 117–126.
35. Tabor, E., Aronson, D. L., and Gerety, R. J. (1980) Removal of hepatitis-B-virus infectivity from factor-IX complex by hepatitis-B immune-globulin. Experiments in chimpanzees. *Lancet* **2**, 68–70.
36. Brummelhuis, H. G., Over, J., Duivis-Vorst, C. C., et al. (1983) Contributions to the optimal use of human blood. IX. Elimination of hepatitis B transmission by (potentially) infectious plasma derivatives. *Vox Sang.* **45**, 205–216.
37. Stephan, W., Berthold, H., and Prince, A. M. (1981) Effect of combined treatment of serum containing hepatitis B virus with beta-propiolactone and ultraviolet irradiation. *Vox Sang.* **41**, 134–138.
38. Tabor, E., Buynak, E., Smallwood, L. A., Snoy, P., Hilleman, M., and Gerety, R. J. (1983) Inactivation of hepatitis B virus by three methods: treatment with pepsin, urea, or formalin. *J. Med. Virol.* **11**, 1–9.
39. Vnek, J., Prince, A. M., Hashimoto, N., and Ikram, H. (1978) Association of normal serum protein antigens with chimpanzee hepatitis B surface antigen particles. *J. Med. Virol.* **2**, 319–333.
40. Prince, A. M., Stephan, W., Kotitschke, R., and Brotman, B. (1983) Inactivation of hepatitis B and non-A, non-B viruses by combined use of Tween 80, beta-propiolactone, and ultraviolet irradiation. *Thromb. Haemost.* **50**, 534–536.
41. Prince, A. M., Stephan, W., and Brotman, B. (1983) Beta-propiolactone/ultraviolet irradiation: a review of its effectiveness for inactivation of viruses in blood derivatives. *Rev. Infect. Dis.* **5**, 92–107.
42. Feinstone, S. M., Mihalik, K. B., Kamimura, T., Alter, H. J., London, W. T., and Purcell, R. H. (1983) Inactivation of hepatitis B virus and non-A, non-B hepatitis by chloroform. *Infect. Immun.* **41**, 816–821.
43. Prince, A. M., Horowitz, B., Brotman, B., Huima, T., Richardson, L., and van den Ende, M. C. (1984) Inactivation of hepatitis B and Hutchinson strain non-A, non-B hepatitis viruses by exposure to Tween 80 and ether. *Vox Sang.* **46**, 36–43.
44. Kobayashi, H., Tsuzuki, M., Koshimizu, K., et al. (1984) Susceptibility of hepatitis B virus to disinfectants or heat. *J. Clin. Microbiol.* **20**, 214–216.
45. Hollinger, F. B., Dolana, G., Thomas, W., and Gyorkey, F. (1984) Reduction in risk of hepatitis transmission by heat-treatment of a human factor VIII concentrate. *J. Infect. Dis.* **150**, 250–262.
46. Purcell, R. H., Gerin, J. L., Popper, H., et al. (1985) Hepatitis B virus, hepatitis non-A, non-B virus and hepatitis delta virus in lyophilized antihemophilic factor: relative sensitivity to heat. *Hepatology* **5**, 1091–1099.
47. Lelie, P. N., Reesink, H. W., Niessen, J., Brotman, B., and Prince, A. M. (1987) Inactivation of 10(15) chimpanzee-infectious doses of hepatitis B virus during preparation of a heat-inactivated hepatitis B vaccine. *J. Med. Virol.* **23**, 289–295.

48. Zolton, R. P., Padvelskis, J. V., and Kaplan, P. M. (1985) Removal of hepatitis B virus infectivity from human gamma-globulin prepared by ion-exchange chromatography. *Vox Sang.* **49**, 381–389.
49. Alter, H. J., Creagan, R. P., Morel, P. A., et al. (1988) Photochemical decontamination of blood components containing hepatitis B and non-A, non-B virus. *Lancet* **2**, 1446–1450.
50. Prince, D. L., Prince, H. N., Thraenhart, O., Muchmore, E., Bonder, E., and Pugh, J. (1993) Methodological approaches to disinfection of human hepatitis B virus. *J. Clin. Microbiol.* **31**, 3296–3304.
51. Maynard, J. E., Krushak, D. H., Bradley, D. W., and Berquist, K. R. (1975) Infectivity studies of hepatitis A and B in non-human primates. *Dev. Biol. Stand.* **30**, 229–235.
52. Krugman, S. (1975) Viral hepatitis type B: prospects for active immunization. *Am. J. Med. Sci.* **270**, 391–393.
53. Drucker, J., Tabor, E., Gerety, R. J., Jackson, D., and Barker L. F. (1979) Simultaneous acute infections with hepatitis A and hepatitis B virus viruses in a chimpanzee. *J. Infect. Dis.* **139**, 338–342.
54. Bradley, D. W., Maynard, J. E., McCaustland, K. A., Murphy, B. L., Cook, E. H., and Ebert, J. W. (1983) Non-A, non-B hepatitis in chimpanzees: interference with acute hepatitis A virus and chronic hepatitis B virus infections. *J. Med. Virol.* **11**, 207–213.
55. Brotman, B., Prince, A. M., Huima, T., Richardson, L., van den Ende, M. C., and Pfeifer, U. (1983) Interference between non-A, non-B and hepatitis B virus infection in chimpanzees. *J. Med. Virol.* **11**, 191–205.
56. Kos, T., Molijn, A., van Doorn, L. J., van Belkum, A., Dubbeld, M., and Schellekens, H. (1991) Hepatitis delta virus cDNA sequence from an acutely HBV-infected chimpanzee: sequence conservation in experimental animals. *J. Med. Virol.* **34**, 268–279.
57. Wilson, S. and Logan, L. M. (1975) Hepatitis B core antigen in the immunosuppressed chimpanzee. *Dev. Biol. Stand.* **30**, 240–243.
58. Trepo, C., Vnek, J., and Prince, A. M. (1975) Delayed hypersensitivity and Arthus reaction to purified hepatitis B surface antigen (HBsAg) in immunized chimpanzees. *Clin. Immunol. Immunopathol.* **4**, 528–537.
59. Negro, F., Shapiro, M., Satterfield, W. C., Gerin, J. L., and Purcell, R. H. (1989) Reappearance of hepatitis D virus (HDV) replication in chronic hepatitis B virus carrier chimpanzees rechallenged with HDV. *J. Infect. Dis.* **160**, 567–571.
60. Ruiz-Opazo, N., Chakraborty, P. R., and Shafritz, D. A. (1982) Characterization of viral genomes in the liver and serum of chimpanzee long-term hepatitis B virus carriers: a possible role for supercoiled HBV-DNA in persistent HBV infection. *J. Cell. Biochem.* **19**, 281–292.
61. Abe, K., Kagei, N., Teramura, Y., and Ejima, H.(1993) Hepatocellular carcinoma associated with chronic *Schistosoma mansoni* infection in a chimpanzee. *J. Med. Primatol.* **22**, 237–239.
62. Lubeck, M. D., Davis, A. R., Chengalvala, M., et al. (1989) Immunogenicity and efficacy testing in chimpanzees of an oral hepatitis B vaccine based on live recombinant adenovirus. *Proc. Natl. Acad. Sci. USA* **86**, 6763–6767.
63. Fujisawa, Y., Kuroda, S., Van Eerd, P. A. C. M., Schellekens, H., and Kakinuma, A. (1990) Protective efficacy of a novel hepatitis B vaccine consisting of M (pre S2+S) protein particles (a third generation vaccine). *Vaccine* **8**, 192–198.
64. Purcell, R. H., Gerin, J. L. (1975) Hepatitis B subunit vaccine: a preliminary report of safety and efficacy tests in chimpanzees. *Am. J. Med. Sci.* **270**, 395–399.
65. Purcell, R. H., London, W. T., McAuliffe, V. J., et al. (1976) Modification of chronic hepatitis-B virus infection in chimpanzees by administration of an interferon inducer. *Lancet* **2**, 757–761.

66. Hilleman, M.R., Buynak, E.B., Roehm, R.R., et al.(1975) Purified and inactivated human hepatitis B vaccine: progress report. *Am. J. Med. Sci.* **270**, 401–404.
67. Gerety, R.J., Tabor, E., Purcell R.H., and Tyeryar, F.J. (1979) Summary of an international workshop on hepatitis B vaccines. *J. Infect. Dis.* **140**, 642–648.
68. Iwarson, S., Tabor, E., Thomas, H.C., et al. (1985) Neutralization of hepatitis B virus infectivity by a murine monoclonal antibody: an experimental study in the chimpanzee. *J. Med. Virol.* **16**, 89–96.
69. Davis, H.L., McCluskie, M.J., Gerin, J.L., and Purcell, R.H. (1996) DNA vaccine for hepatitis B: evidence for immunogenicity in chimpanzees and comparison with other vaccines. *Proc. Natl. Acad. Sci. USA* **93**, 7213–7218.
70. Pancholi, P., Lee, D.H., Liu, Q., et al. (2001) DNA prime/canarypox boost-based immunotherapy of chronic hepatitis B virus infection in a chimpanzee. *Hepatology* **33**, 448–454.
71. Sällberg, M., Hughes, J., Javadian, A., et al. (1998) Genetic immunization of chimpanzees chronically infected with the hepatitis B virus, using a recombinant retroviral vector encoding the hepatitis B virus core antigen. *Hum. Gene Ther.* **9**, 1719–1729.
72. Prince, A.M., Lee, D.H., and Brotman, B. (2001) Infectivity of blood from PCR-positive, HBsAg-negative, anti-HBs-positive cases of resolved hepatitis B infection. *Transfusion* (3), 329–332.
73. Kremsdorf, D., Garreau, F., Duclos, H., et al. (1993) Complete nucleotide sequence and viral envelope protein expression of a hepatitis B virus DNA derived from a hepatitis B surface antigen-seronegative patient. *J. Hepatol.* **18**, 244–250.
74. Bock, C-T., Tillman, H.L., Maschek, H-J., Manns, M.P., and Trautwein, C. (1982) A PreS mutation isolated from a patient with chronic hepatitis B infection leads to virus retention and misassembly. *Gastroenterology* **113**, 1996–1982.
75. Shikata, T., Karasawa, T., and Abe, K. (1980) Two distinct types of hepatitis in experimental hepatitis B virus infection. *Am. J. Pathol.* **99**, 353–363.
76. Federal News Service, (2000) Hearing of the Health and Environment Subcommittee of the House Commerce Committee: Chimpanzees and Biomedical Research, chaired by Rep. Michael Bilirakis (18 May).
77. Hu, X., Margolis, H.S., Purcell, R.H., Ebert, J., and Robertson, B.H. (2000) Identification of hepatitis B virus indigenous to chimpanzees. *Proc. Natl. Acad. Sci. USA* **97**, 1661–1664.
78. Takahashi, K., Brotman, B., Usuda, S., Mishiro, S., and Prince, A.M. (2000) Full-genome sequence analyses of hepatitis B virus (HBV) strains recovered from chimpanzees infected in the wild: implications for an origin of HBV. *Virology* **267**, 58–64.
79. MacDonald, D.M., Holmes, E.C., Lewis, J.C., and Simmonds, P. (2000) Detection of hepatitis B virus infection in wild-born chimpanzees (*Pan troglodytes verus*): phylogenetic relationships with human and other primate genotypes. *J. Virol.* **74**, 4253–4257.
80. Vartanian, J-P., Pineau, P., Henry, M., et al. (2002) Identification of a hepatitis B virus genome in wild chimpanzees (Pan troglodytes schweinfurth:) from East Africa indicates a wide geographical dispersion among equatorial African primates. *J. Virol.* **76**, 11, 155–11,158.
81. Zuckerman, A.J., Thornton, A., Howard, C.R., Tsiquaye, K.N., Jones, D.M., and Brambell, M.R. (1978) Hepatitis B outbreak among chimpanzees at the London Zoo. *Lancet* **2**, 652–654.
82. Vaudin, M., Wolstenholme, A.J., Tsiquaye, K.N., Zuckerman, A.J., and Harrison, T.J. (1989) The complete nucleotide sequence of the genome of a hepatitis B virus isolated from a naturally infected chimpanzee. *J. Gen. Virol.* **69**, 1383–1389.

83. Grethe, S., Heckel, J. O., Rietschel, W., and Hufert, F. T. (2000) Molecular epidemiology of hepatitis B virus variants in nonhuman primates. *J. Virol.* **74**, 5377–5381.
84. Norder, H., Ebert, J. W., Fields, H. A., Mushahwar, I. K., and Magnius, L. O. (1996) Complete sequencing of a gibbon hepatitis B virus genome reveals a unique genotype distantly related to the chimpanzee hepatitis B virus. *Virology* **218**, 214–223.
85. Fares, M. A., and Holmes, E. C. (2002) A revised evolutionary history of hepatitis B virus (HBV) *J. Mol. Evol.* **54**, 807–814.
86. Lanford, R. E., Chavez, D., Brasky, K. M., Burns, R. B. 3rd, and Rico-Hesse, R. (1998) Isolation of a hepadnavirus from the woolly monkey, a New World primate. *Proc. Natl. Acad. Sci. USA* **95**, 5757–5761.
87. Ghany, M. G., Ayola, B., Villamil, F. G., et al. (1998) Hepatitis B virus S mutants in liver transplant recipients who were reinfected despite hepatitis B immune globulin prophylaxis. *Hepatology* **27**, 213–222.
88. Bowyer, S. M., and Sim, J. G. (2000) Relationships within and between genotypes of hepatitis B virus at points across the genome: footprints of recombination in certain isolates. *J. Gen. Virol.* **81**(Pt 2), 379–392.
89. Hannoun, C., Norder, H., and Lindh, M.(2000) An aberrant genotype revealed in recombinant hepatitis B virus strains from Vietnam. *J. Gen. Virol.* **81**(Pt 9), 2267–2272.
90. Kils-Hutten, L., Cheynier, R., Wain-Hobson, S., and Meyerhans, A. (2001) Phylogenetic reconstruction of intrapatient evolution of human immunodeficiency virus type 1: predominance of drift and purifying selection. *J. Gen. Virol.* **82**(Pt 7), 1621–1627.
91. Bollyky, P. L. and Holmes, E. C. (1999) Reconstructing the complex evolutionary history of hepatitis B virus. *J. Mol. Evol.* **49**, 130–141.
92. Sibley, C. G., and Ahlquist, J. E. (1984) The phylogeny of the hominoid primates, as indicated by DNA–DNA hybridization. *J. Mol. Evol.* **20**, 2–15.
93. Chen, F. C., and Li, W. H. (2001) Genomic divergences between humans and other hominoids and the effective population size of the common ancestor of humans and chimpanzees. *Am. J. Hum. Genet.* **68**, 444–456.
94. Hodson, H. H., Jr., Lee, B. D., Wisecup, W. G., and Fineg, J. (1967) Baseline blood values of the chimpanzee. I. The relationship of age and sex and hematological values. *Folia Primatol. (Basel)* **7**, 1–11.
95. Adams, E. J., and Parham, P. (2001) Species-specific evolution of MHC class I genes in the higher primates. *Immunol. Rev.* **183**, 41–64.
96. Adams, E. J., Cooper, S., Thomson, G., and Parham, P. (2000) Common chimpanzees have greater diversity than humans at two of the three highly polymorphic MHC class I genes. *Immunogenetics* **51**, 410–424.
97. McAdam, S. N., Boyson, J. E., Liu, X., et al. (1995) Chimpanzee MHC class I A locus alleles are related to only one of the six families of human A locus alleles. *J. Immunol.* **154**, 6421–6429.
98. de Groot, N. G., Otting, N., Arguello, R., et al. (2000) Major histocompatibility complex class I diversity in a West African chimpanzee population: implications for HIV research. *Immunogenetics* **51**, 398–409.
99. de Groot, N. G., Otting, N., Doxiadis, G. G. M., et al. (2002) An ancient selective sweep in the MHC class I gene repertoire of chimpanzees. *Proc. Natl. Acad. Sci. USA* **99**, 11748–11753.
100. Bertoni, R., Sette, A., Sidney, J., et al. (1998) Human class I supertypes and CTL repertoires extend to chimpanzees. *J. Immunol.* **161**, 4447–4455.
101. Bontrop, R. E., Otting, N., de Groot, N. G., and Doxiadis, G. G. (1999) Major histocompatibility complex class II polymorphisms in primates. *Immunol Rev.* **167**, 339–350.

102. Balla-Jhagjhoorsingh, S. S., Koopman, G., Mooij, P., et al. (1999) Conserved CTL epitopes shared between HIV-infected human long-term survivors and chimpanzees. *J. Immunol.* **162**, 2308–2314.
103. Andrieu, M., Chassin, D., Desoutter, J. F., et al. (2001) Downregulation of major histocompatibility class I on human dendritic cells by HIV Nef impairs antigen presentation to HIV-specific CD8+ T lymphocytes. *AIDS Res. Hum. Retroviruses* **17**, 1365–1370.
104. Adams E.J., Cooper, S., and Parham, P. (2001) A novel, nonclassical MHC class I molecule specific to the common chimpanzee. *J. Immunol.* **167**, 3858–3869.
105. Khakoo, S. I., Rajalingam, R., Shum, B. P., et al. (2000) Rapid evolution of NK cell receptor systems demonstrated by comparison of chimpanzees and humans. *Immunity* **12**, 687–698.
106. Muchmore, E. A., Diaz, S., and Varki, A. (1998) A structural difference between the cell surfaces of humans and the great apes. *Am. J. Phys. Anthropol.* **107**, 187–198.
107. Brinkman-Van der Linden, E. C., Sjoberg, E. R., Juneja, L. R., Crocker, P. R., Varki, N., and Varki, A. (2000) Loss of *N*-glycolylneuraminic acid in human evolution. Implications for sialic acid recognition by siglecs. *J. Biol. Chem.* **275**, 8633–8640.
108. Angata, T., Varki, N. M., and Varki, A. (2001) A second uniquely human mutation affecting sialic acid biology. *J. Biol. Chem.* **276**, 40282–40287.
109. Crocker, P. R. and Varki, A. (2001) Siglecs in the immune system. *Immunology* **103**, 137–145.
110. Mehta, A., Block, T. M., and Dwek, R. A. (1998) The role of *N*-linked glycosylation in the secretion of hepatitis B virus. *Adv. Exp. Med. Biol.* **435**, 195–205.
111. Rother, R. P. and Galili, U. (1999) Alpha-Gal epitopes on viral glycoproteins. *Subcell. Biochem.* **32**, 143–172.
112. Atkins, G. J., Qiao, M., Coombe, D. R., Gowans, E. J., and Ashman, L. K. (1997) Hepatitis B virus binding to leucocyte plasma membranes utilizes a different region of the preS1 domain to the hepatocyte receptor binding site and does not require receptors for opsonins. *Immunol. Cell Biol.* **75**, 259–266.
113. Budkowska, A., Quan, C., Groh, F., et al. (1993) Hepatitis B virus (HBV) binding factor in human serum: candidate for a soluble form of hepatocyte HBV receptor. *J. Virol.* **67**, 4316–4322.
114. Neurath, A. R., Kent, S. B., Strick, N., and Parker, K.(1986) Identification and chemical synthesis of a host cell receptor binding site on hepatitis B virus. *Cell* **46**, 429–436.
115. Check, E. (2002) Bank wants money back from troubled chimp facility. *Nature* **415**, 248.
116. Santiago, M. L., Rodenburg, C. M., Kamenya, S., et al. (2002) SIVcpz in wild chimpanzees. *Science* **295**, 465.
117. Lichter, E. A. (1969) Chimpanzee antibodies to Australia antigen. *Nature* **224**, 810–811
118. Maynard, J. E., Hartwell, W. V., and Berquist, K. R. (1971) Hepatitis-associated antigen in chimpanzees. *J. Infect. Dis.* **123**, 660–664.
119. Lander, H. J., Holland, P. V., Alter, H. J., Chanock, R. M., and Purcell, R. H. (1972) Antibody to hepatitis-associated antigen. Frequency and pattern of response as detected by radioimmunoprecipitation. *JAMA* **220**, 1079–1082.
120. Eichberg, J. W. and Kalter, S. S. (1980) Hepatitis A and B: serologic survey of human and nonhuman primate sera. *Lab. Anim. Sci.* **30**, 541–543.
121. Murphy, B. L., Maynard, J. E., and Le Bouvier, G. L. (1974) Viral subtypes and cross-protection in hepatitis B virus infections of chimpanzees. *Intervirology* **3**, 378–81
122. Bradley, D. W., Maynard, J. E., Berquist, K. R., and Krushak, D. H. (1974) Hepatitis B and serum DNA polymerase activities in chimpanzees. *Nature* **251**, 356–357.

123. Markenson, J. A., Gerety, R. J., Hoofnagle, J. H., and Barker, L. F. (1975) Effects of cyclophosphamide on hepatitis B virus infection and challenge in chimpanzees. *J. Infect. Dis.* **131**, 79–87.
124. Berquist, K. R., Peterson, J. M., Murphy, B. L., Ebert, J. W., Maynard, J. E., and Purcell, R. H. (1975) Hepatitis B antigens in serum and liver of chimpanzees acutely infected with hepatitis B virus. *Infect. Immun.* **12**, 602–605.
125. Alter, H. J., Purcell, R. H., Gerin, J. L., et al. (1977) Transmission of hepatitis B to chimpanzees by hepatitis B surface antigen-positive saliva and semen. *Infect. Immun.* **16**, 928–933.
126. Shikata, T., Karasawa, T., Abe, K., et al. (1977) Hepatitis B e antigen and infectivity of hepatitis B virus. *J. Infect. Dis.* **136**, 571–576.
127. Tabor, E., Gerety, R. J., Barker, L. F., Howard, C. R., and Zuckerman, A. J. (1978) Effect of ethanol during hepatitis B virus infection in chimpanzees. *J. Med. Virol.* **2**, 295–303.
128. Ling, C. M., Mushahwar, I. K., Overby, L. R., Berquist, K. R., Maynard, J. E. (1979) Hepatitis B e-antigen and its correlation with other serological markers in chimpanzees. *Infect. Immun.* **24**, 352–356.
129. Sly, D. L., London, W. T., and Purcell, R. H. (1979) Illness in a chimpanzee inoculated with hepatitis B virus. *J. Am. Vet. Med. Assoc.* **175**, 987–988.
130. Takahashi, K., Miyakawa, Y., Gotanda, T., Mishiro, S., Imai, M., and Mayumi, M. (1979) Shift from free "small" hepatitis B e antigen to IgG-bound "large" form in the circulation of human beings and a chimpanzee acutely infected with hepatitis B virus. *Gastroenterology* **77**, 1193–1199
131. Tabor, E., Frosner, G., Deinhardt, F., and Gerety, R. J. (1980) Hepatitis B e antigen and antibody: detection by radioimmunoassay in chimpanzees during experimental hepatitis *Br. J. Med. Virol.* **6**, 91–99
132. Bond, W.W., Peterson, N. J., Favero, M. S., Ebert, J. W., Maynard, J. E. (1982) Transmission of type B viral hepatitis via eye inoculation of a chimpanzee. *J. Clin. Microbiol.* **15**, 533–534.
133. Will, H., Darai, G., Deinhardt, F., Schellekens, H., and Schaller, H. (1983) Hepatitis B after infection of a chimpanzee with cloned HBV DNA. *Dev. Biol. Stand.* **54**, 131–133.
134. Will, H., Cattaneo, R., Darai, G., Deinhardt, F., Schellekens, H., and Schaller, H. (1985) Infectious hepatitis B virus from cloned DNA of known nucleotide sequence. *Proc. Natl. Acad. Sci. USA* **82**, 891–895.
135. Wands, J. R., Fujita, Y. K., Isselbacher, K. J., et al. (1986) Identification and transmission of hepatitis B virus-related variants. *Proc. Natl. Acad. Sci. USA* **83**, 6608–6612
136. Acs, G., Sells, M. A., Purcell, R. H., et al. (1987) Hepatitis B virusvirus produced by transfected Hep G2 cells causes hepatitis in chimpanzees. *Proc. Natl. Acad. Sci. USA* **84**, 4641–4644.
137. Sureau, C., Eichberg, J. W., Hubbard, G. B., Romet-Lemonne, J. L., and Essex, M. (1988) A molecularly cloned hepatitis B virus produced in vitro is infectious in a chimpanzee. *J. Virol.* **62**, 3064–3067.
138. Thiers, V., Nakajima, E., Kremsdorf, D., et al. (1988) Transmission of hepatitis B from hepatitis-B-seronegative subjects. *Lancet* **2**, 1273–1276.
139. Shih, C., Yu, M. Y., Li, L. S., and Shih, J. W. (1990) Hepatitis B virus propagated in a rat hepatoma cell line is infectious in a primate model. *Virology* **179**, 871–873.
140. Ogata, N., Zanetti, A. R., Yu, M., Miller, R. H., and Purcell, R. H. (1997) Infectivity and pathogenicity in chimpanzees of a surface gene mutant of hepatitis B virus that emerged in a vaccinated infant. *J. Infect. Dis.* **175**, 511–523

141. Ibrahim, A. B., Vyas, G. N., and Prince, A. M. (1974) Studies on delayed hypersensitivity to hepatitis B antigen in chimpanzees. *Clin. Exp. Immunol.* **17**, 311–318.
142. Buynak, E. B., Roehm, R. R., Tytell, A. A., Bertland, A. U, 2nd, Lampson, G. P., and Hilleman, M. R.(1976) Vaccine against human hepatitis B. *JAMA* **235**, 2832–2834.
143. Hollinger, F. B., Gitnick, G. L., Aach, R. D., et al. (1978) Non-A, non-B hepatitis transmission in chimpanzees: a project of the transfusion-transmitted viruses study group. *Intervirology* **10**, 60–68.
144. Prince, A. M. (1977) Prevention of hepatitis B infections by passive immunization. *Ric. Clin. Lab.* **7**, 198–208.
145. Hilleman, M. R., Provost, P. J., Villarejos, V. M., et al. Infectious hepatitis (hepatitis A) research in nonhuman primates. *Bull. Pan Am. Health Org.* **11**, 140–152.
146. Purcell, R. H. and Gerin, J. L. (1978) Hepatitis B vaccines. On the threshold. *Am. J. Clin. Pathol.* **70**(1 Suppl), 159–169.
147. Prince, A. M., Ikram, H., and Hopp, T. P. (1982) Hepatitis B virus vaccine: identification of HBsAg/a and HBsAg/d but not HBsAg/y subtype antigenic determinants on a synthetic immunogenic peptide. *Proc. Natl. Acad. Sci. USA* **79**, 579–583.
148. Prince, A. M., Vnek, J., and Stephan, W. (1983) A new hepatitis B vaccine containing HBeAg in addition to HBsAg. *Dev. Biol. Stand.* **54**, 13–22.
149. Karasawa, T., Shikata, T., Abe, K., et al. (1983) Efficacy of hepatitis B vaccine in chimpanzees given transfusions of highly infective blood. *J. Infect. Dis.* **147**, 327–335.
150. Tabor, E., Purcell, R. H., and Gerety, R. J.(1983) Primate animal models and titered inocula for the study of human hepatitis A, hepatitis B, and non-A, non-B hepatitis. *J. Med. Primatol.* **12**, 305–318.
151. Berthelot, P., Courouce, A. M., Eyquem, A., et al. (1984) Hepatitis B vaccine safety monitoring in the chimpanzee: interpretation of results. *J. Med. Primatol.* **13**, 119–133.
152. Moss, B., Smith, G. L., Gerin, J. L., and Purcell, R. H. (1984) Live recombinant vaccinia virus protects chimpanzees against hepatitis B. *Nature* **311**, 67–69.
153. Stephan, W., Prince, A. M., and Brotman, B. (1984) Modulation of hepatitis B infection by intravenous application of an immunoglobulin preparation that contains antibodies to hepatitis B e and core antigens but not to hepatitis B surface antigen. *J. Virol.* **51**, 420–424.
154. Ohmura, T., Ohmizu, A., Sumi, A., et al. (1987) Properties of recombinant hepatitis B vaccine. *Biochem. Biophys. Res. Commun.* **149**, 1172–1178.
155. Bitter, G. A., Egan, K. M., Burnette, W. N., et al. (1988) Hepatitis B vaccine produced in yeast. *J. Med. Virol.* **25**, 123–140.
156. Prince, A. M., Whalen, R., and Brotman, B. (1997) Successful nucleic acid based immunization of newborn chimpanzees against hepatitis B virus. *Vaccine* **15**, 916–919.
157. Pride, M. W., Bailey, C. R., Muchmore, E., and Thanavala, Y. (1998) Evaluation of B and T-cell responses in chimpanzees immunized with Hepagene, a hepatitis B vaccine containing pre-S1, pre-S2 gene products. *Vaccine* **16**, 543–550.

25

Hepatitis B in Liver Transplant Recipients as a Special Model of Antiviral Drug Development

Robert G. Gish and Adil Wakil

1. Introduction

Treatment of patients before and after liver transplantation diagnosed with chronic hepatitis B virus (HBV) infection represents a special model of treatment with antiviral therapy that has important implications for individuals involved in drug development and designing clinical trials. The high rate of graft infection and early graft failure shortly after orthotopic liver transplantation (OLT), as well as frequent patient death, led to restricted use or abandonment in the early 1990s of OLT for chronic hepatitis B virus (HBV). Marked improvements in long-term survival in the mid-1990s resulted from the use of low-dose immunosuppressive therapy and administration first of short-term and then of long-term (indefinite) hepatitis B immune globulin (HBIG) after OLT with the subsequent introduction of nucleoside therapy both before and after OLT (**Fig. 1**) ***(1–15)***. Graft infection is proportional to the serum level of HBV DNA (replication), type of liver failure (fulminant versus chronic) and presence of hepatitis delta virus (HDV) infection before transplantation (**Fig. 2**). Also, for maximum efficacy, HBIG injections require a strict compliance with measurable serum titers of anti-HBs. It is important to recognize not only that HBIG is a polyclonal antibody preparation initially derived from blood donors who have been exposed to and cleared HBV infection, but also that HBIG was designed to prevent *de novo* infection in individuals exposed to HBV in high-risk settings. In the case of liver transplantation, HBIG binds circulating virus and presumably prevents infection of the hepatocytes in the new graft and may prevent interhepatocyte viral transfer as well.

It is important to understand that the immune system in cirrhotic patients and liver transplant recipients is abnormal with evidence of cellular and immune dysfunction ***(16,16–20)***. Patients with cirrhosis as well as liver transplant recipients have an increased risk of bacterial and viral infections and may not mount a fever in response to infectious problems. The immune system after solid organ transplantation is also abnor-

From: *Methods in Molecular Medicine, vol. 96: Hepatitis B and D Protocols, volume 2*
Edited by: R. K. Hamatake and J. Y. N. Lau © Humana Press Inc., Totowa, NJ

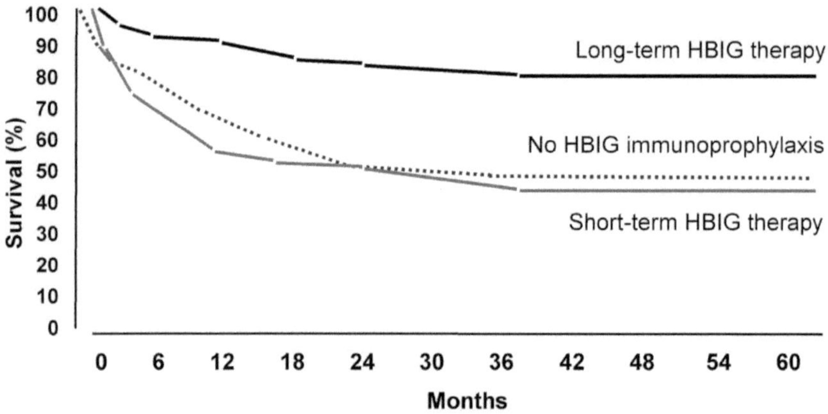

Fig. 1. Survival of patients treated without and with hepatitis B immune globulin (HBIG) therapy after liver transplantation. (Adapted from ref. ***10***.)

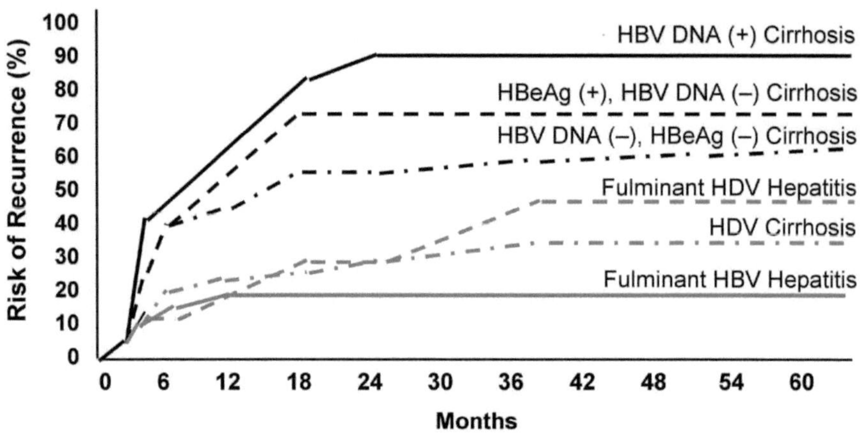

Fig. 2. Risk of recurrence of hepatitis B virus (HBV) after liver transplantation depending on viral status before transplant. HDV, Hepatitis D virus; HBeAg, hepatitis B envelope antigen, (+), positive; (–), negative. (Adapted from ref. ***10***.)

mal due to the introduction of immunosuppressive therapy ***(21,22)***. Both of these milieus provide a favorable host for chronic HBV infection and decrease the chance of clearing or curing the disease due either to high levels of viral replication or to lack of response (or risks) to administration of medication such as interferon. The immunosuppressive medications used for OLT, including prednisone, can cause an increase in HBV levels in serum and liver tissue by directly enhancing HBV viral replication through attachment to putative steroid receptors. The family of immunosuppressive medications used after transplantation change both T- and B-cell function, inhibit the native or normal response to infectious insults, and promote chronic HBV infection and in many cases more aggressive liver disease due to HBV *(23–25)*.

2. The Prevention and Treatment of HBV Infection After Liver Transplantation

2.1. The Use of Antibody Therapy Hepatitis B Immune Globulin (HBIG) to Bind Circulating Virus

Samuel et al. were the first to describe the use of HBIG in a large clinical trial to prevent recurrent liver disease after liver transplantation in patients with liver failure due to HBV infection *(10,11)*. The concept was first to bind the circulating virus during the anhepatic phase when the recipient's liver, as the critical source of HBV replication, was removed and second to administer and maintain high serum levels of anti-HBs to continuously bind all circulating HBV *(26)*. Overall survival and disease-free survival rates were markedly improved, compared to historical controls, and other centers subsequently demonstrated improved survival (>80%) at 1 yr after liver transplant *(26–30)*. Thus, HBIG administration became the standard of care at most centers worldwide that provide liver transplantation. The cost of HBIG was high with per-unit costs increasing dramatically starting in 1994, and total costs relative to the transplant cost itself have been high since the early 1990s (**Figs. 3** and **4**) *(26–30)*.

HBIG therapy is more effective (a lower graft infection rate) when the patient's serum is negative for hepatitis B surface antigen (HBsAg) and HBV DNA is unmeasurable by quantitative testing before liver transplantation. Also, if the HBIG dose is adjusted to maintain antibody to hepatitis B surface antigen (anti-HBs), with blood levels of at least 20 IU/mL, preferably >100 IU/mL or (according to some authors) 500 IU/mL, graft infection rate is lower *(15,31)*. High-dose HBIG (serum levels of HBs: >100 IU/mL or >500 IU/mL) prophylaxis has also been used with a high level of efficacy for patients with high HBV DNA serum level at the time they undergo OLT. There is less than a 40% graft reinfection rate using these serum targets compared to nearly universal graft reinfection in previous series *(15,32,33)*. Fixed dosing schedules, regardless of serum anti-HBs titers, have also been studied with only a modest failure rate of 19% *(4)*.

One major question to answer has been to discover if and when patients can be discontinued from HBIG therapy, that is, once most circulating virus is bound, is the risk of viral infection of hepatocytes/graft lower long-term? We know that the recurrence rates of HBV infection in the liver graft are in excess of 60% with short-term HBIG and 10–20% if HBIG is stopped more than 6 mo to 1 yr after OLT, even with the continuation of a nucleoside such as lamivudine *(7,34,35)*. Some investigators find HBV replication evident in patients who undergo sensitive molecular testing and who are being treated with HBIG and are HBsAg negative in serum *(36)*. It also appears possible to control reinfection and viral replication in patients with core mutations after liver transplantation using HBIG and lamivudine therapy *(37)*. The use of low-dose intramuscular HBIG is also evolving. Studies, including those at California Pacific Medical Center, have shown that dosing and cost can be decreased by 50–300% *(38–42)*. Immediate intra- and perioperative use of intramuscular HBIG is unlikely to be effective in supply-

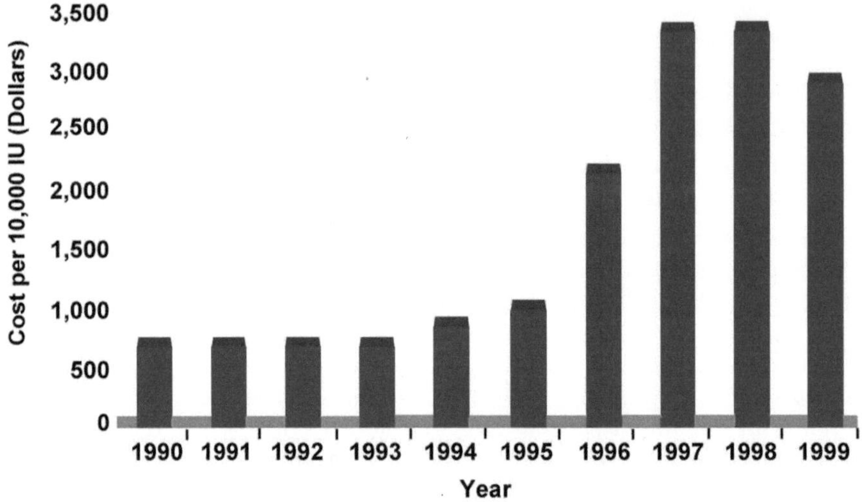

Fig. 3. Cost of therapy with hepatitis B immune globulin (HBIG) during the 1990s.

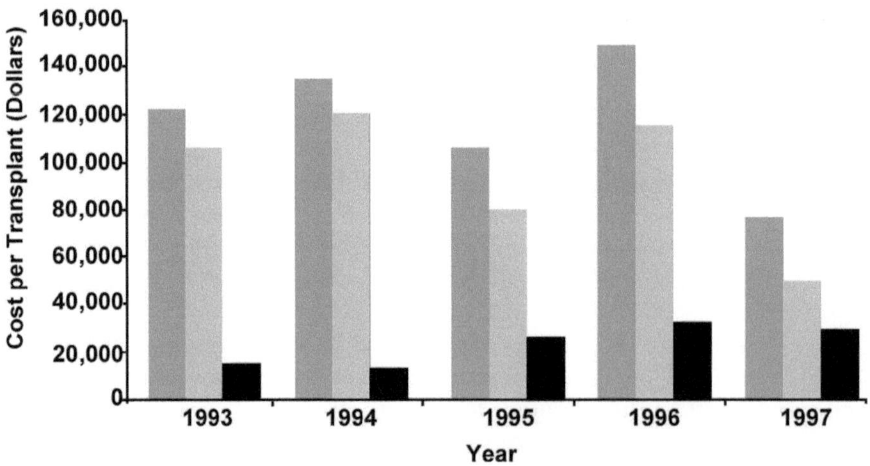

Fig. 4. Cost of therapy with hepatitis B immune globulin (HBIG) relative to the cost of orthotopic liver transplantation (OLT) itself. Medium shading: total cost; light *(gray)* shading: cost of OLT; dark *(black)* shading: cost of HBIG.

ing sufficient antibody to bind and neutralize virus, especially in patients with a moderate to high viral load. Intramuscular dosing (after an initial period of intravenous HBIG) should be customized, using increased doses and frequency, depending on the levels of

HBV DNA before liver transplantation and by following serum levels of anti-HBs after transplantation ***(15,43)***. Attempts to find sources of high-titered HBIG that are less expensive have led to the innovative process of studying fresh frozen plasma as a possible substitute for standard HBIG ***(44)***.

HBIG also aids in managing post-OLT patients coinfected with HBV and HDV before transplantation as well because the binding of circulating particles that contain HBsAg includes those packages that contain delta virus. Cases have been described of fulminant HBV due to HBV/HDV coinfection after liver transplantation in patients who received a liver transplant for end-stage liver disease, which emphasizes the importance of HBIG in these patients as well. In some patients with HBV/HDV coinfection, if graft reinfection occurs after HBIG is discontinued or fails, a benign disease course is often seen, probably as a result of the delayed onset of disease and lower doses of immunosuppression. Some pharmaceutical companies have been trying to develop new products, such as OMRI-Hep-B, that may have improved pharmacokinetic profiles and may achieve either higher titers of anti-HBs or longer half-life of the administered product ***(45)***.

From a historical perspective, the use of a monoclonal HBIG to prevent graft infection has also been described in the setting of liver transplantation ***(46)***. An initial study with a monoclonal antibody directed at the HBV surface protein was conducted in 1990 and resulted in the appearance of an HBV surface antigen mutant form in two liver transplant recipients. These escape mutants were associated with rapidly progressive liver disease ***(47–51)***. These results imply that monoclonal antibody may have selected a genetic drift or allowed emergence of a defective virus that was extremely pathogenic. Alternatively, the presence of this highly conserved antibody may have allowed an existing mutant virus to escape immune surveillance and destroy the liver graft and may require the development of special tests to detect the virus ***(52)***. Studies with this monoclonal antibody were halted and it was never used in any further clinical trials.

Further emphasis of the point that transplant patients are a special population occurred when the use of a polyclonal HBIG preparation resulted in the emergence of HBV with surface antigen mutations ***(49,53,54)***. Changes in the surface region on the HBV genome may result in "escape" from binding to HBIG and allow active and measurable viral replication with HBsAg becoming positive in serum, which explains some of the treatment "failures." Other mutant hepatitis B viruses, not associated with the use of HBIG therapy, have recently been described in a number of transplantation and nontransplantation settings ***(55)*** including HBsAg mutants ***(34,56)***. These newly described viruses have widely varied pathogenic potentials ***(57–59)***.

2.2. The Use of Oral Antiviral Therapy

2.2.1. Lamivudine

Lamivudine [3TC, 3-thiacytadine, (–)2'-deoxy-3'-thiacytadine 5' triphosphate, BCH-189, Epivir ®, Epivir-HBV ®, Glaxo Wellcome, Research Triangle Park, NC] clearly decreases HBV replication in patients who are not immunosuppressed and leads to triple seroconversion (HBeAg positive to negative, anti-HBe negative to positive, and HBV DNA from >2 pg/mL to <2 pg/mL) in 17% of patients treated for a minimum of at least 1 yr ***(60)***. An exciting report of the administration of lamivudine before and continued after liver transplantation revealed that all patients with cirrhosis could have a marked reduction in HBV DNA serum levels (greater than a 3-log reduction in HBV DNA serum levels) prior to transplantation and two of the five patients treated cleared HBsAg long-term after liver transplantation without the use of postoperative HBIG ***(61)***. Further reports have demonstrated that liver disease activity could be controlled, serum levels of liver enzymes decreased, liver function test results improved, in some cases liver enzyme levels as well as liver function test results returned to normal, and time to death or transplantation was delayed by the use of lamivudine before transplantation ***(62–71)***.

Direct antiviral therapy using lamivudine after liver transplantation was shown in a major clinical trial to decrease HBV DNA levels in patient awaiting liver transplantation, resulting in excellent control (suppression) of serum levels of HBV DNA after OLT ***(72–78)***. Also, it now appears possible that patients who develop *de novo* or recurrent HBV infection after OLT (HBIG untreated or treatment failures) can also be managed with nucleoside analogs ***(6,74,75,79–84)***.

Lamivudine pretransplantation combined with lamivudine and HBIG posttransplantation has also been shown in clinical trials to be effective in the long-term management of recipients of liver transplants, but combination with HBIG remains quite expensive (**Figs. 3** and **4**) ***(75,77,85,86)*** including in patients with the precore mutation ***(87)***. Stopping all therapy after liver transplantation is fraught with the danger of severe liver disease and death and must be avoided ***(88)***. This combination administration of lamivudine pretransplantation with indefinite administration both of lamivudine and HBIG after liver transplantation is probably the best current therapy and is considered the standard of care at most institutions. As stated above, lamivudine monotherapy, especially in the setting of immunosuppression, has a significant reinfection (recurrence) rate (>20%) and a very high mutation rate, once reinfection has occurred, leading to nucleoside resistance (*YMDD* motif mutation as well as others). Viral replication in patients even after 2 yr of therapy post-OLT can lead to severe liver disease and death or need for retransplantation ***(74,76,85,89–100)***. Although conversion from HBIG/lamivudine to lamivudine monotherapy is emerging as an alternative option, it is very important to recognize that recurrence rates are approx 10–20%, and any recurrence could be deemed unacceptable with the high risk of progressive liver disease ***(34,35)***.

Unlike patients not undergoing immunosuppression who develop resistance to lamivudine, patients with lamivudine-resistant mutants after transplant may have aggressive liver disease ***(92,97,100)***. The likelihood of recurrence after liver transplant, during administration of lamivudine monotherapy, was related to the serum levels of HBV DNA pretransplant ***(101)***. Interestingly, patients who are immunosuppressed in this clinical setting may still respond to interferon, at least with some levels of viral reduction ***(102)***. If lamivudine therapy is stopped, the lamivudine-resistant mutant virus often reverts to the wild-type virus. Nevertheless, even after the emergence of the viral mutations, lamivudine is often continued in patients after liver transplant because of the overall perception that liver disease is milder, in general, than that seen with the wild-type virus. This circumstance also appears to be the rule in nonimmunosuppressed patients ***(74)***. It is important to note that the lamivudine-resistant mutant can cause severe liver disease and result in patient death due to graft failure ***(88)***. Some authors have proposed that the virus with lamivudine or nucleoside resistance is "less pathogenic," but many reports in the literature have attributed rapidly progressive liver disease to this mutant virus after liver transplantation, or for that matter in the setting of a normal immune system ***(99,103–107)***. The natural history of the lamivurdine-resistant-mutants has not been clearly established in the transplant patient but may well be pathogenic and the best step may be to avoid the possibility of the development of mutants by using HBIG in combination with a nucleoside analog. To date, patients undergoing such therapy have not been reported to develop the emergence of either a nucleoside-resistant mutant or HBIG-resistant viruses but may fail therapy due to inadequate HBIG dosing. Low-dose intramuscular HBIG is also useful, in combination with lamivudine, for patients with the pre-core mutations who undergo liver transplantation ***(96)***.

2.2.2. Famciclovir

Other nucleoside analogs have been used in liver transplant recipients after liver transplantation with modest levels of success (less than a 2-log reduction in HBV DNA levels) such as famciclovir (Famvir ®, SmithKline Beecham Pharmaceutical, Philadelphia, PA), which is the prodrug of penciclovir (BRL 39123; [9-(4-hydroxy-3-hydroxymethylbut-1-yl) guanine]) ***(82,108–116)***. Famciclovir appears to be a less potent nucleoside analog than lamivudine with only a 1- to 2-log reduction in HBV DNA levels in patients treated. Resistance is now being described with a number of variant mutations having been identified in patients treated with famciclovir ***(82,95,109,113,114,117–128)***. There is considerable cross-resistance between virus infections that are resistant to famciclovir and lamivudine.

2.2.3. Ganciclovir

From a historical perspective, ganciclovir (DHPG, Cytovene, Roche Pharmaceuticals, Nutley, NJ) was the first nucleoside to treat post-OLT HBV graft infection ***(6)***. Ganciclovir is a nucleoside analog that has been shown to have efficacy for the treatment of cytomegalovirus infections in HIV-infected patients and patients who are immunosuppressed after organ transplantation. Unfortunately, ganciclovir must be used intravenously to achieve maximum levels of concentration in the blood and only reduces viral levels by 1–2 logs ***(129,130)***. Molecular sequencing has identified the mutation points in the HBV genome that lead to resistance to ganciclovir (Mizokami, *submitted for publication*). The role of valganciclovir (Valcyte ®, Roche Pharmaceuticals, Nutley, NJ) in controlling HBV infection before liver transplantation or treating recurrent disease is not yet defined and is predicted to have a weak antiviral effect.

2.2.4. Adefovir and Entecavir

Future therapy of post-OLT HBV infection will likely include adefovir (Gilead Sciences, Foster City, CA), and entecavir (Bristol Meyers Squibb, Princeton, NJ) may evolve as a "rescue" drug for patients with HBV resistant to lamivudine ***(131,132)***. Resistance to adefovir is also expected, although this has not yet been described, and the ultimate management of immunosuppressed patients will evolve with the development of combination antiviral drug strategies ***(122,133–135)***.

2.3. Fibrosing Cholestatic Hepatitis

The high morbidity and mortality after liver transplantation for HBV infection has been attributed to an increased rate of viral replication as a result of the use of immunosuppression ***(136)*** and accelerated disease resulting from cirrhosis or the development of early liver failure. Once activation of viral replication takes place, this aggressive hepatitis and the subsequent rapid development of liver failure includes a syndrome described as fibrosing cholestatic hepatitis (FCH). FCH is defined as a rapidly progressive liver disease with cholestasis, jaundice, hepatic fibrosis, and liver failure, often complicated by sudden and severe multiorgan dysfunction ***(79,137–147)***.

Both lamivudine and ganciclovir have been used to treat FCH ***(6,148)***. Initially, patients respond well as defined by the marked decline in concentration of serum bilirubin and decrease in serum liver enzyme levels. The international normalized ratio (INR) declines and ascites, if present, often resolves. Famciclovir may also be useful for managing such patients although the efficacy is significantly less than lamivudine and may only have a role as a rescue medication or as part of a combination protocol ***(149)***. The long-term management of patients with severe recurrent disease is more complex. The risk clearly exists not only for development of viral mutations that are resistant to nucleoside analogs but also for development of subsequent more rapidly progressive liver disease. Future management of patients who have accelerated disease after the initiation of nucleoside analogs may include the use of combination nucleoside medications, including the addition of oral valganciclovir or famciclovir to lamivudine early in the course of treatment. This new form of ganciclovir, valganciclovir, has been developed by Roche Pharmaceuticals and is FDA approved for cytomegalovirus infection or prophylaxis. Retransplantation has been performed in patients with fibrosing cholestatic hepatitis (FCH), unfortunately patients who have rapid liver failure shortly after OLT have much poorer survival ***(150,151)***. If recurrence of hepatitis B infection is suspected after OLT, immunoperoxidase staining for the HBV core (HBc) and surface (HBs) antigens is useful to document disease severity and to differentiate recurrent HBV disease from rejection ***(26,152)***. A lobular form of hepatitis has also been described in patients who have a recurrence of HBV infection ***(138,148,153)***.

2.4. Interferon Therapy

From a historical perspective, therapy with interferon just before and continued after transplantation appears to modify the aggressive postoperative course of HBV when HBIG therapy is not commonly used ***(154)*** but does not clear or prevent graft infection ***(155)***. Interferon in the setting of cirrhosis is considered risky from the perspective of potential for decompensation, death, bacterial infections, flare of HBV disease, and need for dose reductions due to side effects ***(155–161)***. These studies demonstrated rare cases in which patients cleared virus and where control of HBV replication was achievable in a minority of patients ***(161)***. Once interferon has reduced viral replication, liver transplantation can take place safely using HBIG with excellent control of HBV replication after liver transplantation. Interferon, even in the setting of cirrhosis, appears to significantly modulate the immune system including increases in the expression of human leukocyte antigen DR and in intrahepatic natural killer cells that may have a role in suppressing or clearing HBV infection ***(160,162)***.

Application of interferon to control recurrent HBV infection after liver transplantation appears to have an effect on disease severity in a minority of patients, although viral suppression can be obtained in some patients ***(102,163–168)***. Also one may expect rejection to take place in the setting of immune stimulations and up-regulation of major histocompatibility complex class 1 molecules ***(169)***. Interestingly, in rare cases, HBsAg seroconversion has been reported after the use of interferon in transplant recipients. At this time, interferon therapy for the post-OLT patient is used but only recommended in rare and closely monitored circumstances. One report of the use of interferon in patients with a lamivudine-resistant mutant infection reported optimistic results ***(102)***.

3. Altering the Immune System Through Modifications in Immunosuppression

Management of liver transplant recipients who have chronic HBV infection can also be enhanced by the use of low-dose immunosuppressive therapy ***(5,7,22,136,170–174)***. Patients who have chronic HBV disease have undergone alterations in their immune system and appear to be at a lower risk of rejection, leading to this innovative approach of posttransplant management.

A recent interesting proposal that has not been used often is simultaneous transplantation of liver with bone marrow from a vaccinated donor or immune donor ***(175)***. One must be careful in defining "immunity," as patients who are both anti-HBc and anti-HBs positive have been reported to transmit HBV to organ transplant recipients. This method of transferring cellular immunity was originally pioneered in bone marrow transplant patients ***(176,177)***, leading to HBV clearance in the recipient of the bone marrow transplant.

4. Hepatitis Delta Infection

Patients with HDV infection who undergo liver transplantation are interesting from the perspective that they often have low or very low serum levels of HBV (low replication) and have an overall good survival rate after liver transplantation due to the "antiviral" effect of delta on HBV replication. Early reports revealed that suppression of HBV replication by delta hepatitis led to better survival in the setting of coinfection compared to HBV infection alone after liver transplantation ***(9,26,178,179)***, probably as a result of the effect of HDV on HBV viral replication (suppression). The importance of the use of HBIG is not well defined in patients coinfected with HDV/HBV, although most centers would use a peri- and post-OLT protocol that included the use of HBIG and potentially lamivudine to serve as "triple" therapy to minimize the risk of HBV reactivation; however, these two treatments will have no effect on delta virus replication. The effect of immunosuppressant drugs on delta infection is unknown and poses a series of interesting questions for the bedside and laboratory. The requirement for post-OLT lamivudine is also not clear in these patients with HDV coinfection, although this combination (lamivudine and HBIG) is used at most centers.

5. Anti-HBc-Positive Donors and *De Novo* HBV After Transplantation

If a liver transplant is not immediately available, the use of a donor who is anti-HBc positive (high-risk donor) (**Table 1**) is considered at many centers, although donors who are anti-HBc positive pose a significant risk (ranging from 34% to 86%) of transmitting HBV infection to the liver transplant recipient ***(180–182)***. The use of anti-HBc-positive donors presents a special problem to the transplant and infectious disease clinician and is an interesting model of the compartmentation of HBV infection ***(183–185)***. Patients who are anti-HBc positive often have molecular evidence of viral replication including covalently closed circular DNA (cccDNA) and pregenomic RNA in liver but have no circulation HBV by the most sensitive molecular tests ***(186)***. Unfortunately, the recipient may develop very aggressive liver disease if preemptive treatment is not initiated. The management of patients who receive a liver from an anti-HBc-positive donor, either intentionally (through informed consent) or inadvertently, is being refined with the immediate prophylactic use of lamivudine, with or without the use of intravenous or intramuscular HBIG ***(187,188)***. These anti-HBc positive grafts are typically given to patients with known HBV infection and the organ recipient will be treated with the same protocol as would be used for a donor liver that is anti-HBc negative, as the recipient is already infected. One point on the use of HBIG, it must be remembered, is to stop infection of the new graft! In the clinical setting of an anti-HBc donor, the liver is or may be infected yet HBIG and lamivudine are used together and rare HBV infection is seen. Additional questions are yet to be answered: Could lamivudine be used alone? Does HBIG modify the activation or movement of HBV in the liver?

6. Other Special Issues

There has been some speculation that Asian patients with chronic HBV infection may do worse than non-Asians after liver transplantation (**Table2**) ***(189,190)***(California Pacific Medical Center data, internal communication) ***(191)***. The decreased survival at some centers in this ethnic group may be based on late referral or need for alternative immunosuppressive therapy. The use of immunosuppressive medications such as mycophenolate mofetil (CellCept, Roche Pharmaceuticals, Nutley, NJ) has an antiviral effect against Epstein–Barr virus, human immunodeficiency virus, and some HCV-like viruses, but it has no role in HBV management and is theoretically problematic because it is an immunosuppressant and may increase viral replication and damage ***(192)***. Children can be safely treated with lamivudine after liver transplantation as well ***(193)***.

7. Vaccination for HBV

The administration of standard HBV vaccine to liver transplant recipients who are infected with HBV probably has no effect on viral replication or clearance, although some authors claim that lower doses of HBIG can be used or eliminated in patients who are surface-antigen negative ***(194–196)***. Some patients have been reported to clear HBV after transplantation following the use of a high dose of HBV vaccination ***(194,196)***.

Table 1
Liver Transplantation Anti-HBc Positive Donors

	Number of patients				
Author of study	Study Participants	Recipients HBsAg positive	Tissue donor positive DNA	Received therapy	Type of therapy (percent protection)
Roque	16	4	14	10	HBIG Post-OLT (100%)
Dickson	23	18	NA	0	—
Wachs	6	3	NA	0	—
Dodson	25	18	NA	0	[a]
Prieto	30	14	NA	5	Anti-HBc pre-OLT (100%)

[a]Four of 18 donors positive for anti-HBs.

Table 2
Hepatitis B Survival

		Survival (percent)		
Survival category	Number of patients	1 yr	3 yr	5 yr
Patient				
Asians	32	74	66	58
Non-Asians	37	97	82	76
Overall	69	86	75	68
Graft				
Asians	32	74	66	53
Non-Asians	37	97	78	74
Overall	69	86	72	64

Patients with cirrhosis are less likely to respond to HBV vaccine, which is attributed to the relative immune-suppressed state of the cirrhotic patient ***(197–201)***. New forms of HBV vaccine being developed by Chiron and GlaxoSmithKline are highly immunogenic and may, alone or in combination, allow a more vigorous T-cell response to bring about a durable seroconversion and may be useful as immunotherapy as well as prophylaxis.

8. Summary

By recognizing the special models of chronic viral disease, great advances in the management of HBV infection have taken place in the treatment of patients who are undergoing OLT for both acute and chronic liver disease due to HBV. Combination therapy with nucleoside analogues and HBIG has emerged as the current standard of care, in spite of the duration of therapy, especially for HBIG, required to minimize recurrent disease. The emergence of new oral medications, especially nucleotide analogues such as adefovir will further advance our ability to control HBV disease. Lessons learned from customizing immunosuppression and preemptive peritransplant treatment have allowed us to achieve superb long-term survival in this group of patients that were nearly abandoned as transplant candidates in the early 1990s.

9. Conclusion

Advances in pre- and post-liver transplant management for HBV-infected patients has resulted in exceptional survival. The future for managing these complex patients will probably involve the use of combination nucleosides and or nucleotides as well as the combination of interferon with these medications, with caveats on the use of interferon in patients with end-stage liver disease and after liver transplantation. Hopefully, early intervention, before the development of liver failure will markedly decrease the need for liver transplant in patients with chronic HBV infection.

References

1. McGory, R. W., Ishitani, M. B., Oliveira, W. M., et al. (1996) Improved outcome of orthotopic liver transplantation for chronic hepatitis B cirrhosis with aggressive passive immunization. *Transplantation* **61**, 1358–1364.
2. Nymann, T., Shokouh-Amiri, M. H., Vera, S. R., Riely, C. A., Alloway, R. R., and Gaber, A. O. (1996) Prevention of hepatitis B recurrence with indefinite hepatitis B immune globulin (HBIG) prophylaxis after liver transplantation. *Clin. Transplant.* **10**, 663–667.
3. Sawyer, R. G., McGory, R. W., Gaffey, M. J., et al. (1998) Improved clinical outcomes with liver transplantation for hepatitis B-induced chronic liver failure using passive immunization. *Ann. Surg.* **227**, 841–850.
4. Terrault, N. A., Zhou, S., Combs, C., et al. (1996) Prophylaxis in liver transplant recipients using a fixed dosing schedule of hepatitis B immunoglobulin. *Hepatology* **24**, 1327–1333.
5. Ingelman-Sundberg, M., Johansson, I., Yin, H., et al. (1993) Ethanol-inducible cytochrome P4502E1: genetic polymorphism, regulation, and possible role in the etiology of alcohol-induced liver disease. *Alcohol* **10**, 447–452.
6. Gish, R. G., Lau, J. Y., Brooks, L., et al. (1996) Ganciclovir treatment of hepatitis B virus infection in liver transplant recipients. *Hepatology* **23**, 1–7.
7. Gish, R. G., Keeffe, E. B., Lim, J., Brooks, L. J., and Esquivel, C. O. (1995) Survival after liver transplantation for chronic hepatitis B using reduced immunosuppression. *J. Hepatol.* **22**, 257–262.
8. Lake, J. R. (1993) Changing indications for liver transplantation. *Gastroenterol. Clin. North Am.* **22**, 213–229.
9. Devlin, J., Smith, H. M., O'Grady, J. G., Portmann, B., Tan, K. C., and Williams, R. (1994) Impact of immunoprophylaxis and patient selection on outcome of transplantation for HBsAg-positive liver recipients. *J. Hepatol.* **21**, 204–210.
10. Samuel, D., Muller, R., Alexander, G., et al. (1993) Liver transplantation in European patients with the hepatitis B surface antigen. *N. Engl. J. Med.* **329**, 1842–1847.

11. Samuel, D., and Bismuth, H. (1993) Liver transplantation for hepatitis B. *Gastroenterol. Clin. North Am.* **22**, 271–283.
12. Shapiro, L. R., Redner, W. J., and Innella, F. P. (1971) Australia antigen and Down's syndrome. *Lancet* **2**, 215–216.
13. Grazi, G. L., Mazziotti, A., Sama, C., et al. (1996) Liver transplantation in HBsAg-positive HBV-DNA—negative cirrhotics: immunoprophylaxis and long-term outcome. *Liver Transplant. Surg.* **2**, 418–425.
14. Girdwood, R. H. (1971) Modern drug treatment and potential hazards to health. *Scott. Med. J.* **16**, 350–356.
15. Pruett, T. L. and McGory, R. (2000) Hepatitis B immune golbulin: the US experience. *Clin. Transplant.* **14 (Suppl 2)**, 7–13.
16. O'Keefe, S. J., El Zayadi, A. R., Carraher, T. E., Davis, M., and Williams, R. (1980) Malnutrition and immuno-incompetence in patients with liver disease. *Lancet* **2**, 615–617.
17. Vega Robledo, G. B., Guinzberg, A. L., Ramos, G. C., and Ortiz, O. L. (1994) Patients with hepatic cirrhosis: altered lymphocyte response to mitogens and its relation with plasmatic zinc, albumin and transferrin. *Arch. Med. Res.* **25**, 5–9.
18. Cheadle, W. G., Mercer-Jones, M., Heinzelmann, M., and Polk, H. C., Jr. (1996) Sepsis and septic complications in the surgical patient: who is at risk? Shock 6 (**Suppl 1**), S6–S9.
19. Chung, R. T., Jaffe, D. L., and Friedman, L. S. (1995) Complications of chronic liver disease. *Crit Care Clin.* **11**, 431–463.
20. Navasa, M., Fernandez, J., and Rodes, J. (1999) Bacterial infections in liver cirrhosis. *Ital. J. Gastroenterol. Hepatol.* **31**, 616–625.
21. de, M. A., Olyaei, A. J., and Bennett, W. M. (1996) Pharmacology of immunosuppressive medications used in renal diseases and transplantation. *Am. J. Kidney Dis.* **28**, 631–667.
22. McMaster, P., Gunson, B., Min, X., Afonso, R., and Bastos, J. (1998) Liver transplantation: changing goals in immunosuppression. *Transplant. Proc.* **30**, 1819–1821.
23. Caselitz, M., Link, H., Hein, R., Maschek, H., Böker, K., Poliwoda, H., and Manns, M. P. (1997) Hepatitis B associated liver failure following bone marrow transplantation. *J. Hepatol.* **27**, 572–577.
24. Clementi, M., Bagnarelli, P., and Pauri, P. (1983) Effect of steroids and adenine-arabinoside (araA) on growth and HBsAg production of a human hepatoma cell line. *Arch. Virol.* **75**, 137–141.
25. Giacchino, R., Facco, F., Loy, A., (1989) [Reactivation of virus replication during immunosuppressive therapy in children with chronic hepatitis B]. *Boll. Ist. Sieroter. Milan* **68**, 24–27.
26. Samuel, D., Bismuth, H., and Benhamou, J. P. (1993) Liver transplantation in cirrhosis due to hepatitis D virus infection. *J. Hepatol.* **17 (Suppl 3),** S154–156.
27. McGory, R. (2000) Pharmacoeconomic analysis of HBV liver transplant therapies. *Clin. Transplant.* **14 (Suppl 2),** 29–38.
28. David, E., Rahier, J., Pucci, A., et al. (1993) Recurrence of hepatitis D (delta) in liver transplants: histopathological aspects. *Gastroenterology* **104**, 1122–1128.
29. Lucey, M. R., Graham, D. M., Martin, P., et al. (1992) Recurrence of hepatitis B and delta hepatitis after orthotopic liver transplantation. *Gut* **33**, 1390–1396.
30. Ottobrelli, A., Marzano, A., Smedile, A., et al. (1991) Patterns of hepatitis delta virus reinfection and disease in liver transplantation. *Gastroenterology* **101**, 1649–1655.
31. Gugenheim, J., Baldini, E., Ouzan, D., and Mouiel, J. (1997) Absence of initial viral replication and long-term high dose immunoglobulin administration improve results of hepatitis B virus recurrence prophylaxis after liver transplantation. *Transplant. Proc.* **29**, 517–518.

32. McGory, R., Ishitani, M., Oliveira, W., Stevenson, W., McCullough, C., and Pruett, T. (1996) Hepatitis B immune globulin dose requirements following orthotopic liver transplantation for chronic hepatitis B cirrhosis. *Transplant. Proc.* **28**, 1687–1688.
33. McGory, R. W., Ishitani, M. B., Oliveira, W. M., et al. (1996) Improved outcome of orthotopic liver transplantation for chronic hepatitis B cirrhosis with aggressive passive immunization. *Transplantation* **61**, 1358–1364.
34. Terrault, N. A., Zhou, S., McCory, R. W., et al. (1998) Incidence and clinical consequences of surface and polymerase gene mutations in liver transplant recipients on hepatitis B immunoglobulin. *Hepatology* **28**, 555–561.
35. Dodson, S. F., de Vera, M. E., Bonham, C. A., Geller, D. A., Rakela, J., and Fung, J. J. (2000) Lamivudine after hepatitis B immune globulin is effective in preventing hepatitis B recurrence after liver transplantation. *Liver Transplant.* **6**, 434–439.
36. Marzan, A., Salizzoni, M., Debernardi-Venon, W., et al. (2001) Prevention of hepatitis B virus recurrence after liver transplantation in cirrhotic patients treated with lamivudine and passive immunoprophylaxis. *J. Hepatol.* **34**, 903–910.
37. Meisel, H., Preikschat, P., Reinke, P., et al. (1999) Disappearance of hepatitis B virus core deletion mutants and successful combined kidney/liver transplantation in a patient treated with lamivudine. *Transplant. Int.* **12**, 283–287.
38. Yao, F. Y., Osorio, R. W., Roberts, J. P., et al. (1999) Intramuscular hepatitis B immune globulin combined with lamivudine for prophylaxis against hepatitis B recurrence after liver transplantation. *Liver Transplant. Surg.* **5**, 491–496.
39. Yoshida, E. M., Erb, S. R., Partovi, N., et al. (1999) Liver transplantation for chronic hepatitis B infection with the use of combination lamivudine and low-dose hepatitis B immune globulin. *Liver Transplant. Surg.* **5**, 520–525.
40. Yoshida, E. M. and Sherlock, C. H. (2000) Assessing virologic efficacy of combination lamivudine and low-dose hepatitis B immune globulin posttransplantation with the ultrasensitive digene hybrid capture II assay (letter). *Liver Transplant.* **6**, 386.
41. Cirera, I., Mas, A., Salmeron, J. M., et al. (2001) Reduced doses of hepatitis B immunoglobulin protect against hepatitis B virus infection recurrence after liver transplantation. *Transplant. Proc.* **33**, 2551–2553.
42. Rosenau, J., Bahr, M. J., Tillmann, H. L., et al. (2001) Lamivudine and low-dose hepatitis B immune globulin for prophylaxis of hepatitis B reinfection after liver transplantation possible role of mutations in the YMDD motif prior to transplantation as a risk factor for reinfection. *J. Hepatol.* **34**, 895–902.
43. Nery, J. R., Nery-Avila, C., Berho, M., et al. (2001) Preliver transplant viremic status and the choice of anti-HBV regimens. *Transplant. Proc.* **33**, 1428–1429.
44. Mentha, G., Giostra, E., Negro, F., et al. (1997) High-titered anti-HBs fresh frozen plasma for immunoprophylaxis against hepatitis B virus recurrence after liver transplantation. *Transplant. Proc.* **29**, 2369–2373.
45. Adler, R., Safadi, R., Caraco, Y., et al. (1999) Comparison of immune reactivity and pharmacokinetics of two hepatitis B immune globulins in patients after liver transplantation. *Hepatology* **29**, 1299–1305.
46. McMahon, G., Ehrlich, P. H., Moustafa, Z. A., et al. (1992) Genetic alterations in the gene encoding the major HBsAg: DNA and immunological analysis of recurrent HBsAg derived from monoclonal antibody-treated liver transplant patients. *Hepatology* **15**, 757–766.
47. McCaughan, G., Angus, P., Bowden, S., et al. (1996) Retransplantation for precore mutant-related chronic hepatitis B infection: prolonged survival in a patient receiving sequential ganciclovir/famciclovir therapy. *Liver Transplant. Surg.* **2**, 472–474.

48. Sterneck, M., Gunther, S., Gerlach, J., et al. (1997) Hepatitis B virus sequence changes evolving in liver transplant recipients with fulminant hepatitis. *J. Hepatol.* **26**, 754–764.
49. Ghany, M. G., Ayola, B., Villamil, F. G., Gish, R., Vierling, J. M., and Lok, A.S.F. (1995) S gene escape mutants as a cause of HBV reinfection in patients who received HBIG post-OLT. *Hepatology* **22**, 150A.
50. Ghany, M. G., Ayola, B., Villamil, F. G., et al. (1998) Hepatitis B virus S mutants in liver transplant recipients who were reinfected despite hepatitis B immune globulin prophylaxis (see comments). *Hepatology* **27**, 213–222.
51. Fischer, L., Sterneck, M., Muller-Ruchholtz, C., Gish, R., and Will, H. (1999) Hepatitis B virus variants associated with clinically severe recurrence after liver transplantation. *Transplant. Proc.* **31**, 492–493.
52. Ijaz, S., Torre, F., Tedder, R. S., Williams, R., and Naoumov, N. V. (2001) Novel immunoassay for the detection of hepatitis B surface "escape" mutants and its application in liver transplant recipients. *J. Med. Virol.* **63**, 210–216.
53. Carman, W. F., Owsianka, A., Wallace, L. A., Dow, B. C., and Mutimer, D. J. (1999) Antigenic characterization of pre- and post-liver transplant hepatitis B surface antigen sequences from patients treated with hepatitis B immune globulin. *J. Hepatol.* **31**, 195–201.
54. Shields, P. L., Owsianka, A., Carman, W. F., et al. (1999) Selection of hepatitis B surface "escape" mutants during passive immune prophylaxis following liver transplantation: potential impact of genetic changes on polymerase protein function. *Gut* **45**, 306–309.
55. Carman, W. F., Trautwein, C., van Deursen, F. J., et al. (1996) Hepatitis B virus envelope variation after transplantation with and without hepatitis B immune globulin prophylaxis. *Hepatology* **24**, 489–493.
56. Rodriguez-Frias, F., Buti, M., Jardi, R., et al. (1999) Genetic alterations in the S gene of hepatitis B virus in patients with acute hepatitis B, chronic hepatitis B and hepatitis B liver cirrhosis before and after liver transplantation. *Liver* **19**, 177–182.
57. Hawkins, A. E., Gilson, R. J., Gilbert, N., et al. (1996) Hepatitis B virus surface mutations associated with infection after liver transplantation. *J. Hepatol.* **24**, 8–14.
58. McMillan, J. S., Bowden, D. S., Angus, P. W., McCaughan, G. W., and Locarnini, S. A. (1996) Mutations in the hepatitis B virus precore/core gene and core promoter in patients with severe recurrent disease following liver transplantation. *Hepatology* **24**, 1371–1378.
59. Trautwein, C., Schrem, H., Tillmann, H. L., et al. (1996) Hepatitis B virus mutations in the pre-S genome before and after liver transplantation. *Hepatology* **24**, 482–488.
60. Grellier, L., Mutimer, D., Ahmed, M., et al. (1996) Lamivudine prophylaxis against reinfection in liver transplantation for hepatitis B cirrhosis. *Lancet* **348**, 1212–1215.
61. Bain, V. G., Kneteman, N. M., Ma, M. M., et al. (1996) Efficacy of lamivudine in chronic hepatitis B patients with active viral replication and decompensated cirrhosis undergoing liver transplantation. *Transplantation* **62**, 1456–1462.
62. Barcena, R., Dominguez-Antonaya, M., Lopez-Sanroman, A., et al. (1999) Lamivudine therapy of hepatitis B virus-related liver disease: cirrhosis, posttransplantation recurrence, and de novo infection. *Transplant. Proc.* **31**, 2457–2458.
63. Fontana, R. J. and Lok, A. S. (2000) Lamivudine treatment in patients with decompensated hepatitis B cirrhosis: for whom and when? *J. Hepatol.* **33**, 329–332.
64. Johnson, M. A., Horak, J., and Breuel, P. (1998) The pharmacokinetics of lamivudine in patients with impaired hepatic function. *Eur. J. Clin. Pharmacol.* **54**, 363–366.
65. Kapoor, D., Guptan, R. C., Wakil, S. M., et al. (2000) Beneficial effects of lamivudine in hepatitis B virus-related decompensated cirrhosis. *J. Hepatol.* **33**, 308–312.

66. Keeffe, E. B. (2000) End-stage liver disease and liver transplantation: role of lamivudine therapy in patients with chronic hepatitis B. *J. Med. Virol.* **61**, 403–408.
67. Leung, N. (2000) Liver disease-significant improvement with lamivudine. *J. Med. Virol.* **61**, 380–385.
68. Van Thiel, D. H., Friedlander, L., Kania, R. J., et al. (1997) Lamivudine treatment of advanced and decompensated liver disease due to hepatitis B. *Hepatogastroenterology* **44**, 808–812.
69. Villeneuve, J. P., Condreay, L. D., Willems, B., et al. (2000) Lamivudine treatment for decompensated cirrhosis resulting from chronic hepatitis B. *Hepatology* **31**, 207–210.
70. Zavaglia, C., Airoldi, A., and Pinzello, G. (2000) Antiviral therapy of HBV- and HCV-induced liver cirrhosis. *J. Clin. Gastroenterol.* **30**, 234–241.
71. Kitay-Cohen, Y., Ben Ari, Z., Tur-Kaspa, R., Fainguelernt, H., and Lishner, M. (2000) Extension of transplantation free time by lamivudine in patients with hepatitis B-induced decompensated cirrhosis. *Transplantation* **69**, 2382–2383.
72. Perrillo, R. P., Wright, T., Rakela, J., et al. (2001) A multicenter United States-Canadian trial to assess lamivudine monotherapy before and after liver transplantation for chronic hepatitis B. *Hepatology* **33**, 424–432.
73. Perrillo, R. P., Schiff, E. R., Dienstag, J. L., et al. (1999) Lamivudine for prevention of recurrent hepatitis B after liver transplantation: final results of a U.S./Candaian multicenter trial. *Hepatology* **3**, A245.
74. Fontana, R. J., Hann, H. W., Wright, T., et al. (2001) A multicenter study of lamivudine treatment in 33 patients with hepatitis B after liver transplantation. *Liver Transplant.* **7**, 504–510.
75. Ben-Ari, Z., Shmueli, D., Mor, E., et al. (1997) Beneficial effect of lamivudine pre- and post-liver transplantation for hepatitis B infection. *Transplant. Proc.* **29**, 2687–2688.
76. Mutimer, D., Dusheiko, G., Barrett, C., et al. (2000) Lamivudine without HBIg for prevention of graft reinfection by hepatitis B: long-term follow-up. *Transplantation* **70**, 809–815.
77. Perrillo, R. P., Rakela, J., Dienstag, J., et al. (1999) Multicenter study of lamivudine therapy for hepatitis B after liver transplantation.Lamivudine Transplant Group. *Hepatology* **29**, 1581–1586.
78. Perrillo, R. P., Kruger, M., Sievers, T., and Lake, J. R. (2000) Posttransplantation: emerging and future therapies (In Process Citation). *Semin. Liver Dis.* **20 (Suppl 1),** 13–17.
79. Angus, P., Richards, M., Bowden, S., et al. (1993) Combination antiviral therapy controls severe post-liver transplant recurrence of hepatitis B virus infection. *J. Gastroenterol. Hepatol.* **8**, 353–357.
80. Ben-Ari, Z., Shmueli, D., Mor, E., Shapira, Z., and Tur-Kaspa, R. (1997) Beneficial effect of lamivudine in recurrent hepatitis B after liver transplantation. *Transplantation* **63**, 393–396.
81. Ben Ari, Z., Mor, E., Shapira, Z., and Tur-Kaspa, R. (2001) Long-term experience with lamivudine therapy for hepatitis B virus infection after liver transplantation. *Liver Transplant.* **7**, 113–117.
82. Boker, K. H., Ringe, B., Krüger, M., Pichlmayr, R., and Manns, M. P. (1994) Prostaglandin E plus famciclovir—a new concept for the treatment of severe hepatitis B after liver transplantation. *Transplantation* **57**, 1706–1708.
83. Broomë, U., Glaumann, H., Hellers, G., Nilsson, B., Sörstad, J., and Hultcrantz, R. (1994) Liver disease in ulcerative colitis: an epidemiological and follow up study in the county of Stockholm. *Gut* **35**, 84–89.
84. Klein, M., Geoghegan, J., Schmidt, K., et al. (1997) Conversion of recurrent delta-positive hepatitis B infection to seronegativity with famciclovir after liver transplantation. *Transplantation* **64**, 162–163.

85. Naoumov, N. V., Lopes, A. R., Burra, P., et al. (2001) Randomized trial of lamivudine versus hepatitis B immunoglobulin for long-term prophylaxis of hepatitis B recurrence after liver transplantation. *J. Hepatol.* **34**, 888–894.
86. Marzano, A., Devernardi-Venon, W., Ciardo, V., et al. (1999) Lamivudine therapy with low dose passive immunoprophylaxis in preventing the recurrence of hepatitis B in liver transplant recipients. *Hepatology* **30**, A337.
87. Ben Ari, Z., Zemel, R., Kazetsker, A., Fraser, G., and Tur-Kaspa, R. (1999) Efficacy of lamivudine in patients with hepatitis B virus precore mutant infection before and after liver transplantation. *Am. J. Gastroenterol.* **94**, 663–667.
88. Petry, W., Adams, O., and Haussinger, D. (2000) Fatal hepatitis B reinfection after orthotopic liver transplantation in an HBsAg negative patient following withdrawal of lamivudine. *J. Hepatol.* **33**, 514–515.
89. Gutfreund, K. S., Williams, M., George, R., et al. (2000) Genotypic succession of mutations of the hepatitis B virus polymerase associated with lamivudine resistance. *J. Hepatol.* **33**, 469–475.
90. Malkan, G., Cattral, M. S., Humar, A., et al. (2000) Lamivudine for hepatitis B in liver transplantation: a single-center experience. *Transplantation* **69**, 1403–1407.
91. Schiff, E. R. (2000) Lamivudine for hepatitis B in clinical practice. *J. Med. Virol.* **61**, 386–391.
92. Yoshida, E. M., Ma, M. M., Davis, J. E., et al. (1998) Postliver transplant allograft reinfection with a lamivudine-resistant strain of hepatitis B virus: long-term follow-up. *Can. J. Gastroenterol.* **12**, 125–129.
93. Bartholomew, M. M., Jansen, R. W., Jeffers, L. J., et al. (1997) Hepatitis-B-virus resistance to lamivudine given for recurrent infection after orthotopic liver transplantation. *Lancet* **349**, 20–22.
94. Aye, T. T., Bartholomeusz, A., Shaw, T., et al. (1997) Hepatitis B virus polymerase mutations during antiviral therapy in a patient following liver transplantation. *J. Hepatol.* **26**, 1148–1153.
95. De Man, R. A., Bartholomeusz, A. I., Niesters, H. G., Zondervan, P. E., and Locarnini, S. A. (1998) The sequential occurrence of viral mutations in a liver transplant recipient re-infected with hepatitis B: hepatitis B immune globulin escape, famciclovir non-response, followed by lamivudine resistance resulting in graft loss. *J. Hepatol.* **29**, 669–675.
96. McCaughan, G. W., Spencer, J., Koorey, D., et al. (1999) Lamivudine therapy in patients undergoing liver transplantation for hepatitis B virus precore mutant-associated infection: high resistance rates in treatment of recurrence but universal prevention if used as prophylaxis with very low dose hepatitis B immune globulin. *Liver Transplant. Surg.* **5**, 512–519.
97. Ben Ari, Z., Pappo, O., Zemel, R., Mor, E., and Tur-Kaspa, R. (1999) Association of lamivudine resistance in recurrent hepatitis B after liver transplantation with advanced hepatic fibrosis. *Transplantation* **68**, 232–236.
98. Honkoop, P., Niesters, H. G., de, M. R., Osterhaus, A. D., and Schalm, S. W. (1997) Lamivudine resistance in immunocompetent chronic hepatitis B. Incidence and patterns. *J. Hepatol.* **26**, 1393–1395.
99. Lai, C. L., Chien, R. N., Leung, N. W., et al. (1998) A one-year trial of lamivudine for chronic hepatitis B. Asia Hepatitis Lamivudine Study Group. *N. Engl. J. Med.* **339**, 61–68.
100. Mutimer, D., Pillay, D., Shields, P., et al. (2000) Outcome of lamivudine resistant hepatitis B virus infection in the liver transplant recipient. *Gut* **46**, 107–113.
101. Mutimer, D., Pillay, D., Dragon, E., et al. (1999) High pre-treatment serum hepatitis B virus titre predicts failure of lamivudine prophylaxis and graft re-infection after liver transplantation. *J. Hepatol.* **30**, 715–721.

102. Seehofer, D., Rayes, N., Berg, T., et al. (2000) Additional interferon alpha for lamivudine resistant hepatitis B infection after liver transplantation: a preliminary report. *Transplantation* **69**, 1739–1742.
103. Seta, T., Yokosuka, O., Imazeki, F., Tagawa, M., and Saisho, H. (2000) Emergence of YMDD motif mutants of hepatitis B virus during lamivudine treatment of immunocompetent type B hepatitis patients. *J. Med. Virol.* **60**, 8–16.
104. Allen, M. I., DesLauriers, M., Andrews, C. W., et al. (1998) Identification and characterization of mutations in hepatitis B virus resistant to lamivudine. Lamivudine Clinical Investigation Group. *Hepatology* **27**, 1670–1677.
105. Allen, M. I., Gauthier, J., DesLauriers, M., et al. (1999) Two sensitive PCR-based methods for detection of hepatitis B virus variants associated with reduced susceptibility to lamivudine. *J. Clin. Microbiol.* **37**, 3338–3347.
106. Atkins, M. and Gray, D. F. (1998) Lamivudine resistance in chronic hepatitis B (letter). *J. Hepatol.* **28**, 169.
107. Liaw, Y. F., Chien, R. N., Yeh, C. T., Tsai, S. L., and Chu, C. M. (1999) Acute exacerbation and hepatitis B virus clearance after emergence of YMDD motif mutation during lamivudine therapy. *Hepatology* **30**, 567–572.
108. Wibell, L., Akerblom, O., Hogman, C., and Jameson, S. (1971) [Autologous blood transfusions in uremia]. *Nord. Med.* **86**, 834.
109. Bartholomeusz, A., Groenen, L. C., and Locarnini, S. A. (1997) Clinical experience with famciclovir against hepatitis B virus and the development of resistance. *Intervirology* **40**, 337–342.
110. Han, S. H., Kinkhabwala, M., Martin, P., et al. (1998) Resolution of recurrent hepatitis B in two liver transplant recipients treated with famciclovir. *Am. J. Gastroenterol.* **93**, 2245–2247.
111. Krüger, M., Tillmann, H. L., Trautwein, C., et al. (1995) Famciclovir treatment of hepatitis B viurs recurrence after orthotopic liver transplantation—a pilot study. *Hepatology* **22**, a.
112. Krüger, M., Tillmann, H. L., Trautwein, C., et al. (1996) Famciclovir treatment of hepatitis B virus recurrence after liver transplantation: a pilot study. *Liver Transplant. Surg.* **2**, 253–262.
113. Main, J., Brown, J. L., and Karayianis, P. (1994) A double-blind, placebo-controlled study to assess the effect of famciclovir on virus replication in patients with chronic hepatitis B virus infection. *J. Hepatol.* Abst.
114. Piqueras, B., Salcedo, M., Bañares, R., et al. (1997) [Famciclovir plus interferon in the treatment of a patient with chronic hepatitis B and severe liver failure]. *Rev. Esp. Enferm. Dig.* **89**, 217–221.
115. Krugman, S. (1971) Viral hepatitis and Australia antigen. *J. Pediatr.* **78**, 887–891.
116. Manns, M. P., Neuhaus, P., Atkinson, G. F., et al. (2001) Famciclovir treatment of hepatitis B infection following liver transplantation: a long-term, multi-centre study. *Transplant. Infect. Dis.* **3**, 16–23.
117. Cane, P. A., Mutimer, D., Ratcliffe, D., et al. (1999) Analysis of hepatitis B virus quasispecies changes during emergence and reversion of lamivudine resistance in liver transplantation. *Antivir. Ther.* **4**, 7–14.
118. Gunther, S., Von Breunig, F., Santantonio, T., et al. (1999) Absence of mutations in the YMDD motif/B region of the hepatitis B virus polymerase in famciclovir therapy failure. *J. Hepatol.* **30**, 749–754.
119. Hussain, M. and Lok, A. S. (1999) Mutations in the hepatitis B virus polymerase gene associated with antiviral treatment for hepatitis B. *J. Viral Hepatol.* **6**, 183–194.
120. Mutimer, D., Pillay, D., Cook, P., et al. (2000) Selection of multiresistant hepatitis B virus during sequential nucleoside-analogue therapy. *J. Infect. Dis.* **181**, 713–716.

121. Seigneres, B., Pichoud, C., Ahmed, S. S., Hantz, O., Trepo, C., and Zoulim, F. (2000) Evolution of hepatitis B virus polymerase gene sequence during famciclovir therapy for chronic hepatitis B. *J. Infect. Dis.* **181**, 1221–1233.
122. Xiong, X., Yang, H., Westland, C. E., Zou, R., and Gibbs, C. S. (2000) In vitro evaluation of hepatitis B virus polymerase mutations associated with famciclovir resistance. *Hepatology* **31**, 219–224.
123. Rayes, N., Neuhaus, R., Naumann, U., et al. (1999) Treatment of hepatitis B-reinfection or de novo-infection after liver transplantation with famciclovir—how effective is it? *Transplant. Proc.* **31**, 481–482.
124. Lander, J. J., Giles, J. P., Purcell, R. H., and Krugman, S. (1971) Viral hepatitis, type B (MS-2 strain). Detection of antibody after primary infection. *N. Engl. J. Med.* **285**, 303–307.
125. Shaw, T., Amor, P., Civitico, G., Boyd, M., and Locarnini, S. (1994) In vitro antiviral activity of penciclovir, a novel purine nucleoside, against duck hepatitis B virus. *Antimicrob. Agents Chemother.* **38**, 719–723.
126. Shaw, T., Mok, S. S., and Locarnini, S. A. (1996) Inhibition of hepatitis B virus DNA polymerase by enantiomers of penciclovir triphosphate and metabolic basis for selective inhibition of HBV replication by penciclovir. *Hepatology* **24**, 996–1002.
127. Tsiquaye, K. N., Slomka, M. J., and Maung, M. (1994) Oral famciclovir against duck hepatitis B virus replication in hepatic and nonhepatic tissues of ducklings infected in ovo. *J. Med. Virol.* **42**, 306–310.
128. Zoulim, F., Dannaoui, E., and Trépo, C. (1995) Inhibitory effect of penciclovir, the active metabolite of famciclovir, on the priming of hepadnavirs reverse transcription. *Hepatology* **22**, A.
129. Roche, B., Samuel, D., Gigou, M., et al. (1999) Long-term ganciclovir therapy for hepatitis B virus infection after liver transplantation. *J. Hepatol.* **31**, 584–592.
130. Chossegros, P., Pouteil-Noble, C., Samuel, D., et al. (1993) Ganciclovir is an effective antiviral agent for post-transplantation chronic HBV infections, maintenance therapy may be required in some cases. *Gastroenterolgy* **104**, A888.
131. Peters, M. G., Singer, G., Howard, T., et al. (1999) Fulminant hepatic failure resulting from lamivudine-resistant hepatitis B virus in a renal transplant recipient: durable response after orthotopic liver transplantation on adefovir dipivoxil and hepatitis B immune globulin. *Transplantation* **68**, 1912–1914.
132. Perrillo, R., Schiff, E., Yoshida, E., et al. (2000) Adefovir dipivoxil for the treatment of lamivudine-resistant hepatitis B mutants. *Hepatology* **32**, 129–134.
133. Lau, G. K. K., Tsiang, M., Jilin, H., and Gibbs, C. S. (1999) Clearance kinetics of HBV infection in Chinese patients: lamivudine versus lamivudine plus famciclovir. *Hepatology* **30**, A732.
134. Gilson, R. J., Chopra, K. B., Newell, A. M., et al. (1999) A placebo-controlled phase I/II study of adefovir dipivoxil in patients with chronic hepatitis B virus infection. *J. Viral Hepat.* **6**, 387–395.
135. Ono-Nita, S. K., Kato, N., Shiratori, Y., et al. (1999) Susceptibility of lamivudine-resistant hepatitis B virus to other reverse transcriptase inhibitors. *J. Clin. Invest* **103**, 1635–1640.
136. Gonzalez, R. A., de la Mata, M., de la Torre, J., et al. (2000) Levels of HBV-DNA and HBsAg after acute liver allograft rejection treatment by corticoids and OKT3. *Clin. Transplant.* **14**, 208–211.
137. Al, F. K., Yoshida, E. M., Davis, J. E., Vartanian, R. K., Anderson, F. H., and Steinbrecher, U. P. (1997) Alteration of the dismal natural history of fibrosing cholestatic hepatitis secondary to hepatitis B virus with the use of lamivudine. *Transplantation* **64**, 926–928.

138. Benner, K. G., Lee, R. G., Keeffe, E. B., Lopez, R. R., Sasaki, A. W., and Pinson, C. W. (1992) Fibrosing cytolytic liver failure secondary to recurrent hepatitis B after liver transplantation. *Gastroenterology* **103**, 1307–1312.
139. McCaughan, G. W., O'Brien, E., and Sheil, A. G. (1993) A follow up of 53 adult patients alive beyond 2 years following liver transplantation. *J. Gastroenterol. Hepatol.* **8**, 569–573.
140. Cooksley, W. G. and McIvor, C. A. (1995) Fibrosing cholestatic hepatitis and HBV after bone marrow transplantation. *Biomed. Pharmacother.* **49**, 117–124.
141. Fang, J. W., Tung, F. Y., Davis, G. L., Dolson, D. J., Van Thiel, D. H., and Lau, J. Y. (1993) Fibrosing cholestatic hepatitis in a transplant recipient with hepatitis B virus precore mutant. *Gastroenterology* **105**, 901–904.
142. Fang, J. W., Wright, T. L., and Lau, J. Y. (1993) Fibrosing cholestatic hepatitis in patient with HIV and hepatitis B (letter). *Lancet* **342**, 1175.
143. Hung, Y. B., Liang, J. T., Chu, J. S., Chen, K. M., and Lee, C. S. (1995) Fulminant hepatic failure in a renal transplant recipient with positive hepatitis B surface antigens: a case report of fibrosing cholestatic hepatitis. *Hepatogastroenterology* **42**, 913–918.
144. Kairaitis, L. K., Gottlieb, T., and George, C. R. (1998) Fatal hepatitis B virus infection with fibrosing cholestatic hepatitis following renal transplantation. *Nephrol. Dial. Transplant.* **13**, 1571–1573.
145. McIvor, C., Morton, J., Bryant, A., Cooksley, W. G., Durrant, S., and Walker, N. (1994) Fatal reactivation of precore mutant hepatitis B virus associated with fibrosing cholestatic hepatitis after bone marrow transplantation. *Ann. Intern. Med.* **121**, 274–275.
146. Munoz, D. B., Ibarrola, C., Andres, A., Colina, F., and Morales, J. M. (1998) Hepatitis-B-virus-related fibrosing cholestatic hepatitis after renal transplantation with acute graft failure following interferon-alpha therapy. *Nephrol. Dial. Transplant.* **13**, 1574–1576.
147. Angus, P. W., Locarnini, S. A., McCaughan, G. W., Jones, R. M., McMillan, J. S., and Bowden, D. S. (1995) Hepatitis B virus precore mutant infection is associated with severe recurrent disease after liver transplantation. *Hepatology* **21**, 14–18.
148. Jamal, H., Regenstein, F., Farr, G., and Perrillo, R. P. (1996) Prolonged survival in fibrosing cholestatic hepatitis with long-term ganciclovir therapy. *Am. J. Gastroenterol.* **91**, 1027–1030.
149. Rayes, N., Seehofer, D., Hopf, U., et al. (2001) Comparison of famciclovir and lamivudine in the long-term treatment of hepatitis B infection after liver transplantation. *Transplantation* **71**, 96–101.
150. Kim, W. R., Wiesner, R. H., Poterucha, J. J., et al. (1999) Hepatic retransplantation in cholestatic liver disease: impact of the interval to retransplantation on survival and resource utilization. *Hepatology* **30**, 395–400.
151. Crippin, J., Foster, B., Carlen, S., Borcich, A., and Bodenheimer, H., Jr. (1994) Retransplantation in hepatitis B—a multicenter experience. *Transplantation* **57**, 823–826.
152. Colina, F., Mollejo, M., Moreno, E., et al. (1991) Effectiveness of histopathological diagnoses in dysfunction of hepatic. *Arch. Pathol. Lab. Med.* **115**, 998–1005.
153. Hirschberger, J., Goldberg, M., and Sauer, U. G. (1993) Glutamine and glutamate in ascitic fluid of dogs. *Eur. J. Clin. Chem. Clin. Biochem.* **31**, 103–106.
154. Hassanein, T., Colantoni, A., De Maria, N., and Van Thiel, D. H. (1996) Interferon-alpha 2b improves short-term survival in patients transplanted for chronic liver failure caused by hepatitis B. *J. Viral Hepat.* **3**, 333–340.
155. Rakela, J., Wooten, R. S., Batts, K. P., Perkins, J. D., Taswell, H. F., and Krom, R. A. (1989) Failure of interferon to prevent recurrent hepatitis B infection in hepatic allograft. *Mayo Clin. Proc.* **64**, 429–432.

156. Hoofnagle, J. H., Di Bisceglie, A. M., Waggoner, J. G., and Park, Y. (1993) Interferon alfa for patients with clinically apparent cirrhosis due to chronic hepatitis B. *Gastroenterology* **104**, 1116–1121.
157. Steininger, R., Muhlbacher, F., Langle, F., et al. (1991) [Experiences with liver transplantation in hepatitis B antigen positive liver cirrhosis]. *Wien. Klin. Wochenschr.* **103**, 573–576.
158. Teuber, G., Dienes, H. P., Meyer zum Buschenfelde, K. H., and Gerken, G. (1996) Long-term follow-up of patients with chronic hepatitis B after interferon treatment. *Z. Gastroenterol.* **34**, 230–236.
159. Tong, M. J., Terrault, N. A., and Klintmalm, G. (2000) Hepatitis B transplantation: special conditions (In Process Citation). *Semin. Liver Dis.* **20 Suppl 1**, 25–28.
160. Yoo, Y. K., Gavaler, J. B., Chen, K., Whiteside, T. L., and Van Thiel, D. H. (1990). The effect of recombinant interferon-alpha on lymphocyte subpopulations and HLA-DR expression on liver tissue of HBV-positive individuals. *Clin. Exp. Immunol.* **82**, 338–343.
161. Nevens, F., Goubau, P., van Eyken, P., Desmyter, J., Desmet, V., and Fevery, J. (1993) Treatment of decompensated viral hepatitis B-induced cirrhosis with low doses of interferon alpha. *Liver* **13**, 15–19.
162. Yoo, Y. K., Gavaler, J. S., Chen, K. N., et al. (1989) Alpha-interferon. Its effect upon lymphocyte subpopulations and HLA-DR expression within the liver. *Dig. Dis. Sci.* **34**, 1758–1764.
163. Ben-Ari, Z., Shmueli, D., Shapira, Z., Mor, E., and Tur-Kaspa, R. (1997) Loss of serum HBsAg after interferon-A therapy in liver transplant patients with recurrent hepatitis-B infection. *Liver Transplant. Surg.* **3**, 394–397.
164. Lavine, J. E., Lake, J. R., Ascher, N. L., Ferrell, L. D., Ganem, D., and Wright, T. L. (1991) Persistent hepatitis B virus following interferon alfa therapy and liver transplantation. *Gastroenterology* **100**, 263–267.
165. Marcellin, P., Samuel, D., Areias, J., et al. (1994) Pretransplantation interferon treatment and recurrence of hepatitis B virus infection after liver transplantation for hepatitis B-related end- stage liver disease. *Hepatology* **19**, 6–12.
166. Wright, H. I., Gavaler, J. S., and Van Thiel, D. H. (1992) Preliminary experience with alpha-2b-interferon therapy of viral hepatitis in liver allograft recipients. *Transplantation* **53**, 121–124.
167. Terrault, N. A., Holland, C. C., Ferrell, L., et al. (1996) Interferon alfa for recurrent hepatitis B infection after liver transplantation. *Liver Transplant. Surg.* **2**, 132–138.
168. Neuhaus, P., Steffen, R., Blumhardt, G., et al. (1991) Experience with immunoprophylaxis and interferon therapy after liver transplantation in HBsAG positive patients. *Transplant. Proc.* **23**, 1522–1524.
169. Jain, A., Demetris, A. J., Manez, R., et al. (1998) Incidence and severity of acute allograft rejection in liver transplant recipients treated with alfa interferon. *Liver Transplant. Surg.* **4**, 197–203.
170. Matthew, E. B., Dietzman, D. E., Madden, D. L., Sever, J. L., al Aish, M. S., and Dodson, W. E. (1971) Possible absence of Australia antigen in G-G translocation-type Down's syndrome. *Lancet* **1**, 702.
171. Behbehani, A. M. (1971) The hepatitis story. Search for a cause. *J. Kans. Med. Soc.* **72**, 227–231.
172. Szmuness, W., Prince, A. M., and Cherubin, C. E. (1971) Serum hepatitis antigen (SH) carrier state: relation to ABO blood groups. *Br. Med. J.* **2**, 198–199.
173. Caccamo, L., Rossi, G., Gridelli, B., Maggi, U., Reggiani, P., Colledan, M., and Fassati, L. R. (1998) High-rate hepatitis and low-rate rejection induced late morbidity and mortality in long-term follow-up after liver transplantation. *Transplant. Proc.* **30**, 1828–1829.

174. Yoshida, H., Iwabuchi, S., Murayama, M., and Uchikoshi, T. (1995) [Long-term prognosis of the interferon-treated patients with chronic hepatitis C]. *Nippon Rinsho* **53 Suppl**, 675–679.
175. Ilan, Y., Nagler, A., Shouval, D., et al. (1994) Development of antibodies to hepatitis B virus surface antigen in bone marrow transplant recipient following treatment with peripheral blood lymphocytes from immunized donors. *Clin. Exp. Immunol.* **97**, 299–302.
176. Lau, G. K., Lok, A. S., Liang, R. H., et al. (1997) Clearance of hepatitis B surface antigen after bone marrow transplantation: role of adoptive immunity transfer. *Hepatology* **25**, 1497–1501.
177. Lau, G. K., Wu, P. C., Liang, R., Yuen, S. T., and Lim, W. L. (1997) Persistence of hepatic hepatitis B virus after serological clearance of HBsAg with autologous peripheral stem cell transplantation. *J. Clin. Pathol.* **50**, 706–708.
178. Muller, R., Wonigeit, K., Bahlmann, J., et al. (1971) [Significance of Australia antigen in patients after kidney transplantation]. *Klin. Wochenschr.* **49**, 768–769.
179. Lerut, J. P., Donataccio, M., Ciccarelli, O., et al. (1999) Liver transplantation and HBsAg-positive postnecrotic cirrhosis: adequate immunoprophylaxis and delta virus co-infection as the significant determinants of long-term prognosis. *J. Hepatol.* **30**, 706–714.
180. Meinick, J. L., Boucher, D. W., Craske, J., and Boggs, J. (1971) Properties of a virus isolated from patients with MS-1 infectious hepatitis. *J. Infect. Dis.* **124**, 76–85.
181. Funabashi, S., Matsumoto, Y., Shikage, K., and Kawai, K. (1971) [Antibody for detection of Australia antigen]. *Rinsho Byori* **19 (Suppl)**
182. Crespo, J., Fabrega, E., Casafont, F., et al. (1999) Severe clinical course of de novo hepatitis B infection after liver transplantation. *Liver Transplant. Surg.* **5**, 175–183.
183. (1971) Hepatitis immunity. *Br. Med. J.* **3**, 442–443.
184. Heisto, H., Julsrud, A. C., Ulstrup, J. C., and Fagerhol, M. K. (1971) [Hepatitis associated antigen (HAA) and the blood transfusion. A follow-up study of recipients of blood from donors with HAA and antibody]. *Tidsskr. Nor Laegeforen.* **91**, 1530–1531.
185. Kim, C. Y. and Bissell, D. M. (1971) Stability of the lipid and protein of hepatitis-associated (Australia) antigen. *J. Infect. Dis.* **123**, 470–476.
186. Marusawa, H., Uemoto, S., Hijikata, M., et al. (2000) Latent hepatitis B virus infection in healthy individuals with antibodies to hepatitis B core antigen. *Hepatology* **31**, 488–495.
187. Dodson, S. F., Bonham, C. A., Geller, D. A., Cacciarelli, T. V., Rakela, J., and Fung, J. J. (1999) Prevention of de novo hepatitis B infection in recipients of hepatic allografts from anti-HBc positive donors. *Transplantation* **68**, 1058–1061.
188. Dodson, S. F. (2000) Prevention of de novo hepatitis B infection after liver transplantation with allografts from hepatitis B core antibody positive donors. *Clin. Transplant.* **14 (Suppl 2)**, 20–24.
189. Ho, B. M., So, S. K., Esquivel, C. O., and Keeffe, E. B. (1997) Liver transplantation in Asian patients with chronic hepatitis B. *Hepatology* **25**, 223–225.
190. Jurim, O., Martin, P., Shaked, A., et al. (1994) Liver transplantation for chronic hepatitis B in Asians. *Transplantation* **57**, 1393–1395.
191. Teo, E. K., Han, S. H., Terrault, N., et al. (2001) Liver transplantation in patients with hepatitis B virus infection: outcome in asian versus white patients. *Hepatology* **34**, 126–132.
192. Ben Ari, Z., Zemel, R., and Tur-Kaspa, R. (2001) The addition of mycophenolate mofetil for suppressing hepatitis B virus replication in liver recipients who developed lamivudine resistance—no beneficial effect. *Transplantation* **71**, 154–156.
193. Smith, H. and Gibbs, P. (2000) Hepatitis B, the hidden danger in cadaveric organ donors (letter; comment). *Transplantation* **69**, 458–459.

194. Barcena, R., Fernandez-Braso, M., Urman, J., et al. (1999) Response to hepatitis B virus vaccine in patients transplanted for HBV- related liver disease under specific gammaglobulin prophylaxis. *Transplant. Proc.* **31**, 2459–2460.
195. Sanchez-Fueyo, A., Rimola, A., Grande, L., et al. (2000) Hepatitis B immunoglobulin discontinuation followed by hepatitis B virus vaccination: a new strategy in the prophylaxis of hepatitis B virus recurrence after liver transplantation. *Hepatology* **31**, 496–501.
196. Weiss, P. (2000) Safe vaccination against hepatitis B virus and discontinuation of hepatitis B immune globulin treatment in a liver transplanted patient. *Transplant. Proc.* **32**, 712–713.
197. Dominguez, M., Barcena, R., Garcia, M., Lopez-Sanroman, A., and Nuno, J. (2000) Vaccination against hepatitis B virus in cirrhotic patients on liver transplant waiting list. *Liver Transplant* **6**, 440–442.
198. Horlander, J. C., Boyle, N., Manam, R., et al. (1999) Vaccination against hepatitis B in patients with chronic liver disease awaiting liver transplantation. *Am. J. Med. Sci.* **318**, 304–307.
199. Sokal, E. M., Ulla, L., and Otte, J. B. (1992) Hepatitis B vaccine response before and after transplantation in 55 extrahepatic biliary atresia children. *Dig. Dis. Sci.* **37**, 1250–1252.
200. Villeneuve, E., Vincelette, J., and Villeneuve, J. P. (2000) Ineffectiveness of hepatitis B vaccination in cirrhotic patients waiting for liver transplantation. *Can. J. Gastroenterol.* **14 (Suppl B)**, 59B–62B.
201. Wiedmann, M., Liebert, U. G., Oesen, U., et al. (2000) Decreased immunogenicity of recombinant hepatitis B vaccine in chronic hepatitis C. *Hepatology* **31**, 230–234.

26

Hepatitis Delta Virus Transfection for the Mouse In Vivo Model

Jinhong Chang, Anthony Lerro, and John M. Taylor

1. Introduction

1.1. Previous Studies of HDV in Mice

Over the years different strategies have been used to achieve the expression of hepatitis delta virus (HDV) sequences in mice. The first studies used cDNA clones of HDV sequences to make mice transgenic for the expression of the small or the large forms of the delta protein *(1)*. Subsequently, three lines of mice transgenic for a cDNA expressing the entire HDV genome were made; these mice demonstrated accumulation of HDV RNA transcripts, but the majority were in the skeletal muscle with only relatively small amounts in the liver *(2)*. At about the same time it was demonstrated that direct injections of HDV cDNA into the skeletal muscle of a mouse led to the accumulation of HDV RNA transcripts *(3)*.

As an approach to achieving infection in the liver of a mouse, Netter et al. injected mice either intraperitoneally or intravenously with HDV particles from the serum of an infected woodchuck and were able to demonstrate at 5–10 d HDV replication within mouse hepatocytes; however, <0.6% of the hepatocytes were infected in such animals *(4)*. A quite different approach has been to engraft primary human hepatocytes adjacent to the mouse kidney capsule; the associated technological difficulty of this system contrasts with the high efficiency with which the hepatocytes can be infected *(5)*.

In 1999 Liu et al. described a most unusual procedure, referred to as "hydrodynamics based transfection," by which it was possible to achieve transient cDNA transfection of as many as 40% of mouse hepatocytes *(6)*. It is the extension of this concept to the use of cDNA for HDV, leading to HDV genome replication in the liver, which is the topic of this chapter.

1.2. General Principles of Hydrodynamics-Based Transfection

Before going into the protocols it is worthwhile to describe the general principle of this procedure. Liu et al. had previously considered mouse intravenous injections with

From: *Methods in Molecular Medicine, vol. 96: Hepatitis B and D Protocols, volume 2*
Edited by: R. K. Hamatake and J. Y. N. Lau © Humana Press Inc., Totowa, NJ

various cDNA, with and without transfection-enhancing agents, but in each case they observed a low efficiency of hepatocyte transfection. In control experiments they showed that the cDNA was rapidly degraded following injection. To obviate this problem, they moved to testing cDNA transfections using larger volumes and delivered in much shorter times. They thus empirically found that when the volume injected was about 10% of the mass of the mouse, and when this volume was injected via the tail vein over a very short time, 5–10 s, then transient transfection efficiencies reached as much as 40%. They and others have since tried to explain the success as follows ***(6–8)***. The volume and speed of the injection produce a pressure that forces the flow of the cDNA solution into tissues directly linked to the inferior vena cava in a direction opposite to the regular circulation. The liver is the organ most affected by this. There is reversal of the blood flow in the hepatic vein. In addition, the pressure exerted might increase the permeability of liver fenestra.

1.3. Application to HDV

We recently reported that with HDV cDNA or even cRNA we could achieve hydrodynamic transfection of mouse hepatocytes, leading to HDV genome replication with all of the characteristics expected ***(9)***.

1.3.1. Evidence of HDV Genome Replication

Three lines of evidence indicate that HDV replication was occurring in the transfected mouse liver ***(9)***. (1) Northern analyses of the RNA extracted from the liver demonstrated the presence of unit-length HDV genomic RNA. This RNA is complementary to the antigenomic RNA transcribed from the DNA of the input expression plasmid. **Figure 1** shows the quantitation of such genomic RNA at a series of times after transfection. After a peak at around d 9 the amount decreased. At d 30 the amount was significantly reduced but still readily discernable. In addition to the unit-length genomic RNA, we also detected the less abundant polyadenylated RNA that acts as mRNA for the translation of the delta protein ***(10)***. (2) Immunoblot assays for the delta protein showed a similar initial increase and ultimate decrease. This assay demonstrated not only the small 195-amino-acid form of the delta protein but also small amounts of the large 214-amino-acid form of the delta protein. The appearance of this large species supported the interpretation that in the mouse, as in cultured cells and infected human and woodchucks, there was posttranscriptional RNA editing of some of the HDV RNA species ***(11)***. (3) The third line of evidence was from immunomicroscopy, to detect the delta protein in fixed sections from the transfected liver. As shown in **Fig. 2**, at d 5, a significant fraction of liver cells showed staining for the delta antigen. Note that this staining was nuclear and in hepatocytes. In addition, these hepatocytes seemed associated with a central vein, as was expected considering the hydrodynamic mechanism of transfection. By d 9, up to approx 4% of the hepatocytes demonstrated HDV replication ***(9)***.

1.3.2. Transfection with RNA Rather than DNA

For cells in culture, HDV replication can be initiated not only by transfection with DNA contructs but also with RNA ***(12,13)***. Thus, we tested whether mice could be transfected with RNA rather than DNA. Surprisingly, the result was not only positive

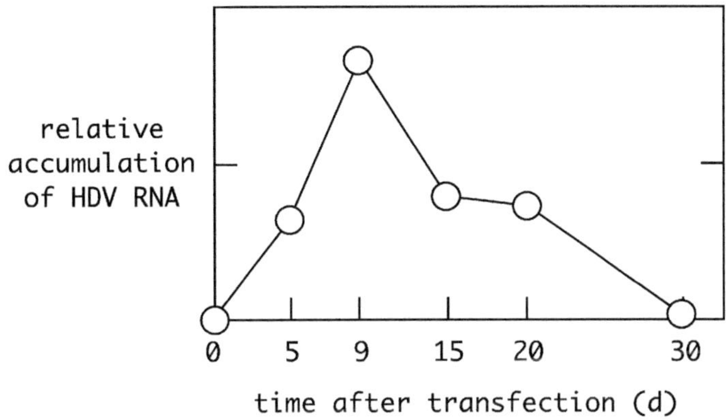

Fig. 1. Time course of accumulation of HDV genomic RNA species following hydrodynamic transfection with HDV cDNA construct.

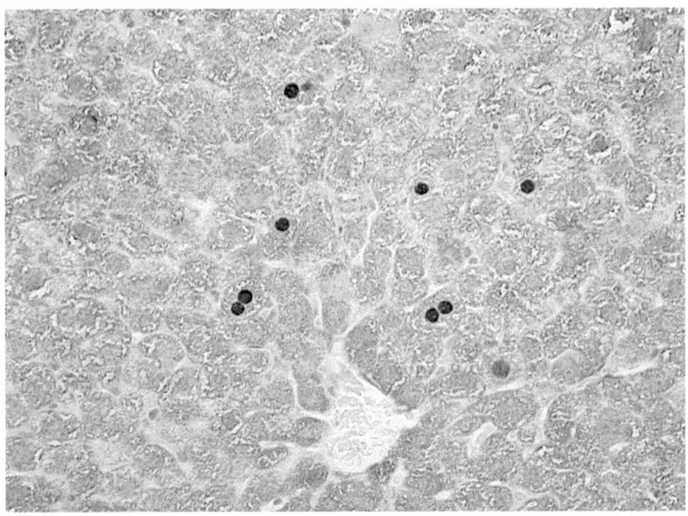

Fig. 2. Immunostaining to detect HDV protein in liver of mouse at 5 d after hydrodynamic transfection with HDV cDNA.

but also of an efficiency comparable to that achieved with cDNA constructs ***(9)***, presumably because the hydrodynamic transfection essentially cleared the way through the venous system so that intact RNA, still in saline, was able to reach the liver cells.

1.3.3. Comparison with Injection into Skeletal Muscle

As mentioned in **Subheading 1.1.**, others have shown that injection of HDV cDNA directly into the skeletal muscle of a mouse will lead to the accumulation of HDV RNA-directed transcripts *(3)*. We have confirmed such studies (data not shown), and compared the efficiency relative to the transfection of mouse liver. We find that the HDV replication in muscle is significant, but still less than what can he achieved with the liver. In addition, the muscle injections use 20 times more cDNA, and in terms of an animal model for HDV, the liver is the better choice.

1.4. Future HDV and Non-HDV Applications

The method has great potential for use in studying liver-tropic virus replication in this small well-characterized animal model. Consider some of the following examples. (1) The studies with HDV have recently been extended by others to HBV (P. Yang and F. Chisari, *personal communication*) and there are plans to do the same with HCV. (2) The transfection can be into mice with specific transgenes or knockouts; for example, we are currently testing the role of an RNA-editing gene on HDV replication. (3) If DNA is transfected, that DNA construct can be one that facilitates integration into the hepatocyte chromosomes *(14)*. (4) The recent discovery that small interfering RNA's can be transfected into cultured cells and achieve gene-specific posttranscriptional gene silencing might be extended to transfected mice and used in many different ways to reveal the host and viral genes needed for replication, pathogenesis, and so forth *(15)*.

We might expect that with time there will be significant enhancements to this hydrodynamics-based procedure. For example, maybe with better choices for the size of animal and the injection conditions, the fraction of transfected hepatocytes might be increased. Also, it is possible that with the additional use of agents such as cationic lipid formulations, the efficiency might even reach as much as >80%, just as for cultured cells.

2. Materials

2.1. Solutions

1. DNA: Expression vectors containing HDV sequences directed by either an SV40 late promoter or a CMV immediate–early promoter were amplified in bacteria and then purified either by a cesium chloride equilibrium density centrifugation or by a Midi-Prep procedure (QIAGEN).
2. RNA: In some experiments the DNA construct was replaced by two HDV RNA species as transcribed in vitro *(16)*.
3. Saline: Dissolve 0.85 g of sodium chloride in 100 mL of distilled water. Sterilize by autoclaving. Store at room temperature.
4. 10% Formalin: Dissolve 10 mL of formalin in 90 mL of distilled water. Store at room temperature.
5. Tri Reagent: Molecular Research Center (cat. no. TR-118). Store at 2–25°C.

2.2. Equipment

1. Injection: disposable 27-gauge × ½-inch needle and 3-mL syringe.
2. Restraining device: Harvard Apparatus mouse restrainer (cat. no. 52-0882).
3. Heat lamp to warm the mice prior to injection.
4. Homogenizer: Brinkmann Instruments, model PT 10/35.
5. 15- or 30-mL Corex glass centrifuge tubes, sterilized.

2.3. Tissues for Study

1. At selected times after injection the animals were killed, and the livers collected and divided into samples of about 50–100 mg, for subsequent extraction or embedding and immunostaining. In some experiments we also collected samples of thigh or calf muscle, heart, spleen, kidney, and lung.
2. For subsequent embedding and immunostaining, a liver sample was fixed in 10% formalin overnight.
3. The remaining tissue samples were transferred to 1.5-mL tubes. These were rapid-frozen with liquid nitrogen, and later stored at −70°C.

3. Methods

3.1 Mice

Typically, we used female Balb/c mice that were about 4 wk old and 16 g at the time of injection (*see* **Note 1**). The strain of mouse is probably not significant. However, as Liu et al. have empirically shown, the mass of the mouse is an important variable for the transfection efficiency of the subsequent injection ***(6)***.

3.2. Injection (See Note 2)

1. For each mouse to be injected, prepare a syringe containing 5 μg of DNA (*see* **Note 3**) or RNA diluted into 1.4 ml of saline (*see* **Note 4**).
2. Warm several mice for about 10 min using a heat lamp.
3. For each mouse to be injected, immobilize with restraining device.
4. Dip tail of mouse into warm water to dilate tail veins.
5. Inject the needle into the tail vein at a point about 1–1.5 inches from the body.
6. In one smooth injection, over a period of < 7 s, deliver the entire volume to the mouse (*see* **Notes 5** and **6**).

3.3. Homogenization of Liver Tissue and Extraction of RNA and Protein

1. Frozen samples of liver tissue were collected as described in **Subheading 2.3.**
2. The frozen sample was transferred to a Corex tube containing 1 mL of Tri Reagent.
3. Without delay, the sample was homogenized for approx 15 s.
4. The homogenate was transferred back to a 1.5-mL tube and extracted, following the manufacturer's protocol (Molecular Research Center) to obtain samples of total RNA and total protein.

4. Notes

1. Age of mice at time of injection: In our studies we chose as a standard to use exclusively 4-wk-old mice. Liu et al. tested a range of older and larger animals. They showed that larger animals required using larger injection volumes to achieve maximal transfection efficiency ***(6)***. Older animals may have the advantage that the injection is easier.
2. Note-taking: Small variations in the injection procedure, such as in the total volume delivered or the rate at which this volume is delivered, can have a major impact on the efficiency of the transfection. Therefore, it is important to make notes regarding the injection of each mouse. Keep track of the times—measure to an accuracy of 1 s the time for injection. Note down all possibly relevant problems that arise during the injection.

3. Amount of DNA: Liu et al. tested the effect of increasing the amount of DNA used in the transfection. We have confirmed their result that increasing the amount of injected cDNA from 5 to 25 μg has no significant effect.
4. Diluent: In the injection procedure a standard saline is used as the diluent. Others have reported that with such a solution only 60% of animals survive, whereas with a Ringer's solution survival is 100% *(7)*. However, in our hands standard saline was not toxic and survival following >100 injections was >98%.
5. Liver damage: The volume injected represents about 10% of the mass of the mouse. This is even more impressive when you consider that the total blood volume of an uninjected mouse is approx 8% of the total body mass. Nevertheless, we have found that the injection is not life threatening, with the mice exhibiting normal behavior within seconds after being returned to cage. However, in a small fraction of the animals (<5%), the injection does produce some liver damage which is only detected later, when one examines the liver tissue 5–30 d after injection. Several healed lesions may be seen on the surface of the liver. Liu et al. noted this and we also have seen this.
6. Efficiency: The efficiency in our hands has been up to 4%, in terms of cells that go on to carry out obvious HDV replication. We have not tried this, but repeated injections were used by Liu et al., and these gave an arithmetic increase. We are currently attempting to increase the efficiency of a single injection via application of cationic lipids, and so forth.

References

1. Guilhot, S., Huang, S.-N., Xia, Y.-P., La Monica, N., Lai, M. M. C. and Chisari, F. V. (1994) Expression of hepatitis delta virus large and small antigens in transgenic mice. *J. Virol.* **68**, 1052–1058.
2. Polo, J. M., Jeng, K.-S., Lim, B., et al. (1995) Transgenic mice support replication of hepatitis delta virus RNA in multiple tissues, particularly in skeletal muscle. *J. Virol.* **69**, 4880–4887.
3. Polo, J. M., Lim, B., Govindarajan, S., and Lai, M. M. C. (1995) Replication of hepatitis delta virus RNA in mice after intramuscular injection of plasmid DNA. *J. Virol.* **69**, 5203–5207.
4. Netter, H. J., Kajino, K. and Taylor, J. (1993) Experimental transmission of human hepatitis delta virus to the laboratory mouse. *J. Virol.* **67**, 3357–3362.
5. Ohashi, K., Marion, P. L., Nakai, H., et al. (2000) Sustained survival of human hepatocytes in mice: a model for *in vivo* infection with human hepatitis B and hepatitis delta viruses. *Nat. Med.* **6**, 327–331.
6. Liu, F., Song, Y. K., and Liu, D. (1999) Hydrodynamics-based transfection in animals by systemic administration of plasmid DNA. *Gene Ther.* **6**, 1258–1266.
7. Zhang, G., Budker, V. and Wolff, J. A. (1999) High levels of foreign gene expression in hepatocytes after tail vein injections of naked plasmid DNA. *Hum. Gene Ther.* **10**, 1735–1737.
8. Zhang, G., Song, Y. K. and Liu, D. (2000) Long-term expression of human alpha1-antitrypsin gene in mouse liver achieved by intravenous administration of plasmid DNA using a hydrodynamics-based procedure. *Gene Ther.* **7**, 1344–1349.
9. Chang, J., Sigal, L. J., Lerro, A., and Taylor, J. (2001) Replication of the human hepatitis delta virus genome is initiated in mouse hepatocytes following intravenous injection of naked DNA or RNA sequences. *J. Virol.* **75**, 3469–3473.
10. Hsieh, S.-Y., Chao, M., Coates, L., and Taylor, J. (1990) Hepatitis delta virus genome replication: a polyadenylated mRNA for delta antigen. *J. Virol.* **64**, 3192–3198.

11. Luo, G., Chao, M., Hsieh, S.-Y., Sureau, C., Nishikura, K., and Taylor, J. (1990) A specific base transition occurs on replicating hepatitis delta virus RNA. *J. Virol.* **64**, 1021–1027.
12. Glenn, J. S., Taylor, J. M. and White, J. M. (1990) In vitro-synthesized hepatitis delta virus RNA initiates genome replication in cultured cells. *J. Virol.* **64**, 3104–3107.
13. Modahl, L. E. and Lai, M. M. C. (1998) Transcription of hepatitis delta antigen mRNA continues throughout hepatitis delta virus (HDV) replication: a new model of HDV RNA transcription and regulation. *J. Virol.* **72**, 5449–5456.
14. Yant, S. R., Meuse, L., Chiu, W., Ivics, Z., Izsvak, Z., and Kay, M. A. (2000) Somatic integration and long-term transgene expression in normal and haemophilic mice using a DNA transposon system. *Nat. Genet.* **25**, 35–41.
15. Tuschl, T. (2001) RNA interference and small interfering RNAs. *Chembiochem.* **2**, 239–245.
16. Moraleda, G. and Taylor, J. Host RNA polymerase requirements for transcription of the human hepatitis delta virus genome. *J. Virol.*, **75**, 10161–10169.

27

Hepatitis Delta Virus RNA Transfection for the Cell Culture Model

Thomas B. Macnaughton and Michael M. C. Lai

1. Introduction

Much of our current understanding of the replication of hepatitis delta virus (HDV) has been based on transfection studies using plasmid-DNA-based expression of HDV RNA. Although this approach is simple and has provided much useful information, there has always been the possibility that this highly artificial system can generate artifacts unrelated to true HDV RNA replication, as there are no DNA intermediates in natural HDV infections. For example, it is not always certain whether any feature observed in these systems is representative of true HDV RNA replication or reflective of artificial DNA-templated HDV RNA transcription. Moreover, HDV cDNA itself has been shown to contain endogenous promoters that may lead to synthesis of additional (unnatural) transcripts *(1)*. A more reliable approach is by direct transfection of HDV RNA. However, this procedure requires that an independent source of small hepatitis delta antigen (S-HDAg) also be provided, presumably to transport the transfected HDV RNA to the nucleus *(2)*, the site of HDV RNA replication, and/or to initiate RNA replication. For this reason, HDV RNA transfection was first done in cell lines that stably expressed S-HDAg from an integrated cDNA copy *(3,4)*, which, however, still involves some HDV cDNA-templated RNA transcription. The next attempt involved transfection of HDV RNA that had been incubated with recombinant S-HDAg to allow the formation of high-molecular-weight ribonucleoprotein complexes *(5,6)*. Although this approach most closely mimics natural HDV infections, it is very inefficient, requires highly purified S-HDAg, and can be used only for the transfection of genomic-sense HDV RNA *(6)*. The most current method of HDV RNA transfection was developed in our laboratory several years ago *(7)* and has become the method of choice because of its simplicity, efficiency, and almost universal applicability. In this approach, the initial requirement of

From: *Methods in Molecular Medicine, vol. 96: Hepatitis B and D Protocols, volume 2*
Edited by: R. K. Hamatake and J. Y. N. Lau © Humana Press Inc., Totowa, NJ

S-HDAg is met by cotransfection of the HDV RNA together with a capped in vitro transcribed mRNA encoding S-HDAg. The rest of this chapter is devoted to the discussion of this technique.

Three major variables need to be considered to achieve the most efficient HDV RNA transfection. These are the choice of cell line, the length and configuration of the HDV RNA species, and the structure of the S-HDAg mRNA. The choice of cell line is flexible, as our technique has been successful in every mammalian cell line we have tried. However, to date the best results have been obtained using the human hepatoma cell line HuH7 *(8)*, in which transfection efficiencies of up to 80% have been achieved. The next consideration concerns the HDV RNA itself. While a number of HDV RNA species of different lengths can successfully be transfected (provided they are at least unit-length), the most efficient HDV RNAs we have used conform to the general structure depicted in **Fig. 1**. The same configuration is used for both genomic- and antigenomic-sense HDV RNA and comprises an approx 1.2× genome-length species with a short terminal redundancy at the 3'-end, such that a functional HDV ribozyme cleavage element will be present at both ends of the transcript. Why HDV RNA species of this general structure initiates HDV RNA replication with the highest efficiency is unclear but may depend on the rapid circularization of the transfected HDV RNA following cleavage at the two ribozyme domains. However, a recent study using this RNA transfection approach demonstrated that initiation of HDV RNA replication is not absolutely dependent on circularization of the transfected HDV RNA species *(9)*; more likely, circularization of HDV RNA renders the RNA more resistant to nuclease attack. The final consideration concerns the length of the S-HDAg mRNA species (**Fig. 2**). We have tested two capped mRNAs with identical sequences at the 5'-end but with differing lengths of sequence at the 3'-end. Specifically, species 2 terminated approx 20 nucleotides (nt) downstream of the S-HDAg stop codon while species 1 contained an additional 230 nt of HDV RNA sequence downstream (including the antigenomic ribozyme domain; **Fig. 2A**). Neither species contained a poly(A) tail. Both S-HDAg mRNA species supported initiation of HDV RNA synthesis with nearly equal efficiency when cotransfected with 1.2× genome-length genomic-sense HDV RNA (**Fig. 2B**, left panel). In contrast, only the longer mRNA species worked efficiently when cotransfected with 1.2× genome-length antigenomic-sense HDV RNA (**Fig. 2B**, right panel). It is likely that the additional HDV RNA sequence on species 1 increases the intracellular half-life of the mRNA, allowing the synthesis of more HDAg. This observation suggests that more HDAg is required when transfecting antigenomic-sense HDV RNA. We therefore recommend the use of S-HDAg mRNAs similar to species 1 (**Fig. 2A**) for all HDV RNA transfection studies.

2. Materials

2.1. Media and Reagents

1. Dulbecco's modified Eagle's medium (DMEM) with high glucose (Gibco cat. no. 12375–010) containing 10% fetal bovine serum (FBS) and 100 U/mL of penicillin and 100 μg/mL of streptomycin. Store at 4°C.

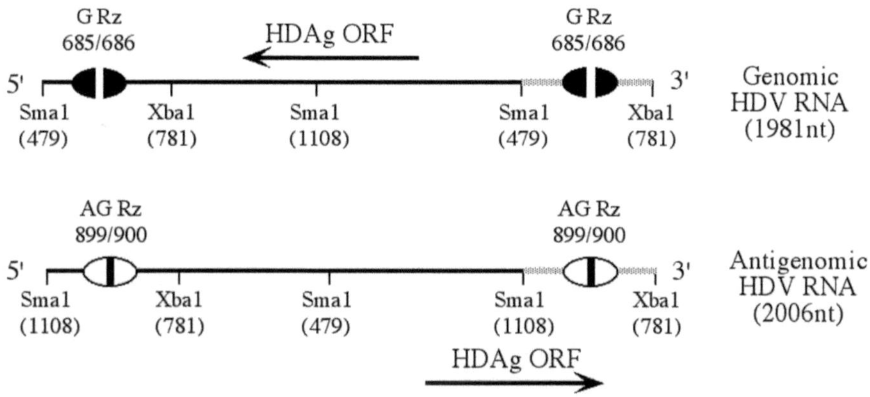

Fig. 1. Genomic and antigenomic HDV RNA species that give optimal results following transfection into HuH7 cells. The numbering and restriction enzyme sites are according to sequence of Wang et al. ***(10)***. Both species are 1.2× genome-length and contain a terminal redundancy at the 3'-end of approx 300 nt (indicated by *shaded line*), which contains an additional ribozyme cleavage site. G Rz and AG Rz indicate the ribozyme cleavage sites on the genomic and antigenomic HDV RNAs, respectively. The arrows indicate the position and orientation of the HDAg open reading frame on each transcript.

2. Opti-MEM 1™ reduced serum media (Gibco cat. no. 31985–070). Antibiotic-free. Store at 4°C.
3. DMRIE-C transfection reagent (Invitrogen cat. no. 10459–014). Store at 4°C. Do not freeze (*see* **Note 1**).
4. 70% Ethanol in distilled water (Gold Shield). Store at room temperature.
5. 100% Ethanol (Gold Shield). Store at room temperature.
6. Phenol–chloroform–isoamyl alcohol (Invitrogen cat. no. 15593–049). Store at 4°C in the dark.
7. 3 *M* Sodium acetate, pH 5.2. Dissolve 24.6 g of sodium acetate (anhydrous) in 75 mL of distilled water. Adjust the pH to 5.2 with glacial acetic acid and bring the volume up to 100 mL with distilled water. Sterilize by autoclaving and store at room temperature.
8. Appropriate restriction enzymes and buffers for linearization of template plasmid DNAs.
9. Nuclease-free water (Ambion cat. no.9930) for the resuspension and dilution of in vitro transcribed HDV RNA.

2.2. Equipment and Kits

1. Good-quality tissue culture ware. Six-well plates, 60-mm Petri dishes, and so forth. We use Falcon brand products throughout (Becton Dickinson).
2. 5-mL (Falcon cat. no. 352058) and 14-mL (Falcon cat. no. 352057) polystyrene tubes for preparing transfection mixtures.
3. RNA transcription kits. We use Ambion brand. In our hands, they give the highest yields and best quality of RNA for transfection. For capped HDAg mRNA production, use mMessage mMachine™ kits (Ambion: SP6 no.1340; T7 no. 1344; T3 no. 1348). For full-length and longer HDV RNA production, use MEGAscript™ kits (Ambion: SP6 no.1330; T7 no.1334; T3 no.1338).

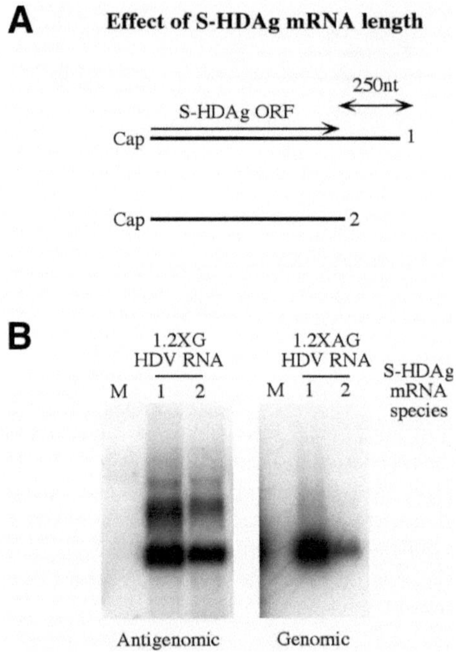

Fig. 2. Initiation of HDV RNA synthesis: Effect of the length of S-HDAg mRNA. (**A**) The diagrammatic structure of the two mRNA species tested. Species 2 terminated approx 20 nt 3' of the S-HDAg stop codon whereas species 1 contained 250 nt of HDV sequence downstream of the HDAg-coding region. Both mRNA species contained a 7-methylguanosine cap at the 5'-end but neither contained a poly(A) tail. (**B**) Northern blot to detect HDV RNA in HuH7 cells 4 d post-transfection. The **left panel** shows antigenomic HDV RNA synthesis following cotransfection of 1.2× genome-length, genomic-sense HDV RNA and either S-HDAg mRNA species 1 or 2. The **right panel** shows genomic HDV RNA synthesis following cotransfection of 1.2× genome-length, antigenomic-sense HDV RNA and either mRNA species. Lane M contains RNA from mock-transfected cells. Probes were ^{32}P-labeled in vitro-transcribed HDV RNA specific for either genomic or antigenomic HDV RNA.

3. Methods

3.1. Preparation of Transcription Templates.

Preparation of good-quality DNA templates for HDV RNA transcription is the single most important factor determining the yield and proportion of the full-length RNA products from the reaction.

1. Use column-purified or CsCl density gradient (twice)-purified plasmid DNA as the starting material. The choice of restriction enzyme used for linearization will depend on the construct. For best results, use enzymes that leave blunt ends or a 5' overhang sequence. Templates containing 3' overhangs may yield sequences that are complementary to the authentic

transcript as well as vector DNA *(11)*. If there is no alternative, include Klenow DNA polymerase in the restriction enzyme digestion step. The 3'–5' exonuclease activity of Klenow DNA polymerase will convert the 3' overhangs to blunt ends.

2. Run an aliquot of the digest from above on an ethidium bromide stained agarose gel to ensure that the plasmid has been cleaved completely. Add an equal volume of the phenol–cloroform–isoamyl alcohol solution to that of the remaining digest, mix vigorously for 1 min, and then centrifuge at 14,000*g* for 5 min. Transfer the upper (aqueous) phase to a fresh Eppendorf tube and precipitate the linearized plasmid DNA by addition of a one-tenth volume of 3 *M* sodium acetate, pH 5.2, and 2 volumes of 100% ethanol. Store at –20°C for at least 1 h.
3. Pellet DNA by centrifugation (14,000*g*, 10 min) and resuspend in 100 μL of distilled water. Transfer the DNA solution to a fresh Eppendorf tube and reprecipitate DNA as above. We have found that this reprecipitation step greatly improves the subsequent RNA transcriptional activity of the DNA templates.
4. Wash the DNA pellet three times with 70% ethanol, carefully removing all the residual ethanol solution after the final wash. Leave the tube open for 10 min at room temperature to dry the pellet partially. Do not dry in a vacuum centrifuge as this may make the DNA hard to resuspend.
5. Finally redissolve the DNA pellet in distilled water and determine the DNA concentration at a 1:100 dilution by measuring the optical density (OD) at 260 nm. Under these conditions, 0.2 OD unit is equivalent to a final DNA concentration of 1 μg/μL in the undiluted solution. It is important to allow the DNA pellet to redissolve for at least 2 h at room temperature (or overnight at 4°C) to ensure that the solution is homogeneous prior to measuring the OD. Adjust the DNA to a final concentration of 0.5 μg/μL with distilled water and store at –20°C.

3.2. Preparation of HDV RNA for Transfection

1. We strongly recommend that in vitro transcription of 1.2× genome-length HDV RNA and S-HDAg mRNA be performed using Ambion MEGAscript™ and mMessage mMachine™ kits, respectively, according to the manufacturer's instructions. Each reaction will generally yield approx 100 μg of the 1.2× genome-length RNA and 25 μg of the S-HDAg mRNA.
2. Precipitate the in vitro transcribed HDV RNA using the lithium chloride reagent and protocol provided in the kit. Store overnight at –20°C.
3. Pellet RNA by centrifugation at 14,000*g* for 10 min at 4°C. Wash the pellet three times with 70% ethanol. The RNA pellet will initially appear translucent and hard to see, but will become white following the wash steps. Remove all residual ethanol following the final wash. There is no need to dry the pellet.
4. Redissolve the pellet in nuclease-free water and determine the RNA concentration at a 1:100 dilution by measuring the OD at 260 nm. Under these conditions, 0.25 OD unit is equivalent to a final RNA concentration of 1 μg/μL in the undiluted solution. Adjust to final concentration of 0.5 μg/μL with nuclease-free water and store at –70°C.
5. The simplest method used routinely in our laboratory to check the quality of RNA transcripts is to run a 1-μL aliquot on a nondenaturing 1% TAE-agarose gel stained with ethidium bromide. The RNA should appear as a single, solid but slightly diffuse band. Degraded or poorly synthesized RNA will appear as a continuous smear from high to low molecular weights. If it is necessary to determine the molecular weight of the RNA accurately, and to run an aliquot on a denaturing agarose gel according to the protocol provided in the Ambion kit. However, we generally find this step unnecessary.

Table 1
Amounts of Reagent Required for Efficient Transfection of Cells Cultured in Different-Size Plates

Culture vessel	Approx area (cm^2)	Opti-MEM (mL)	DMRIE-C (μL)	1.2× HDV RNA (μg)	S-HDAg mRNA (μg)
24-Well plate	2	0.2	2.5	0.5	0.5
6-Well plate	10	1.0	12	2.5	2.5
35-mm Petri dish	10	1.0	12	2.5	2.5
60-mm Petri dish	28	2.0	24	5.0	5.0
100-mm Petri dish	75	5.0	60	12.5	12.5
150-mm Petri dish	175	10.0	120	25.0	25.0

3.3. HDV RNA Transfection

The procedure given is for single 35-mm Petri dishes or six-well plate cultures. Proportions required for culture vessels of different sizes are shown in **Table 1.**

1. For best results, cells should be seeded the previous day and be 70–90% confluent at the time of transfection (*see* **Note 2**).
2. Add 1.0 mL of Opti-MEM 1™ media to a 5-mL polystyrene tube. Then add 12 μL of DMRIE-C reagent directly to the media; do not let it run down the side of the tube. Incubate for 2–5 min at room temperature.
3. Meanwhile, wash cell cultures to be transfected once with 4 mL of Opti–MEM 1 and then drain completely.
4. The next steps need to be performed quickly to prevent the cultures from drying out. Add 5 μL (2.5 μg) of 1.2× genome-length HDV RNA (genomic- or antigenomic-sense) and 5 μL (2.5 μg) of S-HDAg mRNA to the Opti-MEM DMRIE-C mixture, mix briefly with a 1-mL micropipet tip, and transfer immediately to the washed and drained culture. **Do not preincubate the RNA with the DRMIE-C solution.**
5. Incubate culture at 37°C for 4 h in 5% CO_2, then change media to DMEM containing 10% FBS and continue incubation overnight. **Important: Do not incubate cultures overnight without changing media. The DMRIE-C reagent is quite toxic; under these conditions, most cells will be dead by the next day**.
6. Change media again the next day (DMEM containing 10% FBS) and continue incubation for the desired period. Generally, this procedure leads to robust levels of HDV RNA replication which can be detected by Northern blot beginning at 2–3 d posttransfection (*see* **Note 3**).

4. Notes

1. We have also tested a number of other liposomal reagents for HDV RNA transfection, including DOTAP (Roche) and lipofectamine (Gibco), but the best results have always been obtained with DMRIE-C.
2. Do not use cell cultures <50% confluent for this transfection procedure, as the DMRIE-C reagent is quite toxic under these conditions. If cell density is too sparse, incubate the cul-

tures for another day prior to transfection. On the other hand, while 100% confluent cultures can be transfected with this procedure, the efficiency of transfection is much less than that with subconfluent cultures.

3. When analyzing antigenomic HDV RNA synthesis by Northern blot hybridization following transfection with genomic HDV RNA, make sure that the sequence of the probe does not overlap that of the S-HDAg mRNA.

References

1. Macnaughton, T. B., Beard, M. R., Chao, M., Gowans, E. J., and Lai, M. M. C. (1993) Endogenous promoters can direct the transcription of hepatitis delta virus RNA from a recircularized cDNA template. *Virology* **196**, 629–636.
2. Chou, H. C., Hsieh, T. Y., Sheu, G. T., and Lai, M. M. (1998) Hepatitis delta antigen mediates the nuclear import of hepatitis delta virus RNA. *J. Virol.* **72**, 3684–3690.
3. Glenn, J. S., Taylor, J. M., and White, J. M. (1990) *In vitro*-synthesized hepatitis delta virus RNA initiates genome replication in cultured cells. *J. Virol.* **64**, 3104–3107.
4. Macnaughton, T. B., Gowans, E. J., McNamara, S. P., and Burrell, C. J. (1991) Hepatitis δ antigen is necessary for access of hepatitis virus RNA to the cell transcriptional machinery but is not part of the transcriptional complex. *Virology* **184**, 387–390.
5. Dingle, K., Bichko, V., Zuccola, H., Hogle, J. and Taylor, J. (1998) Initiation of hepatitis delta virus genome replication. *J. Virol.* **72**, 4783–4788.
6. Sheu, G. T. and Lai, M. M. (2000) Recombinant hepatitis delta antigen from E. coli promotes hepatitis delta virus RNA replication only from the genomic strand but not the antigenomic strand. *Virology* **278**, 578–586.
7. Modahl, L. E. and Lai, M. M. (1998) Transcription of hepatitis delta antigen mRNA continues throughout hepatitis delta virus (HDV) replication: a new model of HDV RNA transcription and replication. *J. Virol.* **72**, 5449–5456.
8. Nakabayashi, H., Taketa, K., Miyano, K., Yamane, T., and Sato, J. (1982) Growth of human hepatoma cell lines with differentiated function in chemically defined medium. *Cancer Res.* **42**, 3858–3863.
9. Chang, J. and Taylor, J. (2002) In vivo RNA-directed transcription, with template switching, by a mammalian RNA polymerase. *EMBO J.* **21**, 157–164.
10. Wang, K.-S., Choo, Q.-L., Weiner, A. J., et al. (1986) Structure, sequence and expression of the hepatitis δ viral genome. *Nature* **323**, 508–514. Authors' correction (1987) *Nature* **328**, 456.
11. Schenborn, E. T. and Mierendorf, R. C. (1985) A novel transcription property of SP6 and T7 RNA polymerases: dependence on template structure. *Nucl. Acids Res.* **13**, 6223–6236.

III

Antiviral Testing and Clinical Studies

28

Analysis of Hepatitis B Virus Dynamics and Its Impact on Antiviral Development

Manuel Tsiang and Craig S. Gibbs

1. Introduction

Viral dynamics is the study of the population dynamics of viral infection within the body of an infected individual. It describes how viruses spread from cell to cell, with the aim of revealing the basic laws that govern the spread of the virus within the host, their interaction with the immune system, and their response to therapy. For viruses that produce a viremia, changes in the size of the virus population can be measured and followed from blood samples obtained by phlebotomy at various time intervals using very sensitive polymerase chain reaction (PCR)-based assays to quantify viral nucleic acids accurately over a dynamic range of six orders of magnitude.

To analyze these data, mathematical models based on a firm understanding of the biology of the virus and its interaction with the host have been developed. Such models can often provide nonintuitive insights into the dynamics of viral infection. The advent of potent antiviral drugs for the treatment of viral diseases in recent years has facilitated the mathematical analysis of the dynamics of viral infections by providing a means for perturbing the steady state that commonly exists during chronic infection. Such studies have yielded not only insight into our understanding of the establishment, maintenance, and clearance of viral infection, but also predictors of response and principles useful in the design of more effective treatment strategies for human immunodeficiency virus (HIV) ***(1–4)*** and hepatitis C virus (HCV) ***(5,6)*** and promises to do the same for hepatitis B virus (HBV) as well. Importantly, viral dynamics analyses now offer a more sophisticated way of analyzing the response to therapy, particularly in Phase II clinical studies of short duration. Viral dynamics analysis maximizes the use of readily available data and allows different drugs, dosages and regimens to be compared more precisely.

In this chapter, the basic model that has been formulated for HBV dynamics is explained and its application to the analysis of response to antiviral therapy is

From: *Methods in Molecular Medicine, vol. 96: Hepatitis B and D Protocols, volume 2*
Edited by: R. K. Hamatake and J. Y. N. Lau © Humana Press Inc., Totowa, NJ

described. In addition, some limitations and refinements of the model and their future applications are discussed.

2. The Basic Model

2.1. Formulating the Basic Model

The basic model of viral dynamics as conceived by Nowak and Bangham *(7)* has three variables: the population sizes of uninfected cells, x; infected cells, y; and free virus, v (**Fig. 1**). Consistent with good model building practice, the basic model of viral dynamics is constructed with the smallest number of essential assumptions: Uninfected cells are generated at a constant rate λ, die at a rate δx proportional to their own abundance, where δ is the death rate constant, and are infected at a rate bvx, proportional to the product of virus and uninfected cell abundance, where b is the infection rate constant characteristic of the infection efficiency. The infected cells are generated at the same rate bvx as the uninfected cells become infected and die at a rate ay proportional to their own abundance, where a is the death rate constant. The free virus is produced from the infected cells at a rate ky proportional to the abundance of infected cells, where k is the viral production rate constant and is cleared at a rate uv proportional to its own abundance, where u is the clearance rate constant. Taken together, the basic model can be formulated as a system of three differential equations describing the rate of change of x, y, and v:

$$
\begin{aligned}
dx/dt &= \lambda - \delta x - bvx \\
dy/dt &= bux - ay \\
dv/dt &= ky - uv
\end{aligned}
\qquad (1)
$$

2.2. The Basic Reproductive Ratio

Before the start of infection, $v = 0$, $y = 0$ and the uninfected cells are at the steady-state level $x = \lambda/\delta$. When infection is initiated with a nonzero value of v, Eq. (1) becomes a dynamic system describing primary viremia. The system is dynamic in the sense that the three variables are interrelated, and altering the value of one variable will alter the subsequent time course of all the variables. Whether the infection will spread and become established or die out depends on the value of a critical quantity referred to as the basic reproductive ratio R_0 defined as the average number of infected cells that can arise from a single infected cell when most of the cells in the system are still uninfected *(7)*. It is written as the ratio of the rate constants from Eq. (1):

$$R_0 = \frac{\lambda bk}{a\delta u} \qquad (2)$$

If $R_0 < 1$, the infection will not be established, as less than one infected cell will arise from every infected cell. If $R_0 > 1$, the infection will become established with y and v increasing and x decreasing to a steady-state level. In **Subheading 4.2**, we will show how the basic reproductive ratio can be experimentally estimated for HBV infection.

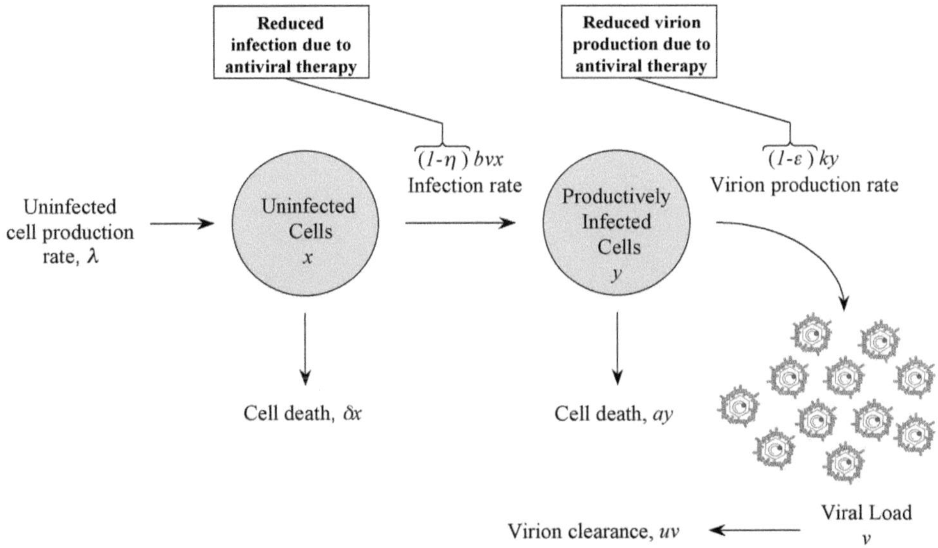

Fig. 1. Flow diagram of the basic model of viral dynamics applied to hepatitis B infection within the host in the presence or absence of adefovir treatment.

2.3. Solving the Basic Model

To test the model or utilize it, Eq. (1) needs to be solved. In general, a system of differential equations can be solved by one of two methods, an analytical method or a numerical method. An analytical solution of x, y, and v will give the mathematical formula of each variable as a function of time. Once the functional forms of the variables are obtained, they can be used to fit the data by regression analysis using software such as SigmaPlot (SPSS® sofware products). However, in most cases, an analytical solution cannot be obtained due to the complexity of the system. A numerical solution, on the other hand, calculates the values of x, y, and v which can be plotted over a specified time period without actually producing a mathematical formula. A numerical solution can always be obtained when the initial conditions x_0, y_0, and v_0 and estimates of the rate constants are supplied. The numerical method is ideal for testing the behavior of the model, but is more challenging to use in regression analysis. For those interested in numerical solutions, a very fast and convenient general purpose differential equation solver, Berkeley Madonna, developed by Robert Macey and George Oster can be purchased at the website www.berkeleymadonna.com.

2.4. Estimation of the Rate Constants

In the case of a primary viremia, Eq. (1) can be solved only numerically. This requires that the initial values for x, y, and v and estimates of all six rate constants be supplied. To obtain a numerical solution of HBV primary viremia to show the time course of x, y, and v (**Fig. 2**), we have attempted to provide realistic estimates for the

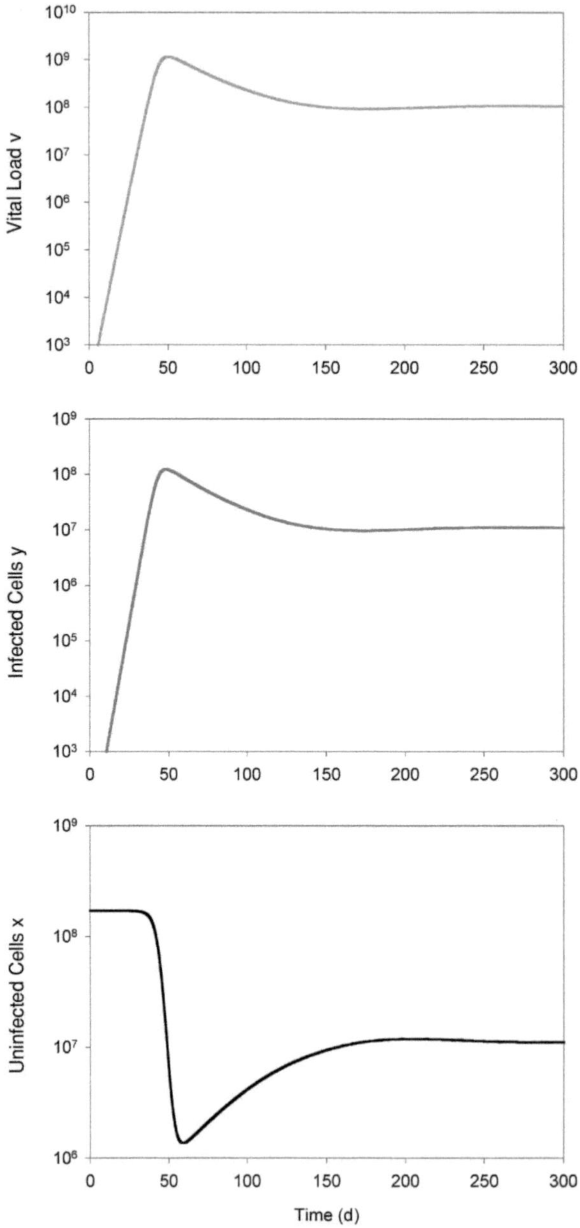

Fig. 2. Numerical solution of viral load, v, infected cells, y, and uninfected cells, x, during primary HBV viremia using the basic model of viral dynamics. Both viral load and uninfected cells display an initial exponential growth followed by a peak and then a decline to a steady-state level. The uninfected cells stay initially constant, then sharply decline to a minimum and recover to a steady-state level. Rate constants used for the simulation: $\lambda = 5 \times 10^5$, $b = 4 \times 10^{-10}$, $k = 6.24$, $a = 0.043$, $d = 0.003$, $u = 0.65$. Initial conditions used for the simulation: $x_0 = 1.7 \times 10^8$, $y_0 = 0$, $v_0 = 400$.

initial conditions and rate constants to Eq. (1). The estimates used here may not be entirely adequate, however, future experimental analyses may provide more accurate determinations.

2.4.1. Number of Cells in Normal Human Liver

The three quantities, x, y, and v are expressed as units of per milliliter of blood. There are no infected cells at the start of an infection, $y_0 = 0$, and the infecting virus can be set at an arbitrarily low quantity of $v_0 = 400$ copies/mL. As to the uninfected cells, the number of cells in an adult liver has been estimated to be approx 10^{12}. Using 6000 mL as the average blood volume of an adult, $x_0 = 10^{12}/6000 = 1.7 \times 10^8$ cells/mL.

2.4.2. Uninfected Cell Growth Rate Constant λ, and Death Rate Constant δ

In rat liver, approx 0.3% of liver cells go through mitosis in any 24-h period *(8,9)*. Assuming the same mitosis rate in human liver, we have $10^{12} \times 0.3\% = 3 \times 10^9$ cells undergoing mitosis every day. Accordingly, the growth rate of uninfected cells per milliter of plasma is $\lambda = 3 \times 10^9/6000 = 5 \times 10^5$ cells/(mL·d). Because before infection the liver is at steady state, the uninfected cell death rate constant δ can be calculated as follows: $dx/dt = 0 \rightarrow \delta = \lambda / x_0 = 5 \times 10^5/(1.7 \times 10^8) = 0.003\ \text{d}^{-1}$ (equivalent to a half-life of 231 d).

2.4.3. Infected Cell Number y, and Viral Production Rate Constant k

It has been reported that approx 5–40% of hepatocytes are infected in chronic HBV patients *(10)*. Therefore, an average value of 22.5% can be used. This allows the estimation of y when the infection has reached a steady state where $y = 10^{12} \times 0.225/6000 = 3.75 \times 10^7$ cells/mL. The clearance rate constants of the virus and infected cells, u and a, can be experimentally determined during antiviral therapy as described in **Subheading 3.3.** For now, we will use those determined values with $u = 0.65\ \text{d}^{-1}$ and $a = 0.043\ \text{d}^{-1}$. Using a mean viral load at steady state of $v = 3.6 \times 10^8$ copies/mL as typically observed in chronic HBV infection, the viral production rate constant k can be calculated. Since $ky = uv$ at steady state, $k = uv/y = 0.65 \times 3.6 \times 10^8/(3.75 \times 10^7) = 6.24\ \text{d}^{-1}$.

2.4.4. Infection Rate Constant b

The infection rate constant b is the most elusive; its value controls the time at which the peak of primary viremia occurs. In the model of acute HBV infection in chimpanzee described by Guidotti et al. *(11)*, the peak of primary viremia occurred at wk 8 or d 56. As b is the only rate constant left to be estimated, different values of b can be tested during the numerical solution of primary viremia. The value of b that gives a viremia peak at day 56 is $b = 4 \times 10^{-10}$ mL/(copies·d).

2.5. Numerical Solution of Primary Viremia

Using the initial conditions and rate constants discussed in **Subheading 2.3.**, a numerical solution to the basic model of viral dynamics described by Eq. (1) can be obtained **(Fig. 2)**. This solution describes the time courses of x, y, and v during primary viremia. Both free virus and infected cells have an initial exponential growth phase followed by a peak and then a decline by damped oscillation to a steady state. Free virus and infected cells cannot continuously grow in number and reach a peak because the supply of uninfected cells is limited. The uninfected cells remain initially constant, allowing for a short exponential growth of both free virus and infected cells, then sharply decline to a valley and slowly recover to a steady-state level by damped oscillation.

3. Antiviral Therapy

In untreated patients with chronic hepatitis B infection, a pretherapy steady state is assumed to have been reached with balance between viral production and viral clearance: $dv/dt = 0 \rightarrow uv_0 = ky_0$, where v_0 and y_0 denote the pretherapy steady-state values of free virus and infected cells. This balance is disturbed when the patient is treated with antivirals such as lamivudine or adefovir, which are potent HBV polymerase inhibitors. Analysis of the rapid decline in viral load during these antiviral therapies has enabled the determination of rate constants critical to viral and infected cells clearance.

3.1. Mechanism of Inhibition

In modeling viral dynamics during antiviral therapy, it is necessary to consider the mechanism by which the virus is being inhibited in order to make reasonable assumptions before solving the basic model. HBV polymerase is necessary for the synthesis of the DNA genome of progeny virions from the pregenomic RNA transcripts; therefore, an HBV polymerase inhibitor should inhibit viral production. In addition, because HBV polymerase may also be involved in completing the synthesis of cccDNA, which migrates into the nucleus to establish a productive infection in the cell, an HBV polymerase inhibitor should also inhibit viral infection. By assuming that lamivudine completely inhibits both viral production ($k = 0$) and viral infection ($b = 0$), Nowak et al. were first to model HBV decline in the plasma of patients under lamivudine treatment ***(12)***.

3.2. Biphasic Solution of HBV Clearance

When we attempted to analyze HBV decline in the plasma of patients during adefovir dipivoxil therapy, we observed a biphasic viral decline with a second slower phase that could not be accommodated by Nowak's solutions. A biphasic solution was obtained from the basic model by modifying the assumptions about the efficacy of inhibition ***(13)***. These efficacy terms were ϵ, the efficacy of inhibiting viral production, and η, the efficacy of inhibiting viral infection such that $(0 \leqslant \epsilon \leqslant 1)$ and $(0 \leqslant \eta \leqslant 1)$. The terms $(1 - \eta)$ and $(1 - \epsilon)$ modify the viral infection rate bvx and the viral production rate ky, respectively (**Fig. 1**). An efficacy of 0 indicates that there is no inhibition, whereas an efficacy of 1 indicates complete inhibition. Values of the efficacy between 0 and 1 indicate partial inhibition. In our solution ***(13)***, we allowed for partial inhibition of viral production $(0 < \epsilon < 1)$, but still assumed complete inhibition of viral infection $(\eta = 1)$. This transformed the basic model into Eq. (3) for the description of HBV viral dynamics during therapy with HBV polymerase inhibitors:

$$\begin{aligned} dx/dt &= \lambda - \delta x \\ dy/dt &= -ay \\ dv/dt &= (1 - \epsilon)ky - uv \end{aligned} \tag{3}$$

An analytical solution for the viral load function *v(t)* can be obtained from Eq. (3):

$$V(t) = v_0 e^{-ut} + \frac{(1-\varepsilon)uv_0}{u-a}(e^{-at} - e^{-ut}) \tag{4}$$

The assumption of complete inhibition of viral infection, although not entirely realistic, does considerably simplify the solution. In **Subheading 5.1.**, we will show that a solution obtained with a more realistic assumption of η yields practically the same dynamic parameters when used to curve fit the same viral load data.

3.3. Curve Fitting the Viral Load Data

The viral load function shown in Eq. (4) can be used to fit the viral load data of HBV patients treated with adefovir dipivoxil or any other HBV polymerase inhibitor **(Fig. 3).** For better accuracy and easier curve fitting, it is recommended to fit $\log(v(t))$ to the logarithm of the viral load data, a detail rarely mentioned in manuscripts. From the nonlinear regression analysis, the clearance rate constants u and a for the virus and for the infected cells and the efficacy of inhibition ϵ of viral production can be determined. The rate constants u and a can also be expressed as the half-lives, $(\ln 2)/u$ and $(\ln 2)/a$ of the virus and infected cells, respectively. In our analysis of 10 patients, $u = 0.65\ d^{-1}$ and $a = 0.043\ d^{-1}$, translating to half-lives of 1.1 d for the virus and 18.2 d for the infected cells, although considerable variation was observed for the half-life of infected cells in different patients. A third way of understanding the rate constants u and a is to express them as $1/u$ and $1/a$, the mean lifespans of HBV virion in plasma and in productively infected cells, respectively. Thus, the mean lifespan of HBV virion in plasma is 36.9 h, and the mean lifespan of productively infected cells is 23.3 d. The mean viral generation time τ is defined as the time from the release of a virion until it infects another cell and causes the release of a new generation of particles; therefore, τ is expressed as $(1/u + 1/a)$, the sum of the mean lifespans of virus and infected cells ***(14).***

3.4. The Meaning of the Two Phases

Counterintuitively, no attempt has been made to predefine the meaning of the two phases during the formulation of the model or the postulation of the assumptions. Instead, it is the analytical solution for the viral load function (Eq. [4]) that provides the meaning for the two phases. The rapid initial phase is controlled by the parameter u, and thus represents the clearance of free virus particles present prior to the initiation of therapy, from patient plasma. The slower second phase is controlled by the parameter a, and thus reflects the clearance of infected cells; it can also be understood as the clearance of newly produced virus particles during antiviral therapy.

3.5. Efficacy of Inhibition of Viral Production

The mean efficacy of inhibition of viral production by adefovir dipivoxil given at a daily dose of 30 mg for the 10 HBV patients shown in **Fig. 3** was determined to be 0.993 ± 0.008. This indicates that 99.3% of viral production was inhibited. It does not mean that 99.3% of baseline viral load has been cleared. Graphically, the efficacy of

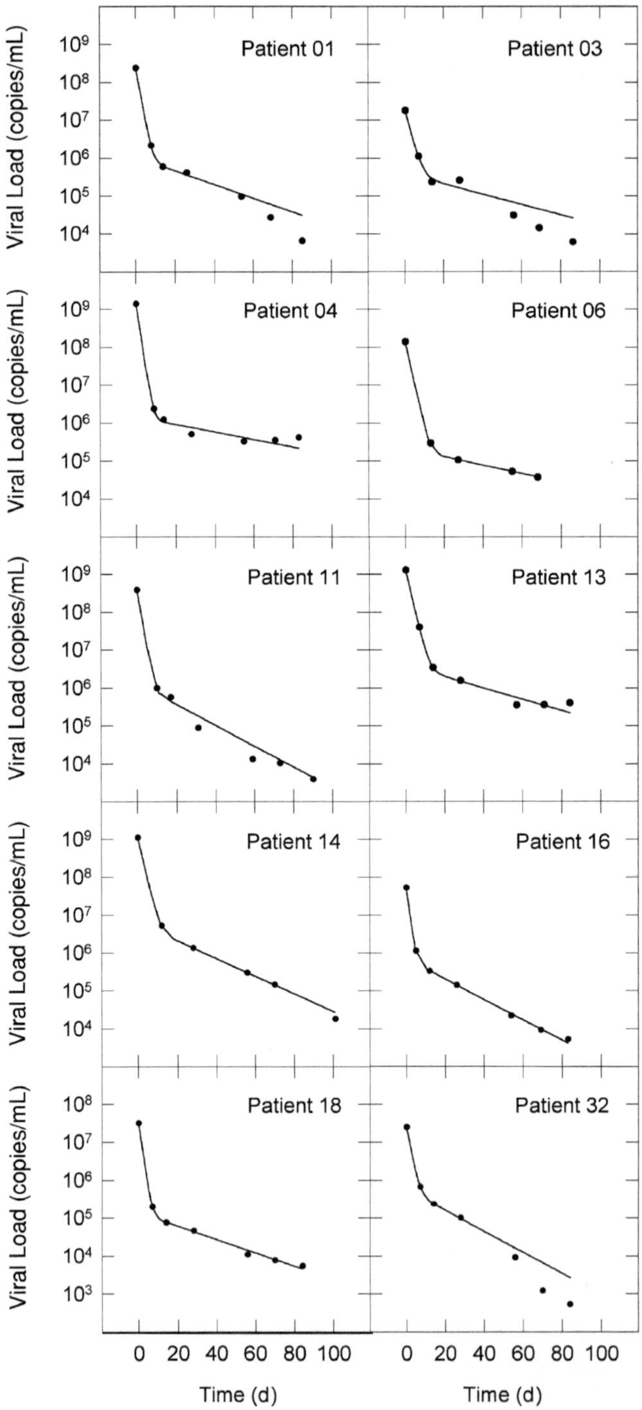

Fig. 3. Plasma viral HBV DNA determinations in 10 patients treated with a 30-mg daily oral dose of adefovir dipivoxil. The *solid lines* represent the best fitted curves using Eq. (4).

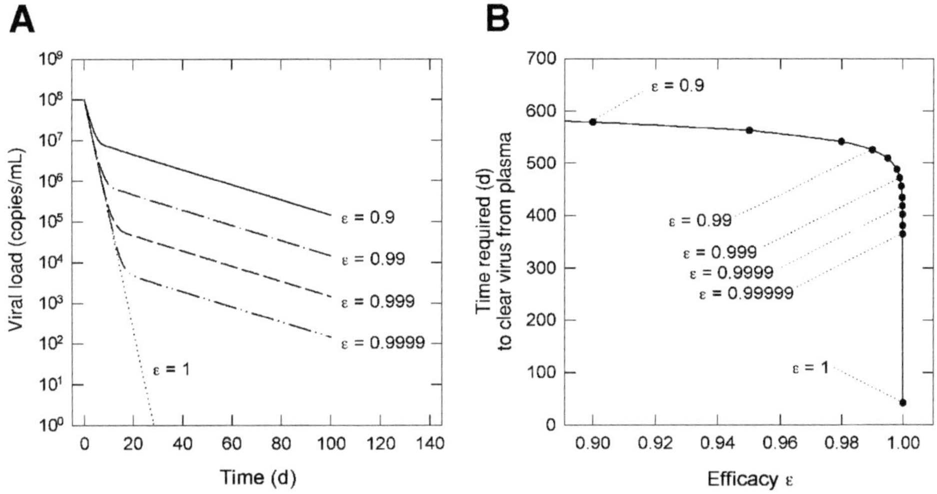

Fig. 4. Effect of efficacy, ϵ, of inhibition of viral production on viral decline. Equation 4 is used in the simulations shown here, with $v_0 = 1 \times 10^8$ copies/mL, $u = 0.65$ d^{-1}, $a = 0.043$ d^{-1}. **(A)** Effect of efficacy, ϵ, on the kinetics of HBV clearance. **(B)** Effect of efficacy, ϵ, on the time required to reduce viral load to clearance level. Clearance level of virus in plasma is defined here as one copy per 6000 mL of plasma.

inhibition of viral production is determined by the time at which the initial phase transitions into the second phase. As shown in the simulation of **Fig. 4A**, the efficacy ϵ affects only the time required to reach the transition from the faster first phase to the slower second phase. Each step between the successive values of ϵ (0.9, 0.99, 0.999, 0.9999, . . .), corresponds to a $\log_{10}$ decrease in the magnitude of the viral production rate constant k and translates into a viral load difference of 54 d in the time required to reduce the total viral load in plasma down to one copy **(Fig. 4B)**.

3.6. Treatment Regimens Affecting Efficacy

In a 12-wk dose escalation study of adefovir at 5, 30, and 60 mg, the mean efficacy ϵ determined from curve fitting with Eq. (4) was 0.8, 0.983, and 0.993 for each dose group, respectively, showing that increasing the dose of adefovir increases the antiviral efficacy. Although the exact relationship between dose and efficacy is unknown, a hyperbolic relationship is a reasonable assumption because the efficacy ϵ can only take values between 0 and 1, and our data are consistent with this assumption. In another study of HBV patients where lamivudine monotherapy (150 mg qd) and combination therapy of lamivudine (150 mg qd) plus famciclovir (500 mg tid) were compared, the efficacies ϵ determined were 0.94 for the monotherapy and 0.988 for the combination therapy *(15)*. The viral declines in both treatment arms were biphasic and famciclovir increased the antiviral efficacy of lamivudine in a manner identical to that observed with increasing doses of adefovir monotherapy.

3.7. Intracellular and Pharmacological Delays

The intracellular delay of the virus is defined as the time between infection of a cell and production of new virus particles. The pharmacological delay is defined as the time required for a drug to be absorbed, distributed, and delivered into target cells after administration *(16)*. Because of these factors, viral load does not decline immediately upon initiation of antiviral therapy, but is preceded by a lag that frequently causes the virus clearance rate constant to be underestimated. To obtain reliable estimates of free virus clearance rate constant u and the combined intracellular and pharmacological delay t_0, frequent sampling of patient blood in the early phase of therapy is necessary. When early data points are available, a viral load function that incorporates this combined delay t_0, shown in Eq. (5), can be used for curve fitting instead of Eq. (4):

$$v(t) = v_0 e^{-u(t-t_0)} + \frac{(1-\varepsilon)uv_0}{u-a}(e^{-a(t-t_0)} - e^{-u(t-t_0)}) \quad (5)$$

This solution is valid for $t > t_0$. For $t < t_0$, the solution is $v(t) = v_0$, where v_0 is the initial viral load. **Figure 5** illustrates the effect of using Eq. (5) for curve fitting when frequent sampling was performed during the first phase. In the absence of frequent sampling during the first phase (**Fig. 5A**), a virus clearance constant of $u = 0.7\ d^{-1}$ was determined using Eq. (4). When five additional points were sampled during the first phase (**Fig. 5B**, *open circles*), a combined pharmacological and intracellular delay $t_0 = 1.9$ d and a larger virus clearance rate constant $u = 1.1\ d^{-1}$ were determined using Eq. (5). In other words, without frequent early samplings, only a lower estimate of the virus clearance rate constant can be determined.

4. Viral Rebound

Like primary viremia, viral rebound after cessation of therapy is also described by the basic model shown in Eq. (1), but an analytical solution of the viral rebound function cannot be obtained.

4.1. Solving the Initial Rebound

However, the initial phase of the viral rebound or initial rebound **(Fig. 6)** can be solved if we assume that, at the end of antiviral therapy, the free virus is practically eradicated ($v \approx 0$) and that during the initial rebound the uninfected cell number remains relatively constant ($dx/dt \approx 0$). With these assumptions, it can be seen that the uninfected cell number is $x_1 \approx \lambda/\delta$ and that Eq. (1) can be simplified to Eq. (6):

$$\begin{aligned} dy/dt &= bvx_1 - ay \\ dv/dt &= ky - uv \end{aligned} \quad (6)$$

Equation (6) can be solved to give the viral load function [Eq. (7)] for the initial rebound where v_1 is the viral load at the end of antiviral therapy and r_0 the rate constant of initial rebound:

$$v(t) = v_1\, e^{r_0 t} \quad (7)$$

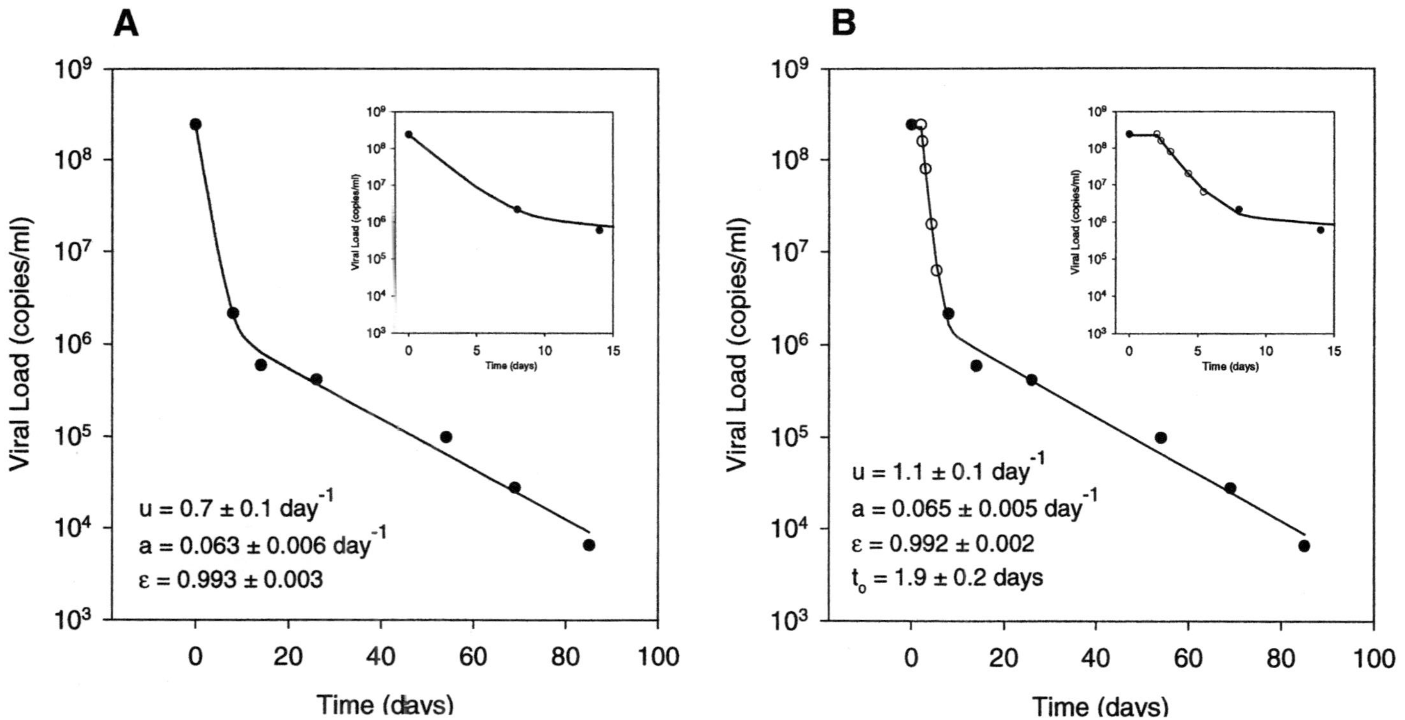

Fig. 5. Frequent early samplings are necessary to determine the delay, t_0 and to avoid overestimation of the virus clearance rate constant, *u*. **(A)** The kinetic parameters were determined by fitting Eq. (4) to the data. **(B)** Five additional points in the initial phase were included in the analysis using eq. (5) to fit the data. A delay of 1.9 d and a larger *u* were determined.

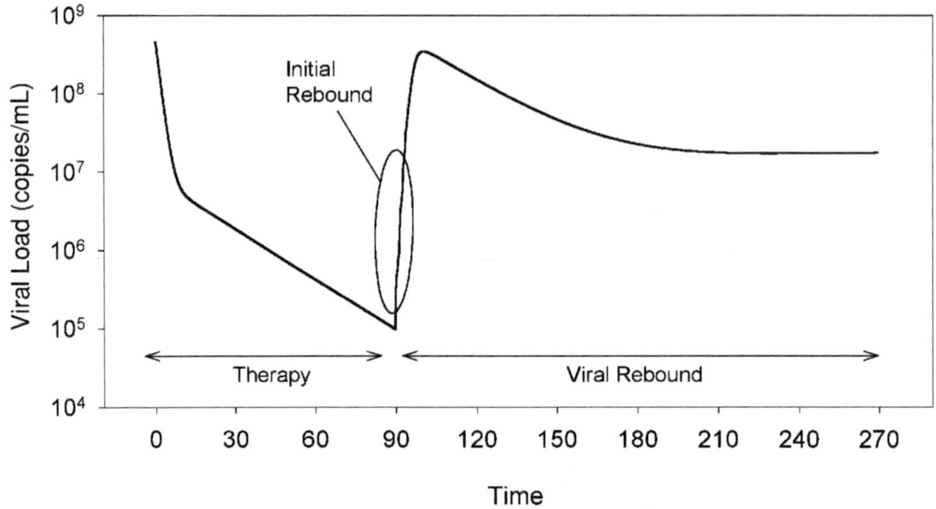

Fig. 6. Simulation of antiviral therapy followed by viral rebound after cessation of therapy.

The rate constant of initial rebound can be determined by fitting Eq. (7) to the viral load data of initial rebound. Another expression for the rate constant of initial viral rebound is the doubling time $t_d = (\ln 2) / r_0$ of the virus in the serum. In our study of HBV patients treated with 30 mg qd adefovir dipivoxil for 12 wk, the initial rebound rate constant r_0 after cessation of therapy was 0.47 d^{-1}, translating to a virus doubling time of 1.5 d in serum. This virus doubling time can also be measured from the initial phase of primary viremia during acute HBV infection in humans. However, the opportunities to study this process in humans are very rare. A virus doubling time of 2.2–5.8 d has been measured from patients with acute HBV infection by Whalley et al. ***(17)*** and is consistent with the result obtained from the initial rebound analysis.

4.2. Determination of the Basic Reproductive Ratio, R_0

The rate constant of initial rebound r_0 is a composite rate constant of all the rate constants in Eq. (1). In the process of solving Eq. (6), its relationship to u, a, and the basic reproductive ratio R_0 can be established and is described by Eq. (8) ***(18)***:

$$R_0 = 1 + \left(\frac{r_0(r_0 + u + a)}{au}\right) \tag{8}$$

Once u, a, and r_0 are determined by curve fitting, the basic reproductive ratio R_0 can be calculated from Eq. (8), which is a more practical three-parameter expression of R_0 in contrast to Eq. (2) (*see* **Subheading 2.2.**). In our study of HBV patients treated with 30 mg qd adefovir, we determined a basic reproductive ratio of 16.

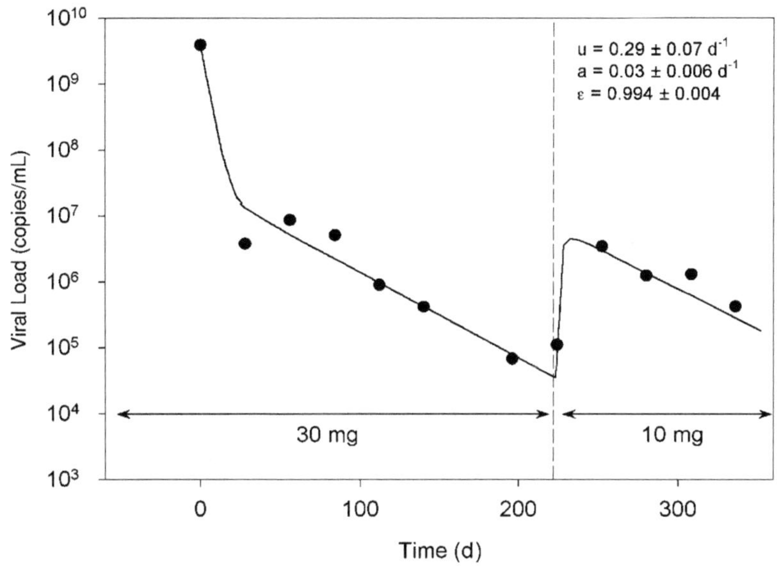

Fig. 7. Partial viral rebound following dose reduction from 30 mg to 10 mg in a single HBV patient.

4.3. Induction/Maintenance Therapy

The observation of rapid HBV viral load decline during the first 2 wk of antiviral therapy (first phase) followed by a period of slow decline (second phase) has led to the proposal that patients might benefit from a treatment regimen involving an initial high induction dose followed by a lower maintenance dose. Numerical simulation of such a dose reduction by reducing the efficacy ϵ predicts that a partial viral rebound will ensue and will be followed by continued second phase clearance identical to that of the lower maintenance dose with unaltered slope. This behavior has been observed ***(19)*** in a single patient dose reduced from 30 mg to 10 mg with a partial viral rebound followed by continued clearance as predicted (**Fig. 7**).

5. Further Refinements

5.1. Partial Inhibition of Infection

In **Subheading 3.2.** we described a biphasic solution for the viral load function obtained by assuming partial inhibition of viral production ($0 < \epsilon < 1$) but complete inhibition of new infections ($\eta = 1$). The assumption that inhibition of new infections was complete provided a simplification that allowed us to obtain an analytical solution describing the biphasic behavior of the viral load decline. However, in reality, complete inhibition of new infections is unlikely. When analyzing the dynamics of HCV under interferon-α therapy, Neumann et al. **(6)** assumed that the inhibition of *de novo* infection were also partial or $0 < \eta < 1$. To allow an analytical solution for the viral load function, they further assumed that the uninfected cells remained constant at the pretreatment steady-state value $x_0 = \frac{ua}{kb}$ during the short period of early treatment. With these assumptions, the basic model was then written as Eq. (9):

$$\begin{aligned} dx/dt &= \lambda - \delta x - (1 - \eta)bvx \\ dy/dt &= (1 - \eta)bvx - ay \\ dv/dt &= (1 - \epsilon)ky - uv \end{aligned} \tag{9}$$

Solving Eq. (9) gave the solution for the viral load function shown in Eq. (10):

$$v(t) = \frac{1}{2}v_0\left[\left(1 - \frac{u + a - 2\varepsilon u}{\theta}\right)e^{-\lambda_1(t-t_0)} + \left(1 + \frac{u + a - 2\varepsilon u}{\theta}\right)e^{-\lambda_2(t-t_0)}\right] \tag{10}$$

where the eigenvalues, λ_1 and λ_2 are given by $\frac{1}{2}(u + a + \theta)$ and $\frac{1}{2}(u + a - \theta)$, respectively, and $\theta = \sqrt{(u - a)^2 + 4(1 - \varepsilon)(1 - \eta)ua}$ and t_0 is the combined delay as defined in **Subheading 3.7.** Again, this solution is valid only for $t > t_0$. For $t < t_0$, the solution is $v(t) = v_0$, where v_0 is the initial viral load.

5.2. Noncytolytic Loss of Infected Cells

In our study of HBV dynamics in patients under adefovir treatment, the half-life for productively infected hepatocytes was as short as 11 d in some patients. This translates to a 6.2% daily loss in this population of cells. Because 5–40% of all hepatocytes in chronic HBV patients can be productively infected ***(4)***, this means that between 0.3% and 2.5% of all hepatocytes are killed daily and must be replenished to maintain a stable liver mass. However, in a study of acute HBV infection in chimpanzees ***(11)***, Chisari and co-workers have demonstrated that >90% of the viral DNA can be eliminated from the liver by noncytolytic processes independent of immune elimination of infected hepatocytes and that the viral cccDNA is also susceptible to noncytolytic control. This means that instead of being killed, the disappearance of productively infected hepatocytes can also occur through a curing mechanism where cured cells reenter the population of uninfected healthy cells. In a recent model for HBV dynamics, Lewin et al. ***(20)*** have introduced a reversion rate constant ρ into Neumann's model (Eq. [9]) to reflect this noncytolytic loss of infected cells through reversion to the uninfected state by loss of all cccDNA from their nucleus. This model is described by Eq. (11):

$$\begin{aligned} dx/dt &= \lambda - \delta x - (1 - \eta)bvx + \rho y \\ dy/dt &= (1 - \eta)bvx - ay - \rho y \\ dv/dt &= (1 - \varepsilon)ky - uv \end{aligned} \tag{11}$$

Thus, the rate constant of infected cell loss is $A = a + \rho$, the sum of the rate constants of cell death and reversion. By assuming that the uninfected cells remained constant at the pretreatment steady-state value $x_0 = \frac{ua}{kb}$ during the short period of early treatment, they obtained the same solution for viral load as the one shown in Eq. (10), except that the death rate constant a of infected cells was now replaced with A the rate constant of infected cell loss.

Hence, the second phase decline could overestimate the actual death rate of infected cells and rather reflect the decay of cccDNA. Again, viral serum kinetics alone does not allow us to dissociate the two rate constants. A separate determination of ρ will be required before the real death rate constant *a* can be estimated.

A recent study of the kinetics of hepadnavirus loss from the liver of woodchucks under L-FMAU therapy by Zhu et al. ***(21)*** pointed to yet a third and even more realistic interpretation of the second phase decline. In that study, the authors compared the rate of loss of replicating genomes, cccDNA, and infected hepatocytes (i.e., cells with at least one molecule of cccDNA) and found that replicating genomes were virtually eliminated from the liver after 6 wk of therapy, while the decline of cccDNA and the actual number of infected cells lagged behind with half-lives longer than 50 d. This suggests that the second phase decline more realistically reflects a decrease in the level of replicating genomes within the infected cells, which themselves are lost at a much slower rate in a third phase decline. This scenario could also reconcile the observations made in the Chisari's chimpanzees where the decline in HBV liver DNA should not be viewed as a loss of infected cells but simply as a loss of replicating genomes within the infected cells. This is a reasonable paradigm, because it is more plausible that the replicating genomes are lost gradually than in an all-or-none fashion within an infected cell. Future models can be developed to accommodate this phenomenon by introducing a fourth variable to denote the replicating genomes.

6. Conclusion

Using mathematical models to analyze the dynamics of HBV viral load during drug therapy or during viral rebound after cessation of therapy can provide quantitative estimates of the rate constants crucial in HBV replication in vivo. Although all mathematical models necessarily rely on simplifications and have certain limitations, their formulation does force all the biological assumptions to be made explicit. Instead of emphasizing accuracy, the current state of HBV dynamic modeling provides a basic, yet not complete, understanding of the underlying processes that allows one to obtain parameter estimates that are invaluable guidelines for therapy planning and comparison of different drugs and drug combinations. As more data are collected on HBV replication and drug action, they can be used to test the conclusions of the model and bring further refinements to the model, which in turn will yield more insight into HBV infection. Furthermore, it is likely that variable factors associated with the virus, such as genotype and host factors, such as the immune response, will influence the specific pattern of viral dynamics observed during the treatment of an individual patient. It is also plausible that the viral dynamic pattern observed may be predictive of treatment outcome. The correlations between baseline parameters, viral dynamic parameters, and treatment outcome remain to be explored for hepatitis B. The challenge for such correlation analyses is the collection of blood samples with the necessary frequency for each phase of viral clearance required for accurate viral dynamic measurements in clinical trials involving sufficient numbers of patients. Another challenge currently facing clinicians treating patients with hepatitis B infection with antiviral therapy is the emergence of resistance to lamivudine ***(22)***. Although the resistance profile of adefovir appears promising with no resistance observed after 1 yr in a Phase III clinical study ***(23)***, experience with anti-HIV therapy warns against complacency. Modeling resistance emergence into HBV viral dynamics could potentially be applied to develop new treatment strategies that may slow down the rate of resistance emergence.

References

1. Wei, X., Ghosh, S. K., Taylor, M. E., et al. (1995) Viral dynamics in human immunodeficiency virus type 1 infection. *Nature* **373,** 117–122.
2. Ho, D. D., Neumann, A. U., Perelson, A. S., Chen, W., Leonard, J. M., and Markowitz, M. (1995) Rapid turnover of plasma virion and CD4 lymphocytes in HIV-1 infection. *Nature* **373,** 123–126.
3. Perelson, A. S., Essunger, P., and Ho, D. D. (1997) Dynamics of HIV-1 and CD4+ lymphocytes in vivo. *AIDS* **11(Suppl A),** S17–S24.
4. Perelson, A. S., Essunger, P., Cao, Y., et al. (1997) Decay characteristics of HIV-1 infected compartments during combination therapy. *Nature* **387,** 188–191.
5. Zeuzem, S., Schmidt, J. M., Lee, J.-H., von Wagner, M., Teuber, G., and Roth W. K. (1998) Hepatitis C virus dynamics in vivo: effect of ribavirin and interferon alfa on viral turnover. *Hepatology* **28,** 245–252.
6. Neumann, A. U., Lam, N. P., Dahari, H., et al. (1998) Hepatitis C viral dynamics in vivo and the antiviral efficacy of interferon-α therapy. *Science* **282,** 103–107.
7. Nowak, M. A. and Bangham, C. R. M. (1996) Population dynamics of immune responses to persistent viruses. *Science* **272,** 74–79.
8. Grisham, J. W. (1962) A morphologic study of deoxyribonucleic acid synthesis and cell proliferation in regenerating rat liver: autoradiography with thymidine-H^3. *Cancer Res.* **22,** 842–849.
9. Blikkendaal-Lieftinck, L. F., Kooij, M., Kramer, M. F., and Den Otter, W. (1977) Cell kinetics in the liver of rats under normal and abnormal dietary conditions. *Exp. Mol. Pathol.* **26,** 184–192.
10. Bianchi, L. and Gudat, F. (1980) Viral antigens in liver tissue and type of inflammation in hepatitis B, in *Virus and the Liver.* (Bianchi, L., Gerok, W., and Sickinger, K., eds.), MTP, Lancaster, UK, pp. 197–204.
11. Guidotti, L. G., Rochford, R., Chung, J., Shapiro, M., Purcell, R., and Chisari, F. V. (1999) Viral clearance without destruction of infected cells during acute HBV infection. *Science* **284,** 825–829.
12. Nowak, M.A., Bonhoeffer, S., Hill, A. M., Boehme, R., Thomas, H.C., and McDade, H. (1996) Viral dynamics in hepatitis B virus infection. *Proc. Natl. Acad. Sci. USA* **93,** 4398–4402.
13. Tsiang, M., Rooney, J. F., Toole, J. J., and Gibbs, C. S. (1999) Biphasic clearance kinetics of hepatitis B virus from patients during adefovir dipivoxil therapy. *Hepatology* **29,** 1863–1869.
14. Perelson, A. S., Neumann, A. U., Markowitz, M., Leonard, J. M., and Ho, D. D. (1996) HIV-1 dynamics in vivo: virion clearance rate, infected cell life-span, and viral generation time. *Science* **271,** 1582–1586.
15. Lau, G. K. K., Tsiang, M., Hou, J., et al. (2000) Combination therapy with lamivudine and famciclovir for chronic hepatitis B-infected Chinese patients: a viral dynamics study. *Hepatology* **32,** 394–399.
16. Herz, A. V. M., Bonhoeffer, S., Anderson, R. M., Ma, R. M., and Nowak, M. A. (1996) Viral dynamics in vivo: limitations on estimates of intracellular delay and virus decay. *Proc. Natl. Acad. Sci. USA* **93,** 7247–7251.

17. Whalley, S. A., Murray, J. M., Brown, D., et al. (2001) Kinetics of acute hepatitis B virus infection in humans. *J. Exp. Med.* **193,** 847–854.
18. Nowak, M. A., Lloyd, A., Vasquez, G. M., et al. (1997) Viral dynamics of primary viremia and antiretroviral therapy in simian immunodeficiency virus infection. *J. Virol.* **71,** 7518–7525.
19. Tsiang, M., Lau, G. K. K., Cheeseman, L. Murray, A., and Gibbs, C. S. (2000) Viral dynamics analysis of HBV clearance under different antiviral treatment regimens using a mathematical model. *Antiviral Res.* **46,** A57.
20. Lewin, S. R., Walters, T., Bowden, S., et al. (2001) Hepatitis B virion (HBV) clearance is extremely rapid in a subset of chronically infected individuals. *Antiviral Res.* **50,** A80.
21. Zhu, Y., Yamamoto, T., Cullen, J., et al. (2001) Kinetics of hepadnavirus loss from the liver during inhibition of viral DNA synthesis. *J. Virol.* **75,** 311–322.
22. Liaw, Y.-F., Leung, N. W. Y., Chang, T.-T., et al. (2000) Effect of extended lamivudine therapy in Asian patients with chronic hepatitis B. *Gastroenterology* **119,** 172–180.
23. Westland, C. E., Yang, H., Delaney IV, W. E., et al. (2001) Week 48 resistance surveillance in chronic hepatitis B patients enrolled in a phase III clinical study of adefovir dipivoxil. *Hepatology* **34(Suppl 4),** 447A.

29

Genotyping Anti-Hepatitis B Virus Drug Resistance

**Eric J. Bourne, Josée Gauthier,
Vincent A. Lopez, and Lynn D. Condreay**

1. Introduction

Agents available or in development for the treatment of chronic hepatitis B virus (HBV) infection fall into two major groups: immunomodulators, such as interferon-α and therapeutic vaccines, and nucleoside/nucleotide analogs, such as lamivudine and adefovir *(1)*. Currently, the only therapies approved in the United States for treatment of chronic HBV infection are IFN-α and lamivudine. However, a number of nucleoside and nucleotide analogs are in development, and it is likely that treatment of chronic HBV infection in the future will involve additional therapies.

Prolonged treatment with antiviral agents can lead to the emergence of drug-resistant virus. Resistance to lamivudine is well documented and is often associated with mutations in the YMDD and FLLAQ loci of the HBV polymerase B and C domains, respectively *(2)*. The primary mutations M552I and M552V are selected in the YMDD locus with L528M in the upstream FLLAQ locus being the most common secondary or compensatory mutation selected. The drug-resistance profiles of investigational drugs such as adefovir, entecavir, L-dT, and ACH-126,443 have yet to be determined. As more drugs become available and combination therapy becomes an option for the treatment of chronic HBV infection, genotyping of clinical samples and assessment of drug-resistance mutations may become an important aspect of disease management.

Methods currently available for genotyping HBV include assays to detect changes throughout the genome (standard sequencing) as well as assays to evaluate identified sites of interest (restriction fragment length polymorphism [RFLP] assays, real-time polymerase chain reaction [PCR]-based assays [Taqman], and the INNO-LiPA HBV DR test). Sequencing of large portions of the viral genome allows detection of changes at multiple sites in the viral genome; however, this methodology does not detect low levels of variants in mixed virus populations without clonal amplification. The site-specific assays permit very sensitive detection of mixed viral populations and thus permit early detection of variants emerging in patients on therapy. Additional assays such as pyrosequencing *(3)*, Luminex *(4)*, and the FLAP endonuclease assay *(5)* could be

From: *Methods in Molecular Medicine, vol. 96: Hepatitis B and D Protocols, volume 2*
Edited by: R. K. Hamatake and J. Y. N. Lau © Humana Press Inc., Totowa, NJ

applied for these purposes, and are currently under development. These site-specific assays have limited utility, if any, in cases where no specific sites of interest have been determined and whole genome sequencing is preferred.

2. Materials

2.1. Lysis and Extraction of HBV DNA from Serum

1. QIAamp® 96 blood kit (cat. no. 351162; QIAGEN, Chatsworth, CA).
2. Tabletop centrifuge and rotor for 96-well plates (Sigma 4-15C, cat. no. 81010; and plate rotor 2 × 96, cat. no. 81031; QIAGEN) or equivalent.
3. Oven for 70°C incubation.
4. Multichannel pipet and filter tips.
5. 95% Ethanol, molecular biology grade.

2.2. PCR Amplification and sequencing

1. Primers ***(6)***:
   Set (i)
   252F (5'-AGACTCGTGGTGGACTTCTCT-3').
   794R (5'-CAAAAGAAAATTGGTAACAGCGGTA-3').
   Set (ii)
   377F (5'-GGA TGT GTC TGC GGC GTT T-3').
   840R (5'-ACC CCA TCT TTT TGT TTT GTT AGG-3') (*see* **Note** 1).
2. SYBR green, 10,000X (Molecular Probes, Eugene, OR) or equivalent for staining of nucleic acids following gel electrophoresis.
3. Thermocycler.
4. 96-Well plates.
5. QIAquick™ PCR purification kit (QIAGEN, cat. no. 28104) or equivalent.
6. Reagents for master mix:10X buffer with 15 m*M* $MgCl_2$ (Perkin Elmer, Foster City, CA), 25 m*M* $MgCl_2$ (Perkin Elmer), 5 U/μL of Ampli*Taq* DNA polymerase (Perkin Elmer), 1.1 μg/μL of Taq Start antibody (ClonTech Laboratories, Palo Alto, CA), DNAse- and RNAse-free sterile water (Sigma, St. Louis, MO), and 20 m*M* dNTPs (Amersham Pharmacia Biotech, Piscataway, NJ).
7. Sequencing reagents (Applied Biosystems, Foster City, CA).
8. DNA sequencer (e.g., ABI 377, ABI 3700, ABI 3100 from Applied Biosystems).

2.3. Reagents for PCR Amplification and RFLP Analysis

1. Primer pairs F1 and B2 (for codon 552 site), F3 and B2 (for codon 528 site) ***(6)***:
   F1 (5'-CAC TGT TTG GCT TTC AGT CAT-3').
   F3 (5'-GTG GGC CTC AGT CCG TTT CTC-3').
   B2 (5'-GTT CAA ATG TAT ACC CAA AG-3').
2. Reagents for master mix: 10X Buffer with 15 m*M* $MgCl_2$ (Perkin Elmer, Foster City, CA), 25 m*M* $MgCl_2$ (Perkin Elmer), 5 U/μL of Ampli*Taq* DNA polymerase, (Perkin Elmer), 1.1 μg/μL of Taq Start antibody (ClonTech Laboratories, Palo Alto, CA), DNAse- and RNAse-free sterile water (Sigma, St. Louis, MO), and 20 m*M* dNTPs (Amersham Pharmacia Biotech, Piscataway, NJ)
3. Restriction endonucleases *Nde*I and *Nla*III (New England Biolabs, Beverly, MA) and *Xho*I (for linearization of control plasmids).
4. Thermocycler.

5. QIAquick™ PCR purification kit (cat. no. 28104).
6. Plasmids pCMVHBV (to generate a standard curve) *(7)* and appropriate control plasmids (e.g., plasmids with L528M/M552V and M552I) *(8)*.
7. Precast 6% TBE-polyacrylamide gel (Invitrogen, Carlsbad, CA).
8. SYBR green, 10,000X (Molecular Probes, Eugene, OR) or equivalent for staining of nucleic acids following gel electrophoresis.
9. Bio-Rad Gel Doc 100 Gel Documentation System and Multi Analyst version 1.1 (Bio-Rad Laboratories, Hercules, CA) or equivalent for capturing gel images.
10. 1000 μg/mL of φX174-*Hae*III digested molecular weight marker (New England Biolabs).
11. 500-V DC power supply.
12. Xcell II gel electrophoresis apparatus (Invitrogen).
13. 5X TBE sample loading buffer (Invitrogen).

2.4. TaqMan Analysis (6)

1. TaqMan Universal PCR master mix (Perkin Elmer).
2. Primers for PCR amplification:
   Codon 528:
   HBVG.F464 (5'-TGT TGC CCG TTT GTC CTC-3').
   HBVG.R711 (5'-AGC CAA ACA GTG GGG GAA-3').
   Codon 552:
   HBVG.F696A (5'-TCA GTG GTT CGT AGG GCT TT-3').
   HBVG.R840A (5'-CCA TCT CTT TGT TTT GTT AGG-3').
3. Fluorescent probes for TaqMan assay: Fluorescently labeled oligonucleotide probes (Genset Corp, Paris, France or Synthetic Genetics, San Diego, CA), containing 6-carboxyfluorescein (FAM), 6-carboxy-4,7,2',7'-tetrachlorofluorescein (TET), or hexachlorofluorescein (HEX) phosphoramidites at the 5' end and the quencher dye 6-carboxytetramethylrhodamine (TAMRA) linked by a phosphate to the 3' end. Different sets of probes are required to encompass various serotypes because of heterogeneity in the HBV DNA sequence within the region.
   Codon 528:
   Set I (*ayw, ayr, adr*)
   528wt (5'-FAM-CCC GTT TCT CCT GGC TCA GTT TAC TAG T-TAMRA-3').
   528mut (5'-TET CCC GTT TCT CAT GGC TCA GTT TAC TAG T-TAMRA-3').
   Set II (*adw2,adw*)
   528wt (5'-FAM-TCCGTTTCTCTTGGCTCAGTTTACTAGTGC-TAMRA 3'.
   528mut (5'-TET-TCCGTTTCTCATGGCTCAGTTTACTAGTGC-TAMRA 3'.
   Codon 552:
   Set I (*ayw, adr*)
   552wt (5'-FAM-TGGCTTTCAGTTATATGGATGATGTGG-TAMRA 3'.
   552mut1 (5'-TET-TGGCTTTCAGTTATGTGGATGATGTG-TAMRA 3').
   552mut2 (5'-HEX-TTGGCTTTCAGTTATATTGATGATGTGG-TAMRA 3').
   Set II (*adw2,adw,ayr*)
   552wt (5'-FAM-TGGCTTTCAGCTATATGGATGATGTG-TAMRA 3').
   552mut1 (5'-TET-TGGCTTTCAGCTATGTGGATGATGT-TAMRA 3').
   552mut2 (5'-HEX-TGGCTTTCAGCTATATTGATGATGTGG-TAMRA 3') *(6)*.
4. Ampli*Taq* Gold (Perkin Elmer).
5. 96-Well optical plates with optical caps (Perkin Elmer).
6. ABI7700 thermocycler-fluorescent plate reader (Perkin Elmer).

2.5. INNO-LiPA Analysis

1. INNO-LiPA HBV DR Amplification kit (cat. no. P-1084, Innogenetics, N.V.).
2. INNO-LiPA HBV DR Detection kit (cat. no. K-1084, Innogenetics, N.V.).

3. Methods

3.1. Lysis and Extraction of HBV DNA from Serum

1. Aliquot serum into a 1.5-mL microcentrifuge tube threaded on the outside containing a screw cap with O-ring, to avoid potential contamination of the original sample. Aliquot only a single tube at a time (*see* **Note 2**).
2. Use appropriate positive (e.g., commercially available HBV-positive serum or control plasmid) and negative (e.g., commercially available HBV-negative serum) controls for determining lysis and extraction efficiency and for detecting possible cross-contamination.
3. Lysis and extraction are performed following the manufacturer's instructions.
4. Store extracted HBV DNA at –20°C for long-term storage and at 4°C for short-term storage.

3.2. Sequencing to Identify Mutation Sites

3.2.1. PCR Amplification (6)

1. PCR primer pairs for amplification are as follows: (1) 252F with 794R to amplify domain B of the HBV polymerase or (2) 377F with 840R to amplify domain C of the HBV polymerase.
2. Set up the following PCR mixture, in a final volume of 50 μL per reaction: 10 μL of extracted HBV DNA, 20 μ*M* Tris-HCl, pH 8.3, 50 m*M* KCl, 2 m*M* $MgCl_2$, 18 m*M* NaCl, 0.2 m*M* of each dNTP (dATP, dCTP, TTP, and dGTP), forward and reverse primers (250 n*M* concentration each), 0.625 U of Ampli*Taq* polymerase, and 0.14 μg Taq Start antibody.
3. Thermocycler conditions: 94°C, 5 min; 40 cycles at 94°C, 30 s; 55°C, 15 s; 72°C, 60 s; 72°C, 60 s; hold at 4°C.
4. Purify the amplicons using the QIAquick™ PCR purification kit (QIAGEN) or equivalent, according to the manufacturer's instructions.
5. Quantify PCR products by using one of the following techniques or equivalent: UV spectroscopy, fluorescence, or visualization following gel electrophoresis and SYBR staining.

3.2.2. DNA Sequencing

1. Perform sequencing reactions using commercially available sequencing reagents and appropriate primers. For sequencing with the ABI377, 40 ng/400 bp of purified DNA is mixed with 3.2 pmol of selected primer in a final reaction volume of 12 μL. For sequencing with the ABI3700, 20 ng/400 bp of purified DNA is mixed with 2.5 pmol of selected primer in a final reaction volume of 6 μL. The primers selected are the same as those used from the initial amplification for each sequencing condition. Sequencing reactions are performed according to manufacturer's suggestions.

3.3. Site-Specific Detection of Mutations

3.3.1. RFLP Assay

1. Generate a standard curve by diluting linearized pCMVHBV and amplifying the linearized DNA using the following concentrations: 10^{10}, 10^9, 10^8, 10^7, 10^4, 10^3, 500, 250, 125, 62.5, and 31.25 copies/mL (*see* **Note 3**).
2. Set up the following PCR mixture, in a final volume of 50 μL per reaction: 10 μL of extracted HBV DNA/positive control/negative control/standard curve; 20 μ*M* Tris-HCl, pH

8.3, 50 m*M* KCl, 2 m*M* $MgCl_2$, 18 m*M* NaCl; 0.2 m*M* of each dNTP (dATP, dCTP, TTP, and dGTP), forward and reverse primers (500 n*M* concentration each), 2.5 U of Ampli*Taq* polymerase, and 0.55 μg of Taq Start antibody. For analysis of the codon 552 site, use primer pairs F1 and B2; for the codon 528 site, F3 and B2 (*see* **Note 4**).

3. Thermocycler conditions: 94°C, 5 min; 40 cycles at 94°C, 30 s; 55°C, 15 s; 72°C, 60 s; 72°C, 60 s; hold at 4°C.
4. Take 5 μL of the amplicon mixture, and digest in a 20-μL volume with *Nde*I or *Nla*III using buffer supplied by the manufacturer.

	Reagents	1 Reaction (μL)
	*Nde*I	*Nla*III
Sterile H_2O	11.8	11.8
10X Buffer 4	2	2
0.293 *M* Spermidine	0.273	N/A
100X Bovine serum albumin (BSA)	N/A	0.2
20 U/μL of *Nde*I	1	N/A
10 U/μL of *Nla*III	N/A	1
PCR sample	5	5
Final volume	20.073	20

5. Add additional enzyme after 30 min of incubation at 37°C. Incubate for an additional 30 min at 37°C.

	Reagents	1 Reaction (μL)
	*Nde*I	*Nla*III
Sterile H_2O	3.5	3.45
10X Buffer 4	0.5	0.5
100X BSA	N/A	0.05
20 U/μL of *Nde*I	1	N/A
10 U/μL of *Nla*III	N/A	1
Final volume	5	5

6. Add and mix 5 μL of 5X TBE sample loading buffer after the 1 h of incubation.
7. Run 5 μL of digestion mixture on a 6% Tris-polyacrylamide gel. Stain with SYBR green for 10 min.
8. Place the gel into a UV light box and capture gel image. Multi Analyst software can be used to quantitate mixtures.

3.3.2. TaqMan Assay (See **Note 5**)

1. Set up PCR reactions in 96-well optical plates. For site 552 reactions, the PCR reaction mixture contained the following (final concentration) in a volume of 50 μL: 1X TaqMan buffer, 4.5 or 4.75 m*M* $MgCl_2$, 200 μ*M* each dNTP, 5% glycerol, 0.01 U of uracil-*N*-glycosylase, 0.04 U of Ampli*Taq* Gold, 200 μ*M* wt fluorescent probe, 200 μ*M* mutant fluorescent probe (for Val or Ile substitution), 800 n*M* forward primer, and 800 n*M* reverse primer. For site 528 reactions, the PCR reaction contained the following in 50 μL: 1X PCR master mix (consisting of buffer, $MgCl_2$, dNTPs, glycerol, uracil-*N*-glycosylase, and Ampli*Taq* Gold), 300 n*M*

forward primer, 900 n*M* reverse primer, 200 n*M* wt fluorescent probe, and 50 or 100 n*M* fluorescent mutant probe.

2. Reaction conditions for site 552 reactions: 50°C, 2 min; 95°C, 10 min; 40 cycles at 95°C, 15s; 65°C, 60 s; hold at 4°C. For site 528 reactions: 50°C, 2 min; 95°C, 10 min; 40 cycles at 95°C, 15 s; 62°C, 60 s; hold at 4°C (*see* **Note 6**).

3.3.3. INNO-LiPA Assay

1. Amplify HBV DNA by PCR using biotinylated primers (*see* above).
2. Perform the assay using the INNO-LiPA HBV DR kit (cat. no. K-1084) according to the manufacturer's instructions.

4. Notes

1. The indicated sequencing primer pairs provide sequences with extensive overlap. However, each set also provides additional sequence information with respect to domain A (set 1) and domain D (set 2).
2. To avoid potential cross-contamination, use filter tips for all pipeting steps.
3. The pCMVHBV plasmid was kindly obtained from Dr. Christoph Seeger. Any plasmid containing the relevant sequence derived from the HBV genome would suffice. Frozen aliquots of the standard curve should be kept at –20°C. This is used to determine the sensitivity of the PCR assay and as a control for the *Nde*I restriction digest reactions. If all members of the standard curve do not completely cut, the restriction digest must be repeated.
4. The RFLP assays detect differences in restriction endonuclease sites between wild-type and drug-resistant viruses. Primer pairs F1 and B2 are designed to examine the methionine codon ATG at position 552 in the YMDD locus. The primer F1 introduces a T → C change in the nucleotide sequence, changing the tyrosine codon at position 551 from TAT to CAT and creating an *Nde*I restriction site (CA↓TATG). If a drug-resistant mutation has occurred that changes the methionine codon to valine (M552V; sequence CATGTG) or isoleucine (M552I; sequence CATATT), the *Nde*I restriction site is destroyed. Substitution of valine for methionine at position 552 creates a new restriction site, *Nla*III (CATG↓). Thus, presence of an *Nde*I site in the codon 552 region indicates a wild-type sequence at codon 552; the presence of an *Nla*III site indicates codon M552V. Primer pairs F3 and B2 are designed to detect a leucine (C/TTG) to methionine (ATG) change at codon 528 in the FLLAQ locus. Substitution of methionine for leucine at that position (L528M) creates an *Nla*III restriction site (CATG↓).
5. Because the TaqMan assay can detect a single basepair mismatch, the presence of polymorphisms in the region to be analyzed may require synthesis of multiple probes to include each expected polymorphism. If information is available in advance indicating serotype, then multiple probe sets may not be necessary.
6. Reaction conditions could be modified slightly based on probe composition ***(6)***.

References

1. Yuen, M-F. and Lai, C-L. (2001) Treatment of chronic hepatitis B. *Lancet Infect. Dis.* **1,** 232–241.
2. Lok, A. and McMahon, B. (2001) Chronic hepatitis B (review). *Hepatology* **34**, 1225–1241.
3. Nordstrom, T., Gharizadeh, B., Pourmand, N., Nyron, P., and Ronaghi, M. (2001) Method enabling fast partial sequencing of cDNA clones. *Analyt. Biochem.* **292**, 266–271.
4. Taylor, J., Briley, D., Nguyen, Q., et al. (2001) Flow cytometric platform for high-throughput single nucleotide polymorphism analysis. *BioTechniques* **30**, 661–666, 668–669.

5. Hsu, T., Law, S., Duan, S., Neri, B., and Kwok, P. (2001) Genotyping single-nucleotide polymorphism by the invader assay with dual-color fluorescence polarization detction. *Clin. Chem.* **47**, 1373–1377.
6. Allen, M., Gauthier, J., DesLauriers, M., et al. (1999) Two sensitive PCR-based methods for the detection of variants associated with reduced susceptibility to lamivudine. *J. Clin. Microbiol.* **37**, 3338–3347.
7. Fallows, D. and Goff S. (1995) Mutations in the epsilon sequences of human hepatitis B virus affect both RNA encapsidation and reverse transcription. *J. Virol.* **69**, 3067–3073.
8. Allen, M., DesLauriers, M., Andrews, C., et al. (1998) Identification and characterization of mutations in hepatitis B virus resistant to lamivudine. *Hepatology* **27**, 1670–1677.

30

A Parsimonious Method for Screening Drug Combinations for Antihepadnaviral Activity Using a Parametric Dose–Response Surface Approach

Tim Shaw and Stephen Locarnini

1. Introduction

Hepatitis B virus (HBV) was identified as a cause of viral hepatitis more than 30 yr ago, and safe and effective hepatitis B vaccines have been available for nearly 20 yr *(1,2)*. Nevertheless, HBV infection continues to be a global health problem, responsible for about 1.2 million deaths every year. It has been estimated that by the end of the year 2000, almost 400 million people—approx 5% of the world's population and more than 10 times the number infected with human immunodeficiency virus (HIV)—were chronically infected with HBV *(1)*. Chemotherapy remains the only option for controlling chronic HBV infection once acquired, but none of the numerous chemotherapeutic strategies used to date has proven consistently successful *(3)*. Prospects for successful treatment of chronic HBV infection have improved dramatically during the past decade as a result of the development of new well-tolerated and efficacious antiviral drugs and to advances in our understanding of HBV replication and pathogenesis. Accumulating knowledge of the mechanisms of antiviral drug action and interaction and drug resistance, together with increasing awareness of their importance, have also contributed *(2,3)*. Although the newer antiviral drugs are capable of reducing viral loads very rapidly, the initial response is invariably followed by a much slower elimination of residual virus *(4)*. As more effective antiviral drugs become available, the emergence of drug resistance during the slower phase of HBV elimination will very likely replace drug-related toxicity as the most significant obstacle in the way of eventual control and ultimately elimination of HBV infection *(3,5)*. Prior experience with HIV indicates that combination chemotherapy has the potential to control or perhaps even eliminate drug resistance, but there is relatively little clinical experience of combination chemotherapy for HBV infection *(3)*. Additional anti-HBV drugs will undoubtedly be needed to con-

From: *Methods in Molecular Medicine, vol. 96: Hepatitis B and D Protocols, volume 2*
Edited by: R. K. Hamatake and J. Y. N. Lau © Humana Press Inc., Totowa, NJ

trol HBV drug resistance in the future *(5)* and methods for preclinical and clinical assessment of anti-HBV drug combinations will also be required *(3)*.

1.1. Combination Chemotherapy

Ideally, combination chemotherapy (the concurrent use of more than one drug to treat disease) offers at least three important advantages over monotherapy. First, provided that appropriate combinations of drugs are used, the dose of each of the individual components of the drug combination will be lower than that required to produce the same desired effect when they are used alone, reducing the risk of troublesome side effects. Second, if the mechanisms or sites of action of each of the individual components of a combination are different or complementary, the duration of treatment required to reach a particular endpoint may be reduced. Finally and most important, it should be possible to minimize the incidence of drug resistance by means of appropriate combination chemotherapy *(3,6)*. Preclinical testing of drug combinations is mandatory even when the individual components of drug combinations have an established history of safety and efficacy. The behavior of drug combinations is not always predictable and they may not interact optimally, especially in chronic HBV-infected patients who may suffer from hepatic and, frequently, from other systemic insufficiency. The aim of preclinical testing of anti-HBV drug combinations is to identify drug combinations that will be safest and most efficacious when used clinically to treat chronic viral infection. How well these aims are satisfied may depend on the choice of assay systems and method used for analysis of results, as we show here.

1.2. Definitions and Terminology

The terms synergy (or synergism) and antagonism are used to describe effects that are, respectively, greater or less than expected. The way in which "expected" results are predicted is therefore crucial to the way in which the outcome of drug interactions is described. Various methods have been used to predict results that are expected if components of a drug combination do not interact *(6–8)*. Here the predicted noninteraction is called a null reference model (NRM). A consensus has yet to be reached regarding the choice of appropriate NRMs, a topic that has fueled controversies for many years *(6)*. Currently there is no universally accepted unambiguous terminology for describing drug interactions *(6)*. The two most widely accepted alternatives for generating NRMs are the empirically based concepts named "Lowe additivity" and "Bliss independence," respectively *(6,8,9)*. It has been proposed that cases in which the observed effects differ from those predicted by the adopted NRM be described as Lowe synergy or Lowe antagonism or Bliss synergy and Bliss antagonism, respectively (*[6]; see* **Table 1**), but even the more specific terminology is misleading. Considering the phenomena that they describe (*see* below), more appropriate descriptions of Lowe additivity and Bliss independence would be "Lowe indifference" and "Bliss interaction," respectively, because only in the former case is the NRM truly null (**Table 1**). Use of the names Lowe and Bliss as adjectives reduces ambiguity and acknowledges the historical origin of the alternatives *(10,11)*, each of which has a logical basis.

Table 1
Terminology for Interactions Between Pairs of Drugs

Activities of individual drugs NRM	Effects of drugs in combination: Greater than predicted	Same as predicted	Less than predicted
Both drugs active			
Lowe NRM	Lowe synergy	Lowe indifference	Lowe antagonism
Bliss NRM	Bliss synergy	Bliss interaction	Bliss antagonism
Only one active drug			
Either NRM	Potentiation	Inertism	Inhibition
Neither drug active			
Either NRM	Coalism	—	—

Modified from *(6)*.

The historically older concept of Lowe additivity is based on the reasonable assumption that a drug cannot interact with itself. The result of a sham combination experiment in which a single agent is used in combination with itself defines Lowe additivity *(11)*. NRMs based on Lowe additivity define noninteraction as conditions that satisfy the equation

$$(d_1/D_1 + d_2/D_2 + \cdots + d_n/D_n) = 1$$

where $D_1, D_2, \ldots, D_n$ are the doses of individual drugs required to produce the same effect as the effect produced by doses $d_1, d_2, \ldots, d_n$ in combination. The sum of this expression is referred to as the interaction or combination index. A combination index of 1 is indicative of no interaction or "Lowe additivity"; combination indices greater or less than 1 indicate antagonism or synergy, respectively. Advantages of this approach are that it is widely applicable and, because it requires no prior knowledge of the mechanisms of action of the individual component drugs, is free of mechanistic restrictions and implications.

The second alternative, Bliss independence, is based on the intuitive notion that each component of a drug combination has the potential to remove targets that would otherwise have been available to the other components. The Bliss independence concept predicts that the effect of two or more drugs should be equal to the product of their fractional effects. Effects can be predicted using the formula

$$E_{1,2,\ldots,n} = E_1 \times E_2 \times \cdots \times E_n$$

where the combined effect $E_{1,2,\ldots,n}$ is the product of the individual fractional effects ($E_1, E_2, \ldots, E_n$). For example, concentrations of two drugs that each reduce replication by 50% of the untreated control level (100%) would be predicted to reduce it to 25% (50% of 50%) when used in combination. The addition of a third drug (at a concentration equivalent to its IC_{50}) to the combination would be predicted to reduce replication to 12.5% of the control (50% of 50% = 25%; 50% of 25% = 12.5%). The main advan-

Table 2
Point-by-Point Analyses of a Simulated Drug Interaction

Raw data			Bliss model			Lowe model		TC-3D analyses					
								Complete data set			Minimal data set		
Data point no.	[Drug 1]	[Drug 2]	Measured effect	Predicted effect	Interaction	Combin. index	Interaction	Predicted	Residual	Interaction	Predicted	Residual	Interaction
1*	0	0	106**					96.6	9.4		100.3	6.4	
2*	0	0	99.2**					96.6	2.6				
3*	0	0	115**					96.6	18.4				
4*	0	0.2	79.2					82.4	–3.2		93.8	–14.6	
5	0	0.5	70.1					60.4	9.7				
6*	0	1	49					38.0	11.0		48.9	0.1	
7	0	2	21					19.5	1.5				
8*	0	5	3.83					6.5	–2.7		6.0	–2.1	
9*	2	0	74.2					89.0	–14.8		81.6	–7.4	
10	5	0	71.5					74.5	–3.0				
11*	10	0	48.1					54.8	–6.7		48.1	0	
12	20	0	30.9					32.6	–1.7				
13*	50	0	16.3					12.3	4.0		16.4	–0.1	
14*	2	0.2	76.3	55.0	ANT.	1.10	ANT.	75.9	0.4	ANT.	76.3	0	BLISS
15	2	0.5	48.8	48.6	ANT.	0.713	SYN.	55.6	–6.8	SYN.			
16*	2	1	44.5	34.0	ANT.	1.10	ANT.	35.0	9.5	ANT.	39.8	4.7	ANT.
17	2	2	15.5	14.6	ANT.	0.901	SYN.	17.9	–2.4	SYN.			
18*	2	5	3.21	2.66	ANT.	0.895	SYN.	6.0	–2.8	SYN.	4.8	–1.7	SYN.
19	5	0.2	56.7	52.9	ANT.	0.944	SYN.	63.5	–6.8	SYN.			
20	5	0.5	47.5	46.9	ANT.	0.978	SYN.	46.5	0.97	ANT.			
21	5	1	26.8	32.7	SYN.	0.811	SYN.	29.3	–2.5	SYN.			
22	5	2	16.9	14.0	ANT.	1.02	ANT.	15.0	1.9	ANT.			
23	5	5	3.25	2.56	ANT.	0.911	ANT.	5.0	–1.8	SYN.			
24*	10	0.2	46.7	35.6	ANT.	1.13	ANT.	46.7	–0.02	SYN.	45.0	1.7	ANT.

25	10	0.5	35.6	31.5	SYN.	0.968	SYN.	34.2	1.37	ANT.			
26*	10	1	21.5	22.1	SYN.	0.818	SYN.	21.6	–0.05	SYN.	23.5	–2.0	SYN.
27	10	2	11.1	9.44	ANT.	0.836	SYN.	11.0	0.06	ANT.			
28*	10	5	2.94	1.72	ANT.	0.878	SYN.	3.7	–0.76	SYN.	2.86	0.08	ANT.
29	20	0.2	24.8	22.9	ANT.	0.809	SYN.	27.8	–3.02	SYN.			
30	20	0.5	21.6	20.3	ANT.	0.844	SYN.	20.4	1.21	ANT.			
31	20	1	17.3	14.1	ANT.	0.899	SYN.	12.8	4.5	ANT.			
32	20	2	7.78	6.07	ANT.	0.751	SYN.	6.6	1.20	ANT.			
33	20	5	1.84	1.10	ANT.	0.698	SYN.	2.2	–0.37	SYN.			
34*	50	0.2	13.6	11.3	ANT.	0.898	SYN.	10.5	3.1	ANT.	15.3	–1.7	SYN.
35	50	0.5	11.1	9.96	ANT.	0.824	SYN.	7.7	3.4	ANT.			
36*	50	1	6.43	7.47	SYN.	0.613	SYN.	4.9	1.6	ANT.	8.0	–1.6	SYN.
37	50	2	3.34	3.20	ANT.	0.539	SYN.	2.5	0.85	ANT.			
38*	50	5	0.89	0.583	ANT.	0.496	SYN.	0.83	0.06	ANT.	0.97	–0.08	SYN.
Control mean = 106.7				Totals	SYN. = 3		SYN. = 21		mean = 0.22	SYN. = 11			SYN. = 5
					ANT. = 22		ANT. = 4		S.D. 2.87	ANT. = 14			ANT. = 3
									S.E. 0.57				IND. = 1

Point-by-point analyses of a simulated drug interaction. The shaded area indicates "surface" (i.e., combination) data points. Columns 1–8 are reproduced from Greco et al. ***(6)***. SYN, Synergy; ANT, antagonism BLISS, exactly as predicted. The measured effects (column 4) were generated from a set of ideal data that described the interaction between a pair of drugs that had maximum effects of 100 (arbitrary units) and IC_{50}s and slope parameters of 10.0 and –1 (drug 1) and 1.0 and –2 (drug 2), respectively. Random errors were introduced into the ideal data set to simulate data that had a relative error characterized by a coefficient of variation of 10%. The Bliss model predictions (column 5) were based on individual calculations for each surface point. If the measured effect was greater than the predicted effect, the interaction was recorded as Bliss synergy (column 6); if less than predicted, it was recorded as Bliss antagonism. Similarly, the combination indices listed in column 7 were calculated for each data point using the dose–effect plots for each drug alone to estimate concentrations required to produce the same effect as the combination. Lowe synergy or Lowe antagonism were recorded in column 8 when the combination index was less or greater than 1.0, respectively. The six right-hand columns show the results of fitting a Bliss model equation to complete sets of data with the aid of TC3D. Columns 9–11 show results for the complete data set; columns 12–14 show the corresponding results for the minimal data set which is identified by **asterisks** in column 1. Synergy and antagonism are recorded if the measured effect is less or greater (respectively) than predicted. **Indicates triplicate controls.

tage of this second approach is its simplicity. The main criticism of the Bliss independence concept seems to be that it is incompatible with Lowe additivity in that it can produce apparently nonsensical results when applied to the sham situation where a single drug is used in combination with itself. Its NRMs involve predictable amounts of drug interaction, hence the description "Bliss Interaction" suggested in **Table 1.**

Another candidate proposed as the basis for NRMs is the "median effect" principle of Chou and Talalay ***(12)***. Despite its lack of statistical rigor, it was rapidly adopted as the basis for assessing drug interactions, especially when anticancer or antiviral drugs were involved. The main reasons for its popularity seem to have been (1) the ease of implementation using commercially available microcomputer software and (2) the ease with which it produces apparently unequivocal results. As a result of frequent citation it has been very influential. Currently, improved, updated software for drug interaction analysis based on the median effect principle remains readily available and now incorporates some statistical functions (*see* **Note 1**). However, for various reasons that are discussed in detail elsewhere ***(6,9)***, it cannot be regarded as a reasonable alternative basis for NRMs, and will not be considered here.

Both Lowe antagonism and Bliss independence concepts have strong advocates. In the antiviral research literature, for example, Prichard and Schipman ***(9)*** favor Bliss independence, whereas Sühnel ***(8)*** advocates Lowe additivity. A comprehensive review of published methods for analysis of drug interactions is provided by Greco et al. ***(6)***, who critically compare different approaches by applying each to analysis of a common data set. The data set consists of 38 datum points that simulate the results of an experiment using two drugs in combination (*see* footnote to **Table 2**). Preference for a simulated rather than a real data set was stated to be determined by the need to have a "true" solution to the drug interaction problem that could provide an absolute standard for comparison of rival analytic approaches. The data set together with some of the results of their analyses is reproduced here in columns 1–8 of **Table 2**. Our reason for appropriating this data set is that it has already been thoroughly analyzed by a variety of other methods with a detailed discussion of both methods and outcomes by Greco and colleagues ***(6)***. Their lucid and comprehensive review, which provides historical and theoretical background as well as mathematical derivation and analyses of 13 different competing analytical approaches, is highly recommended. Here we use the data to demonstrate a parsimonious method of drug interaction analysis that we have developed using the scientific graphics-statistics program TableCurve3D (TC3D; *see* **Note 2**).

2. Dose–Response Surface (DRS) Concepts

As more anti-HBV drugs become available, combination chemotherapy for HBV infection is likely to become routine ***(3)*** and simultaneous development of generally acceptable methods to screen drug combinations for anti-HBV activity and to describe and quantify drug interactions (if any) will be essential. The need for better ways to represent the outcome of drug interactions than by means of conventional two-dimensional (2D) graphs was recognized more than a century ago, when theoretical three-dimensional (3D) models of drug interaction were first developed ***(6,8,9)***. It was recognized that the interaction between two drugs could be represented by plotting the individual drug concentrations on horizontal *X*- and *Y*-axes against the biological effect on the *Z* (vertical) axis to generate a virtual 3D surface. The slope and shape of this DRS would reflect the shapes of sets of 2D profiles produced by cutting the surface vertically or horizontally and viewing only the cut surface. Subsets of these profiles correspond to conventional dose–response plots and conventional isobolograms, respectively. (For detailed discussion, *see [6]* and *[9]*.) However, the technology required for rapid and accurate analysis of data by 3D graphical methods had not been developed until relatively recently. The widespread availability of personal computers and suitable commercially available scientific graphics software now allow 3D graphs to be drawn with ease and make the routine use of 3D graphical analyses feasible. Comparing 2D and 3D graphs that illustrate the same drug interactions should make the main advantage of the latter obvious. Further advantages follow if DRS forms can be described in terms of mathematical and statistical parameters. Parametric DRS methods allow different types of drug interactions to be described quantitatively and ideally include statistical measures of the reliability of parameter estimates. The main advantages of the parametric DRS approach include the following:

1. Large sets of complex data can be reduced to small sets of statistically meaningful parameters.
2. They are relatively objective and rigorous when properly designed.
3. They are flexible and adaptable to a variety of different experimental designs.
4. They facilitate prediction of the effects of particular drug combinations and conversely, prediction of drug doses required to produce a desired effect.
5. They have the potential to provide insights into complex interactions.

Graphical representation of DRS requires only a graphics program capable of producing adequate 3D surface plots; parametric DRS methods require additional statistics capabilities.

The only disadvantage of parametric DRS approaches are associated with the problem of choosing from the variety of credible alternative models available. Furthermore, because these approaches are still evolving, models that are presently satisfactory are likely to be rapidly superseded.

Logical extensions of DRS concepts (both empirical and parametric) entail the subtraction of a predicted surface from the experimentally observed and mapped surface so as to generate 3D difference surfaces. This idea has been championed by Prichard and Shipman (parametric; *[9]*) and Sühnel (empirical; *[8]*) among others. Although the methodology is logical and the results visually appealing, a large number of datum points is required to produce meaningful results. The difference surface that is generated by the extra data processing required by this approach may obscure underlying dose–response relationships and may sometimes lead to spurious conclusions unless rigorous statistical tests for deviation from the predicted reference surface are applied. For example, experimental errors and artifacts may be easily but erroneously interpreted as localized patches of synergy or antagonism.

2.1. Choice of Computer Software

Most modern graphics programs include 3D graphics options, but relatively few offer automated surface fitting and statistical capabilities. Conversely, most statistics programs that are capable of analyzing drug combination data also have the capacity to generate 3D graphs, usually with only limited surface fitting options. Although import and export of data to and from compatible programs is rarely a problem, it is unnecessary with TC3D, a program that is specifically designed for statistical analysis of 3D data (*see* **Note 2**). When we started using TC3D it was—and remains—one of the few such programs readily available. It offers a large number of preprogrammed equations (nearly 4000) and a variety of different curve fitting (error minimization) options, allows the generation and storage of user-defined functions, and is relatively user-friendly compared to others of comparable sophistication and functionality. As shown below, TC3D can be used to model the results of experiments based on real or simulated data and compare expected outcomes based on different models. TC3D will readily import and export data in a variety of common spreadsheet configurations and will export data to other scientific graphics programs. It is also economical compared with much less versatile programs specifically designed for dose–effect analyses such as CalcuSyn (*see* **Note 1**), which has only limited 2D (and no 3D) graphics capacity. The DRS approach outlined here relies heavily on the use of TC3D, but would be readily adaptable to computer software with comparable capabilities.

3. Background to Current Protocol

Our major aim was to develop a method for screening combinations of two or more potential anti-HBV agents that was efficient and economical in terms of materials, labor, and data requirements. It had to be immediately applicable to our existing assays—for example, refs. ***13*** and ***14***—and therefore sufficiently robust to cope with small data sets that were relatively insensitive and inaccurate. At the same time, it had to be sufficiently flexible and forward-looking to be able to handle data generated by more sophisticated, recently developed high-throughput assays—for example, refs. ***15—17***— and others that can reasonably be expected to become routinely available in the near future (*see* **Note 3**). Methods of data analysis had to be as simple as possible, yet sufficiently versatile to adapt to different alternative concepts of drug interaction and, preferably, to different methods of data analysis. The strategy described here was originally developed for application to results obtained from in vitro assays using a duck HBV–primary duck hepatocyte (DHBV-PDH) assay system ***(13)***. It has evolved in parallel with the development of more controllable and reproducible in vitro assays that use recombinant baculovirus vectors to transduce efficiently HepG2 cells with HBV ***(18, 19)***. The latter assay method can also be used to measure the relative sensitivity of drug-resistant strains of HBV ***(7)***. There are no obvious reasons why the concepts and methods outlined here could not be applied to other assay systems and perhaps ultimately to clinical results as more facile and accurate assays become available (***4***; *see also* **Note 3**). Comments on individual aspects of the suggested strategy illustrated by **Table 3** follows.

Table 3
Suggested Strategy for DRS Evaluation of Drug Interactions

1.	Choose an assay system.		
2.	Determine the dose range of interest for each drug.		
3.	Identify the best dose–effect model for each drug when used alone.		
4.	Validate the assay and dose-effect model using replicate experiments.		
5.	Choose a null reference model (NRM).		
6.	Design a combination experiment using appropriate dose ranges for each drug.		
7.	Perform the experiment and collect data.		
8.		EITHER	
	Fit the data to a NRM (Lowe approach)	OR	Fit the preconceived model to the data (Bliss approach)
9.	Form conclusions if possible or repeat starting from appropriate step.		

3.1. Choice of Assay System

Historically, the study of HBV has been hindered by the lack of small animal models and cell culture systems that are able to support complete cycles of HBV infection ***(2,5)***. Besides technical problems, ethical, biosafety, and other constraints restricted the use of primary cultures of human and primate cells, which were the only cell types known to be susceptible to HBV infection. Even after the two main surrogates for study of HBV—duck HBV (DHBV) and woodchuck (WHV)—were established as accepted models, antiviral assays remained (and still remain) difficult. Hepadnaviral infections are generally noncytopathic, so that monitoring viral replication has to depend on assays for virus-specific nucleic acids or their expression products. Transient transfection of cells with HBV is achievable but inefficient and variable in outcome. Stably transfected cell lines continuously producing HBV virions, most notably the HepG2-derived 2.2.15 line, have been generated and widely used for antiviral assays (see ***[17]***, for example), but they are not ideal models of HBV infection because, among other reasons, the viral genome is permanently integrated into the host cells' nuclear DNA. Assays that use primary cell lines (***[13]***, for example) are more closely analogous with natural HBV infections, but they typically produce results that are subject to wide variation and are consequently difficult to standardize. Variability is presumably the result of a variety of factors including differences in initial viral load or efficiency of infection, differences in the cell type makeup of primary cultures, as well as differences in the metabolic state of the cultured cells. A cell-free high throughput assay for DHBV reverse transcriptase assay has been described ***(16)*** but can be expected to be of limited use for drug combination studies. A high-throughput version of the Hep AD38 assay described by King and Ladner ***(15)***, and others like it, appear to have greatest potential for application to future drug combination studies. The protocol described here was developed for application to data obtained using assays based on an in vitro assay system that relies on the use of recombinant baculovirus vectors to introduce replication competent HBV genomes into HepG2 cells with high efficiency ***(19)***. Application of this system for antiviral assays was initially demonstrated using lamivudine *(4)* and later extended for comparing the sensitivities of lamivudine-resistant HBV mutants *(7)*. Most recently, we have used it for drug combination studies *(20)*. Protocols for assays using this recombinant baculovirus (rBV) system have been described in detail elsewhere *(7,18,19)*. As the system is more efficient, controllable, and reproducible than the DHBV-PDH system that we used previously *(13)*, more frugal experimental designs are possible. This is an important advantage because the assays are relatively labor intensive, as they remain ultimately dependent on the efficient isolation and accurate quantification of viral nucleic acids or their expression products (*see* **Note 3**). The suggested protocol should, in principle, be applicable to other assay systems that possess comparable accuracy and sensitivity.

3.2. Assay Validation

The characteristics of the chosen assay system(s) should be established in terms of dynamic range, accuracy, sensitivity, and inter- and intraassay variability using appropriate positive and negative controls. The assay can then be used to determine appropriate drug concentrations for combination experiments. Accuracy may be improved by increasing numbers of replicates and dynamic range and sensitivity increased by altering detection methods. These characteristics will determine the ability of the system to distinguish between possible experimental outcomes of synergy, no interaction, and antagonism.

3.3. Choice of Dose–Effect Models

Pharmacological responses are typically, but not invariably, nonlinear. 2D plots of biological effect (dependent variable, plotted on the *Y* axis) against the drug concentration required to produce it (independent variable, plotted on the *X* axis) usually resemble the profile of the downhill section of an Olympic ski-jump when the *X* axis is linear (*see* **Fig. 2**). Plotting *x* on a logarithmic scale usually reveals upper and lower plateaus connected by an approximately "S"-shaped transition. A variety of mathematical functions can adequately describe such dose–effect relationships. The parameters of the preferred functions have a clear relationship to biological effect(s). Three of the simplest and most useful and widely accepted dose–effect models are described by the logistic dose response (LDR), log normal cumulative (LNC), or single exponential (EXP) functions:

$$\text{LDR: } y = a/[1 + (x/b)^c]$$
$$\text{LNC: } y = a/2^*\text{erfc}[-\ln(x/b)/\sqrt{2c}]$$
$$\text{EXP: } y = a\exp(-x/b)$$

where *y* represents the effect produced and *x* represents the drug concentration required to produce it. For the LNC funtion, erfc is the error function complement.

For LDR and LNC functions *a*, *b*, and *c* determine the amplitude, transition center (*x* at half amplitude), and width, respectively. If a complete (100%) response is achievable, *b* corresponds to drug concentration required to produce a 50% response. This concentration is the reference point for a variety of different types of assays, the most important in the present context being the 50% inhibitory concentration and the 50% cytotoxic concentration (IC_{50} and CC_{50} or alternatively EC_{50} and TC_{50}, respectively). For EXP functions, a is the amplitude and b determines the curve slope; at half the amplitude, $x = \ln(2/b)$.

In the examples used here, the maximum amplitude is the control response (no drug) and response to drug is expressed in terms or the amount of analyte (virus replication) remaining, rather than in terms of inhibition.

4. Analysis of a Set of Simulated Data Using TC3D

Raw data from **Table 2** (columns 2–4) were analyzed using TC3D. First, appropriate dose–response models for each drug were identified separately. LDR, LNC, and EXP functions were fitted to the unweighted raw data and also to data weighted assuming the presence of a 10% fractional error in Z. As shown in **Fig. 1** and **Table 4**, effects of both drugs could be described by LDR, LNC, or EXP functions with varying degrees of accuracy. Weighting data affected "goodness-of-fit" parameters (see below) and equation parameters but not the validity of the models (**Table 4**). The entire data set was then analyzed using TC3D. As the effects of both drug 1 and drug 2 when used alone could be described adequately by LDR equations, preprogrammed equations that had LDR functions in both X (drug 1) and Y (drug 2) were chosen for surface fitting (*see* **Note 4**). Six alternatives were selected. They could be summarized by three basic interaction expressions

$$E_{1,2} = E_1E_2 \text{ (Bliss model)}$$
$$E_{1,2} = E_1 + E_2$$
$$E_{1,2} = E_1 + E_2 + E_1E_2$$

where $E_{1,2}$ represents the effect of the drug combination and E_1 and E_2 represent the effects of the individual drugs when used alone (drugs 1 and 2, respectively, in this example). The three additional equations were identical except that they included a constant that defined a Z-intercept (which determines the position of the surface in the vertical dimension). Further preprogrammed options in which an LDR response was present in X or Y only, as well as a pair of equations (with and without Z-intercept) describing alternatives in which the slope (c) parameters for X and Y were equal were omitted, since they were known to be inappropriate.

4.1. "Goodness-of-Fit" Criteria

Surface fitting using TC3D generates lists of fitted equations ranked in order of four different "goodness-of-fit" criteria, namely: (1) the coefficient of determination (r^2), (2) r^2 adjusted for degrees of freedom (DF adj r^2), (3) fit standard error (FSE), or (4) F-statistic. Each list is arranged in columns showing the following information (in order from left to right): rank number according to nominated criterion; floating point (FP) value; value for selected criterion; TC3D equation number; summary of equation. The number of equation parameters and the FP value can also be used to rank fitted equations. Ranking by r^2 or DF adj r^2 produces the same order in most cases; the same applies to FP value and parameter count. Fitting the complete unweighted data set from **Table 2** gave the results shown in **Panel 1**.

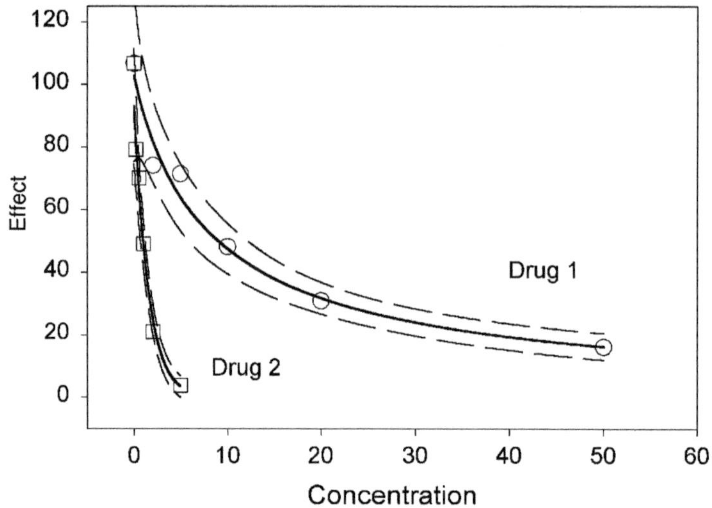

Fig. 1. 2D dose–response plots for drugs 1 and 2 when used alone. The *finer dashed lines* on either side of the each plot represent 95% confidence intervals. Only logistic dose–response (LDR) plots are shown: parameters for these and alternative fits are listed in **Table 4.**

Table 4
Results of Dose–Effect Analysis for Individual Drugs.

	Drug 1			Drug 2		
Equation type	LDR	LNC	EXP	LDR	LNC	EXP
	Raw data *Weighted data*			Raw data *Weighted data*		
Goodness-of-fit parameters						
DF adj r^2	0.94	0.94	0.98	0.94	0.94	0.88
	0.98	*0.98*	*0.97*	*0.97*	*0.97*	*0.84*
FSE	7.4	7.3	4.9	6.3	6.5	9.9
	1.0	*1.0*	*1.16*	*2.9*	*3.0*	*7.1*
F-statistic	65	65	299	65	63	51
	153	*117*	*254*	*123*	*115*	*37*
Equation parameters						
a	102 ± 7	104 ± 7	102 ± 4	105 ± 6	106 ± 6	96 ± 7
	89 ± 7	*92 ± 8*	*93 ± 7*	*103 ± 9*	*104 ± 9*	*77 ± 10*
b	1.1±0.1	0.8 ± 0.2	1.3 ± 0.1	8.1 ± 2.0	8.0 ± 2	17 ± 4
	1.1 ± 0.1	*1.0 ± 0.1*	*1.5 ± 0.1*	*8.5 ± 0.2*	*8.1 ± 2*	*29 ± 5*
c	2.0± 0.2	1.3 ± 0.3		0.8 ± 0.2	1.9 ± 0.3	
	2.0 ± 0.2	*0.93 ± 0.1*		*0.9 ± 0.1*	*1.8± 0.2*	

Data correspond to points 1–13 in **Table 2.** "Goodness-of-fit" parameters and weighting are explained, and formulae are provided in the text.

PANEL 1

Sorted by DF adj r^2				
1	0.9780754629	76	2144	z=a+LDRX(b,c,d)+ LDRY(e,f,g)+LDRX(h,c,d)* LDRY(1,f,g)
2	0.9757918437	37	2133	z=LDRX(a,b,c)*LDRY(1,d,e)
3	0.974087532	38	2134	z=a+LDRX(b,c,d)*LDRY(1,e,f)
4	0.5316786963	37	2137	z=LDRX(a,b,c)+LDRY(d,e,f)
5	−0.045157021	38	2138	z=a+LDRX(b,c,d)+LDRY(e,f,g)
6	−0.233333321	75	2143	z=LDRX(a,b,c)+LDRY(d,e,f)+ LDRX(g,b,c)*LDRY(1,e,f)
Sorted by F-statistic				
1	385.7933297	37	2133	z=LDRX(a,b,c)*LDRY(1,d,e)
2	288.38896748	38	2134	z=a+LDRX(b,c,d)*LDRY(1,e,f)
3	245.11431976	76	2144	z=a+LDRX(b,c,d)+ LDRY(e,f,g)+ LDRX(h,c,d)*LDRY(1,f,g)
4	9.9108310825	37	2137	z=LDRX(a,b,c)+LDRY(d,e,f)
5	0.9302375276	38	2138	z=a+LDRX(b,c,d)+LDRY(e,f,g)
6	5.166667e–08	75	2143	z=LDRX(a,b,c)+LDRY(d,e,f)+ LDRX(g,b,c)*LDRY(1,e,f)
Sorted by Fit Standard Error (FSE)				
1	4.6212057009	76	2144	z=a+LDRX(b,c,d)+ LDRY(e,f,g)+LDRX(h,c,d)* LDRY(1,f,g)
2	4.8635186867	37	2133	z=LDRX(a,b,c)*LDRY(1,d,e)
3	5.0293511537	38	2134	z=a+LDRX(b,c,d)*LDRY(1,e,f)
4	21.381074532	37	2137	z=LDRX(a,b, c)+LDRY(d,e,f)
5	31.924364747	38	2138	z=a+LDRX(b,c,d)+LDRY(e,f,g)
6	34.679412023	75	2143	z=LDRX(a,b,c)+ LDRY(d,e,f)+LDRX(g,b,c)* LDRY(1,e,f)

The F-statistic is a measure of how well a particular equation models the data, with higher values representing better fits. Ranking by F-statistic favors simpler equations over equally effective but more complex equations. If an additional parameter (or data manipulation step) improves the model, the F-statistic increases; otherwise, it decreases. Ranking by F-statistic is recommended for sorting nonlinear equations. The FSE is the least squares error of fit: lower values indicate better fits. It is useful for comparing different fits to a set of data, but it is sensitive to the number and distribution of data points and not appropriate for comparing fits to dissimilar data sets. Because the F-statistic and FSE increase and decrease, respectively, as "goodness-of-fit" improves, it is probably valid to use higher F-statistic/FSE ratios to choose between closely contending equations that describe a particular data set. As a general rule, simpler equations (favored by F-statistic ranking) are preferable. In the example

PANEL 2

Rank 1 Eqn 2133 z=LDRX(a,b,c)*LDRY(1,d,e)

XYZ *	X Value	Y Value	Z Value	Z Value	Residual	Residual%	95% Confidence	Limits	95% Prediction	Limits	Weights
1	0	0	115	100.11645	14.883554	12.942221	95.093391	105.1395	89.019591	111.2133	1
2	0	0	99.2	100.11645	−0.916446	−0.923837	95.093391	105.1395	89.019591	111.2133	1
3	0	0	106	100.11645	5.8835539	5.5505225	95.093391	105.1395	89.019591	111.2133	1
4	0	0.2	79.2	91.126702	−11.9267	−15.05897	86.215257	96.038148	80.07992	102.17348	1
5	0	0.5	70.1	70.434855	−0.334855	−0.477681	64.812464	76.057245	59.054152	81.815557	1
6	0	1	49	44.222104	4.7778964	9.7508089	39.570504	48.873703	33.288372	55.155835	1
7	0	2	21	20.896639	0.1033613	0.4921966	16.344128	25.44915	10.004694	31.788584	1
8	0	5	3.83	5.8227408	−1.992741	−52.02979	3.0813422	8.5641394	−4.444896	16.090378	1
9	2	0	74.2	83.820781	−9.620781	−12.96601	78.786215	88.855346	72.718711	94.92285	1
10	2	0.2	76.3	76.294271	0.0057285	0.0075079	72.108699	80.479844	65.550523	87.03802	1
11	2	0.5	48.8	58.970376	−10.17038	−20.84093	54.635071	63.305681	48.167415	69.773338	1
12	2	1	44.5	37.024199	7.4758008	16.799552	33.324666	40.723732	26.460315	47.588084	1
13	2	2	15.5	17.495353	−1.995353	−12.87325	13.666618	21.324088	6.8855311	28.105175	1
14	2	5	3.21	4.87499	−1.66499	−51.86885	2.5586458	7.1913343	−5.287419	15.037399	1
15	5	0	71.5	66.371863	5.1281371	7.1722198	61.578872	71.164854	55.377234	77.366492	1
16	5	0.2	56.7	60.412142	−3.712142	−6.546988	56.529526	64.294758	49.782758	71.041527	1
17	5	0.5	47.5	46.694551	0.8054489	1.6956818	43.078735	50.310367	36.159693	57.229409	1
18	5	1	26.8	29.316896	−2.516896	−9.391401	26.309905	32.323886	18.975179	39.658612	1
19	5	2	16.9	13.853357	3.0466433	18.027475	10.781362	16.925352	3.4925526	24.214161	2
20	5	5	3.25	3.8601665	−0.610167	−18.77435	2.013483	5.7068501	−6.205585	13.925918	1

21	10	0	48.1	48.787927	−0.687927	−1.430202	44.722697	52.853158	38.090488	59.485367	1
22	10	0.2	46.7	44.407119	2.2928811	4.9098096	41.040967	47.773271	33.955321	54.858917	1
23	10	0.5	35.6	34.323737	1.2762629	3.5850083	31.353347	37.294127	23.992603	44.654871	1
24	10	1	21.5	21.549954	−0.049954	−0.232343	19.189235	23.910672	11.377338	31.722569	1
25	10	2	11.1	10.183179	0.916821	8.2596486	7.8874175	12.478941	0.0254416	20.340916	1
26	10	5	2.94	2.8374904	0.1025096	3.4867211	1.4739172	4.2010636	−7.150925	12.825906	1
27	20	0	30.9	31.51218	−0.61218	−1.981167	27.343722	35.680639	20.775088	42.249273	1
28	20	0.2	24.8	28.682611	−3.882611	−15.65569	24.982378	32.382844	18.118482	39.246741	1
29	20	0.5	21.6	22.169743	−0.569743	−2.637698	19.133442	25.206043	11.819466	32.520019	1
30	20	1	17.3	13.919141	3.3808592	19.542539	11.794138	16.044144	3.7986296	24.039652	1
31	20	2	7.78	6.5773275	1.2026725	15.458516	4.9447435	8.2099114	−3.451353	16.606008	1
32	20	5	1.84	1.8327384	0.0072616	0.3946503	0.9340514	2.7314255	−8.102892	11.768369	1
33	50	0	16.3	14.957469	1.342531	8.2363866	10.97057	18.944368	4.2895513	25.625387	1
34	50	0.2	13.6	13.614395	−0.014395	−0.105844	9.9783552	17.250434	3.0725784	24.156211	1
35	50	0.5	11.1	10.523018	0.5769821	5.1980369	7.64737	13.398666	0.2187246	20.827311	1
36	50	1	6.43	6.6068141	−0.176814	−2.74983	4.7456403	8.4679878	−3.461606	16.675234	1
37	50	2	3.34	3.1219728	0.2180272	6.5277593	2.0590287	4.184917	−6.829859	13.073805	1
38	50	5	0.89	0.8699217	0.0200783	2.2559934	0.4010328	1.3388105	−9.036085	10.775928	1

shown here, the first four equations (2133, 2134, 2143, and 2144) in each list clearly fit the data better than the last two by all criteria. The two leading equations, 2144 and 2133, give similar FSE (4.62 and 4.86, respectively) and DF adj r^2 (0.978 and 0.976, respectively). Inspection of the surface fits (**Fig. 1**) confirms that both equations fit the data well. Equation 2133 gives a better *F*-statistic than 2144 (385.7 compared to 288.4) and a higher *F*-statistic/FSE ratio (approx 79 compared to 53 for Eq. 2144). It is also preferred because it is simpler.

4.2. Data Summary

A list showing the fit for all individual data points can be generated for each fitted equation. Fitting Eq. 2133 to the complete data set produces the data summary shown in **Panel 2**. The default value for parameter estimates is eight digits.

4.3. Numeric Summary

A numeric summary of all fitted parameters and goodness-of-fit statistics for each data set can also be generated, including an estimate of the volume enclosed by the fitted surface (analogous to the area under curve [AUC] parameter for 2D pharmacokinetic plots). In antiviral assays, the volume under the surface ("VUS"; "volume" in numeric summaries) is proportional to the amount of viral replication, smaller volumes indicating greater antiviral activity. As an example, the data summary resulting from fitting Eq. 2133 to the complete data set is shown in **Panel 3**.

4.4. Predictions Based on Fitted DRS

From the fitted surface, it is possible to predict *X, Y*, or *Z* values (or a variety of their derivatives) from input pairs of data. For example, the value of *X* required to give $Z = 50$ in the absence of *Y* and vice versa. Predicting *Z* from these *X* and *Y* estimates gives the *Z* value from the curve fit (in this case, Bliss independence) equation (*see* **Panel 4**). This facility is particularly useful for designing experiments and comparing observed values with those predicted by the model under study.

4.5. Effects of Weighting Data

Because the data set being analyzed was created by introduction of random errors into a set of "perfect" data, we next repeated the procedures outlined above after weighting data by $1/(Z \times 0.1)^2$ to allow for errors of the order of 10% of *Z*. Of the alternative equations, only Eq. 2133 produced an acceptable result by any of the goodness-of-fit criteria, as shown below. Inspection of the new surface modeled by Eq. 2133 showed that the distribution of data points in relation to the surface had changed. There were 13, 5, and 1 points now lying within 1, 2, and 3 standard deviations (SD), respectively, of the surface, with 19 points located beyond 3 SD. Estimated parameters for the surface equation also changed, as summarized in **Table 5**. Although some of the parameters are closer to those that describe the "true" data, the new surface clearly fits the raw data less well than previously, based on lower *F*-statistic and confirmed by visual inspection (*see* **Fig. 2**). *Z* values predicted by the new surface also lead to different conclusions about drug interactions, as summarized in **Tables 2** and **5**. These results, together with the conclusions of Greco et al. ***(6)***,

PANEL 3

Rank 1	Eqn 2133	z=LDRX(a,b,c)*LDRY(1,d,e)

r^2 Coef Det	DF Adj r^2	Fit Std Err	F–val
0.9790632162	0.9757918437	4.8635186867	385.7933297

Parm	Value	Std Error	t–value	95% Confidence	Limits	P>|t|
a	100.1164461	2.468919845	40.55070736	95.09339095	105.1395013	0.00000
b	9.527665422	0.816940493	11.66261864	7.865587493	11.18974335	0.00000
c	−1.04915226	0.088769674	−11.818814	−1.22975552	−0.868549	0.00000
d	0.862589296	0.055651431	15.49985834	0.749365608	0.975812983	0.00000
e	−1.58465568	0.141791388	−11.1759657	−1.87313243	−1.29617894	0.00000

Volume Xmin,Xmax Ymin,Ymax	Volume Precision
2313.3769101	2.1131e–09

X at Fn Zmin	Y at Fn Zmin	Fn Zmin
50	5	0.8699216584
X at Fn Zmax	Y at Fn Zmax	Fn Zmax
0	0	100.11644614

Procedure	Minimization	Iterations	
Lev–Marq	LeastSquares	74	
r^2 Coef Det	DF Adj r^2	Fit Std Err	r^2 Attaina
0.9790632162	0.9757918437	4.8635186867	0.9966304129

Source	Sum of Squares	DF	Mean Square	F Statistic	P>F
Regr	36501.935	4	9125.4837	385.793	0.00000
Error	780.57586	33	23.653814		
Total	37282.511	37			
Lack Fit	654.9492	31	21.127393	0.336352	0.93412
Pure Err	125.62667	2	62.813333		

Description: c:/greco_.prn

X Variable:

Xmin:0	Xmax:50	Xrange: 50
Xmean: 13.736842105	Xstd: 17.244951021	

Y Variable:

Ymin: 0	Ymax: 5	Yrange: 5
Ymean: 1.3736842105	Ystd: 1.7244951021	

Z Variable:

Zmin: 0.89	Zmax: 115	Zrange: 114.11
Zmean: 35.534473684	Zstd: 31.743273618	

PANEL 4

	X	Y	Z	95%Confidence	Intervals	
1.	9.602314904332	0	50	45.33941019975	54.66058980025	X=Root(Z,Y)
2.	0	0.952664382756	50	45.28321662139	54.71678337861	Y=Root(Z,X)
3.	9.602314904	0.952664382	23.96121730108	21.219739990733	26.70503469483	Z=F(X,Y)

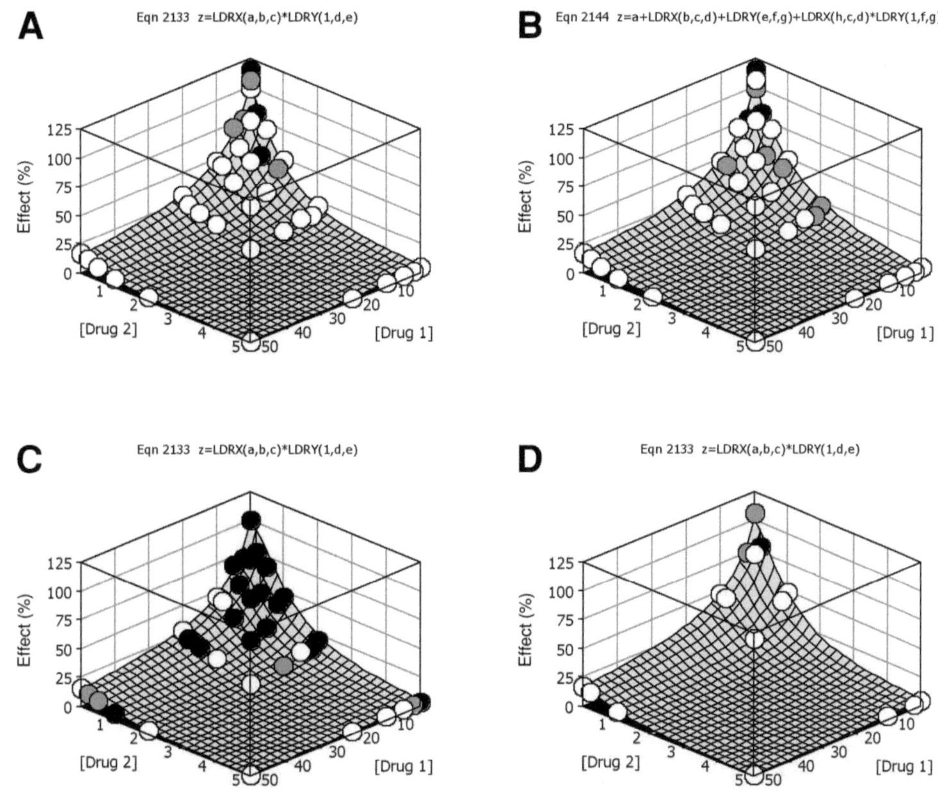

Fig. 2. Dose–response surfaces. Surfaces fitted to raw data by TC3D using Eqs. **(A)** 2133 or **(B)** 2144. **(C)** Surface fitted to weighted data by Eq. 2133. (D) Bliss model (Eq. 2133) fitted to minimal data set. Data points that lie within 1 or 2 standard deviations (SD) from the DRS are in white or gray respectively; those further than 2 SD are in black.

demonstrate how different methods of data treatment and analysis can affect conclusions from experimental data.

5. Frugal Experimental Design

Adoption of the parametric DRS approach for analyses of drug interactions requires three main decisions that determine experimental design: (1) which drug concentrations to use, (2) the number of replicates needed, and (3) the number of experiments required. A minimum of three experiments is usually necessary. A preliminary experiment should establish the responses to individual drugs and identify appropriate drug concentrations for a second "exploratory" experiment aimed at determining how the drugs interact at selected concentrations, and a third confirmatory experiment designed on the basis of results of the second. Whether additional experiments will be required will depend on the nature of the drug interactions (if present) and the degree of stringency required to make conclusions. Interactions that can be approximated by simple models will require less confirmatory data than more complex interactions. Complex interactions may depend not only on absolute drug concentrations but also on concentration ratios. Optimal experimental designs will minimize the number of data points and replicates required while maximizing the possibility of generating conclusive data. Discussion of the concept of "D-optimal" designs, the most frequently used in biological systems, is beyond the scope of this chapter. However, an important consensus observation in this context is noteworthy: the minimum number of experimental data points required for D-optimal designs is usually equal to the number of estimable parameters. Assuming that one or more of the preprogrammed LDR-based equations available in TC3D can adequately describe the 3D combination effects for two drugs, a D-optimal design should require no more than seven data points, equivalent to the maximum number of equation parameters. [The parameters are *a–g* in the most complex equation under consideration, which is: $z = a + \mathrm{LDRX}(a, b, c) + \mathrm{LDRY}(d, e, f) + \mathrm{LDRX}(g, b, c) * \mathrm{LDRY}(1, e, f)$]. Whether this is the case in practice will depend on the accuracy and sensitivity of the particular assay system.

We have devised a parsimonious, essentially empirical, approach bearing these considerations in mind, building mainly on practical experience. For two drug combinations, it requires a minimum of nine drug combination data points, three different concentration controls for each drug separately, and triplicate drug-free controls, a minimum of 18 data points per assay set. This frugal experimental design is recommended for exploratory experiments in which the three different concentrations of each drug should, ideally, be evenly distributed on either side of the (previously estimated) 50% inhibitory concentration (IC_{50}) for each. The nine drug combination data ("surface") points should be able to indicate the type of interaction (if any) in relation to the chosen NRM and indicate what modifications if any are needed for confirmatory experiment(s).

The right-hand columns of **Tables 2** and **4** show the outcome of applying this approach to a subset of the raw data in **Table 2**. The "minimal" data set used the mean value (106.7) as a control (*see* note under raw data columns) and only z data corresponding to x values of 2, 10, and 50 (drug 1) and y values of 1, 2, and 5 (drug 2). The minimal data subset is indicated by asterisks in column 1 of **Table 2**.

6. Selection of Reference Models

The division of suggested strategies into left-hand and right-hand pathways at step 8 in **Table 3** may appear quite trivial, as both pathways later converge. In many cases they lead to the same conclusions. The ostensibly trivial separation is actually based on profound philosophical differences, which have generated endless controversies. The left-hand, Lowe-oriented pathway emphasizes the need for genuinely "null" NRMs that are flexible and independent of preconceived mechanistic and other assumptions. Because these assumptions are absent, it is difficult to specify rigid statistical criteria that might otherwise indicate the degree of compliance with the model. Consequently, its main weakness is that it is prone to accepting aberrant data resulting from technical errors and/or normal biological variation as being "real." The right-hand pathway, by contrast, defines outcomes by reference to a simple, rigidly defined (Bliss interaction) reference model. Its main weakness is that, unless very large sets of data are available, it is prone to regard small but potentially important deviations from the reference model as being due to technical errors or normal biological variation.

6.1. LIM and BIM, the Yin and Yang of Reference Models

Perhaps the simplest way to summarize the difference between Lowe indifference (LIM) and Bliss interaction (BIM) models (our suggested terminology) is that the former fit data to a model whereas the latter fit a model to the data. The defining equations reflect this difference.

LIMs do not predict a combined effect,

$$[d_1/D_1 + d_2/D_2 + \cdots + d_n/D_n] = 1$$

In contrast, BIMs do:

$$E_{1,2,\ldots,n} = E_1 \times E_2 \times \cdots \times E_n$$

Because a parameter equivalent to $E_{1,2,\ldots,n}$ that defines the combined effect cannot be isolated on either side of LIM equations, they cannot be solved directly.

Rather than being regarded as competitors, BIMS and LIMS should be seen as complementary "Yin and Yang" approaches that can't be directly compared.

6.2. A Simple Pragmatic Alternative

Because TC3D requires a combined effect term ($Z = E_{1,2}$ = % viral replication relative to control in the examples used here) to be isolated on the left-hand side of reference equations, fitting data to LIMs is difficult. Although this problem can be overcome by programming a series of user-defined functions, it requires considerable programming skill and is not as efficient as using preprogrammed functions. Consequently, we use the simpler BIMs as the "null" reference. If both drugs are active, but the data do not fit a BIM, it is likely that it can be adequately fitted by either of the alternative general expressions $Z = E_1 + E_2$ or $Z = E_1 + E_2 + E_1 E_2$. The second of these two expressions separates the interaction into separate components: an indifferent (additive or subtractive) component and a separate interactive ("Bliss") component. It is reasonable to identify the major component (the expression—either $E_1 + E_2$ or E_1E_2—that accounts for most of the overall effect in terms of the amplitude of response) as the "real" interaction, and to treat the lesser component as a modifier. However, defining the nature of the interaction on the basis of the ways in which the modifier affects the major component is more complex in practice than it may appear, and beyond the scope of the present discussion. Assuming that a satisfactory alternative fit can be achieved, data can be reexamined to determine whether the predictions of the alternative fit fulfill BIM or LIM criteria for part or all the DRS. If no satisfactory fit can be achieved using TC3D, it is likely that the data are too noisy or that the individual dose–effect models are not valid. In summary, this approach looks for a BIM first, and, if not satisfied, searches for the best alternative from a very large number of possibilities, which is essentially the same as a LIM strategy.

6.3. Interpretation of Data

Choose the simplest best fit model for the data based of F-statistic and/or FSE as described above. Observe how the data are distributed in relation to the DRS and whether residuals are evenly distributed. Look for localized deviations if the data set is large. If a BIM is used, and fits well, a majority of surface points below or above the DRS may indicate synergy or antagonism, respectively. Whether they can justifiably be interpreted as such can be judged from the DRS confidence interval and from the difference in the volumes enclosed by the fitted DRS and a DRS predicted from the individual dose–response equations (*see* **Note 5**).

7. Frugal Experimental Design Applied to Combinations of More Than Two Drugs

The examples above illustrate the application of our preferred DRS method to the analysis of data designed to simulate the results of a combination experiment in which two drugs were used. Essentially the same approach can be used to analyze the results of experiments in which combinations of three or more drugs are used. Before we had access to the rBV system, we showed that combinations of lamivudine, penciclovir, and adefovir acted approximately additively in vitro in the DHBV-PDH assay system ***(13)***. Because of species-dependent differences in drug metabolism, it was necessary to determine whether results obtained using the rBV system would lead to the same conclusion. Raw data and experimental details will appear elsewhere ***(20)***. In summary, we used a frugal experimental design as outlined in the protocol in **Subheading 8**. Each pair of drugs was tested in three parallel combination experiments. The results, which are presented in **Table 5** and illustrated in **Fig. 3A–C**, showed that the activities of each pair of drugs in combination were consistent with BIMs. A second experiment in which the three drugs were used at a fixed concentration ratio of 1:2:300 (lamivudine/adefovir/penciclovir), approximately equivalent to the corresponding IC_{50} ratio, showed that the triple combination also acted as predicted by the Bliss interaction reference model over the concentration ranges used. Because we had already established that the activities of each pair of drugs in combination was consistent with the Bliss interaction RM, we could regard one pair of drugs as "drug 1" and plot the combined effect on a single concentration axis as shown in **Fig. 3D**. With the aid of TC3D, we could also plot the observed results in relation to a Bliss interaction response surface predicted from the individual dose–response equations. This simple approach, which we prefer over alternative methods that require more than one 3D graph to illustrate the results of triple combination experiments, can be extended to multidrug experiments (*see* **Note 6**).

8. Summary Protocol for Parsimonious Combination Analyses

1. If the individual dose–response characteristics of the drugs are unknown, carry out preliminary studies to determine the appropriate concentration ranges for each drug. Upper and lower plateaus of the response as well as the transition should be located. (*See* **Note 7**.)
2. Repeat preliminary experiments using more appropriate drug concentrations if necessary. Use the resulting data to select appropriate dose–response models and to determine whether the assay's sensitivity and accuracy are adequate to justify proceeding to **step 3.** (*See* **note 8**.)

Table 5
Results of Analysis of Data from Table 2

	Bliss model applied to				
	Complete data sets				
	"Ideal" Raw	Raw	Data	Weighted (10% Z)	Minimal data set
Equation parameters					
Goodness-of-fit parameters					
DF Adj r^2	—	—	0.98	0.92	0.97
FSE	—	—	4.9	1.0	5.6
F-statistic	—	—	386	110	130
X parameters (drug 1)					
a	100	107	100 ± 2	105 ± 8	100± 4
b	10	8	9.5 ± 0.8	8.6 ± 1.6	9.2 ± 1.5
c	1	1.0	1.0 ± 0.1	1.0 ± 0.1	1.0 ± 0.1
Y parameters (drug 2)					
a*	100	105	100 ± 2	105 ± 8	103 ± 4
d	1	0.80	0.9 ± 0.1	1.2 ± 0.1	1.0 ± 0.1
e	2	1.5	1.6 ± 0.1	1.9 ± 0.1	1.7 ± 0.4
VUS	2461	2256	2313	2709	2502
Data distribution					
above	—	—	4E, 14S	5E, 2S	4E, 3S
below	—	—	3E, 5S	8E, 23S	3E, 6S
Deviation from surface					
<1 SD	—	—	29	13	13
<2 SD	—	—	4	5	3
<3 SD	—	—	2	1	0
>3 SD	—	—	1	19	0
Overall conclusions based on					
VUS	—	—	ANTAG	ANTAG	ANTAG
Data distribution	—	—	ANTAG	SYN	SYN

Bliss model surfaces were either predicted (from "ideal" data or from individual dose–responses), fitted to the complete weighted or unweighted data set, or fitted to a minimal unweighted data set. Equation parameters, volume under the fitted surface (VUS), and analyses of data distribution are shown. E and S suffixes indicate "edge" and "surface" data points, respectively. Overall conclusions differ depending on criteria on which they are based. If the data points are evenly distributed and the DRS fit the data well (as they do here), the VUS is probably the most objective criterion: volumes greater or less than the expected reference model indicate antagonism and synergy respectively.

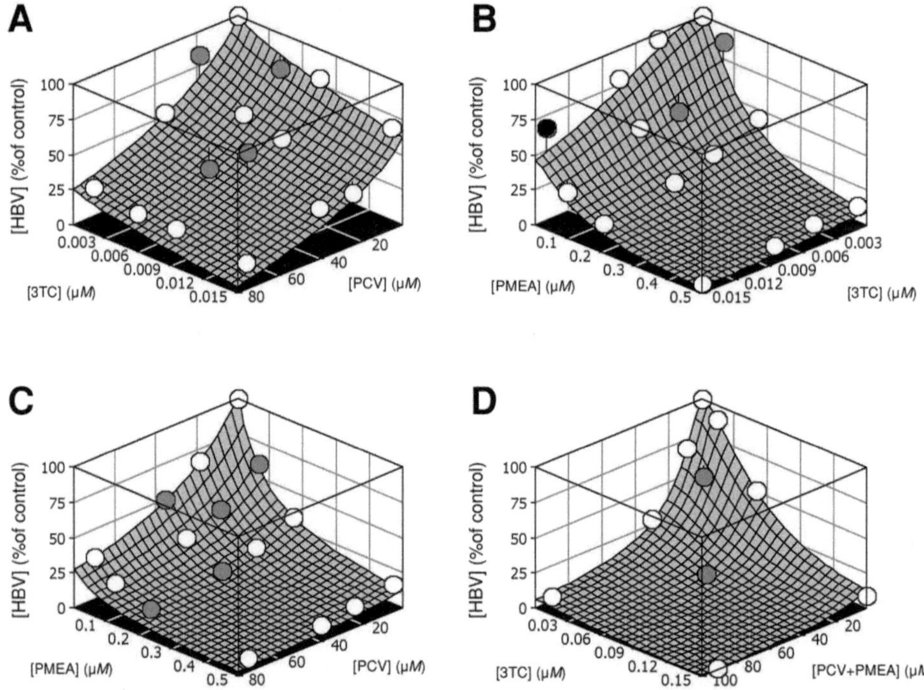

Fig. 3. **A–C**: Bliss model DRS for two drug combinations containing either penciclovir (PCV) and lamivudine (3TC) (**A**); PCV + adefovir (PMEA) (**B**) or 3TC + PMEA (**C**). A frugal experimental design as outlined in the text was used. Effects of each two drug combination closely approximated Bliss interactions. A Bliss interaction also resulted when the three drugs were used in combination at a fixed concentration ratio, as shown in (**D**), in which the PCV + PMEA combination is treated as a single drug. The color code is the same as in **Fig.** 2.

3. From the results of preliminary experiments, determine the approximate concentrations of individual drugs that are required to inhibit viral replication by 25%, 50%, and 75%.
4. Using these estimates as a guide, plan exploratory assays using a "checkerboard" design to test each pair of drugs in combination (*see* **Table 6**). For maximum efficiency and flexibility in later analyses, maintain constant concentration ratios based as closely as possible on IC_{50} ratios of the component drugs. (*See* **Note 9**.)
5. When the exploratory assays have been completed, express the amount of viral replication (or other endpoint) after drug treatment as a percentage of the mean control amount for that particular assay, then calculate mean values for replicate assays.
6. Use the resulting data to generate a DRS for each drug combination with the aid of a TC3D or similar computer software.
7. Using the guidelines for data interpretation suggested above, determine the nature of the drug interaction. If the results are inconclusive, devise and perform additional assays (modified if necessary) to resolve inconsistencies.
8. Once it is possible to reach conclusions about the interactions between pairs of drugs, design

Table 6
Suggested Checkerboard Layout for Testing Two Drug Combinations

Drug 1	Drug 2			
	0	$^2IC_{25}$	$^2IC_{50}$	$^2IC_{75}$
0	100	75	50	25
$^1IC_{25}$	75	56.25	37.5	18.75
$^1IC_{50}$	50	37.5	25	12.5
$^1IC_{75}$	25	18.75	12.5	6.25

Effects of the two drug combination predicted by Bliss models are shown (viral replication as a % of control). ^1IC_x, ^2IC_x, etc. represent individual drug concentrations estimated from preliminary experiments. Shading indicates "surface" data.

additional experiments using subset pairs of drug pairs at appropriate fixed ratio concentrations as one member of a "superpair."

9. Repeat these procedures to confirm the results or to extend the study to combinations that contain additional drugs.

9. Notes

1. CalcuSyn, a PC program that performs dose–effect analyses using the Median Effect principle, is marketed by Biosoft, 2D Dolphin Way, Stapleford, Cambridge, CB2 5DW, UK. It is an update of an earlier Biosoft program, Dose–Effect Analysis with Microcomputers. For more information, *see* http://www.biosoft.com/win/calcusyn.htm
2. We use TableCurve3D, Version 1.0 (and also TableCurve2D, Version 3.0), both of which were originally developed by Jandel Scientific, San Rafael, CA USA. The software company SPSS Inc., 444 North Michigan Avenue, Chicago, IL 60611 has since become the owner and distributor of TableCurve software. For more information see http://www.spssscience.com/tcurve3/index.cfm
3. Several quantititative polymerase chain reaction (PCR) based methods that offer greater accuracy, sensitivity and dynamic range have been developed for HBV (*see* ***[4]*** for example, including a method for assaying HBV cccDNA (*see* Bowden et al., Chapter 5, volume 1).
4. TC3D contains 168 preprogrammed nonlinear functions to describe *Z* in terms of *X* and *Y*. The individual *X* and *Y* functions are also preprogrammed so that the user can reassort to create new user-defined functions (UDFs; e.g., Z = EXPX+LNCY; Z=LDRX*EXPY etc.). TC3D will store up to 15 UDFs.
5. Inventors may cite proof of synergy between drugs as support for the claim of "unobviousness" which can assist in obtaining patents for drug combination formulations in several countries including the United States.
6. Examples of an alternative graphical method can be seen in Snyder et al. ***(21)***.
7. For preliminary studies, it is advisable to use a wide range of concentrations so as to be able to determine the amplitude and transition width of the individual dose–response curves. For example, a 7 $\log_{10}$ concentration range (0.0001–100 μM) would be needed to show the relative activities of lamivudine, adefovir and penciclovir in the rBV assay ***(20)***. Assays should be performed in at least duplicate; triplicates may be needed to achieve statistical acceptability. Because of species- and tissue-dependent differences in expression of the enzymes

responsible for drug metabolism, individual drugs can be expected to show different biological activities in different assay systems.

8. Coefficient of variation $< 10\%$, preferably $< 5\%$.
9. Using fixed concentration ratios facilitates analysis by alternative methods. For most of the newer nucleoside or nucleotide analogs, the IC_{25} and IC_{75} are usually between 2 and 4 times less or greater, respectively, than the IC_{50}. In the example shown in **Fig. 4,** IC_{25}, IC_{50} and IC_{75} concentrations for penciclovir are approx 18, 36, and 72 micromolar, respectively. The corresponding values (in μmol/L) for adefovir are 0.04, 0.12, and 0.36 and for lamivudine are 0.03, 0.06, and 0.12. The order of potency is lamivudine > adefovir > penciclovir, the corresponding IC_{50} ratio (lamivudine/adefovir/penciclovir) being 1:2:600. In this example, the lamivudine/penciclovir, lamivudine/adefovir, and adefovir/penciclovir ratios would be 1:600, 1:2, and 1:300, respectively. Test each drug alone and in combination using approximately equipotent concentrations that correspond as closely as possible to the IC_{25}, IC_{50}, and IC_{75} estimates for each. This will require a total of at least 16 assays for each pair of drugs: three concentrations of each drug alone, at least one untreated control and nine different drug combinations as shown in **Table 6.** We use three six-well tissue culture plates (Becton Dickinson, Franklin Lakes, NJ, USA) for each assay set (a total of 18 wells, allowing triplicate controls), and perform each assay in duplicate or triplicate.

References

1. Medley, G. F., Lindop, N. A., Edmunds, W. J., and Nokes, D. J. (2001) Hepatitis B virus endemicity: heterogeneity, catastrophic dynamics and control. *Nat. Med.* **7,** 619–624.
2. Seeger, C. and Mason, W. S. (2000) Hepatitis B virus biology. *Microbiol. Mol. Biol. Rev.* **64,** 51–68.
3. Shaw, T. and Locarnini, S. (2000) Combination chemotherapy for hepatitis B virus: the path forward? *Drugs* **60,** 517–531.
4. Lewin, S. R., Ribeiro, R. M., Walters, T., et al. (2001) Analysis of hepatitis B viral load decline under potent therapy: complex decay profiles observed. Hepatology **34**, 1012–1020.
5. Delaney, W. E. 4th, Locarnini, S., and Shaw T. (2001) Resistance of hepatitis B virus to antiviral drugs: current aspects and directions for future investigation. *Antiviral Chem. Chemother.* **12,** 1–35.
6. Greco, W. R., Bravo, G., and Parsons, J. C. (1995) The search for synergy: a critical review from a response surface perspective. *Pharmacol. Rev.* **47,** 331–385.
7. Delaney, W. E. 4th, Edwards, R., Colledge, D., et al. (2001) Cross-resistance testing of antihepadnaviral compounds using novel recombinant baculoviruses which encode drug-resistant strains of hepatitis B virus. *Antimicrob. Agents Chemother.* **45,** 1705–1713.
8. Sühnel, J. (1990) Evaluation of synergism or antagonism for the combined action of antiviral agents. *Antiviral Res.* **13,** 23–39.
9. Prichard, M. N. and Shipman, C. Jr. (1990) A three-dimensional model to analyze drug-drug interactions. *Antiviral Res.* **14,** 181–205.
10. Bliss, C. I. (1939) The toxicity of poisons applied jointly. *Ann. Appl. Biol.* **26,** 585–615.
11. Lowe, S. and Muischnek, H. (1926) Effect of combinations: mathematical basis of problem. *Arch. Exp. Pathol. Pharmakol.* **114,** 313–326.
12. Chou, T.-C. and Talalay, P. (1984) Quantitative analysis of dose–effect relationships: The combined effects of multiple drugs or enzyme inhibitors. *Adv. Enzyme Regul.* **22,** 27–55.
13. Colledge, D., Civitico, G., Locarnini, S., and Shaw, T. (2000) In vitro antihepadnaviral activities of combinations of penciclovir, lamivudine, and adefovir. *Antimicrob. Agents Chemother.* **44,** 551–560.

14. Locarnini, S. and Civitico, G. M. (2000) Assays for measuring hepadnaviral supercoiled DNA, in *Methods in Molecular Medicine*, Vol. 24: *Antiviral Methods and Protocols* (Linchington, D. and Schinazi, R. F., eds.), Humana Press, Totowa, NJ, pp. 77–85
15. King, R. W. and Ladner, S. K. (2000) Hep AD38 Assay. A high-throughput, cell-based screen for the evaluation of compounds against hepatitis B virus, in *Methods in Molecular Medicine*, Vol. 24: *Antiviral Methods and Protocols* (Linchington, D. and Schinazi, R. F., eds.), Humana Press, Totowa, NJ, pp. 43–50.
16. Otto, M. J. and Whitaker, R. A. (2000) A rapid microtiter assay for duck hepatitis virus reverse transcriptase, in *Methods in Molecular Medicine*, Vol. 24: *Antiviral Methods and Protocols* (Linchington, D. and Schinazi, R. F., eds.), Humana Press, Totowa, NJ, pp. 69–75.
17. Schmidt, K. and Korba, B. E. (2000) Hepatitis B virus cell culture assays for antiviral activity, in *Methods in Molecular Medicine*, Vol. 24: *Antiviral Methods and Protocols* (Linchington, D. and Schinazi, R. F., eds.), Humana Press, Totowa, NJ, pp. 51–67.
18. Delaney, W. E. 4th, Miller, T. G., and Isom, H. C. (1999) Use of the hepatitis B virus recombinant baculovirus-HepG2 system to study the effects of (–)-beta-2',3'-dideoxy-3'-thiacytidine on replication of hepatitis B virus and accumulation of covalently closed circular DNA. *Antimicrob. Agents Chemother.* **43,** 2017–2026.
19. Delaney, W. E. 4th and Isom, H. C. (1998) Hepatitis B virus replication in human HepG2 cells mediated by hepatitis B virus recombinant baculovirus. *Hepatology* **28**, 1134–1146.
20. Delaney, W. E. 4th, Shaw, T., Edwards, R., Colledge, D., Isom, H. C., and Locarnini, S. (2003) Additive and synergistic inhibition of HBV replication by combinations of lamivudine, adefovir and penciclovir. Submitted for publication.
21. Snyder, S., D'Argenio, D. Z., (2000) *Antimicrob. Agents Chemother.* **44**, 1051–1058.

31

Hepatitis B Virus

Where Are We and Where Are We Going?

Michael P Manns, Johannes Hadem, and Heiner Wedemeyer

1. Introduction

There are few examples in modern medicine that are comparable with the enormous progress in understanding the cause and pathogenesis of viral hepatitis B that has been made in the last three decades leading to efficient therapies and the development of protective vaccines. Nearly one-tenth of the world's population is suffering from viral hepatitis, and it has been estimated that approx 350 million individuals are chronically infected with the hepatitis B virus (HBV). Most important, up to 25% of patients with chronic hepatitis B will eventually die from end-stage liver disease or hepatocellular carcinoma. Thus, HBV is a major health burden especially in high endemic areas where up 15% of the population is infected with HBV.

It is interesting to note that the Australia antigen was first described as a marker of leukemia in the 1960s. However, very soon it was identified as an infectious agent responsible for one of the most frequent infectious diseases in the world. In 1976, Dr. Baruch Blumberg received the Nobel Prize in Physiology/Medicine for his achievements in the identification of HBV, which began with the detection of an immunodiffusion precipitin line between hepatitis B surface antigen (HBsAg) in the serum of an Australian aborigine (later known as the "Australia antigen") and an anti-HBsAg antibody in the blood of a multiply transfused hemophiliac ***(1,2)***. In 1970, David Dane and colleagues first described the 42-nm particles that were later realized to be the hepatitis B particles ***(3)***.

Meanwhile, the diagnosis of HBV is based on serological markers and direct detection of HBV DNA. In vitro models of HBV replication have been established, allowing screening of potential antivirals for anti-HBV activity. In the late 1980s, HBV-transgenic mice were developed that significantly helped our understanding of how

From: *Methods in Molecular Medicine, vol. 96: Hepatitis B and D Protocols, volume 2*
Edited by: R. K. Hamatake and J. Y. N. Lau © Humana Press Inc., Totowa, NJ

HBV-specific T cells control HBV replication. Many investigators have worked with the woodchuck model, which is the only animal model allowing one to study the natural course of hepatitis virus infection in a higher quantity of animals. Finally, recent investigations of HBV infection in chimpanzees dissected the role of innate and adaptive immune responses in different phases of the infection.

The huge boost of research on HBV continued from the 1970s to the 1990s. Even in the new millennium the hepatitis B virus is still among the most intensively investigated viruses. Only HIV and the hepatitis C virus have received similar attention by investigators around the world. Importantly, basic research on HBV not only gave insights into the virus itself but also led to general new concepts in immunology and virology. For example, the so-called noncytolytic clearance of HBV from hepatocytes through release of cytokines by T cells without destroying the infected cell was first described for HBV and now holds true as a general phenomenon in host immune defense against many other infectious agents.

Perhaps the greatest success in hepatitis B research is the fact that the hepatitis B vaccine is the first and currently only vaccine that has been proven to reduce the incidence of cancer. In Taiwan, hepatocellular carcinomas have been a significant problem in children. However, after vaccination of children was introduced in the early 1980s, cases of liver cancer constantly decreased in the next 10 yr. Considering the very high incidence of chronic hepatitis B infection in some areas of the world, with 10% of the population being infected with HBV, the recent development of efficient antivirals not only gives hope for many patients but also potentially has a very significant socioeconomic impact for many countries.

However, many problems still remain and as always in research, in some fields more questions than answers arose in rccent years. Treatment is still not successful in all patients, resistance to the new antivirals can develop, current drugs are very expensive and not affordable for the far majority of infected patients, and the vaccine is effective in only 95% of patients. Research on HBV has to be continued to achieve the ultimate goal: the eradication of HBV in the world.

2. Overview of HBV Virology

HBV belongs to the family of hepadnaviruses. The whole virion, or Dane particle, is a 42-nm sphere that contains a nucleocapsid, enclosing the HBV genome, which is a circular, partially double-stranded DNA of approx 3200 basepairs (bp) in length *(4)*. The HBV genome has a compact organization consisting of four overlapping open reading frames (ORFs) *(5)*. The pre-S/S ORF is divided into pre-S1, pre-S2, and S regions that encode the large (L), middle (M), and small (S) envelope proteins, forming the HBsAg *(6,7)*. These proteins are also capable of assembling into small 22-nm spheres and filaments. The core gene consists of precore and core regions. The core protein can self-assemble into a capsid-like structure *(5)*, whereas the precore polypeptide is posttranslationally modified into a soluble protein, the hepatitis B e antigen (HBeAg) *(7)*. The polymerase has a large ORF (approx 800 amino acids) and overlaps the entire length of the S ORF, consisting of three functional domains: the terminal protein domain, the reverse transcriptase domain, and the RNase H domain. The initial phase of hepadnaviral infection involves the attachment of mature virions onto host cell membranes. Various cellular factors have been shown to bind to the HBV pre-S and S proteins *(5)*. A recent study could identify the QLDPAF sequence within the 21- to 47-amino-acid epitope of pre-S1, expressed on the large HBsAg, as the receptor binding viral domain epitope. Interestingly, a similar sequence is shared by several cellular, bacterial, and viral proteins involved in cell adhesion *(8)*. Duck HBV (DHBV) virions, which have been studied extensively as a model for human HBV, are likely to be initially scavenged by liver sinusoidal endothelial cells, thereafter rescued from lysosomal degradation by binding to carboxypeptidase D, a major DHBV receptor candidate, and finally released to infect adjacent hepatocytes *(9,10)*. Entry of the virus results from fusion of the viral and host membranes as the nucleocapsid is released into the cytoplasm. The covalently closed circular form of HBV DNA in the nucleus serves as the template for transcription *(5)*, which produces a pregenomic RNA that serves both as a template for reverse transcription as well as a messenger RNA for the production of nucleocapsid and polymerase proteins *(7)*. While the newly reverse-transcribed negative-strand DNA in turn serves as template for positive-strand DNA synthesis, interaction of S protein and nucleocapsid at the endoplasmic reticulum leads to the initiation of virion assembly. Both HBeAg and HBX proteins are considered accessory viral gene products. HBeAg might play a role as immunomodulator by inducing a predominant T-helper-2 (Th2) response, which then results in a depletion of HBcAg-specific Th1 cells and could have a profound implication in viral persistence *(11)*. HBX is thought to be an inhibitor of proteasome-mediated proteolysis, thereby interfering with antigen presentation of viral proteins leading to viral evasion of immune response *(5)*.

3. Epidemiology and Transmission of HBV Infection

An estimated 350,000,000 persons worldwide are chronically infected with HBV *(12)*. Areas with low prevalence (0.1–2%) include, for example, the United States, Western Europe, Sri Lanka, Japan, and Australia, intermediate endemic areas (3–5%) are, for example, the Middle East, Central Asia, Korea, Thailand, and South America, whereas prevalence rates can reach up to 10–20% in China and sub-Saharan Africa *(7,13)*. **Figure 1** gives an overview of the worldwide HBV prevalence.

HBV is a parenterally transmitted virus that is acquired from exposure to infected blood or body secretions. The rate of progression from acute to chronic HBV infection is approx 90% for perinatally acquired infection, 20–50% for infections between the age of 1 and 5 yr, and < 5% for adult acquired infection. This has an impact on the wide range in carrier rate in different parts of the world *(7)*. Vertical, that is, perinatal mother-to-infant, transmission with its high rate of chronicity is thought to be an important factor in the rate of HBsAg carriage in high prevalence areas. It accounts for 40–50% of HBsAg carriers in Taiwan and occurs particularly in children born to HBeAg-positive mothers *(14)*. They acquire HBV via maternal–fetal transfusion, exposure to maternal blood in the birth canal, and postnatal close mother–baby contact. Horizontal transmission, on the other hand, plays an important role in early childhood when children may acquire HBV infection via minor skin breaks and mucous membranes or close bodily contact *(7)*. The estimated risk of HBV acquisition within the first 5 yr of life in children

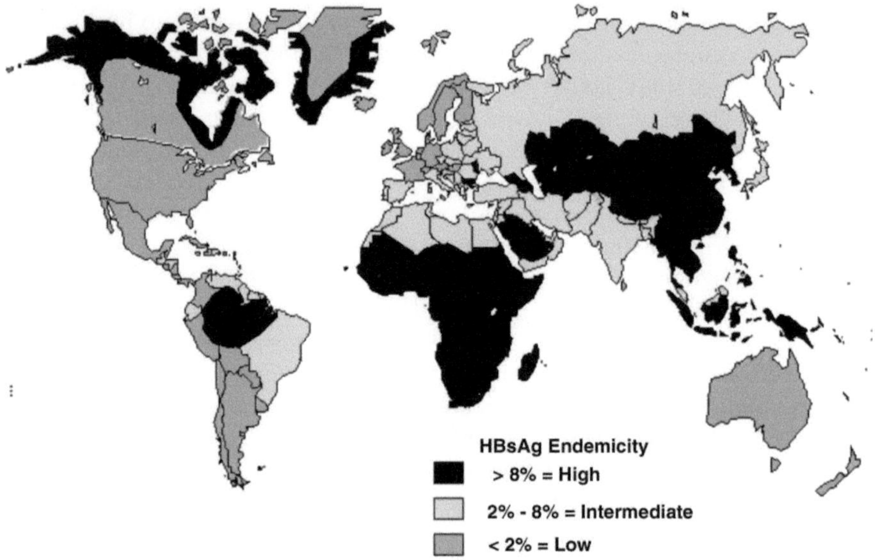

Fig. 1. Geographic pattern of hepatitis B prevalence 1997. (Modified from WHO.)

living in countries with moderate to high HBV prevalence ranges from 5% to 40%. Focused vaccination programs have already proven successful in reducing the prevalence of HBV infection in this age group ***(15)***. Unprotected sexual intercourse and intravenous drug use remain the most frequently identified modes of horizontal infection among adults in low prevalence areas ***(16)***. Sexual transmission accounts for approx 30% of HBV infections in the United States ***(7)***. Serological markers of ongoing or prior HBV infection are almost universal after 5 yr of drug use. Other recognized modes of HBV transmission, including transfusions and dialysis, occur less frequently ***(17)***.

Chronic liver disease, including cirrhosis, represents the 10th most common cause of death in the United States ***(17)***. Viral hepatitis is the most common cause of chronic liver disease with an estimated 1.25 million with chronic HBV infection in the United States ***(4)***. Still, the seroprevalence of HBV is relatively low when compared to other areas of the world. In the National Health and Nutrition Examination Survey (NHANES) III, the age-adjusted seroprevalence of chronic HBV infection, which was defined by the presence of HBsAg and anti-HBc, was 4.9%. Prevalence was low until the age of 12 yr, and increased thereafter in all racial groups, suggesting that sexual contact is likely to be the primary mode of HBV transmission in the United States. Independent predictors of chronic HBV infection after adjustment for age were: (1) non-Hispanic black ethnicity, (2) high number of sexual partners, (3) cocaine use, (4) divorced or separated marital status, (5) foreign birth, and (6) having less than a high school education. Interactions were noted between race, sociodemographic variables, and behavioral risk factors ***(17,18)***.

4. Current Concepts in the Immunopathogenesis of HBV Infection

The ability to mount a coordinated and efficient helper and cytotoxic T cell (CTL) response against different proteins of HBV seems necessary to achieve successful HBV control ***(19)***. Effective viral control does not necessarily imply viral eradication, as it was shown that HBV is still present in patients after recovery of acute viral hepatitis ***(20)***, and that HBV replication persists years in the liver of patients who have cleared serum HBsAg ***(21,22)***. An important parameter associated with viral control is the mounting of a multispecific CTL response, that is, the ability of CD8 cells to recognize different epitopes located in different HBV proteins ***(23,24)***. This requires a strong virus specific $CD4^+$ T cell response (predominantly of the Th1 phenotype) and an efficient presentation of the involved viral antigens. These are presented on HLA class I molecules to be recognized by $CD8^+$ T cells, or on HLA class II molecules within the HLA class II-restricted $CD4^+$ helper pathway. Only a limited array of peptide residues from the HBV proteins (typically from the HBcAg, for example, peptide 18–27 binding to HLA-A2) can gain access to the class I binding groove ***(4)***. The polymorphic nature of the major histocompatibility complex binding sites and differences in the T-cell repertoire among persons leads to highly variable binding affinity for the immunodominant HBV peptides, which in turn determines the outcome after acute HBV infection ***(4,25)***. Not the overall quantity of T cells, but the number of intrahepatic HBV-specific $CD8^+$ cells appears to be associated with an effective inhibition of HBV replication. In contrast, when the HBV-specific CD8 response is unable to control virus replication, it may contribute to liver pathology by causing the recruitment of non-virus-specific T cells ***(26)***. As mentioned above, the HBeAg induces a predominant Th2 response, resulting in a depletion of HBcAg-specific Th1 cells, which may have a profound implication in viral persistence ***(11)***.

Newer evidence indicates that clearance of HBV is not always associated with a cytopathic effect, but that the cellular immune response can resolve acute HBV infection by purging the virus from infected cells without killing them ***(27)***. Studies on HBV transgenic mice showed that cytokines such as interferon-γ (FN γ) and tumor necrosis factor-α (TNF-α), which are released from HBV-specific CTL, and to a lesser extent from helper T cells, natural killer cells, and natural killer T cells, activate hepatocytes to actively degrade viral RNA and inhibit HBV replication by preventing proper assembly. Activation of hepatocytes and nonparenchymal cells of the liver is likely to result in the expression of a complex subset of chemokines that might differ in their antiviral and tissue damaging potential ***(28)***. These intracellular viral inactivation mechanisms could greatly amplify the protective effects of the immune response, while failure of such mechanisms could lead to viral persistence or to the death of the host ***(29)***. Degradation of HBV RNA is tightly associated with the cytokine-induced proteolytic cleavage of La autoantigen, which binds to HBV RNA and might thereafter show endonucleolytic activity ***(30)***. Importantly, viral clearance appears to be due largely to the antiviral effects of cytokines produced by non-T cells while liver disease appears to be due mostly to the destructive effects of the T cells, although the curative effects of cytokines produced by these cells likely contribute to viral clearance as well ***(31)***.

A recent study was able to demonstrate the relevance of the findings in HBV-transgenic mice to natural infection. HBV DNA was shown to largely disappear from the liver and the blood of acutely infected chimpanzees long before the peak of T-cell infiltration and most of the liver disease. These results imply that noncytopathic antiviral mechanisms contribute to viral clearance during acute viral hepatitis by purging HBV replicative intermediates from the cytoplasm and covalently closed circular viral DNA from the nucleus of infected cells ***(32)***.

5. Natural History of HBV Infection

HBV infection is characterized by a wide spectrum of manifestations. Approximately 70% of patients with acute HBV infection have subclinical hepatitis or anicteric hepatitis, whereas 30% become icteric, and 0.1–0.5% develop acute liver failure. The rate of progression from acute to chronic hepatitis B is high in perinatally acquired infection and low in adult-acquired HBV ***(7)***. Rates of progression to cirrhosis and HCC vary according to the state of the immune system, the age of the patient, the serologic stage of infection, and geographic and genetic factors ***(33,34)***.

During the replicative phase of the virus, HBV DNA, HBsAg, and HBeAg are present in the serum, indicating viral replication. As the hallmark of HBV infection, HBsAg is usually detectable 1–10 wk after exposure to HBV, and approx 2–6 wk before the onset of clinical symptoms ***(7)***. HBeAg is thought to be useful as an indicator of relative infectivity, and is rapidly cleared, even before the disappearance of HBsAg ***(35)***. Another serologic marker, detectable 1 mo after the appearance of HBsAg and therefore the first antibody to develop during acute infection, is anti-HBc-IgM. It may be useful to distinguish between acute or recent infection, although its titer may also increase to detectable levels during exacerbations of chronic hepatitis B. Although anti-HBc-IgM is not protective, it is the first indicator of the host's attempt to mount an immune response, which hopefully will be strong enough to clear the virus. This stage of immune clearance occurs soon in adult infection (spontaneous HBeAg seroconversion rate of 10–20% /yr), but relatively late in case of perinatally acquired infections, which are characterized by several decades of immune tolerance, probably as a result of transplacental HBeAg transfer and subsequent T-cell depletion ***(7)***. Typically, immune clearance is accompanied by 3–4 wk of symptomatic hepatitis ***(4)***. But most cases of chronic hepatitis B among adults occur in patients who never had a recognized episode of clinically apparent acute viral hepatitis ***(35)***.

The nonreplicative (or low-replicative) phase is characterized by the presence of anti-HBe and a marked reduction in HBV DNA levels. Where seroconversion to anti-HBs occurs, it indicates the development of full immunity to the virus. However, even in adult infection, there is a small proportion of patients developing chronic hepatitis, most of them with inactive liver disease. Annual rate of HBsAg clearance is estimated to be 0.5–2%, while HBV DNA frequently remains detectable ***(7)***. **Figure 2** illustrates the serologic profile of acute and chronic HBV infection.

During recent years, the direct detection of viral DNA has become a standard parameter within the diagnostic workup. HBV DNA assays include probe hybridization-based and polymerase chain reaction (PCR)-based viral DNA target detection. They are used

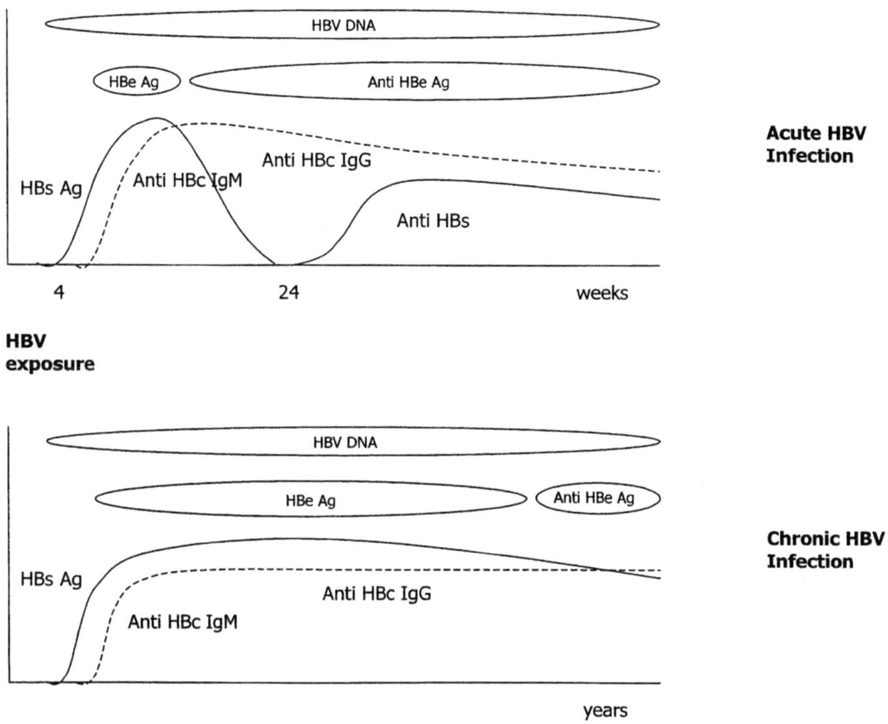

Fig. 2. Serologic profile of acute and chronic HBV infection.

to assess the level of HBV replication, which is particularly helpful in monitoring the response to antiviral therapy in patients with chronic HBV infection. In addition, owing to the high sensitivity of current techniques, they can identify an acute hepatitis B in a patient formerly thought to have cryptogenic liver disease. The recently developed hybridization assay with branched-DNA (bDNA) molecules and signal amplification detects HBV DNA down to 0.7 meq/mL. It has been used as the standard for HBV DNA quantification in more recent antiviral treatment trials ***(36,37)***. Although the Quantiplex bDNA assay, which is the most frequently used method for HBV detection, is characterized by high accuracy and good reproducibility, it may not be suitable for patients with low HBV titers. In contrast, newer quantitative PCR methods, such as the Amplicor and Amplisensor assays, have proven a higher sensitivity, and can detect viral loads as low as 0.002 meq/mL (in comparison: conventional PCR seems to be useful for samples with titers of 1.23 meq/mL or higher). Therefore these tests are particularly useful in HBV surveillance, and perhaps in the posttransplant setting ***(38)***.

6. Chronic HBV Infection and Hepatocellular Carcinoma

Chronic infection with HBV is a major risk factor for the development of hepatocellular carcinoma (HCC). In the United States, the incidence of HCC rose from 1.4 per

100,000 people during the period from 1976 to 1980 to 2.4 during the period 1991 to 1995. This trend was associated with an increased incidence in blacks and older patients, as well as a shift in the incidence rate toward younger age groups ***(39)***. In a meta-analysis of 32 case-control studies, risk estimates of developing HCC appeared to be 20-fold greater in serum HBsAg carriers than in seronegative controls ***(40)***. Annual incidence rates of HCC in prospective studies differ according to geographic characteristics and the severity of liver disease. The largest and longest cohort study available so far examined the clinical outcomes of 1536 Alaska natives chronically infected with HBV. The incidence of HCC was 1.9 per 1000 carrier-years (2.3 in men and 1.2 in women), and was increased in individuals belonging to a certain ethnic group, people of older age, and in case of switches in HBeAg status ***(12)***.

HCC arises almost exclusively in patients with cirrhosis ***(4)***. Its incidence reached 6.6% in 234 Asian cirrhotics during a follow-up of 3 yr ***(41)***. Persistent proliferation of liver cells seems to be a key factor of hepatitis progression to HCC, which is independent of disease etiology ***(42)***, and typically occurs after 25–30 yr of infection ***(4)***. Measured by immunostaining for proliferating cell nuclear antigen (PCNA) in patients with compensated cirrhosis, high liver cell proliferative activity was associated with a higher risk of developing cancer (5% in 80 patients) as compared to 1% in 208 patients with lower liver cell proliferative activity. Not surprisingly, survival was significantly lower in patients with high liver cell proliferation rates than in those with low proliferation rates (10% vs 75%) ***(43)***. Although the majority of patients in the latter study had chronic hepatitis C as underlying liver disease, the situation is likely to be similar in chronic HBV infection, once cirrhosis has developed.

It still remains controversial whether HBV plays a direct or merely an indirect role in the process of carcinogenesis. Although continued cell death and regeneration associated with chronic hepatitis appear to be major factors in hepatocarcinogenesis, HBX protein, to which an oncogenic potential is attributed, may allow some of the multiple stages to be skipped. HBV infection may therefore be capable of inducing HCC in the absence of a complete set of genetic aberrations ***(44)***. The integration of viral DNA into the host-cell chromosomal DNA is regarded as a key event, as it might lead to the activation or suppression of cellular genes involved in cell growth and proliferation ***(45)***.

Once HCC has been diagnosed, treatment options are often limited owing to the advanced stage of the tumor. This underlines the importance of preventive measures to avoid HBV infection. Recent data from Taiwan, an area of hyperendemic HBV infection, provides crucial evidence that universal hepatitis B immunization in children leads to a marked reduction of the reservoir of HBV carriers and a concomitant decline in HCC incidence ***(46)***. The reduction in the prevalence of HBsAg was accompanied by a decline in the average annual incidence of HCC in children 6–9 yr of age from 0.53 per 100,000 for those born between 1974 and 1984 to 0.13 for those born between 1984 and 1986. The adoption of universal HBV vaccination for infants and adolescents throughout the world, as has been recommended by the World Health Organization (WHO), is likely to represent a milestone in the annals of preventive medicine ***(45)***. HBV vaccination should be regarded as a vaccine against cancer.

7. HBV Genotypes and Mutants in Untreated Patients

HBV is classified into four serotypes (adr, adw, ayr, and ayw) based on antigenic determinants of HBsAg, which can be further subdivided into nine subtypes. Direct sequencing, restriction fragment length polymorphism, and other techniques can distinguish seven HBV genotypes (A–G) on the basis of a complete or partial sequence analysis ***(47)***. Genotype A is predominant in Europe, North America, and Africa, whereas genotypes B and C appear to be highly prevalent in Southeast Asia, which might be related to the endemicity of HBV infection in these areas. It has been estimated that the heterogeneity in disease manifestations and response to antiviral therapy among patients with chronic hepatitis B in different parts of the world may, at least in part, be attributed to differences in HBV genotypes ***(48)***. A study of 466 Japanese patients demonstrated a much higher rate of HBeAg positivity in those infected with genotype C than in genotype B, suggesting that HBV genotype B might be associated with a higher HBeAg clearance rate ***(49)***. In addition, there is evidence that patients with long-lasting and high level replication of HBV genotype C might develop advanced liver disease more frequently ***(50)***. The relationship between HBV genotypes and hepatocellular carcinoma is still unclear ***(48)***.

Recent studies have speculated that mutations in specific regions of the HBV genome may influence the clinical course and severity of liver damage, among them precore stop codon and core mutations ***(51,52)***, defective pre-S2-start codon and S-mutations ***(53)***, as well as therapy escape mutations in the polymerase gene. This could happen by altering the level of viral replication or the expression of more immunogenic epitopes.

HBeAg synthesis is most commonly prevented by the precore mutation 1898 (G → A), which results in a stop codon (TGG → TAG) at the end of the precore region, but does not interfere with HBcAg synthesis ***(54)***. This implies that viral replication persists despite blockage of HBeAg expression and subsequent anti-HBe seroconversion. There is a wide variation in the prevalence of the stop codon mutant (high in the Mediterranean basin and Asia, low in North America and northern Europe). This might be due to the preponderance of HBV genotypes B, C, and D in southern Europe and Southeast Asia, which have—in contrast to genotype A—been associated with the appearance of the premature stop codon ***(48,55)***. Whereas former reports suggested an association of the precore mutation with a fulminant course of hepatitis, later studies have not been able to demonstrate a specific mutation predicting fulminant disease ***(54,56)***.

Naturally occurring core promoter mutants have been found to increase viral replication in vitro via various mechanisms, such as (1) up-regulated transcription of pregenomic RNA resulting from alterations in binding sites for transcription factors, (2) enhanced encapsidation by an increase in core protein expression, and (3) by a reduction in the expression of precore protein, which can interrupt the encapsidation process ***(57)***. However, the fact that these mutations have also been found in patients with acute self-limited or chronic hepatitis B without liver disease and in asymptomatic HBV carriers suggests that they are not necessarily pathogenic ***(7)***. A recent study could not find a significant correlation between core promoter mutations, viral replication, and liver damage in patients with chronic hepatitis B infection. Promoter and replication activities of the predominant core promoter mutants were equivalent to those of wild-type virus, despite diverse sequence variation. In addition, no clear correlation between HBeAg status and viral load was visible. Deletion mutants within the core promoter and core gene, as well as variants with large deletions, spanning precore/core and preS/S reading frames, have been detected in highly viremic carriers *(58)*. Interestingly, a number of these mutants seem to need the presence of wild-type virus for replication, which might be due to a dependence on HBVX protein for infection of hepatocytes, as shown for the woodchuck hepatitis virus *(59)*. Core mutations have been demonstrated to influence HBV clearance by the expression of cytotoxic epitopes that act as T-cell receptor antagonists *(60)*. Their correlation with a diminished IFN response remains unclear.

Vaccine-induced S-gene mutations can lead to loss of the common "a" determinant of HBsAg, and are therefore known as "vaccine escape mutants" *(61)*. Mutations in the polymerase gene secondary to nucleoside analog treatment are discussed below.

In summary, HBV genotypes are likely to influence HBeAg seroconversion rates, mutational patterns, and the severity of liver disease *(48)*. But it is still unclear to what degree different HBV mutants can change the outcome of HBV infection. The coexistence of several mutations within the same genome, the cooperation of different HBV-mutant strains, and, perhaps most importantly, the host immune response might all participate in the modulation of disease activity *(62)*.

8. Therapy of Chronic HBV Infection

Among the various factors influencing the histological progression of chronic hepatitis B to cirrhosis, active HBV replication is thought to play a major role, and its reduction is therefore the target of therapeutic interventions. The initial goal of HBV therapy is to suppress viral replication and subsequently induce remission of liver disease. The ultimate goal is to eliminate HBV and prevent progression to cirrhosis *(7)*. In compensated patients with chronic hepatitis B, antiviral therapy is indicated for active viral replication, elevated aminotransferase activity, and histologic evidence of chronic hepatic injury *(63)*.

8.1. Role of IFN-α

Effective therapies against hepatitis B were first introduced in the mid-1980s when it became apparent that prolonged therapy with IFN-α resulted in sustained loss of HBV replication (HBeAg and HBV DNA undetectable) in 30–40% of treated patients compared with only 10–12% of controls *(64,65)*. Once HBeAg loss and HBV negativity are established, the frequency of persistently normal alanine aminotransferase (ALT) approaches 80% *(66)*. HBeAg/anti-HBeAg seroconversion after treatment with IFN-α is likely to be associated with an increase in survival after 6 yr of follow-up in patients with chronic hepatitis B *(67)*. Similarly, the incidence of HCC was significantly reduced in chronic HBV patients after IFN-α in comparison to untreated controls *(68)*. Approximately 10% of patients develop a consecutive HBsAg seroconversion, when IFN-α is given subcutaneously at a daily dose of 5 million units or three times a week at a dose of up to 10 million units for 4–6 mo ***(63)***. Patients who remain HBeAg-positive at wk 16 with low HBV-DNA levels should probably receive treatment beyond 6 mo to improve the rate of response ***(69)***. Successful interferon therapy is more likely in patients with low-level HBV DNA and substantial elevations of aminotransferase activity. Recent studies found that the rate of interferon-induced HBeAg seroconversion was higher in German patients with genotype A than in those with genotype D (37% vs 6%) and in Taiwanese patients with genotype B compared to those with genotype C (41% vs 15%) ***(70,71)***. On the other hand, immunosuppression and the existence of precore mutants are markers of a poor treatment response. It is important to mention that IFN therapy is potentially harmful once complications of end-stage liver disease, such as ascites, bleeding varices, or hepatic encephalopathy, have occurred ***(63)***. IFN therapy is associated with a wide spectrum of side effects, such as flulike symptoms, anorexia, weight loss, mild myelosuppression, psychiatric problems, and autoimmune thyroiditis ***(7)***. This is also true for long-acting interferon modified with polyethylene glycol (PEG-IFN), which might present new opportunities for the treatment of chronic HBV infection ***(72)***.

Combination therapies of IFN-α and steroids have recently been thought to have little additional benefit on the short- and long-term follow-up of patients with chronic HBV infection ***(73,74)***. A meta-analysis of seven trials comparing prednisone-IFN with IFN treatment in adults with chronic hepatitis B could not show a significant steroid-induced increase in the efficacy of IFN treatment, when analyzing HBeAg, HBV DNA, HBsAg loss, and serum ALT at the end of follow-up. However, the combination therapy was significantly more effective in the subgroup of patients with low ALT levels ***(75)***. Interestingly, a recent prospective randomized controlled trial on 42 HBeAg- and HBV-DNA-positive patients suggested an efficacy of corticosteroid withdrawal therapy (CSWT). HBeAg seroconversion rates at wk 104 after 3 wk of CSWT alone were twice those following a combination therapy of 3 wk of CSWT plus 4 wk of IFN-α (38.9% vs 18.8%) ***(76)***. The reasons for these results have to await further investigation. Perhaps the weak response to IFN was related to the fact that HBV genotype C, which has been reported to be relatively IFN-resistant, comprised more than 90% of all cases ***(71)***. Additional studies are needed to clarify the role of a steroid priming therapy, especially in combination with subsequent use of nucleoside analogues ***(77)***.

8.2. Efficacy of Lamivudine and the Role of Resistant Viral Mutations

Lamivudine (β-L-(−)-2',3'-dideoxy-3'-thiacytidine [3TC]) recently has been licensed in the United States, Canada, Europe, and Asia for the treatment of chronic hepatitis B. It is administered orally, and inhibits HBV reverse transcriptase with negligible side effects. Two large multicenter studies, one from the United States and the other one from Asia, showed that 12 mo of lamivudine therapy result in almost universal suppression of hybridization-assay-detectable HBV DNA. HBeAg loss occurs in 30–33%, HBeAg seroconversion in 16–18%, sustained ALT normalization in 41–49%, and liver histologic improvement (i.e., a reduction in histologic activity index [HAI] of ≥2 points) in 52% ***(78,79)***. Prolonged duration of treatment might be able to improve these results further ***(80,81)***. After 3 yr of continuous therapy with 100 mg of lamivudine daily, there are enhanced HBeAg seroconversion rates of 40%, rising up to 65% in the subgroup of patients with baseline serum ALT > 2 × upper limit of normal (ULN) ***(82)***. Prolonged therapy with lamivudine also improves the histological activity index, despite the higher rate of YMDD mutant emergence ***(83)***. ALT flares are not uncommon during therapy, probably representing altered T-cell functions, as it has been suggested that lamivudine therapy can restore T-cell responses against HBV ***(84)***. Posttreatment ALT elevations, although asymptomatic and transient, are likely to reflect a return of liver inflammation associated with resumption of unsuppressed wild-type HBV replication. In fact, HBV DNA reappears in the majority of patients without partial seroconversion after discontinuation of treatment, and this is probably based on residual covalently closed circular DNA (cccDNA) inside the nucleus of the hepatocyte, which is not affected by lamivudine ***(85)***. A more gradual reemergence of wild-type HBV by a stepwise withdrawal of lamivudine over several weeks might be able to minimize the possibility of a clinically significant ALT flare in cirrhotic patients ***(72)***.

Patients with precore HBV mutations (i.e., HBeAg-negative and HBV DNA positive) show normalization of ALT and loss of HBV DNA in > 60%, and are characterized by an improved necroinflammatory activity, independent of the development of YMDD mutations so that they also might be regarded as candidates for long-term therapy (***86***). Another subgroup of patients for whom lamivudine therapy might be beneficial are those with decompensated cirrhosis and actively replicating hepatitis B infection awaiting liver transplantation. A small pilot study pointed toward an improvement of hepatic function in this selected subgroup of patients during lamivudine therapy (150 mg daily), which abrogated the urgent need of orthotopic liver transplantation and suggested a survival advantage. Nevertheless, the significance of these results is still questionable, because a retrospective control cohort was used ***(87)***. Finally, recent evidence from pilot studies strongly suggests that lamivudine can be lifesaving in the setting of a fulminant course of acute HBV infection ***(88)***.

Under lamivudine selection pressure, the high viral production rate and the low fidelity viral polymerase contribute to frequent development of polymerase mutants ***(89)***. Two types of polymerase gene mutations are most frequently observed: group 1 contains two mutations at amino acids 528 and 552 (L528M and M552V), which invariably occur together. Group 2 contains a mutation only at amino acid 552 (M552I). M552V (YVDD) and M552I (YIDD) are mutations in the YMDD motif of the polymerase gene, and are equally resistant to lamivudine ***(90)***. The resistance is thought to arise from the side groups of isoleucine (YIDD) and valine (YVDD) sterically preventing lamivudine from appropriately configuring into the nucleotide binding site of the reverse transcriptase ***(89)***. YMDD mutations occur in approx 15% after 1 yr ***(79)*** and in up to 76% after 4 yr of lamivudine treatment ***(83)*** in initially HBeAg-positive patients. Data on the rate of YMDD mutant emergence in HBeAg-negative chronic hepatitis B are still controversial: 10% after 2–4 yr ***(83)*** vs 56% after 2 yr ***(91)***. Recent data suggested that patients with the adw serotype were more likely to develop resistance to lamivudine than those with the ayw serotype ***(92)***. The clinical ramifications of a YMDD-mutant breakthrough are incompletely characterized ***(87)***, but severe or even fatal flares and progressive disease with graft loss have been reported ***(93,94)***.

To date, there is evidence that lamivudine therapy continues to benefit most patients even in development of breakthrough mutations *(82)*. Nevertheless, because of the uncertain long-term prognosis of YMDD-mutant infection, concern has been voiced about the use of lamivudine monotherapy in patients with mild disease and about prolonged use of this drug in individuals who may ultimately need liver transplantation *(72)*. A dilemma that emerges is whether to delay orthotopic liver transplantation in patients who have significantly improved on lamivudine, thereby prolonging their waiting time, or to proceed with transplantation despite stable hepatic function because of the potential risk for YMDD mutation and subsequent deterioration *(87)*.

8.3. Nucleoside Analogues Under Development

First tested in HIV patients, adefovir dipivoxil is a nucleotide analog that has been shown to have activity against lamivudine-resistant mutants as well as against wild-type HBV. A daily dose of 30 mg given over 12 wk results in a 4 $\log_{10}$ reduction in HBV DNA in patients infected with wild-type HBV *(37)*. Similar responses have recently been demonstrated in five patients with chronic hepatitis B (four after liver transplantation, one with stable cirrhosis) who had developed lamivudine resistance. HBV DNA suppression was sustained during a mean adefovir dipivoxil treatment period of 13 mo, including one patient in whom lamivudine was discontinued *(95)*. Patients with decompensated liver disease and YMDD mutations are also likely to benefit from a combination of lamivudine and adefovir *(96)*. Renal toxicity that has been noted under adefovir dipivoxil treatment is probably minimal with a 10-mg dose, but might limit its use as a first-line drug. Adefovir might therefore be used in combination with lamivudine to prevent the emergence of YMDD mutants *(72)*. **Figure 3** provides recent data on the efficacy of adefovir in HBeAg-negative patients.

Another promising, orally administered deoxyguanine nucleoside analog is entecavir, which has antiherpes and antihepadnaviral activity. It was shown to suppress viral replication 30 times more potently than lamivudine in HepG 2.2.15 cell lines *(97)*, and there is evidence that entecavir also has a direct effect on cccDNA, as shown for the woodchuck model *(98)*. Definite assessment of this drug has been delayed because of concern about pancreatic adenomas in mice *(72)*. In a 28-d study of entecavir, there was a 2.55 mean $\log_{10}$ reduction of viral load without significant side effects *(99)*. Like adefovir dipivoxil, entecavir seems to inhibit both wild-type and lamivudine-resistant forms of HBV *(100)*.

β-L-2'-Deoxythymidine (LdT) belongs to the group of "unnatural" L-nucleosides that are characterized by a highly potent, relatively selective inhibition of HBV polymerase in vitro. This is likely to be conferred by the 3'-OH group of the β-L-2'-deoxyribose *(101)*. A daily dose of 400 mg given over 24 d could induce a median decrease of 3.6 $\log_{10}$ copies/mL *(102)*.

Emtricitabine (FTC) is a fluorinated derivative of lamivudine that is anticipated to have a similar resistance pattern. In a dose-escalating study (98 patients treated over 24 wk), there was HBV DNA level reduction of up to 3 $\log_{10}$ *(103)*, and to date this nucleoside has been well tolerated *(72)*.

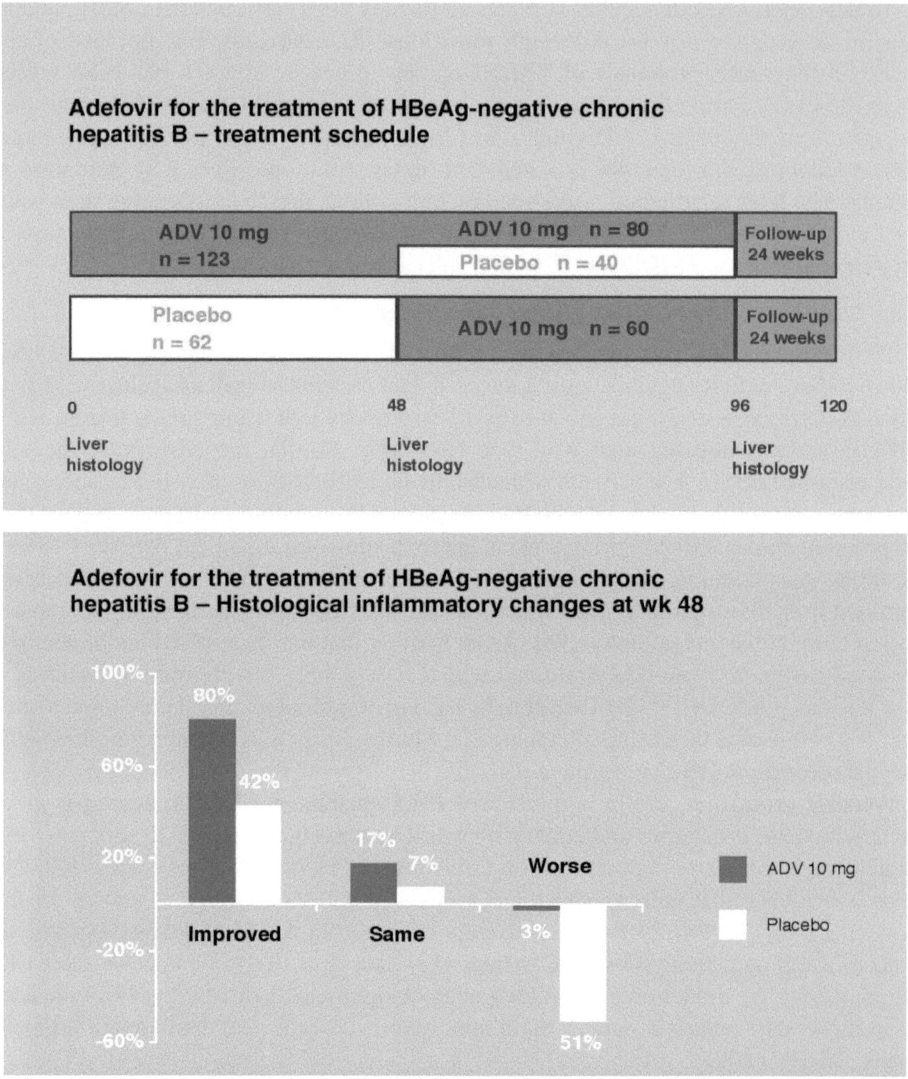

Fig. 3. Preliminary results from a double-blind randomized placebo-controlled trial of adefovir for the treatment of patients with HBeAg-negative chronic hepatitis B. (Modified from Hadziyannis and the GS-98-438 Study Investigator Group, presented at the EASL 2002.)

Clevudine (L-FMAU) is a pyrimidine analog with activity against HBV replication ***(104)*** whose efficacy against YMDD variants might be incomplete (100). Fialuridine (FIAU), a related agent, has been demonstrated to mediate severe toxicity in a significant proportion of patients participating in a Phase II study, and has therefore not achieved further clinical application. Adverse events included nausea, painful paresthesia, hepatic failure, and lactic acidosis, probably resulting from mitochondrial injury and pyruvate oxidation inhibition ***(105)***.

Glucosidase inhibitors have been proposed to exert antiviral effects in woodchuck animal model by altering specific steps in the *N*-linked glycosylation pathway ***(106)***. Even in case they lack potency against HBV by themselves, these drugs might be effective when used in combination with a nucleoside analog ***(64)***.

8.4. Combination Therapy with IFNs and Multiple Nucleoside Analogues

The combination of IFN-α with lamivudine is currently one of the most appealing treatment options for chronic hepatitis B ***(64)***. IFNs induce a targeted immune destruction, which up-regulates the second phase of viral load decay that is observed during nucleoside analog therapy ***(72)***. In one of the largest combination studies, 230 patients with HBeAg-positive chronic hepatitis B were randomized to IFN alone (10 million units three times a week for 16 wk), lamivudine alone (100 mg daily for 52 wk), or a combination (16 wk, preceded by an 8-wk course of lamivudine) ***(107)***. The HBeAg seroconversion rates after 52 wk were 19% with IFN alone, 18% with lamivudine alone, and 29% with the combination. Concern has been voiced about the uneven treatment periods, although the response to therapy was measured at 52 wk from the start of treatment ***(64)***. The concept of reducing HBV replication to very low levels with nucleoside analogs and then delivering a "death blow" to the virus with the addition of IFN seems to make sense ***(64)***. On the other hand, it is possible that an IFN lead-in phase or overlapping treatments could be more effective. This opinion is based on the assumption that a rapid inhibition of viral peptide synthesis during lamivudine therapy may lead to a diminished antigen display on the hepatocyte surface and therefore reduce the IFN efficacy ***(72)***.

Many experts have postulated that combination antiviral therapy, that is, the use of multiple nucleosides in combination, represents the future for treatment of chronic hepatitis B ***(64)***. By providing greater suppression of HBV replication, multidrug therapy could shorten the period of treatment necessary to induce a virologic response, and as a result diminish the rate of acquisition of drug-resistant mutants. Synergistic antiviral effects have been assumed to cause the significantly enhanced HBV inhibition, which was observed with a 12-wk course of lamivudine plus famciclovir, when compared with lamivudine alone ***(108)***. But it is likely that more potent drugs will replace famciclovir, including adefovir dipivoxil, entecavir, L-dT, L-dC, FTC, and L-FMAU, among others. Adefovir seems to be a promising combination partner for lamivudine-induced YMDD variants ***(96)***. Besides, combination regimes may also allow minimization of the toxicity of nucleoside analogs ***(64)***. **Figure 5** summarizes the current treatment options of chronic HBV infection in HBeAg-positive patients and provides an outlook for how we might treat these patients in the coming years.

8.5. Molecular Treatment Approaches to HBV

Innovative antiviral approaches, which are in the early stages of development and have not proven their clinical utility yet, include antisense oligonucleotides and ribozymes among others. Theoretically, these molecules could be targeted to multiple regulatory sites within the viral DNA or RNA, thereby preventing the emergence of viral mutations. Antisense molecules have been shown to inhibit DHBV replication ***(109)***, but their degradation by nucleases in vivo is a problem that has to be solved before clinical implementation. Synthetic nuclease-resistant ribozymes could efficiently be delivered to the liver of mice ***(110)***, and clinical trials are on the way to evaluate this potential treatment option ***(103)***.

9. Liver Transplantation and HBV Infection

Prior to the availability of effective treatment options throughout the 1970s and 1980s, HBV infection was considered to be a contraindication for transplantation. The implementation of nucleoside analogs in patients has led to significant improvements in the outcome of patients transplanted for HBV-induced end-stage liver disease. However, because of the wide range of possible complications, liver transplantation remains an ultima-ratio treatment option, which can be applied safely only at experienced centers.

HBV recurs in approx 80% 3 yr after transplantation without immunoprophylaxis ***(111)***, and is associated with a 5-yr survival rate of approx 50% that is significantly lower than in other forms of chronic liver disease ***(112)***. The highest risk of recurrent HBV infection and mortality is seen in patients with active viral replication prior to transplant (detectable HBeAg and HBV-DNA in serum), whereas the lowest recurrence rates are associated with a negative HBV-DNA and HBeAg prior to transplant, long-term administration of HBIg, hepatitis D virus (HDV) superinfection (fulminant hepatitis or related cirrhosis with a 3-yr recurrence rate of approx 10%), and severe acute liver failure ***(111, 113)***.

The use of HBV immune globulin (HBIG) intraoperatively and following transplantation has reduced the frequency and severity of recurrent HBV and improved survival ***(114)***. In a large multicenter European study of 372 patients, a 6-mo course of HBIG could lower the recurrence rate 3 yr posttransplant to 35%, thereby increasing the survival ***(111)***. Further improvements can be achieved by maintaining anti-HBs levels above 300–500 IU/L ***(115)***. There is evidence that even patients with active viral replication before transplantation benefit from passive immunization with HBIG by reduction of HBV antigenemia, although PCR assays can detect HBV DNA after 1 yr in a considerable proportion ***(116)***. Indefinite, long-term HBIG therapy may therefore be necessary in these patients ***(114)***.

Lamivudine has proven its efficacy in the transplant setting in a multicenter trial from the United States and Canada. Seventy-seven HBsAg-positive liver transplant candidates received treatment with 100 mg of lamivudine daily, which was continued after liver transplantation (60% of patients). At treatment wk 156, 13 of 22 (59%) of the posttransplant patients remained HBsAg negative, with HBV DNA polymerase mutants appearing in 21%. When compared with historical controls, lamivudine significantly decreased the rate of recurrent HBV infection ***(117)*** to an extent that was similar to that reported for long-term HBIG treatment ***(111)***. Because the discontinuation of lamivudine in posttransplant patients with YMDD mutations can be associated with clinical deterioration due to the reappearance of high-replicating wild-type HBV, the common clinical practice is to continue lamivudine in these patients despite the development of this mutation ***(114)***.

Combination prophylaxis with HBIG and lamivudine is very effective in preventing recurrent HBV, may protect against the emergence of resistant mutants, and is significantly more cost effective than HBIG monotherapy ***(118)***. In one study, 23 patients were given lamivudine starting up to 6 mo prior to transplantation and in addition put on HBIG for the first 6 mo after transplantation. No treatment failures were reported after a median follow-up of 13.8 mo ***(119)***. Another study suggested that sequential regimens might be an alternative option for patients with a low HBV recurrence risk. Six months of passive immunoprophylaxis with HBIG followed by lamivudine, 100 mg/d, for 52 wk was effective in preventing HBV recurrence ***(120)***. YMDD mutations have been reported in a small proportion of patients receiving combination prophylaxis. Their appearance prior to transplantation might pose a risk for HBV reinfection ***(121)*** and has even been regarded as contraindication to orthotopic liver transplantation (OLT) in some transplant centers ***(122)***. Therefore, consideration should be given to the risk-vs-benefit ratio of pretransplant lamivudine therapy. Some authors suggest treating HBsAg-positive transplant patients with 10,000 IU/mo of HBIG and lamivudine, 100 mg/d, starting in the anhepatic phase and maintaining anti-HBs titers 500 IU/L for high-risk patients (HBV DNA or HBeAg positivity at transplant) and 100 IU/L for low-risk patients (negativity for HBV-DNA and HBeAg) ***(114)***.

Combination therapy of one or more of the above-mentioned new nucleoside analogs and HBV immune globulin is likely to play a key role for further improvements in posttransplant therapy of HBV-infected patients in the future. Patients with YMDD mutations under lamivudine could benefit from a significant HBV-DNA reduction following adefovir dipivoxil treatment ***(123)***. This treatment is associated with a significant decline in viral load ***(Fig. 4)***. The role of high-titer hepatitis B immune plasma formulations needs to be determined in prospective studies ***(114, 124)***.

Another strategy in the prophylaxis of HBV recurrence after liver transplantation might be the discontinuation of HBIG followed by three applications of a double dose HBV vaccination. In 17 selected posttransplant patients (HBeAg negative, HBV DNA negative, completion of a 18-mo course of HBIG, no HBV recurrence, low-grade immunosuppression), 82% developed anti-HBs titers of >10 IU/L (six patients after the first, eight after a second vaccination course), and there was no HBV recurrence during a mean follow-up period of 14 mo in these patients ***(125)***. Although the level of anti-HBs that is needed to protect liver transplant recipients against HBV graft infection recurrence is a matter of debate, this strategy warrants further study in larger groups of patients. However, careful post-immunization testing and booster doses in case of decreases in anti-HBs appear to be mandatory.

Proposed current and future treatment regimens for HBeAg-positive chronic hepatitis B are illustrated in **Fig.5**.

10. Vaccination Strategies in HBV Prophylaxis and Therapy

Current hepatitis B preexposure vaccines consist of recombinant HBsAg, and provide effective prophylaxis against HBV infection. A series of three injections of vac-

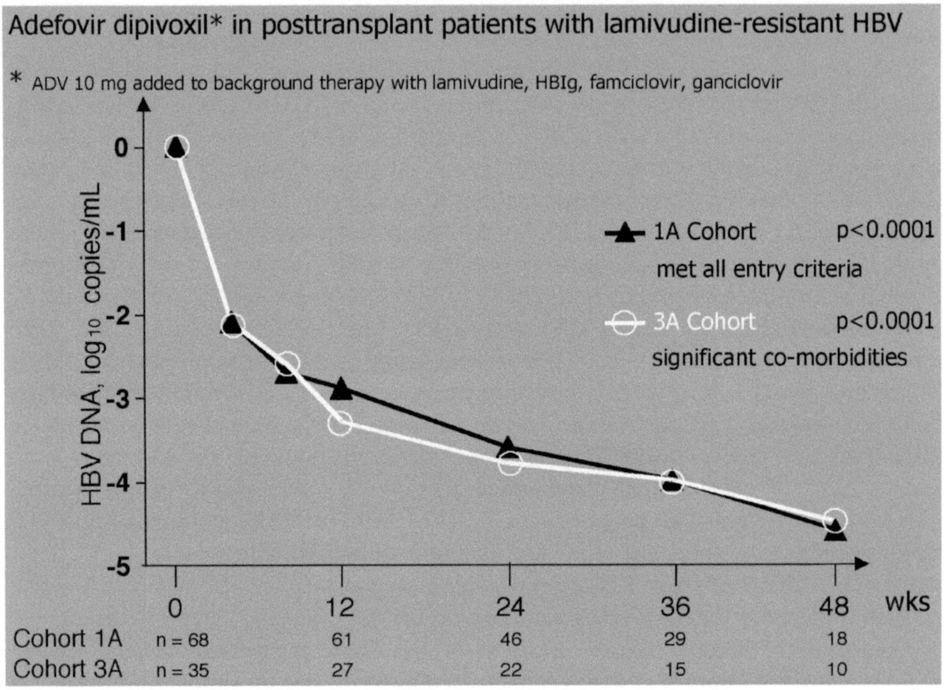

Fig. 4. Safety and efficacy of adefovir dipivoxil (ADV) for the treatment of lamivudine-resistant HBV in patients post-liver transplantation. Inclusion criteria: post-OLT, chronic HBV, clinically relevant lamivudine resistance, HBsAg-positive, HBV DNA $\geqslant 6 \log_{10}$ copies/mL, ALT $\geqslant 1.2 \times$ ULN. (Modified from Schiff and the GS-98-435 Study Investigator Group, presented at EASL 2002.)

cine induces protective levels of anti-HBs (> 10 mIU/mL) in > 95% of infants and children and in 90% of healthy adults. The major determinant of vaccine response is advancing age. By the age of 60 yr, the rate of protective antibody response has declined to 75%. Hepatitis B vaccine is recommended for all newborns, for previously unvaccinated children and adolescents, and for adults in high-risk groups. The latter include health care workers, injection drug users, family members of patients with chronic hepatitis B, patients with chronic renal failure, and recipients of clotting factor concentrates, among others. Vaccine nonresponders show serologic response following up to three additional vaccine doses in 50–75% of cases ***(126)***. They might also benefit from newer vaccine formulations. A recent study in 294 healthy adults from the United Kingdom and the United States demonstrated the efficacy of a new triple antigen HBV vaccine (containing S and pre-S1, and pre-S2 antigens). The two-dose regimen (mo 0, 1) of this vaccine had a similar response (91%) to Engerix B® (GlaxoSmithKline), while the three-dose regimen (mo 0, 1, 6) had a significantly superior response (98%) ***(127)***.

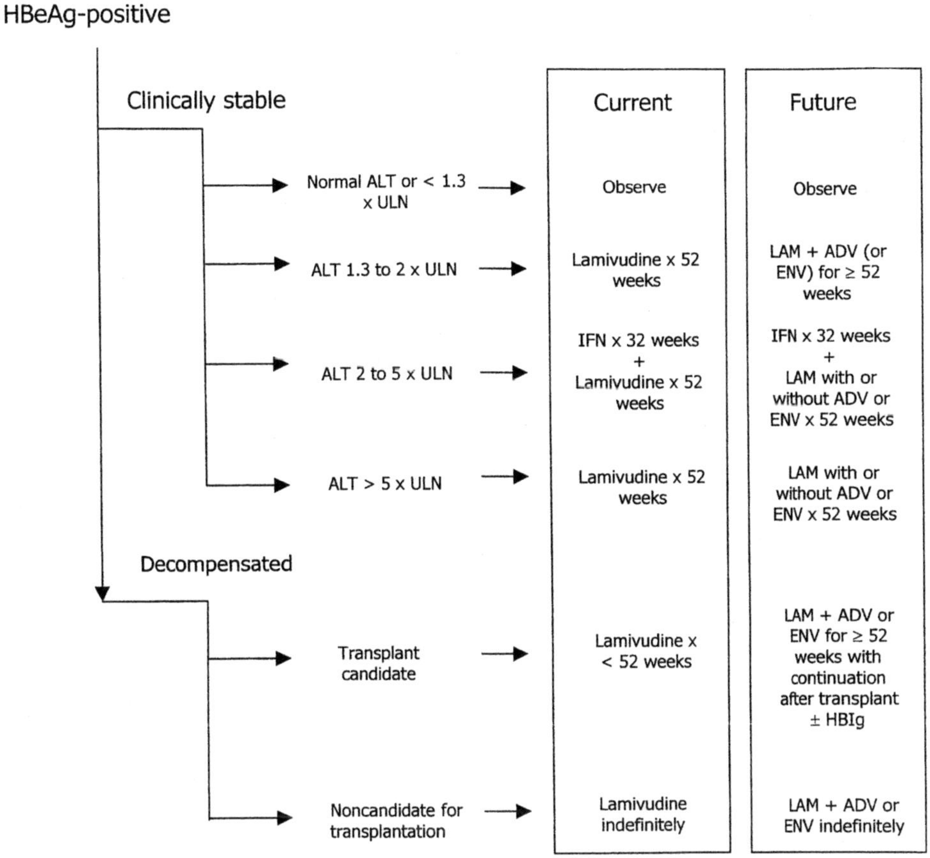

Fig. 5. Nucleoside analogs in current and future treatment regimens for HBeAg-positive chronic hepatitis B. LAM, Lamivudine; ADV, adefovir dipivoxil; ENV, entecavir; ULN, upper limit of normal. (Modified from Perrillo 2002 with kind permission.)

The success of recombinant protein vaccines as a therapeutic option has been less encouraging ***(128)***. Vaccines that contain pre-S portions of HBsAg that serve as additional T- and B-cell epitopes have been attributed to reductions in HBV DNA ***(129)***. Other authors have suggested administering the combination of HBsAg and anti-HBs to enhance cell-mediated immunity via the activation of proinflammatory cytokines ***(130)***.

Bacterial DNA that contains unmethylated CpG sequences within certain base contents (CpG DNA) can induce or enhance the stimulation of a variety of immune cells, and has been found to be one of the strongest Th1-immunomodulating vaccination adjuvants ***(131)***. The addition of CpG DNA to Engerix B® improved the HBsAg-specific CTL activity in chimpanzees ***(128)***, and could overcome Engerix B® hyporesponsiveness in orangutans ***(132)***. Phase I clinical trials are still ongoing, and it is an open question if the results from animal studies can be reproduced in humans.

T-cell tolerance to HBV in HBV-transgenic mice can be broken by immunization with a mixture of lipopeptides encompassing epitopes important in the induction of HBV-specific CTL ***(133)***. These and other results have led to speculations about peptide-based T-cell vaccines. The attraction of this strategy is the ability to identify and combine the very best T-cell epitopes to ensure appropriate T-cell help and CTL generation during immune induction ***(128)***. Administration of CY-1899, a lipopeptide-based HBcAg-epitope T cell vaccine, to subjects chronically infected with HBV initiated CTL activity but was not capable of inducing an immune response strong enough to clear the virus ***(134)***. Interestingly, however, a recent study provided strong evidence that therapeutic immunization with HBV core gene or protein deserves further investigation. Chronic HBsAg carriers who received bone marrow from HLA-identical donors with natural immunity to HBV showed resolution of chronic hepatitis B, which was associated with the transfer of HBcAg-reactive T cells ***(135)***.

The induction of strong T-cell responses might be an advantage of gene-based vaccines that could be demonstrated for several disease entities ***(136,137)***. Using recombinant retroviral vector encoding the HBcAg, gene delivery could trigger the resolution of infection in one of three chronically HBV-infected chimpanzees while activating HBV-specific CTL activity in another ***(138)***. In another example, a chronically HBV-infected chimpanzee received prime immunization with HBsAg encoding plasmid DNA followed by boost immunization with a recombinant HBsAg encoding canarypox, which led to a significant though transient decline of HBV DNA without a corresponding boost in HBV-specific CTL responses ***(139)***. The delivery of DNA vaccines with chimeric antigenes, in which sequences of an epitope of interest are exchanged between different but related viruses ***(140)***, may contribute to the development of more potent DNA vaccines for HBV therapy in the future.

11. HBV: Where Are We Going?

Since the discovery of HBV, enormous efforts have been made to shed light on its epidemiology, mode of transmission, molecular mechanisms of replication, and possible therapeutic intervention strategies. All over the world, physicians, health care workers, scientists, and technicians have applied themselves to help patients suffering from the complications of hepatitis B. Two decades ago, there was no effective intervention for the 300 million people carrying the "Australia antigen" (i.e., with chronic HBV infection). Twenty years on, research and development have changed their outlook. But the primary and ultimate goal is still the same: the eradication of HBV. The WHO has recommended the adoption of universal hepatitis B immunization for infants and adolescents. It is our policy to participate in the rigorous implementation of worldwide vaccination programs. The results of the Taiwanese immunization trial in infants have provided crucial evidence that HBV prophylaxis is the most powerful tool against HBV-associated morbidity. Further improvements in vaccination strategies will possibly be able to provide effective prophylaxis even to immunosuppressed individuals. Perhaps more importantly, preventive measures such as public information about the disease and its transmission by trained health care workers will play a central role. Prevention programs initiated by the WHO and other organizations to reduce the HBV incidence especially in children living in developing countries cannot be underestimated. These initiatives need our full financial attention.

Once chronic HBV infection has developed, the individual is at risk of developing potentially life-threatening complications. Improvements in the sensitivity of current HBV DNA tests and their wide availability have already provided a good basis for an adequate diagnostic workup. The treatment of chronic hepatitis B continues to evolve. IFN is worthwhile in noncirrhotic patients with mild to moderate disease activity, for it has not been associated with viral resistance, but its use is regularly associated with unpleasant, sometimes severe side effects. Nucleoside analogs, on the other hand, offer the advantage of reduced cost and minimal or no side effects. However, the virologic response is often incomplete and limited by the development of viral resistance. Lamivudine, which can be regarded as a first-line therapy for individuals with markedly elevated ALT, is therefore less suitable for children and patients with only minimal disease activity. More importantly, patients in the liver transplant setting have been shown to develop clinical deterioration secondary to the emergence of YMDD mutations. In the future, adefovir dipivoxil might be useful to maintain long-term clinical response in patients with intact renal function, as no resistance has been noted against this drug so far. With regard to the pros and cons of IFNs and the newer evolving nucleoside analogs, combination therapies have been suggested to represent the future for treatment of chronic HBV, as is already the case for HIV treatment. During recent years, scientists have dissected many details about the immunopathogenesis of HBV infection. We have learned that hepatitis B is an immune-mediated disease and that the competence of the host's immune system to mount a proper response at the right time plays a central role for a subsequent viral eradication. For this reason, IFN is likely to be an important combination partner in the near future, and may provide greater benefit than the combination of multiple nucleosides alone. However, because of its nonspecific action and multiple contraindications, IFN cannot be regarded as the ultimate therapeutic goal. More effective vaccination schedules are currently being developed even for immunocompromised patients post-liver transplant. The combination of viral load reduction by nucleoside analogs or one of the newer molecular treatment options followed by an efficacious immunization regimen might ultimately represent the most elegant and applicable treatment tool. Undoubtedly, it will become more and more important to tailor the treatment regimen to the specific disease features of the individual patient. To provide the basis for these sophisticated clinical decisions and enable further steps toward an eradication of HBV continues to be the future task for researchers all over the world.

References

1. Alter, H. J. (1981) Hepatitis B: a tribute to nondirected medical research. *Semin. Liver Dis.* **1**, 1–6.
2. Blumberg, B. S. (1977) Australia antigen and the biology of hepatitis B. *Science* **197**, 17–25.
3. Purcell, R. H. (1993) The discovery of the hepatitis viruses. *Gastroenterology* **104**, 955–963.
4. Lee, W. M. (1997) Hepatitis B virus infection. *N. Eng. J. Med.* **337**, 1733–1745.

5. Liang, T. J. (2000) The molecular virology of hepatitis B virus—new insights into an old virus, in *Update on Viral Hepatitis*, AASLD, Dallas, pp. 78–82.
6. Lau, J. Y. N. and Wright, T. L. (1993) Molecular virology and pathogenesis of hepatitis B. *Lancet* **342**, 1335–1340.
7. Lok, A. S.-F. and Chan, H. L.-Y. (2000) Viral hepatitis B and D, in *Comprehensive Clinical Hepatology* (O'Grady J. G., Lake J. R., and Howdle P. D., eds.), Mosby, London, pp. 12.1–22.
8. Paran, N., Geiger, B., and Shaul, Y. (2001) HBV infection of cell culture: evidence for multivalent and cooperative attachment. *EMBO J.* **20**, 4443–4453.
9. Breiner, K. M., Urban, S., and Schaller, H. (1998) Carboxypeptidase D (gp 180), a Golgi-resident protein, functions in the attachment and entry of avian hepatitis B viruses. *J. Virol.* **72**, 8098–8104.
10. Breiner, K. M., Schaller, H., and Knolle, P. A. (2001) Endothelial cell-mediated uptake of a hepatitis B virus: a new concept of liver targeting of hepatotropic microorganisms. *Hepatology* **34**, 803–808.
11. Milich, D., Chen, M., Hughes, J., and Jones, J. (1998) The secreted hepatitis B precore antigen can modulate the immune response to the nucleocapsid: a mechanism for persistence. *J. Immunol.* **160**, 2013–2021.
12. McMahon, B. J., Holck, P., Bulkow, L., and Snowball, M. (2001) Serologic and clinical outcomes of 1536 Alaska natives chronically infected with hepatitis B virus. *Ann. Intern. Med.* **135**, 759–768.
13. Andre, F. (2000) Hepatitis B epidemiology in Asia, the Middle East, and Africa. *Vaccine* **18**, S20–S22.
14. Stevens, C. E., Beasley, R. P., Tsui, J., and Lee, W. C. (1975) Vertical transmission of hepatitis B antigen in Taiwan. *N. Engl. J. Med.* **292**, 771–774.
15. Harpaz, R., McMahon, B., Margolis, H., et al. (2000) Elimination of new chronic hepatitis B virus infections: results of the Alaska immunization program. *J. Infect. Dis.* **181**, 413–418.
16. Margolis, H., Alter, M., and Hadler S. (1991) Evolving epidemiology and implications for control. *Semin. Liver Dis.* **11**, 84–92.
17. Terrault, N. (2000) Chronic viral hepatitis in the United States, in *Update on Viral Hepatitis*, AASLD, Dallas, pp. 36–46.
18. McQuillan, G., Coleman, P., Kruszon-Moran, D., et al. (1999) Prevalence of hepatitis B virus infection in the United States: the National Health and Nutrition Examination Surveys, 1976 through 1994. *Am. J. Publ. Hlth* **89**, 14–18.
19. Maini, M. and Bertoletti, A. (2000) How can the cellular immune response control hepatitis B virus replication? *J. Viral Hepat.* **7**, 321–326.
20. Michalak, T., Pasquinelli, S., Guilhot, S., and Chisari, F. (1994) Hepatitis B virus persistence after recovery of acute viral hepatitis. *J. Clin. Invest.* **93**, 230–239.
21. Mason, A., Xu, L., Guo, L., Kuhns, M., and Perrillo, R. (1998) Molecular basis for persistent hepatitis B virus infection in the liver after clearance of serum hepatitis B surface antigen. *Hepatology* **27**, 1736–1742.
22. Rehermann, B., Lau, D., Hoofnagle, J. H., and Chisari, F. V. (1996) Cytotoxic T lymphocyte responsiveness after resolution of chronic hepatitis B virus infection. *J. Clin. Invest.* **97**, 1655–1665.
23. Chisari, F. (1997) Cytotoxic T cells and viral hepatitis. *J. Clin. Invest.* **99**, 1472–1477.
24. Rehermann, B., Person, J., Redecker, A., et al. (1995) The cytotoxic T lymphocyte response to multiple hepatitis B virus polymerase epitopes during and after acute viral hepatitis. *J. Exp. Med.* **181**, 1047–1058.

25. Thursz, M. R., Kwiatkowski, D., Allsopp, C. E. M., Greenwood, B. M., Thomas, H. C., and Hill, A. V. S. (1995) Association between an MHC class II allele and clearance of hepatitis B virus in the Gambia. *N. Engl. J. Med.* **332**, 1065–1069.
26. Maini, M. K., Boni, C., Lee, C. K., et al. (2000) The role of virus—specific CD8+ cells in liver damage and viral control during persistent hepatitis B virus infection. *J. Exp. Med.* **191**, 1269–1280.
27. Chisari, F. V. (1999) Th immunobiology of viral hepatitis, in *T Cells in the Liver: Biology, Immunopathology and Host Defense* (Crispe, N., ed.), John Wiley & Sons, New York, pp. 117–138.
28. Kakimi, K., Lane, T. E., Wieland, S., et al. (2001) Blocking chemokine responsive to gamma-2 / interferon (IFN)-gamma inducible protein and monokine induced by IFN-gamma activity in vivo reduces the pathogenetic but not the antiviral potential of hepatitis B virus-specific cytotoxic T lymphocytes. *J. Exp. Med.* **194**, 1755–1766.
29. Guidotti, L. G., Ishikawa, T., Hobbs, M. V., Matzke, B., Schreiber, R., and Chisari, F. V. (1996) Intracellular inactivation of the hepatitis B virus by cytotoxic T lymphocytes. *Immunity* **4**, 25–36.
30. Heise, T., Guidotti, L. G., and Chisari, F. V. (2001) Characterization of nuclear RNases that cleave hepatitis B virus RNA near the La protein binding site. *J. Virol.* **75**, 6874–6883.
31. Chisari, F. V. (2000) Immunopathogenesis of hepatitis B, in *Update on Viral Hepatitis*, AASLD, Dallas, pp. 92–94.
32. Guidotti, L. G., Rochford, R., Chung, J., Shapiro, M., Purcell, R., and Chisari, F. V. (1999) Viral clearance without destruction of infected cells during acute HBV infection. *Science* **284**, 825–829.
33. Fattovich, G., Guistina, G., Schalm, S., et al. (1995) Occurrence of hepatocellular carcinoma and decompensation in western European patients with cirrhosis type B. *Hepatology* **21**, 77–82.
34. Villeneuve, J. P., Desrochers, M., Infante-Rivard, C., et al. (1994) A long-term follow-up study of asymptomatic hepatitis B surface antigen-positive carriers in Montreal. *Gastroenterology* **106**, 1000–1005.
35. Dienstag, J. L. and Isselbacher, K. J. (1988) Acute viral hepatitis, in *Harrison's Principles of Internal Medicine*, (Fauci, A. S., Braunwald, E., Isselbacher, K. J., (eds.), McGraw-Hill, New York, pp. 1677–1692.
36. Gilson, R. J. C., Murray-Lyon, I. M., Nelson, M. R., et al. (1998) Extended treatment with adefovir dipivoxil in patients with chronic hepatitis B virus infection. *Hepatology* **28**, 491A.
37. Heathcote, E., Jeffers, L., Wright, T., et al. (1998) Loss of serum HBV DNA and HBeAg and seroconversion following short-term (12 weeks) adefovir dipivoxil therapy in chronic hepatitis B: two placebo-controlled phase II studies (Abstract) *Hepatology* **28 (Suppl),** 317A.
38. Chen, T., Luk, J. M., Cheung, S.-T., Yu, W.-C., and Fan S.-T. (2000) Evaluation of quantitative PCR and branched-chain DNA assay for detection of hepatitis B virus DNA in sera from hepatocellular carcinoma and liver transplant patients. *J. Clin. Microbiol.* **38**, 1977–1980.
39. El-Serag, H. B. and Mason, A. C. (1999) Rising incidence of hepatocellular carcinoma in the United States. *N. Engl. J. Med.* **340**, 745–750.
40. Donato, F., Boffetta, P., and Puoti, M. (1998) A meta-analysis of epidemiological studies on the combined effect of hepatitis B and C virus infections in causing hepatocellular carcinoma. *Int. J. Cancer* **75**, 347–354.
41. Tsai, J. F., Jeng, J. E., Ho, M. S., et al. (1997) Effect of hepatitis C and B virus infection on risk of hepatocellular carcinoma: a prospective study. *Br. J. Cancer* **76**, 968–974.

42. Colombo, M. (2000) Viral hepatitis and cancer, in *Update on Viral Hepatitis*, AASLD, Dallas, pp. 170–178.
43. Donato, M. F., Arosio, E., et al. (2001) High rates of hepatocellular carcinoma in cirrhotic patients with high liver cell proliferative activity. *Hepatology* **34**, 523–528.
44. Koike, K., Tsutsumi, T., Fujie, H., Shintani, Y., and Kyji, M. (2002) Molecular mechanism of viral hepatocarcinogenesis. *Oncology* **62**, S1:29–37.
45. Zuckerman, A. J. (1997) Prevention of primary liver cancer by immunization. *N. Engl. J. of Med.* **336**, 1906–1907.
46. Chang, M., Chen, C., Lai, M., et al. (1997) Universal hepatitis B vaccination in Taiwan and the incidence of hepatocellular carcinoma in children. Taiwan Childhood Hepatoma Study Group. *N. Engl. J. Med.* **336**, 1855–1859.
47. Stuyver, L., De Gendt, S., Van Geyt, C., et al. (2000) A new genotype of hepatitis B virus: complete genome and phylogenetic relatedness. *J. Genet. Virol.* **81**, 67–74.
48. Chu, C. J. and Lok, A.S.F. (2002) Clinical significance of hepatitis B virus genotypes. *Hepatology* **35**, 1274–1276.
49. Orito, E., Mizokami, M., Sakugawa, H., et al. (2001) A case-control study for clinical and molecular biological differences between hepatitis B viruses of genotypes B and C. Japan HBV Research Group. *Hepatology* **33**, 218–223.
50. Kao, J. H., Chen, P. J., Lai, M. Y., and Chen, D. S. (2000) Hepatitis B genotypes correlate with clinical outcomes in patients with chronic hepatitis B. *Gastroenterology* **118**, 554–559.
51. Omata, M., Ehata, T., Yokosuka, O., Hosoda, K., and Ohto, M. (1991) Mutations in the precore region of hepatitis B virus DNA in patients with fulminant and severe hepatitis. *N. Engl. J. Med.* **324**, 1699–1704
52. Ehata, T., Omata, M., Chuang, W. L., et al. (1993) Mutations in core nucleotide sequence of hepatitis B virus correlate with fulminant and severe hepatitis. *J. Clin. Invest.* **91**, 1206–1213.
53. Pollicino, T., Zanetti, A., Cacciola, I., et al. (1997) Pre-S2-defective hepatitis B virus infection in patients with fulminant hepatitis. *Hepatology* **26**, 495–499.
54. Liang, T. J., Hasegawa, K., Munoz, S. J., et al. (1994) Hepatitis B virus precore mutation and fulminant hepatitis in the United States. A polymerase chain reaction-based assay for the detection of specific mutation. *J. Clin. Invest.* **93**, 550–555.
55. Li, J. S., Tong, S. P., Wen, Y. M., Vitsvitski, L., Zhang, Q., Trepo, C. (1993) Hepatitis B virus genotype A rarely circulates as an HBe-minus mutant: possible contribution of a single nucleotide in the precore region. *J. Virol.* **67**, 5402–5410.
56. Sterneck, M., Günther, S., Santantonio, T, et al. (1996) Hepatitis B virus genomes of patients with fulminant hepatitis do not share a specific mutation. *Hepatology* **24**, 300–306.
57. Chun, Y. K., Kim, J. Y., Woo, H. J., et al. (2000) No significant correlation exists between core promoter mutations, viral replication, and liver damage in chronic hepatitis B infection. *Hepatology* **32**, 1154–1162.
58. Schläger, F., Schaefer, S., Metzler, M., et al. (2000) Quantitative DNA fragment analysis for detecting low amounts of hepatitis B virus deletion mutants in highly viremic carriers. *Hepatology* **32**, 1096–1105.
59. Zoulim F. F., Saputelli, J., and Seeger, C. (1994) Woodchuck hepatitis virus X protein is required for viral infection *in vivo*. *J. Virol.* **68**, 2026–2030.
60. Bertolletti, A., Sette, A., Chisari, F. V., et al. (1994) Natural variants of cytotoxic epitopes are T cell receptor antagonists for antiviral cytotoxic T cells. *Nature* **369**, 407–410.
61. Waters, J. A., Kennedy, M., Voet, P., et al. (1992) Loss of the common "a" determinant of hepatitis B surface antigen by a vaccine-induced escape mutant. *J. Clin. Invest.* **90**, 2543–2547.

62. Blum, H. E., Moradpour, D., von Weizsaecker, F., Wieland, S., Peters, T., and Rasenack, J. W. S. (1997) Hepatitis-B-Virusmutanten—Klinische Bedeutung. *Z. Gastroenterol.* **35**, 347–355.
63. Dienstag, J. L. (2000) Therapy of hepatitis B, in *Update on Viral Hepatitis*, AASLD, Dallas, pp. 95–100.
64. Di Bisceglie, A. M. (2002) Combination therapy for hepatitis B. *Gut* **50**, 443–445.
65. Wong, D. K., Cheung, A. M., O'Rourke, K., et al. (1993) Effect of alpha interferon treatment in patients with hepatitis B e antigen-positive chronic hepatitis B. A meta-analysis. *Ann. Intern. Med.* **119**, 312–323.
66. Lau, D. T-Y., Everhart, J., Kleiner, D. E., et al. (1997) Long-term follow-up of patients with chronic hepatitis B treated with interferon alfa. *Gastroenterology* **113**, 1660–1667.
67. Niederau, C., Heintges, T., Lange, S., et al. (1996) Long-term follow-up of HbeAg-positive patients treated with interferon alfa for chronic hepatitis B. *N. Eng. J. Med.* **334**, 1422–1427.
68. Lin, S. M., Sheen, I. S., Chien, R. N., et al. (1999) Long-term beneficial effect of interferon therapy in patients with chronic hepatitis B virus infection. *Hepatology* **29**, 971–975.
69. Janssen, H. L. A., Gerken, G., Carreno, V., et al. (1999) Interferon alfa for chronic hepatitis B infection: increased efficacy of prolonged treatment. The European Concerted Action on Viral Hepatitis (EUROHEP). *Hepatology* **30**, 238–243.
70. Erhardt, A., Reineke, U., Blondin, D., et al. (2000) Mutations of the core promoter and response to interferon treatment in chronic replicative hepatitis B. *Hepatology* **31**, 716–725.
71. Kao, J. H., Wu, N. H., Chen, P. J., Lai, M. Y., Chen, D. S. (2000) Hepatitis B genotypes and the response to interferon therapy. *J. Hepatol.* **33**, 998–1002.
72. Perrillo, R. P. (2002) How will we use the new antiviral agents for hepatitis B? *Curr. Gastroenterol. Rep.* **4**, 62–71.
73. Zavaglia, C., Bottelli, R., Bellati, G., et al. (1996) Treatment of chronic hepatitis B (HbeAg-HBVDNA-positive) with lymphoblastoid alpha interferon with or without corticosteroids: short- and long-term follow-up. *Ital. J. Gastroenterol.* **28**, 324–331.
74. Zarski, J. P., Causse, X, Cohard, M., Cougnard, J., and Trepo, C. (1994) A randomized, controlled trial of interferon alfa-2b alone and with simultaneous prednisone for the treatment of chronic hepatitis B. French Multicenter Group. *J. Hepatol.* **20**, 735–741.
75. Cohard, M., Poynard, T., Mathurin P., and Zarki, J. P. (1994) Prednisone-interferon combination in the treatment of chronic hepatitis B: direct and indirect metanalysis. *Hepatology* **20**, 1390–1398.
76. Akuta, N., Suzuki, F., Tsubota, A., et al. (2002) Long-term clinical remission induced by corticosteroid withdrawal therapy (CSWT) in patients with chronic hepatitis B infection—a prospective randomized controlled trial—CSWT with and without follow-up interferon-v therapy. *Dig. Dis. Sci.* **47**, 405–414.
77. Liaw, Y. F., Tsai, S. L., Chien, R. N., Yeh, C. T., and Chu, C. M. (2000) Prednisolone priming enhances Th1 response and efficacy of subsequent lamivudine therapy in patients with chronic hepatitis B. *Hepatology* **32**, 604–609.
78. Dienstag, J. L., Schiff, E. R., Wright, T. L., et al. for the US Lamivudine Investigator Group (1999) Lamivudine as initial treatment for chronic hepatitis B in the United States. *N. Engl. J. Med.* **341**, 1256–1263.
79. Lai, C.L., Chien, R.-N., Leung, N.W.Y., et al. for the Asia Hepatitis Lamivudine Study Group (1998) A one-year trial of lamivudine for chronic hepatitis B. *N. Engl. J. Med.* **339**, 61–68.
80. Dienstag, J.L., Schiff, E.R., Mitchell, M., et al. (1999) Extended lamivudine retreatment for chronic hepatitis B: maintenance of viral suppression after discontinuation of therapy. *Hepatology* **30**, 1082–1087.

81. Gauthier, J., Bourne, E.J., Lutz, M.W., et al. (1999) Quantitation of hepatitis B viremia and emergence of YMDD variants in patients with chronic hepatitis B treated with lamivudine. *J. Infect. Dis.* **180**, 1757–1752.
82. Leung, N. W. Y., Lai, C.-L., Chang, T.-T., et al. on behalf of the Asia Hepatitis Lamivudine Study Group (2001) Extended lamivudine treatment in patients with chronic hepatitis B enhances hepatitis B e antigen seroconversion rates: results after 3 years of therapy. *Hepatology* **33**, 1527–1532.
83. Lau, D. T., Khokhar, M. F., Doo, E., et al. (2000) Long-term therapy of chronic hepatitis B with lamivudine. *Hepatology* **32**, 828–834.
84. Boni, C., Bertoletti, A., Penna, A. et al. (1998) Lamivudine treatment can restore T cell responsiveness in chronic hepatitis B. *J. Clin. Invest.* **102**, 968–975.
85. Moraleda, G., Spautelli, J., Aldrich, C. E., Averett, D., Condreay, L., and Mason, W. (1997) Lack of effect of antiviral therapy in nondividing hepatocyte cultures on the closed circular DNA of woodchuck hepatitis B virus. *J. Virol.* **71**, 9392–9399.
86. Tassopoulos, N. C., Volpes, R., Pastore, G., et al. (1999) Efficacy of lamivudine in patients with hepatitis B e antigen-negative/hepatitis B virus DNA-positive (precore mutant) chronic hepatitis B. Lamivudine Precore Mutant Study Group. *Hepatology* **29**, 889–896.
87. Yao, F. Y., Terrault, N. A., Freise, C., Maslow, L., and Bass, N. M. (2001) Lamivudine treatment is beneficial in patients with severely decompensated cirrhosis and actively replicating hepatitis B infection awaiting liver transplantation: a comparative study using a matched, untreated cohort. *Hepatology* **34**, 411–416.
88. Tillmann, H. L. (2002) Efficacy of lamivudine in fulminant HBV infection. Unpublished observation.
89. Doo, E. and Liang, T. J. (2001) Molecular anatomy and pathophysiologic implications of drug resistance in hepatitis B virus infection. *Gastroenterology* **120**, 1000–1008.
90. Whalley, S. A., Brown, D., Teo, C. G., Dusheiko, G. M., and Saunders N. A. (2001) Monitoring the emergence of hepatitis B virus polymerase gene variants during lamivudine therapy using the lightcycler. *J. Clin. Microbiol.* **39**, 1456–1459.
91. Lok, A. S.-F., Hussain, M., Cursano, C., et al. (2000) Evolution of hepatitis B virus polymerase gene mutations in hepatitis B e antigen-negative patients receiving lamivudine therapy. *Hepatology* **32**, 1145–1153.
92. Zollner, B., Petersen, J., Schroter, M., Laufs, R., Schoder, V., and Feucht, H. (2001) 20-fold increase in risk of lamivudine resistance in hepatitis B virus subtype adw. *Lancet* **357**, 934–935.
93. Liaw, Y., Chien, R., Yeh, C., Tsai, S. L., and Chu, C. M. (1999) Acute exacerbation and hepatitis B virus clearance after emergence of YMDD motif mutation during lamivudine therapy. *Hepatology* **30**, 567–572.
94. Perrillo, R., Rakela, J., Dienstag, J., et al. (1999) Multicenter study of lamivudine therapy for hepatitis B after liver transplantation. *Hepatology* 29, 1581–1586
95. Perrillo, R., Schiff, E., Yoshida, E., et al. (2000) Adefovir for the treatment of lamivudine-resistant hepatitis B mutants. *Hepatology* **32**, 129–134.
96. Perrillo, R., Schiff, E., Hann, H.-W. L., et al. (2001) The addition of adefovir dipivoxil to lamivudine in decompensated chronic hepatitis B patients with YMDD variant HBV and reduced response to lamivudine: preliminary 24 week results (Abstract). *Hepatology* **34**, 349A.
97. Innaimo, S. F., Seifer, M., Bissachi, G. S., et al. (1997) Identification of BMS-200475 as a potent and selective inhibitor of hepatitis B virus. *Antimicrob Agents Chemother.* **41**, 1444–1448.

98. Colonno, R. J., Genovesi, E. V., Median, I., **et al.** (2000) Long-term therapy with entecavir (BMS-200475) in the woodchuck model of chronic hepatitis infection, in *Abstracts of the 40th ICAAC,* **172**.
99. De Man, R. A., Wolters, L. M. M., Nevens, F., et al. (2001) Safety and efficacy of oral entecavir given for 28 days in patients with chronic hepatitis B virus infection. *Hepatology* **34**, 578–582.
100. Ono, S. K., Kato, N., Shiratori, Y., **et al.** (2001) The polymerase L528 mutation cooperates with nucleotide binding site mutations, increasing hepatitis B virus replication and drug resistance. *J. Clin. Invest.* **107**, 449–455.
101. Bryant, M., Bridges, E. G., Placidi, L., et al. (2001) Antiviral L-nucleosides specific for hepatitis B virus infection. *Antimicrob. Agents Chemother.* **45**, 229–235.
102. Lai, C. L., Lam, P. F., Myers, M. W., et al. (2001) Safe and potent suppression of hepatitis B virus (HBV) with L-deoxythymidine (LdT): results of a dose-escalation trial [Abstract]. *Hepatology*, 321A.
103. Lok, A. S., Heathcote, E. J., and Hoofnagle, J. H. (2001) Management of hepatitis B 2000—Summary of a workshop. *Gastroenterology* **120**, 1828–1853.
104. Peek, S. F., Cote, P. J., Jacob, J. R., et al. (2001) Antiviral activity of clevudine [L-FMAU, (1-(2-fluoro-5-methyl-B, L-arabinofuranosyl)uracil)] against woodchuck hepatitis virus replication and gene expression in chronically infected woodchucks (marmota monax). *Hepatology* **33**, 25401–50266.
105. Honkoop, P., Scholte, H. R., de Man, R. A., and Schalm S. W. (1997) Mitochondrial injury. Lessons from the fialuridine trial. *Drug Safety* **17**, 1–7.
106. Block, T. M., Lu, X., Mehta, A. S., et al. (1998) Treatment of chronic hepadnavirus infection in a woodchuck animal model with an inhibitor of protein folding and trafficking. *Nat. Med.* **4**, 610–614.
107. Schalm, S. W., Heathcote, J., Cianciara, J., et al. (2000) Lamivudine and alpha interferon combination treatment of patients with chronic hepatitis B infection: a randomized trial. *Gut* **46**, 562–568.
108. Lau, G. K., Tsiang, M., Hou, J., et al. (2000) Combination therapy with lamivudine and famciclovir for chronic hepatitis B-infected Chinese patients: a viral dynamics study. *Hepatology* **32**, 394–399.
109. von Weizsäcker, F., Wieland, S., Kock, J., et al. (1997) Gene therapy for chronic viral hepatitis: ribozymes, antisense oligonucleotides and dominant negative mutants. *Hepatology* **26**, 251–255.
110. Morrisey, D. V., Johnson, D. A., Macejak, D. G., et al. (2000) Inhibition of HBV protein synthesis by nuclease resistant ribozymes (Abstract). *Hepatology* **32**, 459A.
111. Samuel, D., Müller, R., Alexander, G., et al. (1993) Liver transplantation in European patients with the hepatitis B antigen. *N. Engl. J. Med.* **329**, 1842–1847.
112. Terrault, N. A. (1999) Hepatitis B virus and liver transplantation. *Clin. Liver Dis.* **3**, 389–415.
113. Samuel, D., Zignego, A., Reynes, M., et al. (1995) Long-term clinical and virological outcome after liver transplantation for cirrhosis caused by chronic delta hepatitis. *Hepatology* **21**, 333–339.
114. Sponseller, C. A. and Ramrakhiani, S. (2002) Treatment of hepatitis B and C following liver transplantation. *Curr. Gastroenterol. Rep.* **4**, 52–62.
115. Gugenheim, J., Baldini, E., Ouzan, D., et al. (1997) Absence of initial viral replication and long-term high-dose immunoglobulin administration improve results of hepatitis B virus recurrence prophylaxis after liver transplantation. *Transplant. Proc.* **29**, 517–518.

116. Terrault, N. A., Zhou, S., Combs, C., et al. (1996) Prophylaxis in liver transplant recipients using a fixed dosing schedule of hepatitis B immunoglobulin. *Hepatology* **24**, 1327–1333.
117. Perrillo, R., Wright, T., Rakela, J., et al. (2001) A multicenter United States-Canadian trial to assess lamivudine monotherapy before and after transplantation for chronic hepatitis B. The Lamivudine Transplant Group. *Hepatology* **33**, 424–432.
118. Han, S. H., Ogman, J., Holt, C., et al. (2000) An efficacy and cost-effectiveness analysis of combination hepatitis B immune globulin and lamivudine to prevent recurrent hepatitis B after orthotopic liver transplantation compared with hepatitis B immune globulin monotherapy. *Liver Transplant.* **6**, 741–748.
119. Terrault, N. A., Wright, T. L., Roberts, J. P., et al. (1998) Combined short-term hepatitis B immune globulin (HBIg) and long-term lamivudine versus HBIg therapy as hepatitis B prophylaxis in liver transplant recipients (Abstract). *Hepatology* **28**, 389A.
120. Naoumov, N. V., Ross Lopes, A., Burra, P., et al. (2001) Randomized trial of lamivudine versus hepatitis B immunoglobulin for long-term prophylaxis of hepatitis B recurrence after liver transplantation. *J. Hepatol.* **34**, 888–894.
121. Rosenau J., Bahr, M. J., Tillmann, H. L., et al. (2001) Lamivudine and low-dose hepatitis immune globulin for prophylaxis of hepatitis B reinfection after liver transplantation: possible role of mutations in the YMDD motif prior to transplantation as a risk factor for reinfection. *J. Hepatol.* **34**, 895–902.
122. Villeneuve, J. P., Condreay, L. D., Willems, B., et al. (2000) Lamivudine treatment for decompensated cirrhosis resulting from chronic hepatitis B. *Hepatology* **31,** 207–210.
123. Ahmad, J., Dodson, S. F., Balan, V., et al. (2000) Adefovir dipivoxil suppresses lamivudine-resistant hepatitis B virus in liver transplant recipients. Paper presented at the American Association for the Study of Liver Disease Annual Meeting, Dallas, TX. October 27–31.
124. Dickson, R. C., Terrault, N. A., Ishitani, M. B., et al. (2001) Protective antibody levels and dose requirements of IV 5% NABI hepatitis B immune globulin combined with lamivudine in liver transplantation for hepatitis B induced end stage liver disease. Paper presented at the American Association for the Study of Liver Disease Annual Meeting. Dallas, TX. Novemeber 9–13.
125. Sanchez-Fueyo, A., Rimola, A., Grande, L., et al. (2000) Hepatitis B immunoglobulin discontinuation followed by hepatitis B virus vaccination: a new strategy in the prophylaxis of hepatitis B virus recurrence after liver transplantation. *Hepatology* **31**, 496–501.
126. Margolis, H. (2000) Hepatitis B vaccine, in *Update on Viral Hepatitis*, AASLD, Dallas, pp. 88–91.
127. Young, M. D., Schneider, D. L., Zuckerman, A. J., Du, W., Dickson, B., and Maddrey W. C. for the US Hepacare Study Group(2001) Adult hepatitis B vaccination using a novel triple antigen recombination vaccine. *Hepatology* **34**, 372–376.
128. Payette, P. J. and Davis, H. L. (2001) Are therapeutic vaccines a realistic approach to therapy for chronic hepatitis B? in *Therapy in Hepatology* (Arroyo, V., Bosch, J., Bruix, J., Gines, P., Navasa, M., and Rodes, J., eds.), Ars Medica, Barcelona, pp. 239–244.
129. Couillin, I., Pol, S., Mancini, M., et al. (1999) Specific vaccine therapy in chronic hepatitis B: induction of T cell proliferative response specific for envelope antigens. *J. Infect. Dis.* **180**, 15–26.
130. Wen, Y. M., Qu, D., and Zhou, S. H. (1999) Antigen-antibody complex as therapeutic vaccine for viral hepatitis B. *Int. Rev. Immunol.* **18**, 251–258.
131. Dalpke, A. H., Zimmermann, S., Albrecht, I., and Heeg, K. (2002) Phosphodiester CpG oligonucleotides as adjuvants: polyguanosine runs enhance cellular uptake and improve immunostimulative activity of phosphodiester CpG oligonucleotides in vitro and in vivo. *Immunology* **106**, 102–112.

132. Davis, H. L., Suparto, I. I., Weeratna, R. R., et al. (2000) CpG DNA overcomes hyporesponsiveness to hepatitis B vaccine in orangutans. *Vaccine* **18**, 1920–1924.
133. Sette, A. D., Oseroff, C., Sidney, J., et al. (2001) Overcoming T cell tolerance to the hepatitis B virus surface antigen in hepatitis B virus-transgenic mice. *J. Immunol.* **166**, 1389–1397.
134. Heathcote, J., McHutchison, J., Lee, S., et al. and the CY-1899 T cell vaccine study group (1999) A pilot study of CY-1899 in subjects chronically infected with hepatitis B virus. *Hepatology* **30**, 531–536.
135. Lau, G. K., Suri, D., Liang, R., et al. (2002) Resolution of chronic hepatitis B and anti-HBs seroconversion in humans by adoptive transfer of immunity to hepatitis B core antigen. *Gastroenterology* **122**, 614–624.
136. Calarota, S., Bratt, G., Nordlund, S., et al. (1998) Cellular cytotoxic response induced by DNA vaccination in HIV-I-infected patients. *Lancet* **351**, 1320–1325.
137. Wang, R., Doolan, D. L., Le, T. P., et al. (1998) Induction of antigen specific cytotoxic T lymphocytes in humans by a malaria DNA vaccine. *Science* **282**, 476–480.
138. Sallberg, M., Hughes, J., Javadian, A., et al. (1998) Genetic immunization of chimpanzees chronically infected with the hepatitis B virus, using a recombinant retroviral vector encoding the hepatitis B virus core antigen. *Hum. Gene Ther.* **9**, 1719–1729.
139. Pancholi, P., Lee, D. H., Liu, Q., et al. (2001) DNA prime/canarypox boost- based immunotherapy of chronic hepatitis B virus infection in a chimpanzee. *Hepatology* **33**, 448–454.
140. Schirmbeck, R., Zheng, X., Roggendorf, M., et al. (2001) Targeting murine immune responses to selected T cell- or antibody-defined determinants of the hepatitis B surface antigen by plasmid DNA vaccines encoding chimeric antigen. *J. Immunol.* **166**, 1405–1413.

32

Designing Studies to Evaluate Anti-Hepatitis B Virus Therapies

From the Perspective of Studies for the Registration of Pharmaceutical Products

Alison B. Murray

1. Introduction

The clinical studies that are required to obtain world-wide regulatory approval to market therapies for the treatment of hepatitis B virus (HBV) are lengthy, large, and costly. It is therefore important that those undertaking such studies fully understand the disease, the current therapies available, the requirements of major regulatory authorities, and the role that the new therapy will play in the treatment of the disease before embarking on these studies. The aims of this chapter are to outline some of the factors that should be taken into consideration when planning such studies, to highlight common pitfalls in the design and conduct of these studies, and to provide some suggestions on how these pitfalls might be avoided.

The specific designs of the studies that will form part of the clinical program will differ depending on the phase of development, the type of therapy being evaluated, and the patient population for whom the therapy will be indicated. This chapter focuses on considerations for the design and conduct of the Phase III studies that support the efficacy and safety of a new therapy in international registration dossiers. It is not intended to provide a blueprint for an entire development program for an anti-HBV therapy.

2. Selection of Patients

Selection of the appropriate patient populations for the Phase III studies is key to the success of the development program, and has important implications for how the product under evaluation will ultimately be labeled.

From: *Methods in Molecular Medicine, vol. 96: Hepatitis B and D Protocols, volume 2*
Edited by: R. K. Hamatake and J. Y. N. Lau © Humana Press Inc., Totowa, NJ

2.1. Acute and Chronic HBV Infection

Patients chronically infected with HBV are the most commonly treated group, and should therefore be the focus of the registration studies. The efficacy of anti-HBV therapies is rarely studied among patients with acute HBV infection, as these patients are only transiently affected, are at low risk of progressive liver disease and hepatocellular carcinoma, and are therefore seldom treated ***(1,2)***.

2.2. HBeAg-Positive and HBeAg-Negative Disease

Patients who are hepatitis B virus e antigen (HBeAg) positive are generally the focus of at least one of the pivotal studies that are included in a registration dossier. In addition, consideration should be given to conducting a study among patients who have HBeAg negative chronic hepatitis B, sometimes referred to as precore mutant HBV infection. These patients are HBsAg positive, HBeAg negative, and anti-HBe positive, but can be distinguished from patients who have seroconverted, by having detectable HBV DNA on one of the less sensitive assays, such as hybridization assays (limit of detection approx 10^6 copies/mL) and alanine aminotransferase (ALT) levels that may be intermittently or continuously elevated ***(3)***. It is important to study these patients in the program, as the prevalence of precore mutant HBV disease in increasing in many areas, particularly in southern Europe ***(4)*** and Southeast Asia ***(5)***. In other areas this form of the disease is becoming more widely recognized as clinicians adopt the use of HBV DNA testing in serum into the routine assessment of patients infected with HBV.

2.3. Treatment of Naive Patients and Those Who Have Previously Failed Therapy

It is prudent to focus the pivotal registration studies on treatment-naive patients if possible, unless the new therapy is targeted specifically at patients who have previously failed to respond to other treatments. It is becoming increasingly difficult to conduct studies in treatment-naive patients, as increasing numbers of patients are being offered, and respond to, treatment. The patients remaining in the specialist clinics, where these studies are generally conducted, will be those who have failed to respond to prior therapy. The challenge for future development programs will be to balance studies in a relatively uncomplicated, treatment-naive population where it is relatively simple to evaluate the efficacy and safety of therapy with studies in the more complex, previously treated population, who will be the population requiring treatment in years to come.

The advantages of conducting studies in treatment-naive patients are as follows:

- These patients represent a population with the widest range of potential therapy responses, that is, those with a high and low likelihood of responding to therapy, in particular, on seroconversion endpoints. Patients who have previously failed to seroconvert using other therapies are also less likely to seroconvert on the new therapy. If the majority of patients in the study have previously failed therapy, the chances of the study showing a difference in seroconversion rates between placebo and active treatment are likely to be small ***(6)***.
- For new antiviral therapies, allowing patients who have previously been treated with a different antiviral to be enrolled in the study increases the potential for including patients who have an HBV strain that is resistant to the prior therapy. Including these patients would

make it difficult to assess accurately the antiviral effect of the new therapy, and enrolling patients with preexisting resistance to the comparator could bias the results of the study against the comparator.

- Patients who have failed prior therapy may have more advanced disease than treatment-naive patients. These patients are therefore more likely to experience adverse events during the study than a treatment-naive population. If the study is a placebo-controlled study, including patients with advanced disease is likely to be questioned by Institutional Review Boards or Ethics Committees. If the comparator is an interferon, there may be limitations on using such therapy in patients with advanced disease.

2.4. Cirrhotic and Noncirrhotic Patients and Patients with Compensated and Decompensated Liver Disease

When defining the patient population to be studied, it is important to distinguish between excluding patients with cirrhosis from those who have decompensated liver disease. Many protocols exclude all patients with cirrhosis, often without adequately screening for the presence of cirrhosis in those being considered for enrollment. Rather than excluding patients with cirrhosis, consideration should be given to excluding patients with decompensated liver disease. This allows patients with early stage cirrhosis who have compensated liver disease to be enrolled, and will also facilitate a broader label for the product without necessarily increasing the potential for adverse events in the study.

Adequately controlled trials using new therapies are difficult to conduct in patients with decompensated liver disease and those who are awaiting or have undergone liver transplantation. However, prior to embarking on the clinical program, consideration should be given to how the needs of these patients are to be addressed in the program, as these are the patients in greatest need of new therapeutic options. Although controlled studies may be difficult to conduct in this patient group, an attempt should be made to collect data on efficacy and safety if these patients do receive the new treatment. If a compassionate release program is considered, the scope of the program, the criteria under which patients will be treated, the data to be collected, and the mechanism for such data collection should be prospectively defined before the first patient is treated under such a program. If not adequately planned in advance, an opportunity to collect valuable data may be missed, the compassionate use program can become a major drain on resources, and a point of conflict between the sponsor and treating physicians.

2.5. A Geographically Diverse, Representative Patient Population

To evaluate a new anti-HBV therapy in the populations in which it is most likely to be used, and where the medical need is greatest, consideration should be given to conducting these studies in areas where chronic HBV infection is endemic *(7)*.

2.6. Baseline ALT Levels

Inclusion criteria for pretreatment ALT levels are another important consideration in selecting patients for the study. There is generally agreement that patients with elevated ALT levels should be treated, but the question as to whether patients with normal ALT levels should be treated is still a topic of debate. The advantage of including patients with normal ALT levels in the study is that the study might support a broader label, however, there are disadvantages. Seroconversion rates are lower among patients with normal or only slightly elevated ALT levels *(8,9)*. Therefore, including patients with normal ALT levels in the study is likely to result in a lower seroconversion rate, and hence a larger sample size will be required if statistical significance is sought for this endpoint.

2.7. Other Characteristics of the Patient Population

Patients who are coinfected with other hepatitis viruses such as hepatitis C virus or hepatitis delta virus are generally excluded from the pivotal registration studies. The reason for this is that coinfection makes it difficult to assess the impact of the anti-HBV therapy on the liver disease, if other causes of liver disease are also present. For this reason patients with other liver diseases such as autoimmune or alcoholic hepatitis, Wilson's disease, or hemochromatosis are also generally excluded from the pivotal studies. Patients who are immunosuppressed as a result of human immunodeficiency virus (HIV) infection, or treatment of malignant disease, are also generally excluded, as immunosuppression may alter the behavior of the HBV disease or response of the disease to therapy. In addition, the multiple concomitant medications that immunosuppressed patients may require increase the potential for drug–drug interactions with the new therapy, and make it difficult to assess the safety profile of the new therapy. However, once the safety profile of the therapy has been established in immunocompetent patients, and once the potential for drug interactions has been explored, studies can be considered in these more complex patient groups, in whom the need for new therapeutic options may be significant.

3. Choice of Comparator

Wherever possible randomized, placebo-controlled studies are the optimal studies to assess accurately the efficacy and safety of a new therapy. However, as therapies for HBV improve, and are more widely adopted into clinical practice, it will become increasingly difficult to conduct placebo-controlled trials.

If an active comparator is included, care should be taken to ensure that the study design allows for an unbiased comparison of the treatments. The duration of treatment should be comparable, and endpoints should be evaluated at similar time points for the two therapies. This is particularly important when comparing therapies with different treatment regimens, such as when a nucleoside/nucleotide analog is compared to an interferon. If the endpoints are evaluated at different points, for example at the end of treatment for one group and 6 mo after therapy in another, the study results may be difficult to interpret *(6)*.

4. Choice of Endpoints

The primary endpoint of the study should be appropriate for the population being studied, and the indication to be sought for the product. The study should be adequately powered to determine the efficacy of the therapy using the chosen endpoint. The goal of treating HBV infection is to prevent progressive liver disease, hepatic failure, and primary hepatocellular carcinoma. However, as liver disease due to chronic HBV evolves over decades, it is neither practical nor reasonable to require that studies of new anti-HBV therapies be designed to demonstrate efficacy using these endpoints. Therefore three categories of surrogate endpoints are generally used in registration studies for new anti-HBV therapies: liver histology, seroconversion, and serum or plasma viral load. A fourth endpoint, serum ALT, is also included, although this is seldom a primary endpoint.

4.1. Liver Histology

The most commonly employed endpoint for the Phase III studies that have been used to register pharmaceutical or biological products in the past is an assessment of the impact of therapy on liver histology. This is the endpoint that best evaluates the impact of therapy on the liver, the target organ of the infection, and can be used in patients with HBeAg-positive and HBeAg-negative chronic hepatitis B.

To ensure that studies employing histological endpoints succeed, the following points should be considered. At least two biopsies are required, one prior to commencement of therapy and the second at or near the end of the study. The timing of the second biopsy will vary depending on the type of therapeutic regimen being studied. For interferons, where 4- to 6-mo treatment regimens are approved in most countries, the second biopsy is generally conducted 6 mo after the course of therapy has been completed. For antiviral therapies, such as lamivudine or adefovir, where therapy is administered chronically to suppress viral replication, the second biopsy is generally taken after 1 yr, while patients remain on therapy. These patients generally continue on therapy after the biopsy has been taken, either within the study, or in a "rollover" protocol designed to evaluate long-term safety and efficacy.

The timing of the first biopsy is often the subject of a great deal of discussion with study investigators during study design and start-up activities. Ideally the first biopsy should be taken as close to the commencement of treatment as possible, that is, within the days or weeks before therapy is started. However, as there is both risk and discomfort for patients undergoing the liver biopsy procedure, it is reasonable to accept biopsies that had been taken recently, for example, up to 6 mo prior to enrollment. These prior biopsies should be accepted only if the tissue sections, histological slides, and other specimens required for the study evaluations are available for assessment by the study pathologist. It is important to cap the time allowed between biopsy and enrollment, and make this point very clear to investigators prior to the start of the study. Ideally a limit of 6 mo should be stipulated; however, many sponsors will accept biopsies taken up to a year prior to the commencement of therapy. One year is probably too long, however, as this allows variation of up to a year between the timing of the baseline biopsies of different patients within the study. It also introduces a variation of 1 and 2 yr between baseline and end of study biopsies for different patients within the study. If the design of the study and the statistical analyses do not take this factor into account, there is a potential for bias to be introduced. If the sponsor permits baseline biopsies taken up to 12 mo prior to enrollment, the bias could be reduced by stratifying for timing of the baseline biopsy, for example, $>$ or $\leq$ 6 mo, should be considered.

Two biopsies are essential to be able to evaluate a histological endpoint. Excessive numbers of patients who do not have the second biopsy can have a significant impact on the power of the study to detect a treatment effect. Investigators should therefore be strongly encouraged to enroll only patients who will consent to the second biopsy, and the study should be powered assuming that dropouts will occur.

The assessment of liver histology is somewhat subjective; it is therefore essential to use one central pathologist to evaluate and score the study histology slides to remove the potential for interobserver differences ***(10,11)***. Intraobserver variation in histological scoring can be minimized by having the pathologist assess and score the baseline and end of study biopsies in the same session, which will ensure that the two biopsies from a patient are compared under the same circumstances. To avoid biasing the pathologist, the biopsies should be blinded as to the order in which they were taken. This is particularly important in placebo-controlled studies of highly effective therapies, where the pathologist could easily become unblinded as to treatment group if the order in which the biopsies were taken is known.

The optimal method for studying the effect of treatment of hepatitis using liver histology has been a topic of debate for a number of years ***(12–14)***. Scoring systems have been devised to attempt to quantify the damage to the liver caused by the infection, and measure changes in liver pathology during the course of therapy. The most commonly employed scoring system for registration studies for both HBV and HCV disease has been the Histological Activity Index (HAI) ***(11)***, which assigns a weighted score to each of four categories of the liver pathology as shown in **Table 1**.

This scoring system was later modified by Ishak (**Table 2**), who was one of the authors on the paper describing the original HAI score ***(14)***. This modified HAI score addressed a number of the disadvantages of the original HAI scoring system. The modified system is composed of two separate scores, one used to grade the necroinflammatory activity and the other to stage fibrosis and cirrhosis. The scores for the necroinflammatory and fibrosis components, considered to be quite different pathological processes, were combined in the original HAI score. The original HAI score generated discontinuous variables, whereas the modified HAI score generates continuous variables, and therefore may be analyzed using a number of different statistical methods. The modified score provides a more detailed evaluation of the impact of therapy on fibrosis and cirrhosis. For large, Phase III studies, it is prudent to have the biopsies scored using both the HAI and the modified HAI scores.

The histological data can be analyzed in a number of ways. The most commonly employed method used in past studies was to evaluate the proportion of patients in each treatment group in whom there was at least (i.e., ⩾) a 2-point decrease in the HAI score between the biopsies taken at baseline and the end of treatment/study ***(6,15–19)***. This categorical method provided a means of analyzing the data from the discontinuous variable generated by the HAI score. Although this method of evaluating the impact of therapy on liver histology has been used for years, and was the basis of registration of multiple therapies, there is not consensus among pathologists that this indeed indicates a clinically relevant change in liver histology. Some pathologists and statisticians would prefer a comparison of the median change in the HAI score between treatment groups.

Table 1
HAI Scoring System

Category	Possible scores
I. Periportal necrosis (with or without bridging)	0, 1, 3, 4, 5, 6, 10
II. Intralobular degeneration and focal necrosis	0, 1, 3, 4
III. Portal inflammation	0, 1, 3, 4
IV. Fibrosis	0, 1, 3, 4

Table 2
Modified HAI Scoring

Necroinflammatory Scores (Grading)	
Category	Scores
A. Portal and periseptal interface hepatitis (piecemeal necrosis)	0, 1, 2, 3, 4
B. Confluent necrosis	0, 1, 2, 3, 4, 5, 6
C. Focal lytic necrosis, apoptosis, and focal inflammation	0, 1, 2, 3, 4
D. Portal inflammation	0, 1, 2, 3, 4
Fibrosis and cirrhosis (staging)	
Category	Scores
Fibrosis and cirrhosis	0, 1, 2, 3, 4, 5, 6

This analysis is possible if the continuous variable from the modified HAI scoring system is used. In this case, median changes in the necroinflammatory and fibrosis components can be compared across treatment groups.

4.2. Seroconversion

The endpoint most favored by study investigators is anti-HBe seroconversion. The reason this endpoint is preferred to histology by investigation is that it can be evaluated using blood samples, avoiding the liver biopsy procedure, and it is the endpoint that is used in clinical practice to assess a patient's response to therapy. However, anti-HBe seroconversion should be used with caution as a primary endpoint in registration studies. The most important implication of this endpoint is on the size, and therefore duration of enrollment and cost, of the study. The most common error in the design of past studies using seroconversion as a primary endpoint was that studies were not adequately powered to detect a difference between the treatment and control groups in the populations being studied. This led to years of debate on the efficacy of interferon as a treatment for HBV, the debate being finally resolved in 1993 by the meta-analysis conducted by Wong et al. ***(20)***. Underpowering of studies using a seroconversion primary endpoint may be further compounded if the relationship between seroconversion rates and ALT levels and between seroconversion rates and study duration are not taken into account in the study design. Seroconversion rates increase, with increasing duration of therapy; therefore studies of shorter duration will require larger sample sizes.

In recent studies in treatment-naïve patients with elevated ALT levels (>1.5× the upper limit of the normal range), treated with lamivudine or adefovir for a year, seroconversion rates in the placebo groups were between 4% and 6%, while those in the active groups were between 12% and 17% ***(16,17,19)***. Therefore each study had to be powered to detect a difference of 6–12% between the active and placebo groups. To show a statistically significant difference between active treatment and placebo in this setting, between 120 and 150 patients are required in each treatment group if a 1:1 randomization is employed. If an unequal randomization is employed to reduce the number of patients receiving placebo, the sample size would have to be even larger. Similarly if patients with normal ALT levels were included in the study, or for a study of a shorter duration, both factors that would result in a decrease in the seroconversion rate at the end of the study, the required sample size would be greater ***(8)***.

Seroconversion may be defined in three increasingly rigorous ways: patients who enter the study with a detectable HBeAg are considered to have seroconverted if they become:

1. HBeAg negative.
2. HBeAg negative and anti-HBe positive.
3. HBeAg negative, anti-HBe positive, and have an HBV DNA below the limit of detection of the solution hybridization assay (< approx 10^6 copies of HBV to DNA/mL)***(17)***.

The definition to be used should be discussed during the study design process, as this too can influence the sample size. The rate of HBeAg loss is higher than the rate of HBeAg loss accompanied by acquisition of anti-HBe, and both are higher than the rate of seroconversion using the definition that includes HBV DNA. Only if anti-HBe appears is the seroconversion likely to be sustained when therapy is stopped. As the prevalence of HBeAg-negative chronic hepatitis B increases, the HBV DNA level will become an increasingly important tool for differentiating this population from true seroconverters. The first or second definitions were used in most of the interferon registration studies, but in the recent lamivudine Phase III registration studies seroconversion was evaluated using the third definition listed in the preceding list ***(6,8,16,17)***. This definition may need to be refined further for future studies, in which more sensitive HBV DNA tests (lower limit of detection approx 10^2–10^3 copies/mL) that employ more sensitive polymerase chain reaction technology will be used. Using these assays low levels of HBV DNA can be detected in patients who seroconverted many years previously, and in whom liver disease has not progressed ***(3,21–24)***. Therefore the definition of seroconversion for newer therapies will need to be reviewed, to include a requirement that the HBV DNA level is below some agreed cutoff value (e.g., 10^6 copies/mL) rather than requiring patients to have undetectable HBV DNA levels ***(3)***.

Timing of assessment of anti-HBe seroconversion should be appropriate for the type of therapy being studied. In studies in which different therapy types are being used, care should be taken to ensure that the timing of the measurement of seroconversion does not bias the results in favor of any one therapy or combination of therapies. For example, seroconversion should be assessed either at the end of therapy in all treatment groups, or after 6 mo off therapy in all treatment groups. If seroconversion is measured at the end of treatment in one group and 6 mo after therapy is stopped in another, it is not possible to make an accurate assessment of the relative efficacy of the two treatments ***(6)***.

Anti-HBs seroconversion may also be considered as a study endpoint; however, as this generally follows anti-HBe seroconversion by months or years, this is seldom used as a primary endpoint in the pivotal registration studies, in which patients are followed for a year to 18 mo. As the rate of anti-HBs seroconversion is lower than the rate of anti-HBe seroconversion, studies using an anti-HBs primary endpoint would have to be very large to show differences between active treatment and placebo. Anti-HBs seroconversion is best evaluated in follow on or rollover studies, into which patients from the Phase III studies may be enrolled to assess longer term efficacy and safety.

4.3. Viral Load

The third possible primary endpoint is measurement of changes in HBV DNA levels before and during treatment. To date this endpoint has not been widely accepted as a primary endpoint by regulatory authorities. The major reason for this is that changes in HBV DNA levels have not been fully established as a surrogate marker for disease progression. The data supporting the suitability of HBV DNA as a surrogate marker for the clinical efficacy of a therapy are becoming available. Three antiviral therapies have undergone Phase III testing over the past 5 yr. Lamivudine and adefovir have been shown to suppress HBV DNA levels effectively in all patients undergoing therapy, by between 2 and 4 log, depending on the dynamic range of the test used to measure viral load, and both have been shown to halt or reverse liver damage effectively after 1 yr of therapy ***(6,16–19)***. The third treatment, famciclovir, was less effective at reducing HBV DNA levels; HBV DNA levels fell by < 1 log, and after 1 yr, was shown to be minimally effective at halting or reversing liver disease ***(25,26)***.

HBV DNA levels have a number of advantages as a primary endpoint. Differences in HBV DNA levels between patients receiving active therapy and those receiving placebo are easily demonstrated with a relatively small sample size, and so studies using this primary endpoint can be smaller than those using seroconversion as a primary endpoint. The test is noninvasive, and therefore simpler and cheaper to perform, and can be performed more frequently than histology. The other advantage of HBV DNA as a primary endpoint is that it can be used to detect the development of resistance, as HBV DNA levels that have been suppressed by therapy rise when a resistance develops.

In the future, when therapies will be targeted at management of resistance in previously treated patients, the importance of an HBV DNA endpoint will increase, as has been the case in studies evaluating therapies used to treat HIV infection. Similarly, now that an increasing number of anti-HBV therapies are being approved, placebo-controlled studies will become more difficult to conduct, and active comparators will become the norm. The sample sizes required to be able to detect differences between active comparators using histological or serological endpoints will be prohibitive, and so HBV DNA will become the favored primary endpoint for these studies in the future.

Currently measurement of HBV DNA is the primary endpoint of choice for Phase II studies of antiviral therapies, as this endpoint provides the most suitable and rapid means of comparing the efficacy of various doses of a new therapy. If the therapy has a strong antiviral effect, it is essential to use a sensitive assay (limit of detection 10^2–10^3 copies/mL) to quantify HBV DNA levels. This will maximize the opportunity to select the correct dose. If an insensitive assay (limit of detection 10^5–10^6 copies/mL) is used in the Phase II studies, an opportunity to identify a lower, equally effective dose could be missed, with potential safety consequences at a later stage of the development process.

4.4. ALT Levels

Although changes in ALT levels are seldom used as a primary study endpoint, ALT levels are a useful tool for assessing both the efficacy and safety of new therapies. These can be assessed either by comparing median changes in ALT levels over time, the proportion of patients in each treatment group in whom ALT levels become normal, or time to normalization of ALT levels in each treatment group.

ALT is also a useful indicator of hepatotoxicity, and so patients in whom ALT levels rise on therapy should be monitored carefully. An elevated ALT at study entry and ALT flares during the first 1–3 mo of therapy or after therapy is withdrawn are also indicative of immune responsiveness and may either predict, or accompany, seroconversion *(27)*. ALT flares, provided they remain asymptomatic and anicteric, may indeed be desirable. However, one of the difficulties in assessing new anti-HBV therapies, particularly during the early stages of the development program, is distinguishing this phenomenon from hepatotoxicity *(28)*. Monitoring ALT levels is complicated further in blinded, placebo-controlled studies, in which rising ALT levels or ALT flares in untreated patients may indicate progression of disease. Therefore when designing studies in patients with HBV infection, it is essential for the investigators and the sponsors' medical team to have a mechanism in place for monitoring changes in ALT levels and other safety data during the study on a regular basis. An independent data and safety monitoring board should also be established to review all study safety data on a regular basis.

5. Conclusions

Careful and well-informed design of clinical studies will ensure that the full potential of a new anti-HBV therapy can be demonstrated. Appropriate selection of patients, endpoints and the sample size will help to minimize risk and maximize the cost-effectiveness of the clinical development program.

References

1. Liaw, Y. F., Tai, D. I., Chu, C. M., and Chen T. J. (1988) The development of cirrhosis is patients with chronic type B hepatitis: a prospective study. *Hepatology* **8**, 493–496.
2. de Jongh, F. E., Janssen, H. L., de Man, R. A., Hop, W. C., Schalm, S. W., and van Blankenstein M. (1992) Survival and prognostic indicators in hepatitis B surface antigen positive cirrhosis of the liver. *Gastroenterology* **103**, 1630–1635.
3. Hadziyannis, S. J. and Vassilopoulos, D. (2001) Hepatitis B e antigen negative chronic hepatitis B. *Hepatology* **34**, 617–624.
4. Rizzetto, M., Volpes, R., and Smedile, A. (2000) Response of pre-core mutant chronic hepatitis B infection to lamivudine. *J. Med. Virol.* **61**, 398–402.

5. Chan, H. L. Y, Leung, N. W. Y, Hussain, M., Wong, M. L., and Lok, A. S. F. (2000) Hepatitis B e antigen negative chronic hepatitis B in Hong Kong. *Hepatology* **31**, 763–768.
6. Schalm, S. W., Heathcote, J., Cianciara, J., et al., (2000) Lamivudine and alpha interferon combination treatment with chronic hepatitis B infection: a randomised trial. *Gut* **46**, 562–568.
7. Maddrey, W. C. (2000) Hepatitis B: an important public health issue. *J. Med. Virol.* **61**, 362–366.
8. Farrell, G. (2000) Hepatitis B e antigen seroconversion: effects of lamivudine alone or in combination with interferon alpha. *J. Med. Virol.* **61**, 374–379.
9. Chien, R-N., Liaw, Y-F., Atkins, M., et al. (1999) Pretherapy alanine transaminase level as a determinant for hepatitis B e antigen seroconversion during lamivudine therapy in patients with chronic hepatitis B. *Hepatology* **30**, 770–774.
10. Goldin, R. D., Goldin, J. G., Burt, A. D., et al. (1996) Intra-observer and inter-observer variation in the histopathological assessment of chronic viral hepatitis. *J. Hepatol.* **25**, 649–654.
11. Knodell, R. G., Ishak, K. G., Black, W. C., et al. (1981) Formulation and application of a numerical scoring system for assessing histological activity in asymptomatic chronic active hepatitis. *Hepatology* **1**, 431–435.
12. Scheur, P. J. (1997) Chronic hepatitis: what is activity and how should it be assessed? *Histopathology* **30**, 103–105.
13. Ikawa, H., Hayashi, Y., Ninomiya, T., et al. (2001) Various scoring systems evaluating histologic features of chronic hepatitis C treated with interferon. *Hum. Pathol.* **32**, 910–917.
14. Ishak, K., Baptista, A, Bianchi, L, et al. (1995) Histological grading and staging of chronic hepatitis. *J. Hepatol.* **22**, 696–699.
15. Leung, N. (2000) Liver disease—significant improvement with lamivudine. *J. Med Virol.* **61**, 380–385.
16. Lai, C-L., Chien, R-N., Leung, N. W. Y., et al. (1998) A one-year trial of lamivudine for chronic hepatitis B. *N. Engl. J. Med.* **339**, 61–68
17. Dienstag, J. L., Schiff, E. R., Wright, T. L., et al. (1999) Lamivudine as initial treatment for chronic hepatitis B in the United States. *N. Engl. J. Med.* **341**, 1256–1263.
18. Tassopoulos, N. C., Volpes, R., Pastore, G., et al. (1999) Efficacy of lamivudine in patients with hepatitis B e antigen-negative/hepatitis B virus DNA positive (precore mutant) chronic hepatitis B *Hepatology* **29**, 889–896.
19. Marcellin, P., Chang, T., Lim, S., et al. (2001) GS-98-437 a double-blind, randomized, placebo-controlled study of adefovir dipivoxil (ADV) for the treatment of patients with HBeAg+ chronic hepatitis B infection: 48 week results. *Hepatology* **34 (Suppl)**, 340A.
20. Wong, D. K. H., Cheung, A. M., O'Rourke, K., Naylor, C. D., Detsky, A. S., Heathcote, J. (1993) Effect of alpha-interferon treatment in patients with hepatitis B e antigen—positive chronic hepatitis B—a meta-analysis. *Ann. Intern. Med.* **119**, 312–323.
21. Hiroshi, Y., Yasuda, K., Iino, S, et al. (1998) Persistent viremia after recovery from self limited acute hepatitis B. *Hepatology* **27**, 1377–1382.
22. Mason, A. L., Xu, L., Guo, L., Kuhns, M., and Perrillo, R. P. (1998) Molecular basis for persistent hepatitis B virus infection in the liver after clearance of serum hepatitis B surface antigen. *Hepatology* **27**, 1736–1742.
23. Rehermann, B., Ferrari, C., Pasquinelli, C., and Chisari, F. V. (1996) The hepatitis B virus persists for decades after patients' recovery from acute viral hepatitis despite active maintenance of a cytotoxic T-lymphocyte response. *Nat. Med.* **2**, 1104–1108.
24. Michalak, T. I., Pasquinelli, C., Guilhot, S., and Chisari, F. (1994) Hepatitis B virus persistence after recovery from acute viral hepatitis. *J. Clin. Invest.* **93**, 230–239.

25. de Man, R. A., Marcellin, P., Habal, F., et al. (2000) A randomized, placebo-controlled study to evaluate the efficacy of 12-month famciclovir treatment in patients with chronic hepatitis B e antigen positive hepatitis B. *Hepatology* **32**, 413–417.
26. Chang, T-T., Leung, N. W. Y., Coulden, S., et al. (1999) Famciclovir (FCV) for the treatment of chronic hepatitis b (CHB): results of one-year study in Asian patients. *J. Hepatol.* **30 (Suppl 1)**, 114.
27. Chokshi, S., Papakonstantinou, A., Gilson, R. J. C., et al. (1998) Hepatitis flares in patients treated with adefovir dipivoxil correlate with activation of hepatitis B core-specific T cell reactivity. *Hepatology* **28 (Suppl)**, 588A.
28. McKenzie, R., Fried, M. W., Sallie, R., et al. (1995) Hepatic-failure and lactic-acidosis due to fialuridine (FIAU), an investigational nucleoside analog for chronic hepatitis B. *N. Engl. J. Med.* **333**, 1099–1105.

33

Specific Considerations in the Design of Hepatitis B Virus Clinical Studies in the Far East

Man-Fung Yuen and Ching-Lung Lai

1. Introduction

Seventy-five percent of the world's population of approx 400 million hepatitis B virus (HBV) carriers are Asians *(1,2)*. It is therefore not surprising that the majority of clinical studies of HBV infection is from Asian countries or consists of a large proportion of Asians. Because of the difference in the time of acquiring HBV between patients in the East and West, the profile of the HBV disease and treatment response are significantly different. In the East, nearly all HBV patients acquire the disease at birth or during the perinatal/early childhood period *(3)*. The HBV infection is followed by a prolonged period of immunotolerance that can last for several decades. This is followed by another prolonged period of immune clearance that may result in severe damage to the liver and its architecture. As a consequence of this, hepatitis B e antigen (HBeAg) seroconversion does not necessarily prevent the development of cirrhosis-related complications and hepatocellular carcinoma (HCC) in Asians. In fact, the majority of cirrhosis-related complications and HCC develops after HBeAg seroconversion *(4,5)*. Achieving a relatively low viremia state with HBeAg seroconversion is not enough to stop disease progression in Asians with chronic HBV infection.

Currently, the endpoints for most clinical trials assessing treatment efficacy are short term. These endpoints are as follows:

1. Viral suppression as evidenced by the loss of HBeAg with or without seroconversion to antibody against HBeAg (anti-HBe) and a reduction of HBV DNA to levels undetectable by hybridization-based assays.
2. Reduction in liver damage as evidenced by normalization of serum aminotransferase levels (if these are elevated) and by improvement in histological appearance on liver biopsy.
3. Loss of hepatitis B surface antigen (HBsAg), with seroconversion to antibody against HBsAg (anti-HBs) and lowering of HBV DNA to levels undetectable by polymerase chain reaction (PCR) assays.

From: *Methods in Molecular Medicine, vol. 96: Hepatitis B and D Protocols, volume 2*
Edited by: R. K. Hamatake and J. Y. N. Lau © Humana Press Inc., Totowa, NJ

In practice, few agents can achieve the third endpoint. Whether the achievement of the first two short-term objectives is associated with long-term clinical benefits (i.e., the prevention of cirrhosis-related complications and HCC) would require long-term follow-up studies.

2. Target Population for Clinical Trials

In conducting future clinical trials in Asian hepatitis B patients, the selection criteria of the treatment population should differ in certain aspects from those for the Caucasian population. These will be discussed under the following headings: serum aminotransferase levels, viral serology, HBV DNA levels, liver histology, and patients with liver decompensation

2.1. Alanine Aminotransferase (ALT) Levels

Abnormal ALT is frequently used as a criterion for entry into clinical trials because high ALT is taken to reflect active inflammation of the liver. Trials usually include patients with mild to moderate increase in ALT levels, for example, between 1.3× upper limit of normal (ULN) and 10× ULN. Patients with ALT levels higher than 10× ULN are usually excluded because they have a high chance of HBeAg seroconversion within a short period of follow-up ***(6–8)***.

In designing future trials for Asian patients, however, patients with ALT levels at the high range of the normal limit should probably be considered for treatment. There are two reasons for this. Patients who respond to lamivudine therapy have ALT levels usually at or below 0.5× ULN. This means that patients with completely quiescent disease should have ALT levels below 0.5× ULN, whereas those whose ALT levels are 0.5–1× ULN may still have significant disease. This is confirmed by an ongoing study of the natural history of HBV involving 3433 HBV patients. Patients with ALT levels between 0.5 and 1× ULN have a significantly higher risk for the development of cirrhosis-related complications and HCC when compared with patients with ALT levels less than 0.5× ULN (Yuen and Lai, unpublished data).

2.2. HBeAg/Anti-HBe Status

Loss of HBeAg with or without seroconversion to anti-HBe is frequently used as an endpoint for antiviral therapy. This is probably an adequate endpoint for treatment for Caucasians ***(9,10)***. In Caucasians, the survival rate and complication rate are both significantly reduced after loss of HBeAg irrespective of whether the loss is treatment induced or spontaneous. But the achievement of HBeAg seroconversion alone may not be adequate for Asians. It has been shown that around two-thirds of Asian patients with cirrhosis-related complications and HCC are anti-HBe positive ***(4,5)***. In addition, HBV DNA is detectable in >90% of anti-HBe positive patients using a qualitative PCR assay ***(11)***. The median HBV DNA level is more than 10^6 copies/mL by a quantitative PCR assay (Yuen and Lai, *unpublished data*).

More clinical trials should be performed recruiting anti-HBe positive patients with detectable HBV DNA. Not all of the detectable HBV DNA and/or elevated ALT levels in these patients are caused by the presence of precore mutations ***(12)***. Recent studies show that there are no differences in the rate of HBV exacerbation, development of cirrhosis-related complications, and HCC between patients with wild-type virus and patients with precore mutations ***(12)***. Anti-HBe positive patients with detectable HBV DNA and elevated ALT levels should be considered as candidates for drug trials irrespective of whether they have precore mutants or wild-type HBV, although it is still advisable to stratify the patients into two groups. This will take into account the possibility of a treatment agent being less efficacious for one type of virus, as interferon-α is for precore mutants ***(13)***.

In conclusion, at least in Asian patients, trials should not be restricted to HBeAg positive patients and should not only rely on the HBeAg seroconversion as a successful endpoint for treatment.

2.3. *HBV DNA Level*

There is little doubt concerning the importance of measuring HBV DNA levels in assessing antiviral therapy. Because serum HBV DNA is a reliable and technically feasible measurement to document active replication of HBV, it is universally taken as one of the endpoints in all well-designed clinical trials. Most trials require a minimal HBV DNA level for entrance into the study. This allows a measurable and significant reduction of HBV DNA levels (according to the power of viral suppression by specific trial agents) that can be detected by the chosen HBV DNA assays.

The efficacy of the trial agents in the reduction of HBV DNA levels can be expressed either in terms of median percentage decrease in actual levels or median logarithmic decrease. The latter mode of expressing HBV DNA reduction is to be preferred. The distribution of HBV DNA is skewed in almost all study populations. It is therefore more appropriate to calculate any reduction in HBV DNA levels after logarithmic transformation. Moreover, with the development and testing of more potent therapeutic agents, the difference in efficacy of different agents is mainly in the lower range of viral titers because the lower ranges would reflect the potency of an agent in reducing HBV templates from productively infected cells. Logarithmic transformation would allow a more accurate comparison of differences in the lower ranges. Finally, because, as discussed below, disease progression in the Asian hepatitis B patients can probably occur at a low viral titer, the suppression of even low levels of viral replication may be where therapeutic advances can be made. For these three reasons, we favor the use of median logarithmic reduction in expressing treatment efficacy.

There are two other important issues concerning HBV DNA levels. First, one should aim at achieving target HBV DNA levels that could be expected to have an effect in preventing long-term cirrhosis-related complications and HCC. In a consensus meeting, HBV DNA titers lower than 10^5 copies/mL has been suggested to be the desired level ***(14)***. This arbitrary figure is based on the fact that after HBeAg seroconversion there is usually a decrease in HBV DNA levels from the range of 10^7–10^{10} copies/mL to $< 10^5$ copies/mL, a level not detectable by most commercial hybridization assays ***(15)***. However, the consensus opinion from the meeting is that this target HBV DNA level needs to be verified. There is no study of natural history of hepatitis B in Asians to show that patients with HBV DNA levels below 10^5 copies/mL are free from the development of cirrhosis-related complications and HCC. Future clinical trials should clearly state the levels of HBV DNA achieved by the drugs. Long-term follow up studies are then required to confirm whether the achieved levels of HBV DNA is associated with a significant reduction in the chance of development of cirrhosis-related complications and HCC. This issue is even more important in Asian HBV patients in whom the cirrhosis-related complications and HCC may be the result of prolonged low levels of viremia. For Asians, antiviral therapy in clinical trials should aim at achieving very low levels of HBV DNA, measured by reliable, reproducible, and sensitive HBV DNA assays.

This leads to the second important issue in determining the HBV DNA levels in clinical trials. In the past, there were no standard HBV DNA measurements. The efficacy of different antiviral agents cannot be directly compared from different trials because of the difficulty in evaluating the accuracy of the HBV DNA measurements done either by in-house assays or different commercial assays. Although in general different commercial HBV DNA assays correlate well in the linear range of the detection profile, these assays vary greatly in lower detection limits of HBV DNA levels ***(16–18)***. Correlation between different assays is either impossible or dubious at the lower range. We suggest that in the future, a quantitative PCR assay with the lowest detection limit below 1000 copies/mL should be used. The HBV DNA results should also be standardized against an international standard, for example, the standard set by the Eurohep Pathobiology Group ***(19)***.

With the emergence of more and more powerful nucleoside analogs, measurement of covalently closed circular (ccc) DNA inside the liver may become more important. cccDNA forms the pool of HBV template inside the hepatocytes from which future viral replication may be initiated. It is relatively inert to the nucleoside analogs. The reduction of cccDNA levels is mainly the result of the natural cell death of the infected hepatocytes ***(20)***. To date, clinical trials have not been using cccDNA as one of the endpoints partly because there are no standard methods or assays to quantify the cccDNA levels. In addition, it may require a substantial treatment and follow-up period before there may be a significant reduction of the cccDNA levels. However, it should become one of the important assessments of antiviral therapy in future clinical trials.

2.4. Liver Histology

Liver histology has been a primary short-term endpoint of assessment of antiviral agents in some recent trials. Usually, the histological activity index (HAI) is adopted in assessing mainly two aspects, the necroinflammatory score and fibrosis score. In the first large-scale multicenter trial of lamivudine, a change of more than 2 points of the score is taken to be significant ***(21)***. Taking a change of 2 points in the score as endpoint is arbitrary but the correlation between histological, virological, and biochemical improvement appears to be excellent. This study shows that lamivudine improves necroinflammation and reduces progression of fibrosis when compared to placebo. It is reasonable to believe that there would be a reduction in the progression of cirrhosis if these effects continue on prolonged treatment.

There is some recent debate as to the real necessity of having two biopsies for comparison in newer trials of nucleoside analogs. Many patients, especially Asian patients, do not like to have two, or even one, liver biopsies. Another reason that has been proposed is that the serum ALT levels reflect the degree of necroinflammatory activity quite well *(22)*.

Although it is difficult to change patient's acceptance of liver biopsies, patients with normal ALT levels can still have significant necroinflammatory activity *(23)*. Furthermore, the progression or regression of fibrosis is still best assessed through histological studies.

We suggest that future trials should still include histological comparisons as one of the endpoints even if it is not used as the primary endpoint.

2.5. Patients with Liver Decompensation

It is always a challenge to conduct trials of antiviral agents in patients with liver decompensation. There are mainly two issues to be addressed. First, is it worth studying these patients with irreversible and end-stage liver diseases because their disease may be too advanced to be amenable to treatment? Second, will the antiviral agents further jeopardize the liver functions of these patients?

IFN-α treatment, and presumably other immunomodulatory agents, are contraindicated in patients with liver decompensation because enhancing cell-mediated hepatocyte destruction in a liver in which normal regenerative power to produce normal hepatocytes is already jeopardized can result in severe or even fatal hepatic decompensation. However, clinical trials using lamivudine, which suppresses viral replication, show that it does not increase the risk of liver decompensation. In fact, studies have shown that lamivudine improves the liver function in patients with liver decompensation *(24–26)*. Therefore, further trials for patients with liver decompensation should be performed with newer nucleoside analogs in the future.

3. Trial Monitoring

The liver biochemistry must be monitored very closely once patients are placed on a regimen of any trial agent. Especially with pivotal trials of newer compounds, trial centers should be asked to enforce the guidelines for Good Clinical Practice according to the International Conference of Harmony to ensure high standards of practice even in developing countries with little prior experience in conducting trials. Elevation of ALT levels while patients are on treatment may indicate impending HBeAg seroconversion, hepatic toxicity induced by the trial agents, or emergence of drug-resistant mutants. Normalization of ALT usually signifies improvement of liver inflammation. Prothrombin time and bilirubin levels are the useful indicators of hepatic decompensation and serious adverse events that may happen.

Because nucleotide analogs cause prompt and dramatic reduction of HBV DNA levels, interest has been focused on studying the viral dynamics of HBV during treatment in recent years *(27,28)*. HBV DNA dynamics may be of value in predicting treatment efficacy and clinical benefits. Frequent monitoring of HBV DNA by a sensitive HBV DNA assay should be done in clinical trials.

Monitoring HBV DNA is also important for the early detection of drug resistant mutations as a result of antiviral therapy. Continuous surveillance for the emergence of drug resistant mutants is necessary. Drug resistance has become a major problem in therapy with lamivudine. The common mutation site is in the catalytic domain of the viral polymerase gene. The typical nucleotide changes are at codon 552 where the methionine of the tyrosine-methionine-aspartate-aspartate (YMDD) motif can either change to isoleucine (YIDD) or valine (YVDD). The antiviral effects of lamivudine are greatly reduced in these mutants. These mutants typically become detectable after 9 mo of lamivudine therapy ***(21)***. A study has shown that these mutants may be present 3 mo before HBV DNA breakthrough ***(29)***. Continuous surveillance for these mutants using a sensitive assay, for example, a line probe assay (Innogenetics), PCR restriction fragment length polymorphism (RFLP) assay, is necessary. Other mutations may emerge with newer nucleoside analogues that are now being extensively investigated.

4. Treatment Endpoints

Because of the shortcomings of the short-term endpoints mentioned above, more definitive long-term endpoints are needed to assess the treatment efficacy for HBV. We suggest the following endpoints for clinical trials for Asians:

1. Complete eradication of the virus as evidenced by the loss of hepatitis B surface antigen (HBsAg), with or without seroconversion to antibody against HBsAg (anti-HBs), combined with undetectable HBV DNA in the serum and the liver by PCR assay, endpoints that are practically not possible to date.
2. Eradication of the HBV supercoiled or cccDNA from the nuclei of hepatocytes.
3. Long-term monitoring of HBV DNA levels to define the HBV DNA levels below which the risk of development of cirrhosis-related complications and HCC becomes minimal. The reduction in the development of cirrhosis-related complications and HCC is the ultimate aim in the treatment of chronic hepatitis B diseases.

References

1. Lai, C. L. (1997) Chronic hepatitis B in Hong Kong: immunization strategies for the control of hepatitis B virus infection, in *Hepatitis B in the Asian-Pacific Region*, vol. 1: *Screening, Diagnosis and Control* (Zuckerman, ed.), Royal College of Physicians of London 79–87.
2. Lee, W. M. (1997) Hepatitis B infection. *N. Engl. J. Med.* **337,** 1733–1745.
3. Derso, A., Boxall, E. H., Tarlow, M. J., and Flewett, T. H. (1978) Transmission of HBsAg from mother to infant in four ethnic groups. *Br. Med. J.* **1,** 949–952.
4. Yuen, M. F., Wong, W. M., Cheng, C. C., Wu, C. H., Wu, P. C., and Lai C. L. (1997) Natural History of Chronic hepatitis in the Chinese: prognostic significance of HBeAg/anti-HBe positivity. *Hepatology* (Suppl) **26,** 316A.
5. Yuen, M. F., and Lai, C. L. (2000) Natural history of chronic hepatitis B infection. *J. Gastro. Hepatol.* (Suppl) **15,** 20–25.
6. Liaw, Y. F., Chu, C. M., Su, I. J., Huang, M. J., Lin, D. Y., and Chang-Chien, C. S. (1983) Clinical and histological events preceding hepatitis B e antigen seroconversion in chronic type B hepatitis. *Gastroenterology* **84,** 216–219.
7. Liaw, Y. F., Pao, C. C., Chu, C. M., Sheen, I. S., and Huang, M. J. (1987) Changes of serum hepatitis B virus DNA in two types of clinical events preceding spontaneous hepatitis B e antigen seroconversion in chronic type B hepatitis. *Hepatology* **7,** 1–3.

8. Yuen, M. F., Yuan, H. J., Hui, C. K., et al. (2003) A large population study of spontaneous HBeAg seroconversion and acute exacerbation of chronic hepatitis B infection: implications for antiviral therapy. *Gut* **53,** 416–419.
9. Niederau, C., Heintges, T., Lange, S., et al. (1996) Long-term follow-up of HBeAg-positive patients treated with interferon alfa for chronic hepatitis B. *N. Engl. J. Med.* **334,** 1422–1427.
10. Lau, D. T., Everhart, J., Kleiner, D. E., et al. (1997) Long-term follow up of patients with chronic hepatitis B treated with interferon alfa. *Gastroenterology* **113,** 1660–1667.
11. Yuen, M. F., Hui, C. K., Cheng, C. C., Wu, C. H., Lai, Y. P., and Lai, C. L. (2001) Long-term follow-up of interferon-alpha treatment in Chinese patients with chronic hepatitis B infection: the effect on HBeAg seroconversion and the development of cirrhosis-related complications. *Hepatology* **34,** 139–145.
12. Yuen, M. F., Sablon, E., Yuan, H. J., et al. (2002) Relationship between the development of precore and core promoter mutations and hepatitis B e antigen seroconversion in patients with chronic hepatitis B virus. *J. Infect. Dis.* **186,** 1335–1338.
13. Brunetto, M. R., Giarin, M., Saracco, G., et al. (1993) Hepatitis B virus unable to secrete e antigen and response to interferon in chronic hepatitis B. *Gastroenterology* **105,** 845–850.
14. Lok, A. S., Heathcote, E. J., and Hoofnagle, J. H. (2001) Management of hepatitis B: 2000—summary of a workshop. *Gastroenterology* **120,** 1828–1853.
15. Di Bisceglie, A. M., Waggoner, J. G., and Hoofnagle, J. H. (1987) Hepatitis B virus deoxyribonucleic acid in liver of chronic carriers: correlation with serum markers and changes associated with loss of hepatitis B e antigen after antiviral therapy. *Gastroenterology* **93,** 1236–1241.
16. Lai, V. C. H., Guan, R., Wood, M. L., Lo, S. K., Yuen, M. F., and Lai, C. L. (1999) Nucleic acid-based crosslinking assay for the detection and quantification of hepatitis B virus DNA. *J. Clin. Microbiol.* **37,** 161–164.
17. Ho, S. K., Chan, T. M., Cheng, I. K., and Lai, K. N. (1999) Comparison of the second-generation digene hybrid capture assay with the branched-DNA assay for measurement of hepatitis B virus DNA in serum. *J. Clin. Microbiol.* **37,** 2461–2465.
18. Yuen, M. F. and Lai, C. L. (1999) Debates in hepatitis: how to assess HBV DNA reductions in association with therapy. *Viral Hepat. Rev.* **5,** 159–175.
19. Heermann, K. H., Gerlich, W. H., Chudy, M., Schaefer, S., Thomssen, R., and Eurohep Pathobiology Group (1999) Quantitative detection of hepatitis B virus DNA in two international reference plasma preparations. *J. Clin. Microbiol.* **37,** 68–73.
20. Averett, D. R., Mason, W. S. (1995) Evaluation of drugs for antiviral activity against hepatitis B virus. *Viral Hepat. Rev.* **1,** 129–142.
21. Lai, C. L., Chien, R. N., Leung, N. W. Y., et al. (1998) A one-year trial of lamivudine for chronic hepatitis B. *N. Engl. J. Med.* **339,** 61–68.
22. Van Ness, M. M., and Diehl, A. M. (1989) Is liver biopsy useful in the evaluation of patients with chronically elevated liver enzymes? *Ann. Intern. Med.* **111,** 473–478.
23. Perrillo, R. P. (1997) The role of liver biopsy in hepatitis C. *Hepatology* **(Suppl 1) 26,** 57–61.
24. Yap, F. Y., Terrault, N. A., Freise, C., Maslow, I. and Bass, N. M. (2001) Lamivudine treatment is beneficial in patients with severely decompensated cirrhosis and actively replicating hepatitis B infection awaiting liver transplantation: a comparative study using a matched, untreated cohort. *Hepatology* **34,** 411–416.
25. Kapoor, D., Guptan, R. C., Wakil, S. M., et al. (2000) Beneficial effects of lamivudine in hepatitis B virus-related decompensated cirrhosis. *J. Hepatol.* **33,** 308–312.
26. Yap, F. Y., and Bass, N. M. (2000) Lamivudine treatment in patients with severely decompensated cirrhosis due to replicating hepatitis B infection. *J. Hepatol.* **33,** 301–307.

27. Nowak, M. A., Bonhoeffer, S., Hill, A. M., Boehme, R. Thomas, H. C., and McDade, H. (1996) Viral dynamics in hepatitis B virus infection. *Proc. Natl. Acad. Sci. USA* **93,** 4398–4402.
28. Tsiang, M., Rooney, J. F., Toole, J. J., and Gibbs, C. S. (1999) Biphasic clearance kinetics of hepatitis B virus from patients during adefovir dipivoxil therapy. *Hepatology* **29,** 1863–1869.
29. Yuen, M. F., Sablon, E., Hui, C. K., Yuan, H. J., Decraemer, H., Lai, C. L. (2001) Factors predicting hepatitis B virus DNA breakthrough in patients receiving prolonged lamivudine therapy. *Hepatology* **34,** 785–791.

34

Studying the Treatment of Chronic Hepatitis B Viral Infection in Special Populations

Robert G. Gish and Stephen Locarnini

1. Introduction

There are estimated to be more than 400 million people chronically infected with the hepatitis B virus (HBV) worldwide (**Fig. 1**) *(1)*. At least 20–30% of those chronically infected will die of complications of chronic liver disease including cirrhosis and liver cancer *(2,3)*. The World Health Organization (WHO) places HBV in the top 10 causes of death worldwide *(4)*. The estimated viral burden in the United States is 1.5 million people, with disease concentrated in ethnic subgroups and populations with high-risk behavior, and health care costs to the North American economy that exceed $350 million per year. Although the United States is considered an area of low-prevalence hepatitis B infection, the incidence of new cases, the prevalence of carriers, and the burden of acute and chronic disease maintain hepatitis B high among the important communicable diseases. It is estimated that 300,000 new cases of hepatitis B infection occurred each year in the United States in the 1970s and 1980s. Currently about 125,000 new cases occur each year in North America. These acute infections have led to at least 27,000–42,000 chronic carriers, 17,000 hospitalizations, 300 cases of fulminant liver failure, and ultimately 4000–5500 deaths per year in the United States from cirrhosis and primary liver cancer as well as the morbidity and cost of liver transplantation in approx 350 patients per year *(5–11)*. The age-specific incidence of acute HBV infection is shown in **Fig. 2**. The risk of developing chronic HBV infection after acute exposure ranges from 1% to 5% for adults and 90% for infants born to infected mothers (**Fig. 3**). Once chronic infection has occurred, a heterogeneous group of patients or clinical profiles is evident based on a combination of viral replication, fibrosis progression, host immune response, and presence or evolution of viral mutants. The understanding of clinical research targeted at special subsets of HBV-infected patients is essential to study design and the interpretation of the clinical literature. The purpose of this chapter

From: *Methods in Molecular Medicine, vol. 96: Hepatitis B and D Protocols, volume 2*
Edited by: R. K. Hamatake and J. Y. N. Lau © Humana Press Inc., Totowa, NJ

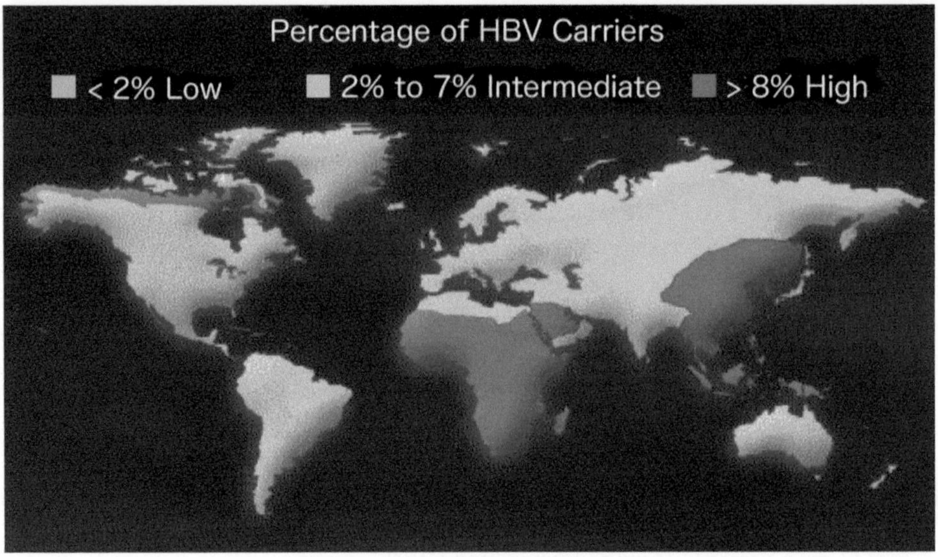

Fig. 1. The 350 million chronic carriers of HBV worldwide account for more than 5% of the world's population. Although widely distributed, the prevalence of HBV varies from a highly endemic disease (>8%) in China, Southeast Asia, and Africa to a disease of low endemicity (>2%) in North America, western Europe, and Australia. Areas with intermediate levels of prevalence (2–7%) are also noted. In most developed countries, the prevalence of chronic HBV infection is <2%. Within these areas reside ethnic groups with HBV infection rates that are significantly higher than those of the general population, for example, Eskimo populations in Alaska and Canada and the Maoris in New Zealand. (WHO Statistics ***[166]***.)

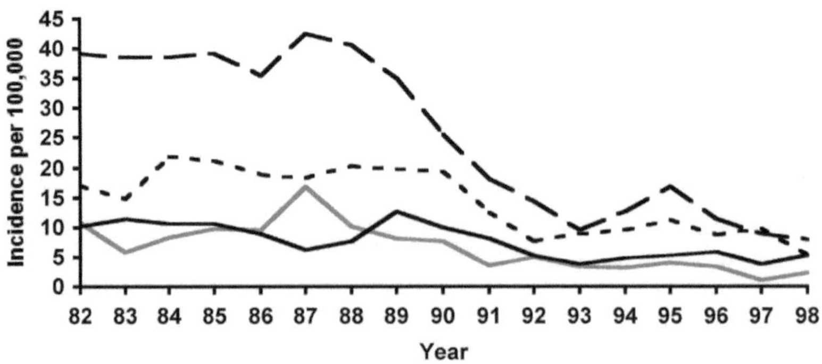

Fig. 2. Age-specific incidence of acute hepatitis B in the United States from 1982 to 1998. The median age increased from 27 to 32 yr, with 61% males. Age groups: *gray line*, 10–19 yr; *dashed line*, 20–29 yrs; *dotted line*, 30–39 yr; *solid line*, 40–49 yr. (Centers for Disease Control, Sentinel Counties Study.)

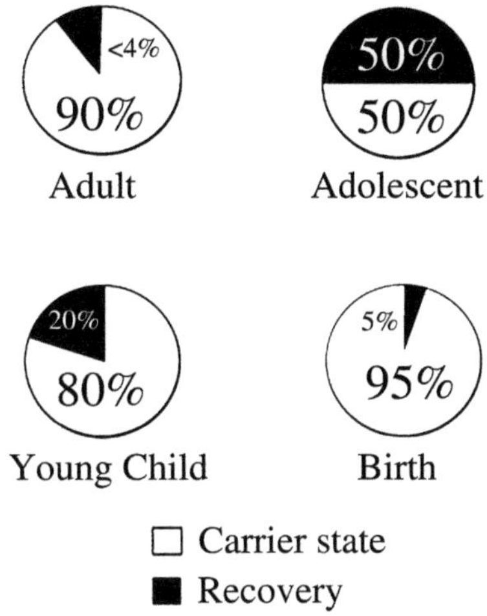

Fig. 3. Carrier state and recovery.

is to discuss the patient populations with chronic HBV infection and aid in the design of clinical trials, clinical assessment, and treatment of patients with HBV.

2. Definitions

To understand the special populations with HBV infection one must understand the terminology and test results for HBV infection. The WHO case definition for a person chronically infected with HBV is the presence of the hepatitis B surface antigen (HBsAg) in serum on two occasions at least 6 mo apart ***(12–14)***. Inconsistent and inaccurate terms such as "healthy carrier" must be removed from our terminology; no patient with HBV infection can be considered healthy. These outdated terms, often used to reassure patients or referring physicians, do not represent the true clinical outcome of HBV.

The liver biopsy remains a very important step in evaluating patients with chronic HBV infection but is not required for all patients. The outpatient liver biopsy is a safe procedure with a risk of serious complications (bleeding) of less than 1:2000 and the risk of death less than 1:10,000 ***(15,16)***. The liver biopsy determines the *stage* of disease (fibrosis) and the extent or level of inflammation (*grade)*. This determination then allows the patient and physician to decide on the necessity and urgency of treatment, the need and frequency of liver cancer screening, as well as monitoring of viral replication and liver panels. The natural history of HBV infection is one of viral evolution or mutation with many presently known variants. These variants are discussed in detail and must be understood, and clinicians must take into account these variants when designing protocols for clinical trials.

With the arrival of new antiviral medications aimed at HBV infection, increasing rates of resistance to medications has been observed. The clinical significance of these resistant viruses is still being evaluated currently. As combination therapy is currently in development, awaiting new information about treatment is reasonable as part of a patient treatment decision for some patients. Conversely, patients with advancing liver disease or impending liver failure usually require immediate treatment with the current best therapy, such as interferon or lamivudine.

Chronic HBV disease is defined as hepatic necroinflammation due to the presence of HBV. These patients are HBsAg (+) and HBV DNA (+) with serum levels of HBV DNA > 100,000 copies/mL or the presence of hepatitis B core antigen staining in the liver. Liver enzymes are either persistently elevated or intermittently elevated over time periods of 6 mo or longer. Liver biopsy is an important component in defining the severity of liver disease (inflammation and fibrosis) in these patients. Abnormal levels of liver enzymes are defined as alanine aminotransferase (ALT) of > 27 IU/mL in women and 30 IU/mL in men when individuals have a normal body mass index ***(17)***. Patients with chronic HBV with ongoing or measurable replication can be divided into two basic subgroups, those who are hepatitis B envelope antigen (HBeAg) (+) and (–), which is discussed further in the section on HBV mutants. Patients with normal ALT levels but high levels of HBV DNA and necroinflammation on liver biopsy are also included in the group owing to a similar natural history ***(8,10,11)***. "Flares" of hepatitis B infection occur in some patients and are defined as intermittent elevations of serum aminotransferases to more than 10 times the upper limit of normal. These events occur in 10–15% of patients each year and may be asymptomatic and undetected.

Inactive HBsAg carrier state is defined as the presence of HBsAg in serum, no detectable HBeAg, low levels of HBV DNA (< 100,000 copies/mL), and persistently normal ALT levels for periods of > 6 mo. A liver biopsy can be performed in such patients, but is not a usual practice, and the hepatitic activity index is typically < 3 on a 1–22 Knodell scale ***(18)*** (hepatitic activity index [HAI]). These patients are often described as immunotolerant and remain at risk for HBV DNA integration into hepatocyte nuclear DNA with the attendant risk of developing liver cancer later in life.

Reactivation of hepatitis B occurs when a person is in the inactive HBsAg carrier state, develops elevated liver enzymes, and DNA levels rise and transition to the state of chronic HBV infection. The HBeAg can become positive in a subset of these patients depending on the presence or absence of a variant virus. The liver biopsy typically has an HAI score of 4 or greater once reactivation has occurred.

Resolved hepatitis B occurs when a person has serologic tests showing HBsAg (–) and HBV DNA (–) with a history of acute or chronic HBV infection and currently normal levels of liver enzymes. These patients are often positive for antibody to HBsAg (anti-HBs) and typically may remain anti-HBc positive for many years. These individuals are at risk for transmission of disease on rare occasions, such as the donation of solid organ tissue, or for reactivation of HBV disease if the patient is treated with immunosuppressive medications. In addition, those patients who appear to have resolved HBV infection may develop active liver disease if they are treated with immunosuppressive medications such as prednisone, methotrexate, or chemotherapy.

3. HBV and Common HBV Mutants

3.1. Viral Particles

Electron microscopy of partially purified preparations of HBV from infected human serum reveal three particle types. By far the most abundant type are 22-nm spherical particles that lack nucleic acid and are therefore noninfectious. These particles are present in serum in a 10,000- to 1,000,000-fold excess over the hepatitis B virions. The 22-nm particles consist exclusively of virus-derived glycoproteins comprising HBsAg as well as host-derived lipids, principally phospholipids, cholesterol, cholesterol esters, and triglycerides. When purified, the 22-nm particles are highly immunogenic and induce a neutralizing anti-HBs antibody response. The second particle type consists of long filamentous particles that are also 22 nm in diameter but of variable length. These particles share properties with the 22-nm particles including envelope content. The virion is a double-shelled particle ranging from 42 to 47 nm in diameter. The outer shell is of similar composition to the spherical and filamentous 22-nm particles ***(19)*** while the inner component, which can be released following treatment with nonionic detergents, consists of an icosahedral nucleocapsid 25–27 nm in diameter. The nucleocapsid comprises multiple subunits of a 21-kDa basic phosphoprotein, the HBcAg, the viral genome ***(20)***, a viral encoded polymerase (POL) protein, and a host-derived serine kinase ***(21,22)***.

3.2. The HBV Genome: Genotypes, Serotypes, and RNA Species

Based on sequence analysis, HBV can be classified into seven genotypes (A–G), with an intergroup divergence in complete nucleotide sequence of $\geqslant 8\%$. Genotype A is found throughout the world but is particularly common in North America and western Europe. Genotypes B and C are distributed over the Asia–Pacific region while genotype D is the dominant form of HBV in southern Europe, around the Mediterranean basin as well as the Middle East. Genotype E is distributed throughout Africa while genotype F has been found in native South American Indians and Polynesians. Genotype G is the most recently discovered genotype and has been found distributed in Europe and North America. The clinical significance of HBV genotypes is only now being appreciated as large databases are developed and utilized in natural history and therapy studies. Genotype assessment may allow epidemiologists to track the historical movement of HBV infections through or within regions of the world and establish other epidemiological behavior of HBV infection. Genotyping may be useful to help define treatment and risk of liver cirrhosis or cancer.

Depending on the predominant HBV genotype in the particular geographical setting, non-genotype A infected patients often present to the liver clinic seropositive for anti-HBe rather than HBeAg. They have the precore G1896A stop codon precore mutation ("precore mutant") and commonly have intermediate serum levels of HBV DNA. Genotype A HBV infected patients still tend to present to the clinic seropositive for HBeAg and so have HBeAg-positive or wild-type chronic hepatitis B.

HBV can also be classified into four major serological subtypes that share one common antigenic determinant called "a," which is a conformational epitope located in the

HBsAg. There are two additional pairs of mutually exclusive subtypic determinants, "d" or "y" and "w" or "r," that constitute the four major antigenic subtypes: adr, ayr, adw, and ayw. Antibodies to the "a" determinant confer protection against all HBV subtypes. The "a" determinant is located on amino acids (aa) 110–160 of the HBsAg small (S) gene product. Changes at aa122 and aa160 of the S region define the subtypes of HBV: at aa122, glutamine (K) or arginine (R) define "d" or "y" subtypes, respectively, and at aa160, K or R define subtypes "w" or "r," respectively.

The HBV genome comprises a 3.2-kb relaxed circular, partially double-stranded DNA species (**Fig. 4**). The minus (–) or long strand is unit length and has the terminal protein (TP) domain of the POL protein covalently attached to the 5'-end. The TP serves as a primer for (–) strand synthesis (*see* below). The plus (+) or shorter genomic strand is 50–80% of unit length with a fixed 5'-end and a variable 3'-end. Attached to the 5'-end of the (+) strand is a capped oligoribonucleotide.

The coding organization of the HBV genome is efficient, with most of the nucleotides having protein coding functions in more than one open reading frame. The viral genome has four open reading frames (ORFs) (**Fig. 5**) that are frameshifted. The POL ORF encompasses 80% of the genome and encodes the viral polymerase (POL). The pre-C/C region encodes HBcAg and the secretable protein HBeAg. The pre-S/S codes for the three components of viral surface glycoproteins. The X ORF encodes the X protein, which is a transcriptional activator ***(23–25)***, and has been shown in the woodchuck model to be essential for viral replication in vivo ***(26–28)***.

The HBV proteins are translated from four mRNA species of 3.5 kb, 2.4 kb, 2.1 kb, and 0.7 kb. All these mRNA species are capped, unspliced, and share a common polyadenylation signal within the core coding region ***(28)***. These RNA transcripts are divided into two major classes based on size: genomic and subgenomic. The transcription of these RNAs is driven by four separate promoters and influenced by two enhancer elements (EI, EII) as well as a glucocorticoid responsive element (GRE, **Fig. 5**). The promoters for the 3.5-kb mRNA species and the 2.4-kb mRNA species are highly liver specific ***(29)***. The 3.5-kb mRNA species is translated into both the core and POL protein and also serves as the template for reverse transcription of (–)-strand DNA ***(28)***. This former species is also referred to as the pregenome (pgRNA). Transcription from the genomic basal core promoter (BCP) also produces a set of transcripts with a longer heterogeneous 5'-end containing a start codon for the pre-C region, which acts as the mRNA for the precore or HBeAg protein. The pre-S1 promoter (SPI) is a weak although liver-specific promoter that drives transcription of a 2.4-kb species of RNA that spans the pre-S1, pre-S2, and S domain and codes for large-surface protein (L-HBsAg) ***(29)***. The pre-S2/S promoter (SPII) directs transcription of a 2.1-kb RNA species with 5'-staggered ends and serves as mRNA for middle- and small-surface antigen (M-HBsAg and S-HBsAg, respectively) ***(30,31)***. Unlike the genomic and SPI promoters, the SPII promoter is functional in a wide variety of cell types ***(31)***. Mammalian hepadnaviruses produce an additional transcript via the X promoter, which is located approx 140 bp upstream of the first ATG codon of the X ORF ***(32)***. This 0.7 kb mRNA species serves as a template for synthesis of the X protein.

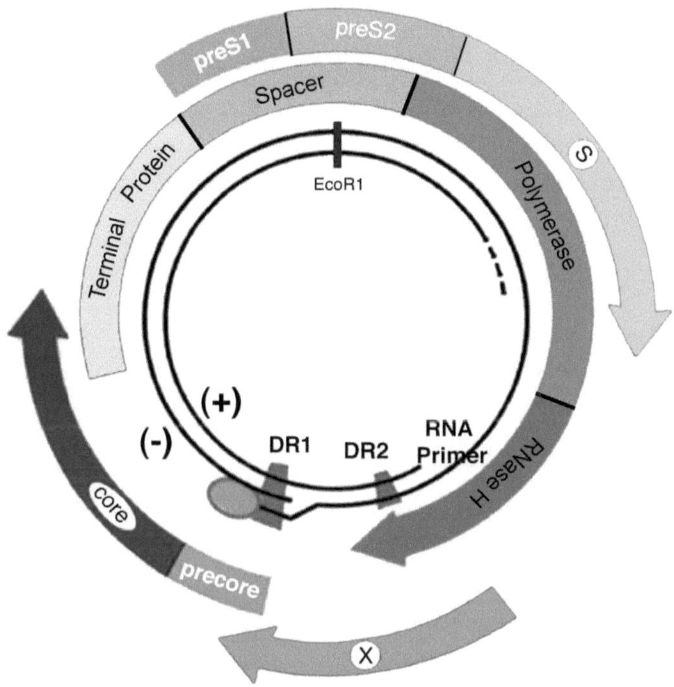

Fig. 4. HBV genome and specific areas of viral protein production.

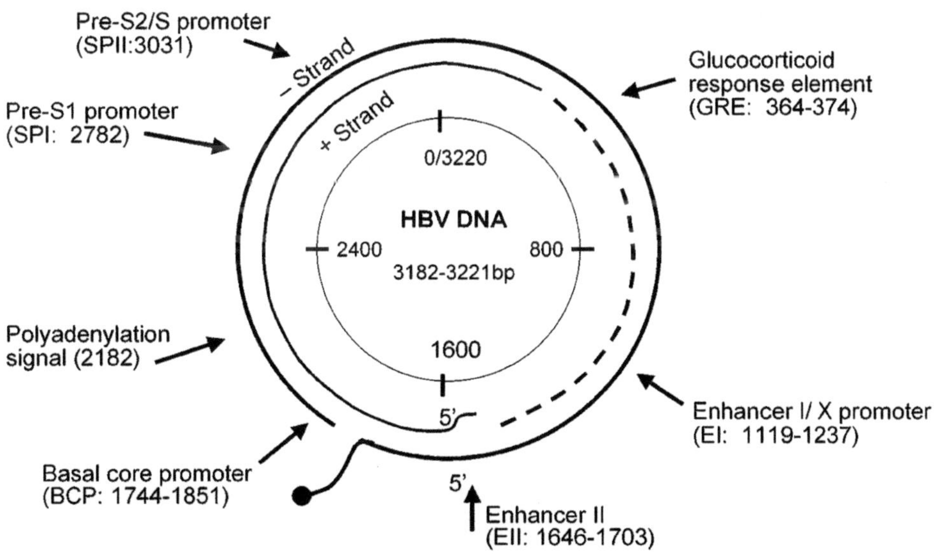

Fig. 5. Hepatitis B virus DNA regulatory elements.

Two *cis*-acting enhancer elements, EI and EII, have been identified within the HBV genome ***(33,34)*** (**Fig. 5**). Both of these elements are able to up-regulate transcription from distally located promoters. EI is approx 200 nucleotide (nt) region adjacent to the X promoter and has the ability to up-regulate transcription from all HBV promoters and appears to contribute to the replication level of HBV ***(35)***. EI is also active in nonhepatic as well as hepatic cell lines. EII partially overlaps the BCP and, unlike EI, is highly liver specific ***(34)***. In addition to the above enhancer elements, HBV transcription is under hormonal control via the GRE ***(36)***. The GRE is located within the S coding region and has been shown to up-regulate S gene expression ***(37)*** (**Fig. 5**).

4. Viral Life Cycle of HBV

4.1. Initial Events

The initial events of hepadnavirus replication are not well understood mainly because of a lack of an authentic cell culture system. Hepadnavirus attachment is thought to be mediated by the pre-S1 domain of L-HBsAg, as pre-S1 synthetic peptides as well as pre-S1 antibodies have been shown to be capable of neutralizing HBV infection in vitro ***(38)***. The region between aa3 and 77 of the pre-S1 domain is involved in the process of HBV attachment but the identity of the cellular receptor for HBV is still unknown ***(39)***.

4.2. Viral cccDNA Generation and Processing

Following receptor binding and virion uncoating, viral cores in the cytoplasm are transported to the nucleus where the partially duplexed, relaxed circular genome is converted into covalently closed circular DNA (cccDNA) that exists as a viral minichromosome (**Fig. 6**). This conversion is carried out by host cell enzymes. Recently it has been shown that the phosphorylated form of HBcAg interacts with the nuclear core complex in a karyopherin-dependent manner, suggesting the possible role of these transport factors in the delivery of the viral genome to the nucleus. The viral minichromosome is the template for transcription of the four viral mRNA species by the host cell RNA polymerase II (*see* **Fig. 6**).

4.3. Early Replicative Events: Viral Genome Replication

Once in the cytoplasm, the mRNAs are translated into POL, precore, core, pre-S, and S as well as X proteins. Nucleocapsid assembly is initiated when sufficient levels of core, POL, and pgRNA have accumulated. The pgRNA is selectively encapsidated via a *cis*-acting packaging signal on the RNA termed epsilon (ϵ) ***(28,40,41)***. This signal spans approx 100 nts from the 5'-end of the RNA and can form a bipartite stem-loop structure ***(42,43)***. The structure of the stem-loop is believed to be essential for encapsidation in vivo, as most disruptions of this structure severely suppress encapsidation ***(43,44)***. The ϵ sequence is present on both the 5'- and 3'-ends of the pgRNA but only the 5' copy is necessary for RNA packaging ***(45)***. Studies indicate that encapsidation of pgRNA occurs following the binding of the POL protein directly to the ϵ element ***(22,46)***. This event triggers the *in trans* addition of low levels of core protein dimers to the preassembly complex, and the capsid shell is completed by addition of more core protein dimers attracted to the RNA via the presence of nonspecific nucleic acid binding domains on core ***(22,47,48)***.

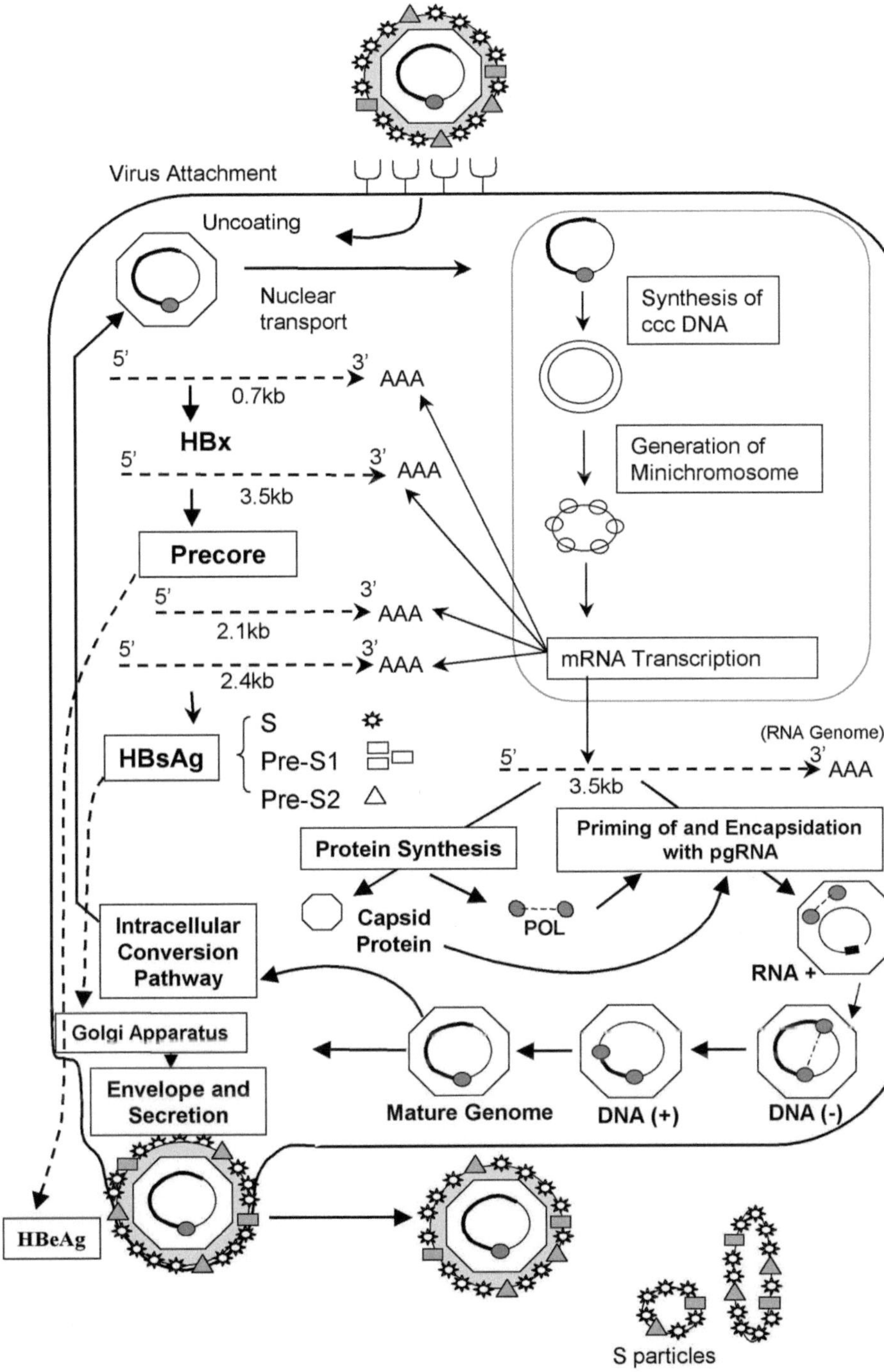

Fig. 6. HBV: intracellular events in viral life cycle.

Within the cytoplasmic core particles, HBV genome replication occurs by a novel discontinuous mechanism of (–)-strand synthesis ***(48,49)***. The template for reverse transcription is the pgRNA species that contains terminally redundant sequences (R) in addition to direct repeat sequences at both 5'- and 3'-ends of 11–12 nts termed DR1 and DR2. Within the terminal redundancy there is an additional copy of DR1 and ϵ. These direct repeat sequences provide sites for priming of (+) and (–)-strand DNA.

The POL protein binds to the bulge region of the 5'-copy of ϵ to initiate reverse transcription, providing the primer for (–)-strand synthesis through covalent linkage between the first nucleotide on DNA and a tyrosine residue in the TP domain of P ***(22,27)***. Minus strand DNA synthesis extends for 3–4 nts followed by transfer of the nascent DNA to the 3' copy of DR1. Following the annealing to DR1, full length (–)-strand DNA is synthesized with the concomitant degradation of the RNA template by the RNaseH activity of POL ***(49,50)***. RNaseH digestion terminates at the 5'-end of the RNA template, leaving a capped RNA oligomer of 15–18 nts consisting of short terminal redundancies of (–)-strand DNA (r) and DR1 sequences ***(22,28)***. This RNA oligomer is transferred and annealed to DR2 where it primes (+)-strand synthesis ***(51,52)***.

Plus strand synthesis proceeds to the 5'-end of the (–)-strand DNA. Because of the exhaustion of (–)-strand template, an intramolecular strand transfer event occurs to circularize the genome, thereby allowing continuation of (+)-strand synthesis. The circularization event is facilitated by the presence of homologous sequences on the 3'-end of both the (–)- and (+)-strand DNA. HBV (+)-strand synthesis does not proceed to completion, resulting in the characteristic partially duplex DNA species. At this stage, DNA-containing nucleocapsids can either be exported from the cell as enveloped virions or be shunted to the nucleus for amplification of cccDNA ***(53,54)*** (*see* **Fig. 6**). Interestingly, genome maturation inside the capsid appears to be coupled to envelopment, as predominately mature, partially double-stranded DNA is found in the secreted virions. It is thought that DNA synthesis inside the capsids induces some conformational change on the capsid exterior that allows for interaction with L protein. This finding could have implications for exploiting and understanding the effects of nucleoside and nucleotide inhibitors of HBV DNA replication (*see* below).

4.4. HBV Morphogenesis: Late Replicative Events

HBV virion formation is thought to require the maturation of the genome prior to envelopment of the cytoplasmic core particles. Studies indicate that all hepadnaviral surface proteins are synthesized as transmembrane proteins in the endoplasmic reticulum (ER) and it follows that virion formation probably proceeds via budding into the ER. Both S- and L-HBsAg proteins but not M-HBsAg are required for virion formation. A short sequence that maps to a region overlapping the pre-S1–pre-S2 domains of L-HBsAg is required for complete virion formation. A number of studies have confirmed that S-HBsAg, in particular regions in the cytosolic loop, is directly involved in nucleocapsid envelopment. However, the question remains as to how the pre-S1 encoded domain, which is exposed on the virion surface (and would presumably be in the ER lumen), interacts with the cytoplasmically disposed nucleocapsids. Evidence suggests that the pre-S1 domain is initially synthesized on the cytoplasmic face of the ER. What follows is a posttranslational translocation of a fraction of pre-S1 domains across the membrane. Hence virion formation is initiated by interaction between the nucleocapsid and cytoplasmic pre-S1 domains. Following budding, the virions are secreted via the constitutive pathway of vesicular transport.

5. Natural History of HBV

To understand the special populations with chronic HBV infection one must understand the natural history of HBV infection. With up to 30% of patients who have chronic HBV infection developing cirrhosis and/or liver cancer, the course of HBV must be defined individually for each patient being evaluated for clinical trials or treatment. The important spontaneous seroconversion from HBeAg to anti-HBe (and a concomitant decrease in HBV DNA levels) occurs in 1–10% of chronic hepatitis B carriers (in patients with wild-type virus) per annum, but seroconversion from HBsAg to anti-HBs, with clearance of HBV from the liver, is very uncommon (at or less than 1% per year).

6. Managing HBeAg Positive (Wild-Type Virus) Infection

6.1. Treatment of Clinical (Serological) Scenarios of HBV Infection

For patients with HBV "wild-type infection" with HBeAg+ and HBV DNA+, definitions of response to antiviral therapy are very important when evaluating patients who are about to undergo antiviral therapy or for those patients who have been previously treated and appear to need subsequent treatment. Definitions of response are defined as biochemical (liver enzymes), virologic (viral replication), and histologic (liver biopsy).

Biochemical response is defined as a fall in liver enzyme levels into the normal range. These events, like the virologic definition below, can be initial (during therapy), end of therapy, or sustained. Sustained response means that the liver enzymes were normal at the end of therapy and at least 6–12 mo following cessation of therapy. Partial biochemical response means a marked fall (50%) in liver enzymes to the near normal range and may be correlated with improvement in histology.

Virologic response means a decrease of HBV DNA to fewer than 100,000 copies/mL when pretreatment levels were greater than 100,000 copies/mL or by a greater than 2-log reduction from baseline. Although earlier HBV DNA assays were barely able to measure 100,000 copies/mL, currently available commercial assays have greatly increased the linear range of sensitivity to enable a more accurate depiction of virologic response (**Table 1**). The reduction in viral levels (commonly to fewer than 10,000) should correlate with HBeAg loss if positive pretreatment and finally anti-HBe conversion from negative to positive would complete what is termed "triple seroconversion." Studies with lamivudine have shown that full HBeAg seroconversion will not occur if the viral load is not reduced to below 10,000 copies/mL *(55)*. Virologic response can also be termed initial, end of treatment, and sustained if there is loss of viral markers or replication for 6–12 mo after treatment. HBeAg seroconversion is used when the HBeAg is lost (negative) long term.

Histological response is defined as an improvement in liver histology on paired liver biopsies. Improvement is typically defined using the HAI, the Ishak *(56)* score, or the

Table 1
Measurement of Hepatitis B DNA Viral Load[a]

Assay[b]	Volume (μL)	Sensitivity (pg/mL)	Copies (no./mL)	Linearity (no. copies/mL)	Genotype effects	Coefficient of variation (%)
Genostics (Abbott)	100	1.6	4.5×10^5 [8×10^6]	5×10^5–10^{10}	D > A	12–22
bDNA (Bayer-Chiron)	10	2.1	7×10^5	7×10^5–5×10^9	A–F	6–15
Naxcor (crosslinking)	50	2.1	7×10^5	—	—	—
Digene	30	0.5	1.4×10^5	2×10^5–1×10^9	ABCD	10–15
(HCII)	1 mL	0.02	5×10^3	5×10^3–3×10^6	ABCD	10–15
Roche MONITOR (quantitative PCR)	50	0.001	4×10^2	2×10^2–1×10^7 COBAS 1×10^5	(A) B–E	14–44
Molecular Beacons (real-time PCR)	10–50	—	<50	50–1×10^9	A–F	5–10

[a]One picogram of HBV DNA = 283,000 copies (approx 3×10^5 vge).
[b]bDNA, = Branched DNA; HCII, Hybrid Capture II.
Modified from Lok and McMahon ***(165)***.

Metavir score ***(57)*** with a reduction in 2 points or more by inflammatory score (grade). There is no international consensus about which liver biopsy scoring method is best. A significant improvement is based on a decrease in number by 1–3 points and is usually based on improvement in necroinflammation, as fibrosis score changes usually lag behind changes in inflammatory cells in the liver.

Complete response means normalization of liver enzyme levels, virologic response (as defined previously), and loss of HBsAg. Both HBeAg and HBV DNA must be negative by the most sensitive serological and molecular test available. For viral DNA tests, this usually means by polymerase chain reaction (PCR)-based assays. This is thereby synonymous with resolved or cured HBV infection. This term does not require the presence of anti-HBs and the patient does not require a follow-up liver biopsy.

6.2. Interferon

Interferon treatment must be considered as the first line of therapy in all patients with HBV, as it is the only medication that may result in a "cure" with HBsAg seroconversion. Approximately 20 natural forms of interferon (IFN) exist in humans including α_{2a} (produced in lymphocytes), α_{2b}, β (produced in fibroblasts), γ (produced in T cells), and ω IFN. A number of these interferons have been isolated and have been shown to have direct antiviral effects on HBV replication in humans ***(58)***. IFN is the only medication that has been proven to reduce and eliminate HBV infection in chronically infected patients in randomized controlled trials ***(59)*** including patients with HBeAg (+) and (–) chronic HBV infection. This appears to benefit patients long-term, with documented improved outcomes in clinical trials that have acumulative increase in patients who are HBV DNA (–) and HBeAg (–) and a decrease in the number of patients developing decompensated liver disease.

Unfortunately, only an "ideal" subset of patients responds to interferon and clears HBsAg (patients with low levels of liver enzyme elevation). Interferon appears to be efficacious in those patients who have an ongoing primed endogenous immune response, although this will probably change as we introduce nucleoside and nucleotide analogs in combination with IFN or we are able to stimulate an immune response with therapeutic vaccines. The presence of elevated liver enzymes and the presence of hepatic inflammation identify these "ideal" patients who have an inherent immune response to chronic HBV infection. One form of IFN, IFN α_{2b} (Intron-A, Schering, Kenilworth, NJ), results in HBeAg clearance in 30–50% of selected patients and HBsAg clearance in up to 30% of patient with long-term follow-up ***(60)***. The new pegylated forms of IFN α_{2a} (PEGASYS®) and α_{2b} (Peg-Intron®) are undergoing Phase III trials to determine if the longer half-life of these compounds imparts any improvement in therapeutic outcome over standard IFN preparations for the treatment of chronic HBV. IFN α_{1n} (Wellferon, GlaxoSmithKline, Research Triangle Park, NC) was approved in some European countries for HBV infection but has since been withdrawn from the market. Prolonged treatment with IFN for up to 32 wk may be useful in patients who have an initial reduction in viral levels of HBV DNA without DNA clearance. IFN is now being used for up to 1 yr in patients with the precore mutant HBV virus or HBeAg-negative hepatitis ***(61–64)***.

6.3. Lamivudine

Currently, lamivudine (3-thiacytidine, 3TC, Epivir™, Epivir™-HBV, GlaxoSmithKline, Research Triangle Park, NC) is the only FDA-approved oral medication that has proven efficacy against HBV including HBeAg seroconversion and triple seroconversion and is the second of the first-line treatments for the "wild-type virus infection." Lamivudine does not result in "cure," clearance of HBsAg, or HBsAg seroconversion at any significant level. Lamivudine is also approved in many other countries including China. A summary of the data concerning efficacy includes a rate of 30–35% HBeAg seroconversion at 1 yr of therapy and 17% triple seroconversion (HBeAg [+] to [–], anti-HBe [–] to [+], and HBV DNA [+] to [–]). Rare (<6%) HBsAg seroconversion to negative has also been reported with most patients remaining HBeAg and HBV DNA negative long term after 1 yr of therapy ***(65–68)***. Resistance to lamivudine is very common after 1 yr of treatment (20%) with mild elevations in liver enzymes and slightly more active liver disease, but few patients return to their baseline levels of liver disease or viral replication. Flares of liver disease with decompensation have been seen in few patients. The YMDD motif of the polymerase mutates to YVDD or YIDD or occasionally to YSDD, resulting in lamivudine resistance. This and other resistant variants are discussed below. This site in the HBV reverse transcriptase or "polymerase" is the catalytic domain and is the most common site of lamivudine resistance, although other sites of mutations associated with resistance have been identified. The rate of viral resistance after 3 yr is 50–70% ***(64,69–74)***. Other nucleosides that confer some level of anti-HBV activity include famciclovir and ganciclovir but these medications have found little use to date because of lower levels of efficacy ***(75)***.

6.4. Future Medications

Future medications that are in development to treat wild-type chronic HBV infection with the wild-type virus and mutants include pegylated interferons, FTC, DAPD, adefovir, tenofovir, entecavir, L-FMAU, L-β thymidine, adenine, and cytosine ***(12,13,76)*** as well as ribozymes and therapeutic vaccines. Other more far-reaching treatments may include dominant negative viral mutants, antisense DNA and RNA, intracellular antibodies, and delivery of current medications via new and advanced delivery methods such as liposomes or other methods that include molecules that bind to specific cellular receptors. Treatment may also take place with DNA vaccines that may provide ongoing internal immune suppression through production of HBV-derived proteins ***(77,78)***. Liposomes may eventually be used to deliver oral prophylactic and therapeutic vaccines such as those originally developed for hepatitis B via intramuscular injections.

7. HBV and Common HBV Mutants

Although HBV is a DNA virus, replication is through an RNA-replicative intermediate requiring an active viral reverse transcriptase/polymerase enzyme. The reverse transcriptase of HBV lacks a conventional proofreading function that is found in other higher order polymerases. Therefore, HBV exhibits a mutation rate more than 10-fold higher than other DNA viruses and has resulted in a number of variants. The rates for nucleotide substitutions vary depending on the stage of disease. The natural evolutionary rate for the HBV genome in chronic hepatitis B is approx $1.4–3.2 \times 10^{-5}$ substitutions per site per year, while in the liver transplant setting, it is almost 100-fold higher. This higher substitution rate may also be a result of the immunosuppression regimen associated with transplantation, especially the use of steroids and the positive enhancing effect on the HBV GRE.

7.1. Pre-S and S Gene Variants

The surface (S) envelope gene contains three in-frame start codons that divide the gene into the three surface proteins of HBV: the pre-S1 region, the pre-S2 region, and the S region. The three corresponding mRNAs formed provide the template for the synthesis of each respective protein. Surface mutations have obvious relevance to clinical practice as well as research ***(12,13,79,80)***. Follow-up studies of several large HBV vaccination programs in endemic regions have revealed a 2–3% incidence of vaccine escape mutants resulting from alterations in the HBsAg protein, indicating that this is an important and emerging special population and this mutant must be considered when developing HBV vaccines. These changes also must be understood to explain liver disease in patients who are HBV DNA positive but HBsAg negative ***(81)***. Generally, the amino acid (aa) substitution of glycine for arginine at aa 145 of the S protein makes this epitope unlikely to bind to antibodies generated to wild-type HBsAg, and hepatitis B immune globulin (HBIG) or natural antibodies may not be protective. The "a" determinant of the HBsAg is a peptide sequence located between aa 110 and 160 of the S protein and represents the major immune target of polyclonal antibody to the HBsAg derived from patients with natural immunity or vaccine recipients. This antibody reactivity is directed mainly against the second loop of this determinant, located in aa 139–147. In patients infected with HBV exhibiting surface mutations affecting the "a" determinant, the mutant HBsAg will be present but will not be detectable by commonly used HBsAg assays, especially if based on monoclonal antibody "capture" reagents leading to false-negative tests. As a result, these mutants do represent a potential public health challenge, as patients harboring HBV with these surface mutants remain infectious but do not exhibit readily detectable HBsAg that can be measured in conventional serological assays. In some cases, infection may result in aggressive liver disease after liver transplantation and will require the development of new assays for their detection ***(81,82)***. No therapeutic trials with interferon or nucleosides have been developed to date for this special group of patients with surface antigen mutants but these infections are rare and will unlikely be the focus of clinical research. The biggest concern is that our current vaccines may not be effective in preventing HBV spread if these infections become more prevalent. Reduced protection by standard HBIG needs to be documented and could potentially justify the development of immune globulin preparation that may be more broad based in terms of targeted epitopes for antibody binding.

7.2. X Gene Mutants

The X-ORF spans nucleotide positions 1380–1842 and encodes a 154-amino-acid polypeptide with a predicted molecular weight of 16–19 kDa. X protein is a nonstructural protein that can transactivate a variety of cellular and viral promoters in vitro by activating signaling pathways ***(83)***. X has been reported to interact with a number of nuclear proteins involved in cell cycle regulation, DNA repair, and transcription including NFkβ, CREB, AP-1, and AP-2 ***(28)***. Persistently high levels of the HBx expression have been associated with the development of liver tumors in transgenic mice and it can transform nontumorigenic cell lines in vitro. Owing to the overlap of the basal core promoter (BCP) with the X gene, the core promoter mutations often affect the structure and possibly the function of the X protein (*see* above). Nearly all deletions/insertions in the BCP shift the X gene frame and lead to the production of truncated X proteins. These X proteins lack a domain in the C-terminus (around aa 130–140) which is essential for transactivation activity. The amino acid changes that are introduced in the X protein by the T1762/A1764 BCP mutations do not affect the transcriptional function of X.

7.3. Pol Gene Mutations

The polymerase ORF is the longest, covering almost 80% of the whole genome, and overlaps the other three ORFs. Translation of the POL gene is thought to occur by leaky scanning of ribosomes on the first AUG in POL ORF ***(84,85)***. The HBV polymerase protein mediates encapsidation of the pgRNA into the core particle and synthesizes the HBV DNA genome therein (*see* **Fig. 6**). It has four enzymatic activities: DNA synthesis priming activity, RNA-dependent (RT) and DNA-dependent DNA polymerase activity, and RNaseH activity ***(86)***. These activities of the POL protein are located in different domains with primase encoded N-terminally, followed by the nonessential spacer region; thereafter follows the polymerase activity domain after which is located the RNaseH domain at the C-terminal end of the protein ***(87)***. The HBV RT contains several regions that are conserved in other RNA-dependent polymerases. These regions have been designated domains A–F, where domain F is located upstream of domain A. The "YMDD" motif of HBV is located in the C domain. The polymerase protein of HBV has not been crystallized, however, there is amino acid similarity with human immunodeficiency virus (HIV) in the conserved domains and these comparable regions may be involved in NTP binding and substrate recognition. In the analysis of the X-ray crystal structure of HIV it was proposed that domains A, C, D, and F may participate directly in nucleotide triphosphate (NTP) binding and catalysis. Domains B and E may be involved in the positioning of the template-primer relative to the active site, in which domain B forms part of the "template grip" and domain E forms the "primer grip" ***(88,89)***.

Hepatitis B virus quasispecies with mutations in the polymerase gene have been detected in patients undergoing antiviral therapy. On exposure to lamivudine therapy, quasispecies with L180M (the template binding site of the polymerase or domain B) as well as codon M204V/I of the YMDD motif (the catalytic site of the polymerase or domain C), or both are selected as the new dominant HBV (**Table 2**). These mutations significantly decrease the in vitro sensitivity of the polymerase to lamivudine-associated chain termination. Similarly, after famciclovir therapy, polymerase mutations in codon L180M markedly decrease famciclovir efficacy ***(90–92)***.

7.4. Precore and Core Gene Variants

The HBV core gene contains two in-frame start codons that control the synthesis of HBcAg and HBeAg. Both proteins are targets for immune-mediated viral clearance mechanisms. The region between the first (pre-C ATG) and second (C ATG) start codons is designated the "pre-C" region. HBeAg translation is initiated from the first AUG of this ORF, giving rise to a 25-kDa polypeptide with the pre-C region encoding a signal peptide. The signal peptide functions by inserting the precursor protein into the ER where the peptide is cleaved, resulting in a 17-kDa protein product that is exported through the secretory pathway. During export, the basic C-terminal domain is cleaved to generate a 15- to 17-kDa soluble protein that is ultimately secreted into the serum, but some is also incorporated into the outer cell membrane. The HBeAg is not required for productive viral replication. HBcAg is a 21-kDa phosphoprotein whose synthesis is initiated from the second in-frame initiation codon and is translated from the shorter of the genomic transcripts. The HBcAg is the major protein component of the nucleocapsid. The C-terminal domain is highly basic and possesses a non-sequence-specific nucleic acid binding domain.

The BCP (nt 1744–1804), residing in the overlapping X-ORF region, controls transcription of both precore and core regions and directs the synthesis of two mRNAs, the precore mRNA and the pregenomic/C mRNA. The precore mRNA encodes HBeAg. The pregenomic/C mRNA encodes the core protein, the DNA polymerase, and itself acts as the pgRNA, the template for reverse transcription.

Table 2
HBV Antiviral Drug-Related Resistance Mutations Listed with the Standardized HBV Polymerase Protein Nomenclature and Numbering System Proposed by Stuyver et al. *(91)*

Antiviral drug	HBV polymerase nomenclature of mutation: Group	Domain	New (old) amino acid number	Drug-resistant isolate sensitive to:
Lamivudine	1	B + C	L180M (526) + M204V (550)	Adefovir dipivoxil[a]
	2	C	M204I (550)	
	3	A + C	L80V/I (426) + M204I (550)	
	4	B + C	L180M (526) + M204I (550)	
Famciclovir		A, B, C	L180M (526)	Lamivudine[b] Adefovir dipivoxil[c]
Adefovir dipivoxil		D	N236T	—[c]

[a]Groups 1–4 isolates resistant to famciclovir. All groups sensitive to adefovir dipivoxil.
[b]Isolates sensitive to lamivudine, but lamivudine resistance emerges more quickly. Isolates sensitive to adefovir dipivoxil.
[c]Ref. ***167***.

The two major groups of mutations that affect HBeAg synthesis are precore protein mutations (G1896A) and mutations in the BCP at nt 1762 and nt 1764, all resulting in diminished production of HBeAg and a resultant increased host immune response, although this may be transient in some patients and does not have a clear correlation with more aggressive liver disease in patients who are not immunosuppressed. Precore mutations frequently occur at a similar time and are often related to core gene mutations/deletions.

It is also important to understand the connection between the precore stop mutation and HBV genotypes. Nucleotide (nt) 1896 is a guanosine (G) and is found within the RNA structural element ϵ, involved in encapsidation. This is base paired with nt 1858 and mutations at nt 1858, in conjunction with the precore stop mutation at nt 1896, can enhance viral base pairing within the stem-loop region of ϵ. In patients with genotype A HBV infections (the most common genotype in North America and parts of Europe), nt 1858 is a C. In this genotype, both a mutation at nt 1896 (G–A) and nt 1858 (C–T) would be required to stabilize the stem-loop structure. Without a compensatory mutation at nt 1858 in genotype A HBV, impaired base pairing results when C-1858 tries to pair with a A-1896, which destabilizes the stem-loop structure of the packaging signal. Without a stable ϵ for packaging, decreased encapsidation and consequently decreased replication may occur, resulting in a replication deficient virus. Thus, precore stop codon mutations may be less frequent in genotype A because of the requirement for two mutational events. In contrast, HBV sequences in more than 70% of chronic HBV carriers from Asia, Africa, the Mediterranean basin, or the Middle East already contain a T at nt 1858. Thus, only a single mutation at nt 1896 is required to yield a precore mutant with stable stem-loop pairing. This higher frequency of precore stop mutant HBV in patients harboring these other genotypes (genotypes B, C, D, and E) where nt 1858 is a T is simply a reflection of the requirement of only a single mutation (G1896A) needed to cause a stop codon and a stable stem-loop structure for epsilon ***(93,94)***.

Mutations in the BCP, especially at nt 1762 and nt 1764, resulting in T1762 and/or A1764, have been detected in a variety of patients with persistent infection and fulminant hepatitis as well as in immunosuppressed patients. The double mutation at T1762 and A1764 together is associated with a decrease in HBeAg (but not disappearance) and an increase in viral load ***(93,95)***. In general, this pattern of precore change is found in some genotype A-infected patients.

The core protein can be divided into two major domains, the N-terminal assembly domain up to amino acid position 144 and the functionally important, arginine-rich C-terminal domain. The C-terminal domain is required for binding of the pregenomic RNA and genome replication, as well as being involved in nuclear transportation. Interestingly, core protein sequences of HBV from patients in the HBeAg-positive immune tolerant phase contain none or very few amino acid changes, suggesting that less immune pressure may result in less clinically evident mutations. The prevalence of HBc/e amino acid changes is very similar to that of pre-C defects and is seen during multiple stages of chronic infection. However, once patients enter the immune reactivation (clearance) phase, the mean rate of HBc/e amino acid changes increase by more than fivefold, clustering onto 36 hot-spot positions possibly influenced by the immune pressure and subsequent virus "selection." These hot-spot positions have been linked to major cytotoxic T lymphocyte (CTL) (aa 18–30) and T-helper (T_H) cell (aa 50–70) regions, and two B-cell (HBc/e1 and HBc/e2) epitopes at aa residues 75–90 and 120–140, respectively ***(93,95)***.

In patients with the HBV "precore type infection" with HBeAg (–) and HBV DNA (+) treatment of precore mutation is less well defined. It appears that at least 1 yr of interferon therapy is required to suppress HBV replication and lamivudine has, at most, an ancillary role since the relapse rate is more than 90% following 1 yr with lamivudine ***(64,96–98)***. There is no information concerning the treatment of core variant viruses or HBsAg mutants with interferon or oral agents.

8. Special Patient Populations

8.1. Coinfected Populations

8.1.1. Hepatitis B and Hepatitis C Virus Coinfection

In patients who are infected with HBV, coinfection with hepatitis C virus (HCV) ***(99)*** and/or HIV exists in certain risk groups, especially those with adult high-risk behavior. All patients with HBV infection, a risk history of sexual exposure, or intravenous drug abuse (IVDA) must be tested for HCV infection. HCV coinfection with HBV results in a higher risk of cirrhosis and a higher risk of liver cancer. Patients often have one dominant viral disease. Treatment focused on the dominant virus, as revealed by blood tests of viral replications, is probably the best management step.

HIV coinfection with HBV results in more aggressive (progression to cirrhosis and liver failure) liver disease in some patients although other patients have minimally active liver disease with little or no evidence of progressive liver disease. The reason(s) why some coinfected patients have progressive liver disease and others do not is unclear and is not correlated with any specific clinical factor or laboratory test. The discrepancies may be explained by an interaction between the host immune system, T-cell types present (T-helper-1 [Th1] vs T-helper-2 [Th2]), host factors that predict fibrosis, and levels of HBV and HIV viral replication. These patients are much less likely to respond to cytokine-based therapies based on our current knowledge of interferon. Also these patients will probably have a higher rate of mutations to nucleoside analogs based on preliminary work completed with lamivudine-resistant populations of HBV, which were also detected in patients who were coinfected with both HBV and HIV and who were receiving lamivudine as part of antiretroviral therapy ***(100–102)***. In HBV and HIV coinfection, HIV infection clearly influences the response to HBV vaccine. Interferon treatment in these populations is not likely to be effective.

8.1.2. Hepatitis B and Hepatitis Delta Virus Coinfection

Hepatitis delta virus (HDV) infection occurs usually as a coinfection (infection initiated at the same time) with HBV or a superinfection imposed on a chronic HBV carrier. HDV infection is limited to the liver and is characterized by an initial phase associated with acute hepatitis that either progresses to a chronic carrier state or is resolved. This infection must be tested for prior to initiation of clinical trials, as the presence of delta infection markedly changes the response to interferon and lamivudine and would probably influence the response to any other new antiviral medication in development. The spectrum of liver disease mediated by HDV ranges from an asymptomatic carrier state to fulminant hepatitis. Simultaneous acute coinfection usually results in an acute, self-limited infection of both HBV and HDV with fewer than 5% of patients developing chronic infection with HBV and HDV. Superinfection with HDV imposed on chronic HBV disease tends to result in a more severe form of acute hepatitis with a short incubation period, which commonly progresses to a chronic carrier state in more than 70% of cases. This chronic carrier state is associated with a more aggressive form of liver disease with a much higher risk of cirrhosis and a faster development of cirrhosis. Superinfection can often be associated with fulminant acute HDV hepatitis.

HDV coinfection is also an important medical and research issue. HDV infection is specific also to certain world regions such as Amerindians in South America and high-risk populations in the Mediterranean area. In the United States, HDV occurs predominantly in IVDA in large cities and among persons involved in high-risk sexual activity and paid sex work ***(103)***. Ethnic populations from the Mediterranean region or Middle East may carry HBV and need to be tested for HDV infection as well. Delta infection leads to much more severe liver disease in those patients who acquire HDV and HBV at the same time (*see* **Subheading 8.1.2.**) ***(104–107)***. These patients with acute coinfection have a very high rate of viral clearance of both HBV and HDV. When HDV infection is superimposed on chronic HBV infection, the disease commonly accelerates to cirrhosis in a much shorter time. Patients with HDV and HBV coinfection may also have a higher risk of liver cancer, probably as a result of the high risk and rate of developing cirrhosis ***(108)***.

HDV superinfection on chronic hepatitis B is defined as primary virus infection on a preexisting persistent HBV replication. Serological markers such as titers of HBsAg and HBV DNA can show transient reduction during superinfection. The typical serological profile is HBsAg (+) as well as anti-HD (IgG and IgM) (+), but (–) for IgM-specific anti-HBc. Again the diagnosis of persistent infection is established by repeated testing for HDV RNA by PCR. The diagnosis of chronic hepatitis D is readily made when HDAg in the nucleus of hepatocytes is detected in the liver biopsy by immunohistochemistry.

Suppression of markers of HBV replication during HDV superinfection has been observed in humans as well as in the woodchuck and chimpanzee animal models. In more than 90% of hepatitis B patients superinfected with HDV, seroconversion occurs from an HBeAg (+) to an HBeAg (–)/anti-HBe (+) state. Serum HBV-specific DNA polymerase activity and intrahepatic HBcAg expression can no longer be detected in many of these patients. On rare occasions, HDV superinfection has been associated with termination of the HBsAg carrier state and seroconversion to anti-HBs. The mechanism for this interference has not been conclusively established and the patient remains delta positive, raising the question about the very low level of HBV replication or presence that is not detected by our current best tests.

HDV is a serious disease including both acute infection simultaneous with HBV and superinfection of HDV superimposed on chronic HBV. Acute infection simultaneously with HBV and HDV commonly results in severe disease with a high risk of fulminant liver failure. If the patient survives the acute disease, viral clearance of both HBV and HDV will probably take place. Liver transplantation for patients with acute HDV infection will often be followed after liver transplant by milder liver disease if HBV and HDV infection persist compared to HBV graft infection without HDV coinfection. HBIG therapy to prevent graft infection with HBV can also prevent HDV infection of the new graft ***(109)***. HDV infection can be treated with interferon, although results are discouraging with rare patients clearing HDV and HBV long term. Therapy requires at least 1 yr of IFN treatment with the hope to suppress disease activity. Nucleoside analogue therapy such as lamivudine does not suppress HDV infection.

Coinfection with other hepatitis viruses, such as delta, poses a major clinic problem to patients with HBV infection and must be determined to exclude these special subgroups of patients from primary clinical trials; however, these special subgroups of patients will eventually need to be evaluated during Phase III or Phase IV studies to determine the role of new medications in the treatment of broader populations. The dilemma is even greater to the clinician trying to help the patient, as therapies are quite limited in such patients. IFN must be used for at least 1 yr to suppress HDV infection and inflammation, and lamivudine appears to have no defined role as there is no major HBV replication during HDV and HBV coinfection.

8.2. Patients with Liver Cancer

Hepatocellular carcinoma (HCC), hepatoma, or primary liver cancer is a serious risk for all HBV carriers and must be screened for before all clinical trial initiation or inclusion. The estimated lifetime risk for HCC in patients with chronic HBsAg (+) is estimated to be about 20% with a higher risk level in the subgroup of patients with cirrhosis. This risk is also increased in patients with active liver disease (inflammation) as demonstrated by biopsy, elevated liver enzymes, coinfection with HCV, strong history of alcohol abuse, more than 50 yr as a carrier of HBV, exposure to aflatoxins, family history of HCC, high serum HBV DNA levels, and those patients with an elevated α-fetoprotein (>7 ng/dL). Issues such as prevention of HCC by vaccine is covered in other sections, and prevention of HCC by use of IFN and new antiviral therapies is discussed in the section on HBV therapies (*see* below). Patients who are chronic HBV carriers need to be informed of the risk of HCC and screened for HCC according to relative risk of HCC in special groups of patients with HBV, most importantly, patients with cirrhosis.

8.3. Pediatric Patients

Clinical research in children infected with HBV is just beginning. The U.S. government mandates pharmaceutical research in children as a part of drug development although the complexity of identifying and treating children must be identified. Theoretically, children should respond better to IFN and nucleoside analogs because of the shorter time of infection and, possibly, higher levels of immune activation ***(110–114)***.

8.4. Elderly Patients

Older patients represent a special subgroup of patients with acute or chronic HBV infection. Acute HBV infection in elderly patients is commonly associated with severe or fulminant hepatitis with a high likelihood of liver failure. Older patients also have a lower response rate to HBV vaccine and may respond poorly to interferon therapy ***(115)***. Analysis of nucleoside analogues in this population has not yet taken place ***(116–118)***.

8.5. Course and Complications

Each subgroup of patients with HBV infection has a different clinical course. The clinical presentation for a given patient must be identified at the time of selection for clinical trials. Heterogeneity of particular patient populations can lead to inconclusive research results. Patients with cirrhosis may develop decompensation or cancer during a treatment trial and would be excluded from the trial results owing to drop out during treatment, although they may have had short- and long-term viral benefit from the medication. The chronic carrier with consistently elevated liver enzymes is the patient with the highest risk of progression to cirrhosis and the subsequent complications. These patients may also be the most likely to respond, short term, to antiviral treatment. The next highest risk patient with risk of progression is the patient who presents with intermittent flares of liver enzyme levels and reactivation of liver disease. Each cycle of liver enzyme elevation is due purportedly to immune activation and attempts, often ill fated, to clear HBV infection. Only about 1% of patients with chronic HBV spontaneously clear infection (convert from HBsAg [+] to [–]) each year. The rate of HBsAg seroconversion is higher in patients with more active liver disease, as determined by liver enzyme levels or by liver biopsy, but is in general < 15% over any 3-yr interval. During these immune "attacks" or flares there is ongoing hepatocellular damage and commonly progressive fibrosis. Thus, in general, the level of liver enzymes and the number of flares often correlate, over time, with the level or severity of liver injury. In specific patients, testing and evaluation by sequential liver biopsies is necessary to time and determine the urgency of treatment. The liver biopsy also allows a medical practitioner to provide a full level of informed consent to patients prior to starting therapy by providing full clinical information on the stage of liver disease. Blood testing for progressive liver disease and cancer will also take place more frequently in those patients with cirrhosis when compared to patients with mild or no fibrosis.

The chronic carrier with persistently normal liver enzymes (<30 IU/mL) is at a much lower risk of progressive liver disease as well as cancer. These patients commonly have minimal liver disease on liver biopsy. The frequency of blood testing of these patients is an important issue, as annual testing probably is insufficient to document a stable patient or define inactive disease (conversely to identify reactivation of disease). The frequency of screening with blood tests for such patients should be at least biannual and a more thorough evaluation could be justified for testing every 3 mo.

During regular laboratory testing for liver function, liver enzyme levels, HBV DNA, anti-HBe, and HBeAg one can define if a patient has developed reactivation, a mutant or variant virus, and decompensated liver disease. Viral variants can be identified by the presence of moderate to high levels of HBV DNA in the absence of HBeAg. This clinical profile would strongly support the presence of a precore variant or mutant virus. Patients who appear to clear HBsAg but do not develop anti-HBs or clear HBeAg but do not develop anti-HBe may have developed core or surface mutant viruses. The clinical significance of these mutant viruses is not clear. Long-term studies are in progress to determine what specific markers might identify or predict which patients are at risk of progressive liver disease. As therapy evolves and becomes much more complex the options to treat such patients will expand.

8.6. Patients Who Develop Lamivudine Resistance

Initial clinical trials established that treatment of chronic HBV infection with lamivudine was (1) safe and well tolerated and (2) caused rapid and substantial decreases in viremia. However, decreases in viremia were not stable and rebounded in the majority of cases after treatment stopped ***(119–122)***. As longer term trials progressed, it became apparent that "rebound" could occur during treatment and this was attributed to the development of drug resistance (**Table 2**). Clinically a variety of drug-resistant HBV variants or mutants have emerged under the selective pressures of oral lamivudine and/or famciclovir therapy. Cross-resistance among these variants has also now been defined with the associated point mutations in the HBV polymerase identified (**Table 2**). Rational design of effective single or combination chemotherapeutic strategies for the future will require the determination of the sensitivities of these mutants to novel nucleoside and nucleotide analogues as they become available. This will be necessary both to provide effective treatment to patients who are already infected with drug-resistant HBV and to prevent, delay, or at least minimize the possibility of drug resistance arising in treatment-naïve individuals.

It has been observed that the viral loads are at least 0.5- to 1.0-log greater after viral breakthrough in this group of patients who develop lamivudine-resistant mutants than at their pretherapy level. The HBV DNA characterized from these patients usually have multiple mutations in the polymerase and envelope genes. As with lamivudine resistance, efforts to determine the molecular basis of famciclovir resistance focused predominately on sequencing the reverse transcriptase portion of the polymerase. In contrast to lamivudine resistance, which is almost invariably associated with mutation of the codon M204, famciclovir resistance does not affect the active site (YMDD) motif, nor does it map predominately to a single locus. Mutations associated with famciclovir resistance occur most frequently in the A and B motifs for POL and the intermotif sequence that separates them. However, mutations have also been observed in motifs C, D, E, and G of the reverse transcriptase, as well as in the terminal protein region. In comparison to lamivudine-resistant mutations, considerably less is known about famciclovir-resistant mutations.

Fortunately there is convincing evidence that indicates that adefovir dipivoxil and entecavir inhibit replication of lamivudine- and famciclovir-resistant HBV. Knowing the patient's previous treatment and possible resistance patterns is very important and promotes patient management, as all new HBV therapies will be tested against the wild-type virus infection as well as drug-resistant variants. Cell-free polymerase assays show that the sensitivity of wild-type and genetically engineered mutant HBV polymerases to adefovir diphosphate is not significantly different from the wild HBV virus level ***(123,124)***. Analyses from several independent laboratories have confirmed that adefovir dipivoxil and entecavir are equally effective as inhibitors of wild-type and lamivudine-resistant HBV in cell culture. Furthermore, recent clinical experience shows that treatment with adefovir dipivoxil can suppress the replication of lamivudine-resistant HBV in vivo ***(125,126)***.

8.7. Patients with Alcohol Dependency

Alcohol use in patients chronically infected with HBV increases the risk for progression to cirrhosis, results in more rapidly progressive liver disease, and also increases the risk of liver cancer ***(12,13,127)***. Patients with chronic liver disease should not drink alcohol and patients with documented chronic HBV infection should be educated about the risks of alcohol use and advised not to drink any alcohol, as the threshold for complications of alcohol use are unknown.

8.8. Patients on Renal (Hemo-) Dialysis

Dialysis patients need to be tested for HBV infection and those without evidence of immunity need to be vaccinated with a double dose of vaccine in the usual time course of vaccinations of 0, 1, and 6 mo, as they generally are poor responders to vaccine. Patients who are chronically infected have been historically isolated from other patients in dialysis centers, but more recently, with sterile techniques used, the exchange of equipment in dialysis centers, and other advances in dialysis therapy, we do not mandate complete separation or isolation of such patients. Treatment of dialysis patients with chronic HBV infection should focus on the presence or absence of progressive liver disease as demonstrated by biopsy. Interferon probably has less efficacy in dialysis patients owing to the relative state of immunosuppression in these patients ***(128)***. Lamivudine can also be used in renal failure but dose adjustments must take into account the dominant renal clearance of these medications. Close inspection of the pharmacokinetics of drug metabolites in renal insufficiency needs to take place during drug development of other nucleoside or nucleotide medications to determine correct dosing profiles and avoid renal and systemic toxicity.

9. HBV and Liver Transplantation

The management of posttransplant HBV infection after liver transplant is complex ***(12)*** and is discussed in a separate chapter in great detail. The most important step is to prevent graft infection or reinfection, which can start before liver transplantation by screening donors for anti-HBc and recipients for HBV DNA replication and suppressing HBV replication to low levels using nucleoside or nucleotide analogs before the patient enters the operating room. After transplantation, HBIG is used to bind circulating virus and prevent graft infection ***(129)*** and results in improved survival and a much lower rate of HBV graft infection, thereby preventing aggressive liver disease. Ganciclovir was the nucleoside analogue first used to treat posttransplantation HBV infection with documented reversal of liver dysfunction and reduced HBV protein expression in hepatocytes ***(130)***. Lamivudine can also be used in the setting of liver transplantation and is now considered the standard of care for decompensated liver disease in patients awaiting orthotopic liver transplantation (OLT) and for prevention of graft reinfection after liver transplantation, especially in combination with HBIG ***(12,125,131–144)***.

Lamivudine maintains viral replication at a very low level initially, both before and after liver transplantation, and when used in combination with HBIG, after liver transplantation, results in a risk of 5% of graft infection in compliant patients ***(144)***. Newer nucleoside and nucleotide analogs may also be used in a similar clinical setting. The use of two oral agents such as lamivudine and famciclovir or lamivudine and adefovir dipivoxil may obviate the need for HBIG use, which is quite costly. The emergence of mutant viruses that are resistant to lamivudine are a major problem after liver transplantation with more than 30–40% of patients developing resistance and more aggressive liver disease once resistance emerges ***(145)***. This resistance was also observed in both the transplant setting ***(146–148)*** and in immunocompetent patients ***(149–152)***. Although varying frequencies of resistance and different times preceding the detection of resistance were reported, the incidence of resistance clearly correlated with treatment duration. During the first year of lamivudine therapy, resistance developed in 14–32% of cases studied ***(153–155)***, a frequency that increased to 50% after 2 yr ***(151)***.

As outlined above, changes in the HBV POL gene can result in a concomitant change to the overlapping S gene. Similarly, changes in the envelope gene selected by pressure of treatment with HBIG or therapeutic vaccination can affect the polymerase gene. Treatment of HBV recurrence post-OLT with either passive immunoprophylaxis using HBIG monotherapy or with antiviral agents such as famciclovir or lamivudine has improved the outcome for a number of patients post-OLT. Unfortunately, viral breakthroughs are common and the liver-disease associated with the emergence of drug-resistant virus can be more aggressive than the wild-type HBV form.

10. Other Organ Transplant Recipients

All organ transplant recipients are at risk for reactivation of HBV disease after receiving organ transplants such as bone marrow, heart, and kidney ***(156–160)***. An expert in hepatitis B management must evaluate these patients before they undergo transplantation. If active HBV replication is present, avoiding or delaying organ transplantation is advised. Some transplant centers historically would not perform organ transplantation on patients who were HBsAg (+), although currently almost all programs will offer transplantation with HBIG and lamivudine as a method to prevent graft reinfection. Another clinical setting is the transmission of HBV from the organ donor to the recipient. There is nearly a 100% risk of recipient infection with HBV if the donor is HBsAg (+) and liver transplantation in this setting is rarely performed. Another risk is the presence of anti-HBc in the donor, which poses a small risk of HBV transmission for organ transplant recipients other than liver ***(161,162)***. Finally, recipients who are anti-HBc positive can reactivate nascent HBV disease once immunosuppression is initiated ***(163)***. Any patient who develops acute liver disease after solid organ transplant needs to be assessed by HBsAg testing. Conversely, bone marrow transplants have resulted in HBsAg clearance by adoptive immunity from the donor's immune cells ***(164)***.

11. Conclusion

The best management of patients with HBV can be studied and instituted with the knowledge and definition of the special populations who are chronically infected with HBV. Each group needs to be approached separately and when pharmaceutical medication development takes place, population subgroups need to be studied separately.

References

1. Maynard, J. E. (1990) Hepatitis B: global importance and need for control. *Vaccine* **8 (Suppl)**, S18–S20.
2. Dodd, R. Y. and Nath, N. (1987) Increased risk for lethal forms of liver disease among HBsAg-positive blood donors in the United States. *J. Virol. Methods* **17**, 81–94.
3. Lee, W. M. (1997) Hepatitis B virus infection. *N. Engl. J. Med.* **337**, 1733–1745.
4. Hoofnagle, J. H. (1990) Chronic hepatitis B. *N. Engl. J. Med.* **323**, 337–339.
5. Moyer, L. A. and Mast, E. E. (1994) Hepatitis B: virology, epidemiology, disease, and prevention, and an overview of viral hepatitis. *Am. J. Prev. Med.* **10 (Suppl)**, 45–55.
6. Kane, M. (1995) Epidemiology of hepatitis B infection in North America. *Vaccine* **13 (Suppl 1)**, S16–S17.
7. McMahon, B. J., Lanier, A. P., and Wainwright, R. B. (1998) Hepatitis B and hepatocellular carcinoma in Eskimo/Inuit population. *Int. J. Circumpolar. Health* **57 (Suppl 1)**, 414–419.
8. Chu, C. M. (2000) Natural history of chronic hepatitis B virus infection in adults with emphasis on the occurrence of cirrhosis and hepatocellular carcinoma. *J. Gastroenterol. Hepatol.* **15 (Suppl)**, E25–E30.
9. de Franchis, R., Meucci, G., Vecchi, M., et al. (1993) The natural history of asymptomatic hepatitis B surface antigen carriers. *Ann. Intern. Med.* **118**, 191–194.

10. Fattovich, G., Brollo, L., Giustina, G., et al. (1991) Natural history and prognostic factors for chronic hepatitis type B. *Gut* **32**, 294–298.
11. Lok, A. S. (1992) Natural history and control of perinatally acquired hepatitis B virus infection. *Dig. Dis.* **10**, 46–52.
12. Angus, P. W. (1997) Review: hepatitis B and liver transplantation. *J. Gastroenterol. Hepatol.* **12**, 217–223.
13. Arevalo, J. A. and Washington, A. E. (1988) Cost-effectiveness of prenatal screening and immunization for hepatitis B virus. *JAMA* **259**, 365–369.
14. Blumberg, B. S. (1977) Australia antigen and the biology of hepatitis B. *Science* **197**, 17–25.
15. Perrault, J., McGill, D. B., Ott, B. J., and Taylor, W. F. (1978) Liver biopsy: complications in 1000 inpatients and outpatients. *Gastroenterology* **74**, 103–106.
16. Younossi, Z. M., Teran, J. C., Ganiats, T. G., and Carey, W. D. (1998) Ultrasound-guided liver biopsy for parenchymal liver disease: an economic analysis. *Dig. Dis. Sci.* **43**, 46–50.
17. Piton, A., Poynard, T., Imbert-Bismut, F., et al. (1998) Factors associated with serum alanine transaminase activity in healthy subjects: consequences for the definition of normal values, for selection of blood donors, and for patients with chronic hepatitis C. MULTIVIRC Group. *Hepatology* **27**, 1213–1219.
18. Knodell, R. G., Ishak, K. G., Black, W. C., et al. (1981) Formulation and application of a numerical scoring system for assessing histological activity in asymptomatic chronic active hepatitis. *Hepatology* **1**, 431–435.
19. Hruska, J. F. and Robinson, W. S. (1977) The proteins of hepatitis B Dane particle cores. *J. Med. Virol.* **1**, 119–131.
20. Summers, J., O'Connell, A., and Millman, I. (1975) Genome of hepatitis B virus: restriction enzyme cleavage and structure of DNA extracted from Dane particles. *Proc. Natl. Acad. Sci. U.S.A* **72**, 4597–4601.
21. Albin, C. and Robinson, W. S. (1980) Protein kinase activity in hepatitis B virus. *J. Virol.* **34**, 297–302.
22. Nassal, M. (1999) Hepatitis B virus replication: novel roles for virus–host interactions. *Intervirology* **42**, 100–116.
23. Spandau, D. F. and Lee, C. H. (1988) Trans-activation of viral enhancers by the hepatitis B virus X protein. *J. Virol.* **62**, 427–434.
24. Twu, J. S. and Robinson, W. S. (1989) Hepatitis B virus X gene can transactivate heterologous viral sequences. *Proc. Natl. Acad. Sci. USA* **86**, 2046–2050.
25. Twu, J. S., Chu, K., and Robinson, W. S. (1989) Hepatitis B virus X gene activates kappa B-like enhancer sequences in the long terminal repeat of human immunodeficiency virus 1. *Proc. Natl. Acad. Sci. USA* **86**, 5168–5172.
26. Chen, H. S., Kaneko, S., Girones, R., et al. (1993) The woodchuck hepatitis virus X gene is important for establishment of virus infection in woodchucks. *J. Virol.* **67**, 1218–1226.
27. Zoulim, F., Saputelli, J., and Seeger, C. (1994) Woodchuck hepatitis virus X protein is required for viral infection in vivo. *J. Virol.* **68**, 2026–2030.
28. Ganem, D. (1996). *Hepadnaviridae* and their replication. In: "*Virology*," 3rd Ed. (Fields, B. N., Eds.). New York: Lippincott-Raven Publishers, pp. 2703–2737
29. Raney, A. K., Milich, D. R., Easton, A. J., and McLachlan, A. (1990) Differentiation-specific transcriptional regulation of the hepatitis B virus large surface antigen gene in human hepatoma cell lines. *J. Virol.* **64**, 2360–2368.
30. Cattaneo, R., Will, H., Hernandez, N., and Schaller, H. (1983) Signals regulating hepatitis B surface antigen transcription. *Nature* **305**, 336–338.

31. Standring, D. N., Rutter, W. J., Varmus, H. E., and Ganem, D. (1984) Transcription of the hepatitis B surface antigen gene in cultured murine cells initiates within the presurface region. *J. Virol.* **50**, 563–571.
32. Siddiqui, A., Jameel, S., and Mapoles, J. (1987) Expression of the hepatitis B virus X gene in mammalian cells. *Proc. Natl. Acad. Sci. USA* **84**, 2513–2517.
33. Shaul, Y., Rutter, W. J., and Laub, O. (1985) A human hepatitis B viral enhancer element. *EMBO J.* **4**, 427–430.
34. Yee, J. K. (1989) A liver-specific enhancer in the core promoter region of human hepatitis B virus. *Science* **246**, 658–661.
35. Bock, C., Malek, N. P., Tillmann, H. L., Manns, M. P., and Trautwein, C. (2000) The enhancer I core region contributes to the replication level of hepatitis B virus In vivo and In vitro. *J. Virol.* **74**, 2193–2202.
36. Tur-Kaspa, R., Burk, R. D., Shaul, Y., and Shafritz, D. A. (1986) Hepatitis B virus DNA contains a glucocorticoid-responsive element. *Proc. Natl. Acad. Sci. USA* **83**, 1627–1631.
37. Tur-Kaspa, R., Shaul, Y., Moore, D. D., et al. (1988) The glucocorticoid receptor recognizes a specific nucleotide sequence in hepatitis B virus DNA causing increased activity of the HBV enhancer. *Virology* **167**, 630–633.
38. Neurath, A. R., Kent, S. B., Parker, K., et al. (1986) Antibodies to a synthetic peptide from the preS 120–145 region of the hepatitis B virus envelope are virus neutralizing. *Vaccine* **4**, 35–37.
39. Le Seyec, J., Chouteau, P., Cannie, I., Guguen-Guillouzo, C., and Gripon, P. (1999) Infection process of the hepatitis B virus depends on the presence of a defined sequence in the pre-S1 domain. *J. Virol.* **73**, 2052–2057.
40. Jung, M. C., Diepolder, H. M., Spengler, U., et al. (1995) Activation of a heterogeneous hepatitis B (HB) core and e antigen-specific CD4+ T-cell population during seroconversion to anti-HBe and anti-HBs in hepatitis B virus infection. *J. Virol.* **69**, 3358–3368.
41. Chiang, P. W., Jeng, K. S., Hu, C. P., and Chang, C. M. (1992) Characterization of a cis element required for packaging and replication of the human hepatitis B virus. *Virology* **186**, 701–711.
42. Junker-Niepmann, M., Bartenschlager, R., and Schaller, H. (1990) A short cis-acting sequence is required for hepatitis B virus pregenome encapsidation and sufficient for packaging of foreign RNA. *EMBO J.* **9**, 3389–3396.
43. Pollack, J. R. and Ganem, D. (1993) An RNA stem-loop structure directs hepatitis B virus genomic RNA encapsidation. *J. Virol.* **67**, 3254–3263.
44. Pollack, J. R. and Ganem, D. (1994) Site-specific RNA binding by a hepatitis B virus reverse transcriptase initiates two distinct reactions: RNA packaging and DNA synthesis. *J. Virol.* **68**, 5579–5587.
45. Hirsch, R. C., Loeb, D. D., Pollack, J. R., and Ganem, D. (1991) cis-acting sequences required for encapsidation of duck hepatitis B virus pregenomic RNA. *J. Virol.* **65**, 3309–3316.
46. Bartenschlager, R. and Schaller, H. (1992) Hepadnaviral assembly is initiated by polymerase binding to the encapsidation signal in the viral RNA genome. *EMBO J.* **11**, 3413–3420.
47. Nassal, M. and Schaller, H. (1993) Hepatitis B virus replication. *Trends Microbiol.* **1**, 221–228.
48. Tavis, J. E., Perri, S., and Ganem, D. (1994) Hepadnavirus reverse transcription initiates within the stem-loop of the RNA packaging signal and employs a novel strand transfer. *J. Virol.* **68**, 3536–3543.

49. Summers, J. and Mason, W. S. (1982) Replication of the genome of a hepatitis B—like virus by reverse transcription of an RNA intermediate. *Cell* **29**, 403–415.
50. Oberhaus, S. M. and Newbold, J. E. (1995) Detection of an RNase H activity associated with hepadnaviruses. *J. Virol.* **69**, 5697–5704.
51. Lien, J. M., Aldrich, C. E., and Mason, W. S. (1986) Evidence that a capped oligoribonucleotide is the primer for duck hepatitis B virus plus-strand DNA synthesis. *J. Virol.* **57**, 229–236.
52. Loeb, D. D., Hirsch, R. C., and Ganem, D. (1991) Sequence-independent RNA cleavages generate the primers for plus strand DNA synthesis in hepatitis B viruses: implications for other reverse transcribing elements. *EMBO J.* **10**, 3533–3540.
53. Tuttleman, J. S., Pourcel, C., and Summers, J. (1986) Formation of the pool of covalently closed circular viral DNA in hepadnavirus-infected cells. *Cell* **47**, 451–460.
54. Wu, T. T., Coates, L., Aldrich, C. E., Summers, J., and Mason, W. S. (1990) In hepatocytes infected with duck hepatitis B virus, the template for viral RNA synthesis is amplified by an intracellular pathway. *Virology* **175**, 255–261.
55. Gauthier, J., Bourne, E. J., Lutz, M. W., et al. (1999) Quantitation of hepatitis B viremia and emergence of YMDD variants in patients with chronic hepatitis B treated with lamivudine. *J. Infect. Dis.* **180**, 1757–1762.
56. Ishak, K. G. (1994) Chronic hepatitis: morphology and nomenclature. *Mod. Pathol.* **7**, 690–713.
57. Bedossa, P. and Poynard, T. (1996) An algorithm for the grading of activity in chronic hepatitis C. The METAVIR Cooperative Study Group. *Hepatology* **24**, 289–293.
58. Eddleston, A. (1986) Interferons in the treatment of chronic hepatitis B virus infection. *Med. Clin. North Am.* **Suppl**, 25–30.
59. Di Bisceglie, A. M. (1995) Long-term outcome of interferon-alpha therapy for chronic hepatitis B. *J. Hepatol.* **22**, 65–67.
60. Korenman, J., Baker, B., Waggoner, J., Everhart, J. E., Di Bisceglie, A. M., and Hoofnagle, J. H. (1991) Long-term remission of chronic hepatitis B after alpha-interferon therapy. *Ann. Intern. Med.* **114**, 629–634.
61. Hadziyannis, S. (1995) Hepatitis Be Antigen Negative Chronic Hepatitis B: from Clinical Recognition to Pathogenesis and Treatment. *Viral Hepat. Rev.* **1**, 7–36.
62. Brunetto, M. R., Oliveri, F., Rocca, G., et al. (1989) Natural course and response to interferon of chronic hepatitis B accompanied by antibody to hepatitis B e antigen. *Hepatology* **10**, 198–202.
63. Hadziyannis, S., Bramou, T., Makris, A., Moussoulis, G., Zignego, L., and Papaioannou, C. (1990) Interferon alfa-2b treatment of HBeAg negative/serum HBV DNA positive chronic active hepatitis type B. *J. Hepatol.* **11 Suppl 1(S133–136)**.
64. Santantonio, T., Mazzola, M., Iacovazzi, T., Miglietta, A., Guastadisegni, A., and Pastore, G. (2000) Long-term follow-up of patients with anti-HBe/HBV DNA-positive chronic hepatitis B treated for 12 months with lamivudine. *J. Hepatol.* **32**, 300–306.
65. Dusheiko, G. (1999) Lamivudine therapy for hepatitis B infection. *Scand. J. Gastroenterol.* **230 (Suppl)**, 76–81.
66. Dienstag, J. L. (1997) Sexual and perinatal transmission of hepatitis C. *Hepatology* **26**, 66S–70S.
67. Dienstag, J. L., Schiff, E. R., Mitchell, M., et al. (1999) Extended lamivudine retreatment for chronic hepatitis B: maintenance of viral suppression after discontinuation of therapy. *Hepatology* **30**, 1082–1087.

68. Liaw, Y. F., Leung, N. W., Chang, T. T., et al. (2000) Effects of extended lamivudine therapy in Asian patients with chronic hepatitis B. Asia Hepatitis Lamivudine Study Group. *Gastroenterology* **119**, 172–180.
69. Hadziyannis, S. J., Papatheodoridis, G. V., Dimou, E., Laras, A., and Papaioannou, C. (2000) Efficacy of long-term Lamivudine monotherapy in patients with hepatitis B e antigen-negative chronic hepatitis B. *Hepatology* **32**, 847–851.
70. Fischer, K. P., Gutfreund, K. S., and Tyrrell, D. L. (2001) Lamivudine resistance in hepatitis B: mechanisms and clinical implications. *Drug Resist. Updat.* **4**, 118–128.
71. Gutfreund, K. S., Williams, M., George, R., et al. (2000) Genotypic succession of mutations of the hepatitis B virus polymerase associated with lamivudine resistance. *J. Hepatol.* **33**, 469–475.
72. Kobayashi, S., Ide, T., and Sata, M. (2001) Detection of YMDD motif mutations in some lamivudine-untreated asymptomatic hepatitis B virus carriers. *J. Hepatol.* **34**, 584–586.
73. Leung, N. W., Lai, C. L., Chang, T. T., et al. (2001) Extended lamivudine treatment in patients with chronic hepatitis B enhances hepatitis B e antigen seroconversion rates: results after 3 years of therapy. *Hepatology* **33**, 1527–1532.
74. Perrillo, R., Rakela, J., Dienstag, J., et al. (1999) Multicenter study of lamivudine therapy for hepatitis B after liver transplantation.Lamivudine Transplant Group. *Hepatology* **29**, 1581–1586.
75. De Man, R. A., Heijtink, R. A., Niesters, H. G., and Schalm, S. W. (1995) New developments in antiviral therapy for chronic hepatitis B infection. *Scand. J. Gastroenterol.* **212 (Suppl)**, 100–104.
76. Bridges, E. G. and Cheng, Y. C. (1995) Use of novel beta-L(−)-nucleoside analogues for treatment and prevention of chronic hepatitis B virus infection and hepatocellular carcinoma. *Prog. Liver Dis.* **13**, 231–245.
77. Cossart, Y. E. (1972) Australia antigen and hepatitis in renal units. *Proc. Eur. Dial. Transplant. Assoc.* **9**, 235–242.
78. Davis, H. L. (1999) DNA vaccines for prophylactic or therapeutic immunization against hepatitis B virus. *Mt. Sinai J. Med.* **66**, 84–90.
79. Tiollais, P., Pourcel, C., and Dejean, A. (1985) The hepatitis B virus. *Nature* **317**, 489–495.
80. Carman, W. F. (1997) The clinical significance of surface antigen variants of hepatitis B virus. *J. Viral Hepat.* **4 (Suppl 1)**, 11–20.
81. Yoshida, E. M., Ramji, A., Erb, S. R., et al. (2000) De novo acute hepatitis B infection in a previously vaccinated liver transplant recipient due to a strain of HBV with a Met 133 Thr mutation in the "a" determinant. *Liver* **20**, 411–414.
82. Ijaz, S., Torre, F., Tedder, R. S., Williams, R., and Naoumov, N. V. (2001). Novel immunoassay for the detection of hepatitis B surface 'escape' mutants and its application in liver transplant recipients. *J.Med.Virol.* **63**, 210–216.
83. Rossner, M. T. (1992). Review: hepatitis B virus X-gene product: a promiscuous transcriptional activator. *J.Med.Virol.* **36**, 101–117.
84. Jean-Jean, O., Weimer, T., de Recondo, A. M., Will, H., and Rossignol, J. M. (1989). Internal entry of ribosomes and ribosomal scanning involved in hepatitis B virus P gene expression. *J.Virol.* **63**, 5451–5454.
85. Lin, C. G. and Lo, S. J. (1992). Evidence for involvement of a ribosomal leaky scanning mechanism in the translation of the hepatitis B virus pol gene from the viral pregenome RNA. *Virology* **188**, 342–352.
86. Lanford, R. E., Kim, Y. H., Lee, H., Notvall, L., and Beames, B. (1999). Mapping of the hepatitis B virus reverse transcriptase TP and RT domains by transcomplementation for nucleotide priming and by protein-protein interaction. *J.Virol.* **73**, 1885–1893.

87. Bartenschlager, R. and Schaller, H. (1988). The amino-terminal domain of the hepadnaviral P-gene encodes the terminal protein (genome-linked protein) believed to prime reverse transcription. *EMBO J.* **7**, 4185–4192.
88. Jacobo-Molina, A., Ding, J., Clark, A. D., Jr., Lu, X., Williams, R. L., Williams, R. L., Kamer, G., Ferria, A. L., and Clark, P. (1993). Crystal structure of human immunodeficiency virus type 1 reverse transcriptase complexed with double-stranded DNA at 3.0 A resolution shows bent DNA. *Proc.Natl.Acad.Sci.U.S.A* **90**, 6320–6324.
89. Bartholomeusz, A. and Thompson, P. (1999). Flaviviridae polymerase and RNA replication. *J.Viral Hepat.* **6**, 261–270.
90. Locarnini, S. and Birch, C. (1999). Antiviral chemotherapy for chronic hepatitis B infection: lessons learned from treating HIV-infected patients. *J.Hepatol.* **30**, 536–550.
91. Stuyver, L. J., Locarnini, S. A., Lok, A., Richman, D. D., Carman, W. F., Dienstag, J. L., and Schinazi, R. F. (2001). Nomenclature for antiviral-resistant human hepatitis B virus mutations in the polymerase region. *Hepatology* **33**, 751–757.
92. Das, K., Xiong, X., Yang, H., Westland, C. E., Gibbs, C. S., Sarafianos, S. G., and Arnold, E. (2001). Molecular modeling and biochemical characterization reveal the mechanism of hepatitis B virus polymerase resistance to lamivudine (3TC) and emtricitabine (FTC). *J.Virol.* **75**, 4771–4779.
93. Hunt, C. M., McGill, J. M., Allen, M. I., and Condreay, L. D. (2000). Clinical relevance of hepatitis B viral mutations. *Hepatology* **31**, 1037–1044.
94. Lok, A. S., Akarca, U., and Greene, S. (1994). Mutations in the pre-core region of hepatitis B virus serve to enhance the stability of the secondary structure of the pre-genome encapsidation signal. *Proc.Natl.Acad.Sci.U.S.A* **91**, 4077–4081.
95. Gunther, S., Fischer, L., Pult, I., Sterneck, M., and Will, H. (1999). Naturally occurring variants of hepatitis B virus. *Adv.Virus Res.* **52**, 125–137.
96. Cabrerizo, M., Bartolome, J., Ruiz-Moreno, M., Otero, M., Lopez-Alcorocho, J. M., and Carreno, V. (1996). Distribution of the predominant hepatitis B virus precore variants in hepatitis B e antigen-positive children and their effect on treatment response. *Pediatr.Res.* **39**, 980–984.
97. Lampertico, P., Manzin, A., Rumi, M. G., Paolucci, S., Del Ninno, E., Clementi, M., and Colombo, M. (1995). Hepatitis B virus precore mutants in HBeAg carriers with chronic hepatitis treated with interferon. *J.Viral Hepat.* **2**, 251–256.
98. Lopez-Alcorocho, J. M., Cabrerizo, M., Bartolome, J., Cotonat, T., and Carreno, V. (1995). Analysis of hepatitis B virus precore variants in hepatitis B e antibody-positive patients treated with prednisone plus interferon. *J.Viral Hepat.* **2**, 279–284.
99. Alberti, A., Pontisso, P., Chemello, L., Fattovich, G., Benvegnu, L., Belussi, F., and De Mitri, M. S. (1995). The interaction between hepatitis B virus and hepatitis C virus in acute and chronic liver disease. *J.Hepatol.* **22**, 38–41.
100. Benhamou, Y., Bochet, M., Thibault, V., Di, M., V, Caumes, E., Bricaire, F., Opolon, P., Katlama, C., and Poynard, T. (1999). Long-term incidence of hepatitis B virus resistance to lamivudine in human immunodeficiency virus-infected patients. *Hepatology* **30**, 1302–1306.
101. Bessesen, M., Ives, D., Condreay, L., Lawrence, S., and Sherman, K. E. (1999) Chronic active hepatitis B exacerbations in human immunodeficiency virus-infected patients following development of resistance to or withdrawal of lamivudine. *Clin. Infect. Dis.* **28**, 1032–1035.

102. Thibault, V., Benhamou, Y., Seguret, C., et al. (1999) Hepatitis B virus (HBV) mutations associated with resistance to lamivudine in patients coinfected with HBV and human immunodeficiency virus. *J. Clin. Microbiol.* **37**, 3013–3016.
103. Bonino, F. and Smedile, A. (1986) Delta agent (type D) hepatitis. *Semin. Liver Dis.* **6**, 28–33.
104. Hadziyannis, S. J. (1983) Delta antigen positive chronic liver disease in Greece: clinical aspects and natural course. *Prog. Clin. Biol. Res.* **143**, 209–217.
105. Rizzetto, M., Shih, J. W., Gocke, D. J., Purcell, R. H., Verme, G., and Gerin, J. L. (1979) Incidence and significance of antibodies to delta antigen in hepatitis B virus infection. *Lancet* **2**, 986–990.
106. Rizzetto, M., Purcell, R. H., and Gerin, J. L. (1980) Epidemiology of HBV-associated delta agent: geographical distribution of anti-delta and prevalence in polytransfused HBsAg carriers. *Lancet* **1**, 1215–1218.
107. Rizzetto, M. (1993) Hepatitis delta virus disease: an overview. *Prog. Clin. Biol. Res.* **382**, 425–430.
108. Cenac, A., Pedroso, M. L., Djibo, A., et al. (1995) Hepatitis B, C, and D virus infections in patients with chronic hepatitis, cirrhosis, and hepatocellular carcinoma: a comparative study in Niger. *Am. J. Trop. Med. Hyg.* **52**, 293–296.
109. Mion, F., Boillot, O., Gille, D., Chevallier, P., and Paliard, P. (1993) Liver transplantation for posthepatic B-delta cirrhosis: prevention of recurrence with high-dose anti-HBs immunoglobulins. *Transplant. Proc.* **25**, 2638–2639.
110. Alvarez, F. (1996) Therapy for chronic viral hepatitis. *Clin. Invest Med.* **19**, 381–388.
111. Bortolotti, F., Jara, P., Barbera, C., et al. (2000) Long term effect of alpha interferon in children with chronic hepatitis B [see comments]. *Gut* **46**, 715–718.
112. Carreno, V., Porres, J. C., Ruiz-Moreno, M., Gutiez, J., and Bartolome, F. J. (1991) [A controlled study of treatment with recombinant interferon alpha of chronic hepatitis due to the B virus in childhood]. *Rev. Esp. Enferm. Dig.* **79**, 24–28.
113. Castaneda, G. C., Sotto, E. A., and Lopez, S. P. (1990) Antiviral effect of interferon: the interferon in viral hepatitis. *Rev. Roum. Virol.* **41**, 171–179.
114. Jara, P. and Bortolotti, F. (1999) Interferon-alpha treatment of chronic hepatitis B in childhood: a consensus advice based on experience in European children. *J. Pediatr. Gastroenterol. Nutr.* **29**, 163–170.
115. (1996) Hepatitis B immunization/prophylaxis: recommendations for adults/older adults. *Nurse Pract.* **21**, 64, 67–64, 70.
116. Mahon, M. M. and James, O. F. (1994) Liver disease in the elderly. *J. Clin. Gastroenterol.* **18**, 330–334.
117. Malaguarnera, M., Restuccia, S., Ferlito, L., Mazzoleni, G., Giugno, I., and Pistone, G. (2001) Antiviral drugs in chronic hepatitis B: review and meta-analysis. *Int. J. Clin. Pharmacol. Ther.* **39**, 4–11.
118. Chiaramonte, M., Floreani, A., and Naccarato, R. (1987) Hepatitis B virus (HBV) in the elderly: an underestimated problem? *Biomed. Pharmacother.* **41**, 121–123.
119. Dienstag, J. L., Perrillo, R. P., Schiff, E. R., Bartholomew, M., Vicary, C., and Rubin, M. (1995) A preliminary trial of lamivudine for chronic hepatitis B infection. *N. Engl. J. Med.* **333**, 1657–1661.
120. Lai, C. L., Ching, C. K., Tung, A. K., et al. (1997) Lamivudine is effective in suppressing hepatitis B virus DNA in Chinese hepatitis B surface antigen carriers: a placebo-controlled trial. *Hepatology* **25**, 241–244.

121. Nevens, F., Main, J., Honkoop, P., et al. (1997) Lamivudine therapy for chronic hepatitis B: a six-month randomized dose-ranging study. *Gastroenterology* **113**, 1258–1263.
122. Honkoop, P., De Man, R. A., Niesters, H. G., et al. (1998). Quantitative hepatitis B virus DNA assessment by the limiting-dilution polymerase chain reaction in chronic hepatitis B patients: evidence of continuing viral suppression with longer duration and higher dose of lamivudine therapy. *J. Viral Hepat.* **5**, 307–312.
123. Xiong, X., Flores, C., Yang, H., Toole, J. J., and Gibbs, C. S. (1998) Mutations in hepatitis B DNA polymerase associated with resistance to lamivudine do not confer resistance to adefovir in vitro. *Hepatology* **28**, 1669–1673.
124. Xiong, X., Yang, H., Westland, C. E., Zou, R., and Gibbs, C. S. (2000) In vitro evaluation of hepatitis B virus polymerase mutations associated with famciclovir resistance. *Hepatology* **31**, 219–224.
125. Perrillo, R., Schiff, E., Yoshida, E., et al. (2000) Adefovir dipivoxil for the treatment of lamivudine-resistant hepatitis B mutants. *Hepatology* **32**, 129–134.
126. Peters, M. G., Singer, G., Howard, T., et al. (1999) Fulminant hepatic failure resulting from lamivudine-resistant hepatitis B virus in a renal transplant recipient: durable response after orthotopic liver transplantation on adefovir dipivoxil and hepatitis B immune globulin. *Transplantation* **68**, 1912–1914.
127. Brechot, C., Nalpas, B., and Feitelson, M. A. (1996) Interactions between alcohol and hepatitis viruses in the liver. *Clin. Lab. Med.* **16**, 273–287.
128. Abou-Saif, A. and Lewis, J. H. (2000) Gastrointestinal and hepatic disorders in end-stage renal disease and renal transplant recipients [In Process Citation]. *Adv. Ren. Replace. Ther.* **7**, 220–230.
129. Samuel, D., Zignego, A. L., Reynes, M., et al. (1995) Long-term clinical and virological outcome after liver transplantation for cirrhosis caused by chronic delta hepatitis. *Hepatology* **21**, 333–339.
130. Gish, R. G., Lau, J. Y., Brooks, L., et al. (1996) Ganciclovir treatment of hepatitis B virus infection in liver transplant recipients. *Hepatology* **23**, 1–7.
131. Al, F. K., Yoshida, E. M., Davis, J. E., Vartanian, R. K., Anderson, F. H., and Steinbrecher, U. P. (1997) Alteration of the dismal natural history of fibrosing cholestatic hepatitis secondary to hepatitis B virus with the use of lamivudine. *Transplantation* **64**, 926–928.
132. Andreone, P., Caraceni, P., Grazi, G. L., et al. (1998) Lamivudine treatment for acute hepatitis B after liver transplantation. *J. Hepatol.* **29**, 985–989.
133. Ben-Ari, Z., Shmueli, D., Mor, E., et al. (1997) Beneficial effect of lamivudine pre- and post-liver transplantation for hepatitis B infection. *Transplant. Proc.* **29**, 2687–2688.
134. Ben-Ari, Z., Shmueli, D., Mor, E., Shapira, Z., and Tur-Kaspa, R. (1997) Beneficial effect of lamivudine in recurrent hepatitis B after liver transplantation. *Transplantation* **63**, 393–396.
135. Ben Ari, Z., Zemel, R., Kazetsker, A., Fraser, G., and Tur-Kaspa, R. (1999) Efficacy of lamivudine in patients with hepatitis B virus precore mutant infection before and after liver transplantation. *Am. J. Gastroenterol.* **94**, 663–667.
136. De Man, R. A., Bartholomeusz, A. I., Niesters, H. G., Zondervan, P. E., and Locarnini, S. A. (1998) The sequential occurrence of viral mutations in a liver transplant recipient re-infected with hepatitis B: hepatitis B immune globulin escape, famciclovir non-response, followed by lamivudine resistance resulting in graft loss. *J. Hepatol.* **29**, 669–675.
137. Dodson, S. F., Bonham, C. A., Geller, D. A., Cacciarelli, T. V., Rakela, J., and Fung, J. J. (1999) Prevention of de novo hepatitis B infection in recipients of hepatic allografts from anti-HBc positive donors. *Transplantation* **68**, 1058–1061.

138. Dodson, S. F. (2000) Prevention of de novo hepatitis B infection after liver transplantation with allografts from hepatitis B core antibody positive donors. *Clin. Transplant.* **14 (Suppl 2)**, 20–24.
139. Grellier, L., Mutimer, D., Ahmed, M., et al. (1996) Lamivudine prophylaxis against reinfection in liver transplantation for hepatitis B cirrhosis. *Lancet* **348**, 1212–1215.
140. Gugenheim, J., Baldini, E., Ouzan, D., Sowka, P., and Mouiel, J. (1999) Good results of lamivudine in hepatitis B surface antigen-positive patients with active viral replication before liver transplantation. *Transplant. Proc.* **31**, 554–555.
141. McCaughan, G. W., Spencer, J., Koorey, D., et al. (1999) Lamivudine therapy in patients undergoing liver transplantation for hepatitis B virus precore mutant-associated infection: high resistance rates in treatment of recurrence but universal prevention if used as prophylaxis with very low dose hepatitis B immune globulin. *Liver Transplant Surg.* **5**, 512–519.
142. Mutimer, D., Dusheiko, G., Barrett, C., et al. (2000) Lamivudine without HBIg for prevention of graft reinfection by hepatitis B: long-term follow-up. *Transplantation* **70**, 809–815.
143. Perrillo, R. P. (1997) Treatment of posttransplantation hepatitis B. *Liver Transplant. Surg.* **3**, S8–12.
144. Perrillo, R. P., Rakela, J., Dienstag, J., et al. (1999) Multicenter study of lamivudine therapy for hepatitis B after liver transplantation.Lamivudine Transplant Group. *Hepatology* **29**, 1581–1586.
145. Terrault, N. A., Holland, C. C., Ferrell, L., et al. (1996) Interferon alfa for recurrent hepatitis B infection after liver transplantation. *Liver Transplant. Surg.* **2**, 132–138.
146. Bartholomew, M. M., Jansen, R. W., Jeffers, L. J., et al. (1997) Hepatitis-B-virus resistance to lamivudine given for recurrent infection after orthotopic liver transplantation. *Lancet* **349**, 20–22.
147. Ling, R., Mutimer, D., Ahmed, M., et al. (1996) Selection of mutations in the hepatitis B virus polymerase during therapy of transplant recipients with lamivudine. *Hepatology* **24**, 711–713.
148. Tipples, G. A., Ma, M. M., Fischer, K. P., Bain, V. G., Kneteman, N. M., and Tyrrell, D. L. (1996) Mutation in HBV RNA-dependent DNA polymerase confers resistance to lamivudine in vivo. *Hepatology* **24**, 714–717.
149. Honkoop, P., Niesters, H. G., De Man, R. A., Osterhaus, A. D., and Schalm, S. W. (1997) Lamivudine resistance in immunocompetent chronic hepatitis B. Incidence and patterns. *J. Hepatol.* **26**, 1393–1395.
150. Chayama, K., Suzuki, Y., Kobayashi, M., et al. (1998) Emergence and takeover of YMDD motif mutant hepatitis B virus during long-term lamivudine therapy and re-takeover by wild type after cessation of therapy. *Hepatology* **27**, 1711–1716.
151. Liaw, Y. F., Chien, R. N., Yeh, C. T., Tsai, S. L., and Chu, C. M. (1999) Acute exacerbation and hepatitis B virus clearance after emergence of YMDD motif mutation during lamivudine therapy. *Hepatology* **30**, 567–572.
152. Seta, T., Yokosuka, O., Imazeki, F., Tagawa, M., and Saisho, H. (2000) Emergence of YMDD motif mutants of hepatitis B virus during lamivudine treatment of immunocompetent type B hepatitis patients. *J. Med. Virol.* **60**, 8–16.
153. Lai, C. L., Chien, R. N., Leung, N. W., et al. (1998) A one-year trial of lamivudine for chronic hepatitis B. Asia Hepatitis Lamivudine Study Group. *N. Engl. J. Med.* **339**, 61–68.
154. Dienstag, J. L., Schiff, E. R., Wright, T. L., et al. (1999) Lamivudine as initial treatment for chronic hepatitis B in the United States. *N. Engl. J. Med.* **341**, 1256–1263.
155. Tassopoulos, N. C., Volpes, R., Pastore, G., et al. (1999) Efficacy of lamivudine in patients with hepatitis B e antigen-negative/hepatitis B virus DNA-positive (precore mutant) chronic hepatitis B.Lamivudine Precore Mutant Study Group. *Hepatology* **29**, 889–896.

156. Wedemeyer, H., Pethig, K., Wagner, D., et al. (1998) Long-term outcome of chronic hepatitis B in heart transplant recipients. *Transplantation* **66**, 1347–1353.
157. Chen, P. M., Chiou, T. J., Fan, F. S., et al. (1999) Fulminant hepatitis is significantly increased in hepatitis B carriers after allogeneic bone marrow transplantation. *Transplantation* **67**, 1425–1433.
158. Cooksley, W. G. and McIvor, C. A. (1995) Fibrosing cholestatic hepatitis and HBV after bone marrow transplantation. *Biomed. Pharmacother.* **49**, 117–124.
159. Fan, F. S., Tzeng, C. H., Yeh, H. M., and Chen, P. M. (1992) Reverse seroconversion of hepatitis B virus infectious status after allogeneic bone marrow transplantation from a carrier donor. *Bone Marrow Transplant.* **10**, 189–191.
160. Fornairon, S., Pol, S., Legendre, C., et al. (1996) The long-term virologic and pathologic impact of renal transplantation on chronic hepatitis B virus infection. *Transplantation* **62**, 297–299.
161. Uemoto, S., Inomata, Y., Sannomiya, A., et al. (1998) Posttransplant hepatitis B infection in liver transplantation with hepatitis B core antibody-positive donors. *Transplant. Proc.* **30**, 134–135.
162. Wachs, M. E., Amend, W. J., Ascher, N. L., et al. (1995) The risk of transmission of hepatitis B from HBsAg(–), HBcAb(+), HBIgM(–) organ donors. *Transplantation* **59**, 230–234.
163. Fabia, R., Levy, M. F., Crippin, J., et al. (1998) De novo hepatitis B infection after liver transplantation: source of disease, incidence, and impact. *Liver Transplant. Surg.* **4**, 119–127.
164. Lau, G. K., Liang, R., Lee, C. K., et al. (1998) Clearance of persistent hepatitis B virus infection in Chinese bone marrow transplant recipients whose donors were anti-hepatitis B core- and anti-hepatitis B surface antibody-positive. *J. Infect. Dis.* **178**, 1585–1591.
165. Lok, A. S. F. and McMahon, B. J. (2001) Chronic hepatitis B. *Hepatology* **34**, 1225–1241.
166. Margolis, H. S., Alter, M. J., and Hadler, S. C. (1991) Hepatitis B: evolving epidemiology and implications for control. *Semin. Liver Dis.* **11**, 84–92.
167. Angus, P., Vaughan, R., Xiong, S., et al. (2003) Resistance to adefovir dipivoxil therapy associated with the selection of a novel mutation in the HBV polymerase. *Gastroenterology* **125**, 292–297.

35

Designing Clinical Development Programs for Anti-Hepatitis B Virus Drugs

Nathaniel A. Brown

Introduction and Background

Hepatitis B virus (HBV) infection remains one of the leading infectious causes of chronic liver disease and death in the world ***(1,2)***. With the advent of universal HBV vaccination and with the availability of antiviral therapeutics, HBV infection is increasingly preventable and treatable. Substantial progress has been achieved with vaccination programs, but the current social and economic impediments to full global implementation of universal HBV vaccination render it likely that many people will continue to be afflicted with chronic HBV infection for several more decades. Hence antiviral treatment for clinically significant HBV infection will continue to be needed for the foreseeable future. Current treatment modalities for chronic hepatitis B—interferon, lamivudine, and adefovir—allow clinical management of some patients but are associated with frequent nonresponse (interferon), frequent viral resistance (lamivudine), or potential safety issues (adefovir), so additional treatment options are needed before optimal clinical management can be assured for most patients.

Chronic HBV infection, usually defined as HBV infection persisting more than 6–12 mo, is termed the HBV carrier state; chronic HBV infection is clinically established by documenting persistent hepatitis B surface antigen (HBsAg) antigenemia. Chronic HBV carriage is associated with the development of chronic necroinflammatory liver disease, termed chronic hepatitis B, in a proportion of carriers. The severe clinical sequelae of chronic hepatitis B, that is, decompensated cirrhosis and hepatocellular carcinoma, develop in 15–40% of chronic HBV carriers and account for most of the severe morbidity and mortality associated with HBV infection. Consequently, antiviral development programs for HBV infection are focused on treating chronic HBV infection and its associated chronic liver disease. Acute hepatitis B, associated with acute (primary) HBV infection, is most often asymptomatic but can be severe and is occasionally fatal. Most often, however, acute hepatitis B is a self-resolving clinical condition.

From: *Methods in Molecular Medicine, vol. 96: Hepatitis B and D Protocols, volume 2*
Edited by: R. K. Hamatake and J. Y. N. Lau © Humana Press Inc., Totowa, NJ

Many chronic HBV carriers have low-level HBV viremia detectable by polymerase chain reaction (PCR) or other DNA amplification methods, for example, serum HBV DNA levels averaging 2–5 $\log_{10}$ genome copies/mL. Most of these low-level carriers remain healthy with minimal or no liver disease, albeit with a lifelong risk of potentially developing HBV-associated liver disease if HBV replication recrudesces to higher levels ***(1–3)***. In contrast, chronic HBV carriers with persistently high levels of HBV replication—that is, who are HBeAg seropositive and/or have high levels of HBV viremia (e.g., serum HBV DNA levels > 4–6 $\log_{10}$ genomes/mL)—are at risk for developing progressive necroinflammatory liver disease, which can lead to cirrhosis and liver failure or to hepatocellular carcinoma ***(1–7)***. Hence, antiviral development programs for chronic HBV infection usually focus on the subgroup of HBsAg carriers who have the greatest risk for developing severe long-term clinical consequences of HBV infection, that is, patients with established necroinflammatory liver disease (chronic hepatitis B) and persistent high levels of HBV replication, documented by the persistent presence of hepatitis B "e" antigen (HBeAg) and/or levels of HBV DNA in the bloodstream that exceed 4–6 $\log_{10}$ copies/mL ***(1–3)***.

As a disease entity, chronic hepatitis B can be divided into two disease variants: HBeAg-seropositive and HBeAg-seronegative. Persistent high replication of wild-type HBV is associated with persistent detectability of HBeAg in serum. After prolonged HBV infection, usually decades, a proportion of such patients develop HBV genomic variants containing mutations in the precore, core promoter, or core gene regions, by which production of detectable HBeAg is abrogated or reduced below detectable levels ***(1–3,8,9)***. Clinically, such patients may continue to experience progressive liver injury if HBV replication remains at high levels. The phenotype of such patients with chronic "precore mutant" hepatitis B (more correctly called precore/core mutant) comprises variably elevated serum aminotransferases, progressive necroinflammatory changes on liver biopsy, and serum HBV DNA levels which are usually detectable by unamplified hybridization assays (e.g., > 6 $\log_{10}$ copies/mL) but which sometimes dip into the 4–5 $\log_{10}$ copies/mL range, particularly as the disease advances ***(1–3,10)***.

In patients with wild-type (HBeAg-positive) chronic hepatitis B, HBeAg loss and HBeAg seroconversion (HBeAg loss and gain of detectable anti-HBe) comprise a poorly understood transition to a state of substantially lower HBV replication, associated with a multilog reduction in serum HBV DNA, usually to levels below 6 $\log_{10}$ copies/mL, that is, to levels that are typically undetectable in unamplified hybridization assays ***(1–3,11)***. Such HBeAg responses (HBeAg loss or seroconversion) can occur spontaneously, at a rate of 2–15%/yr, depending on age and ethnic group derivation. Because it comprises a usually durable transition to a state of lower HBV replication and decreased liver inflammation, HBeAg loss/seroconversion is usually clinically beneficial if it occurs prior to the development of cirrhosis. As a corollary, one of the principal beneficial effects of antiviral therapy for chronic HBV infection can be to increase the rate of HBeAg loss and seroconversion in patients with HBeAg-positive chronic hepatitis B. However, a note of caution is warranted. HBeAg/loss/seroconversion appears to be immunologically mediated and is often associated with a concurrent "flare" in hepatic disease, signaled by a period of substantial elevations in serum alanine aminotransferase (ALT) levels. Disease “flare” activity, with or without HBeAg loss/seroconversion, can sometimes result in episodes of severe symptomatic liver disease, including hepatic decompensation and occasionally death. Fortunately, at least in patients treated with anti-HBV antivirals, severe disease flares with hepatic decompensation appear to be relatively rare in noncirrhotic patients treated with anti-HBV drugs. In the Phase III trials of lamivudine and adefovir, although a number of patients had ALT flares associated with HBeAg clearance, there were reportedly no fatal disease flares and no flares with hepatic decompensation in these 1-yr trials involving patients with compensated liver disease. Instead, such severe outcomes appear to be more common in patients with advanced underlying liver disease.

The largest clinical experience in treating chronic viral infection is in the field of HIV therapeutics. Many experts familiar with the need for multidrug regimens for the treatment of HIV infection currently consider that combination antiviral therapy may also be needed for optimal treatment of patients with chronic hepatitis B. However, there are several important disease differences in HIV vs HBV infection that need to be considered before prejudging this notion: (1) HIV is cytopathic to its primary target cells (CD4 lymphocytes), while HBV is essentially a noncytopathic virus with a limited tissue tropism compared to HIV; (2) HBV is less resistance prone, as HBV mutability is about 10-fold less than that of HIV during viral replication cycles; (3) intracellular replication templates for HIV (double-stranded DNA integrants) are maintained by cellular DNA polymerases, while the replication templates for HBV (covalently closed circular DNA [cccDNA] episomes) require ongoing HBV polymerase activity for replenishment; (4) HBV infection, even chronic HBV infection, can be self-resolving, with eventual immune clearance in some patients; (5) the liver is probably a more regenerable (more repairable) target organ than the CD4 lymphocyte compartment; and (6) progression to end-stage disease is, on average, significantly slower for HBV infection compared to HIV infection (e.g., 10–40 yr for HBV infection compared to 5–15 yr for HIV). These considerations, and the clinical results from hepatitis B trials with interferon and lamivudine, collectively suggest that, unlike the HIV circumstance, antiviral monotherapy can have substantial clinical value in treating HBV infection. Thus, although clinical investigation of combination regimens for HBV infection will be important, monotherapy regimens may continue to have a role in the treatment of patients with compensated chronic hepatitis B—especially if newer HBV antivirals, with more profound and more sustained suppression of HBV replication, are found to be associated with increased durable response rates in these patients, compared to interferon, lamivudine, and adefovir. On the other hand, it is already apparent that combination regimens need urgent evaluation in HBV patient subgroups for whom durable response rates are low (e.g., patients with precore mutant HBV infection), or in whom the consequences of disease progression due to resistance-associated viral breakthrough can be severe or fatal (e.g., posttransplant patients or patients with decompensated cirrhosis).

Present antiviral therapies for HBV infection have minimal short-term effect on hepatic cccDNA pools, although a recent small-scale study with adefovir suggests that long-term nucleoside/nucleotide therapy (1 yr or more) can be associated with a reduction in cccDNA ***(12)***. Consequently, current therapies do not usually eradicate HBV infection in the early years of treatment, and clinical treatment guidelines generally restrict treatment recommendations to patients with high-level HBV replication and evidence of underlying chronic liver disease, in whom HBV suppression can be clinically beneficial through amelioration of liver disease even when HBV infection is not fully eradicated. Indeed, the fact that long-term durable responses can be achieved in HBeAg seroconverters, despite the persistence of hepatic cccDNA and low-level HBV viremia, argues that virologic "cures" are not necessary for durable clinical responses in hepatitis B patients. Nonetheless, it can also be said that, if HBV therapy becomes more eradicative, that is, if treatment regimens can be derived that result in HBsAg clearance in a large proportion of patients within the first 1–2 yr of therapy, then antiviral therapy could appropriately be used more widely in chronic HBV carriers. Under these circumstances, the issue of treating the "inactive" HBV carrier state (i.e., HBV chronic carriers with normal ALTs and minimal liver disease) could be readdressed in controlled studies.

It is possible that "direct" antivirals (nucleosides/nucleotides) may not afford maximal HBV clearance rates, even when used in combination. Increasing evidence suggests that type I immune responses are important to natural clearance of HBV infection, and may be important for optimal responses to anti-HBV agents. Hence, for optimal rates of durable HBV clearance, it may be necessary to combine direct antiviral agents (i.e., nucleosides/nucleotides) with immunomodulators. This notion will likely remain an important issue in HBV clinical research, and will be more tractably addressed as the science and pharmaceutics of immunomodulation make parallel progress with antiviral pharmaceutics.

Previous clinical development programs for HBV antivirals, including the groundbreaking clinical trial programs conducted with interferon products and with lamivudine, have resulted in clinicians' current ability to clinically manage some patients with chronic hepatitis B, and have provided important insights relevant to the design of clinical trial programs for new HBV antiviral therapeutics. Phase III adefovir data are available only in abstract form as this chapter goes to press, so much of the paradigm for HBV drug development described here will be drawn from the extensively published clinical trial data for interferon and lamivudine. Key observations to consider from the interferon and lamivudine clinical development programs can be summarized as follows.

1.1. Key Insights from Interferon (IFN) Trials and Follow-Up Studies

- Over study periods of 10–24 mo, HBeAg loss and seroconversion (gain of anti-HBe) were significantly more frequent with IFN treatment compared to no treatment, and were associated with generally durable clinical benefits (ALT normalization and longer term histologic improvement), in patients who responded with loss of HBeAg, who comprised a minority of treated patients.
- The major pretreatment factors favorably associated with HBeAg clearance were elevated serum ALT levels (e.g., $\geq$ 2× upper limit of normal [ULN]) and low serum HBV DNA levels (< 200 pg/mL by an unamplified solution hybridization assay) ***(1–3,13)***.
- Some HBeAg-responding patients lost detectable HBsAg, usually months to years after the loss of detectable HBeAg ***(1–3,14)***.
- In association with HBeAg loss/seroconversion, patients' HBV viremia typically dropped to levels of 2–5 $\log_{10}$ copies/mL, similar to the viremia levels found in inactive carriers, and

remained in this low range if the patient remained HBeAg-seroconverted, except in patients in whom loss of HBeAg was caused by the development of precore mutant HBV strains.

- At the time of HBsAg loss, serum HBV DNA usually became nondetectable (even by PCR methods), but HBV DNA remained detectable in patients' livers, probably mostly in the form of cccDNA but perhaps also with some HBV DNA integrants ***(14)***.
- Although still somewhat controversial, it appears likely that therapeutic induction of HBeAg loss/seroconversion in precirrhotic patients is associated with a reduced long-term risk for decompensated cirrhosis ***(15,16)***.
- One retrospective follow-up study suggested a beneficial effect of IFN treatment on the incidence of hepatocellular carcinoma. This observation needs confirmation in additional studies.
- Treatment of HBeAg-negative patients (with precore mutant HBV infection) appeared potentially beneficial, with ALT normalization and histologic responses in some patients, but most responders relapsed after 4–12 mo of IFN treatment ***(17,18)***.
- IFN treatment of patients with decompensated cirrhosis was found to be risky, with some treated patients experiencing leukopenia-related bacterial sepsis and some experiencing disease flares with hepatic decompensation ***(1–3)***.

1.2. Key Insights from the Lamivudine Trials

- Unlike IFN, lamivudine treatment was associated with nearly universal initial virologic responses (HBV DNA reductions), which were variable but averaged about 3 $\log_{10}$ at 1 yr of treatment ***(19–23)***.
- Lamivudine-related suppression of serum HBV DNA levels was consistently associated with significantly more frequent efficacy responses (histologic response, HBeAg loss/seroconversion, ALT normalization) during the first year of treatment, compared to concurrent placebo control groups ***(19,20,23)***.
- HBeAg responses appeared to be equally frequent for lamivudine and IFN 12 mo after initiation of therapy, using a standard (16-wk) course of IFN ***(23,24)***.
- Like IFN, elevated pretreatment ALT level was significantly associated with HBeAg responses to lamivudine treatment ***(24)***.
- Unlike IFN, pretreatment viral load (HBV DNA level) did not appear to significantly influence HBeAg responses to lamivudine, after multivariate adjustment for other pretreatment covariates ***(24)***.
- Tolerance of lamivudine was found to be good, allowing longer term treatment which can be associated with additional cumulative HBeAg responses after the first year ***(25,26)***.
- Like IFN, lamivudine-related HBeAg responses appeared to be durable posttreatment in most (but not all) HBeAg-responding patients, especially if treatment was continued for at least 6–12 mo after HBeAg loss ***(27,28)***.
- Serum ALT normalization and histologic responses were observed when HBV viremia was reduced to levels persistently below 5–6 $\log_{10}$ copies/mL, but HBeAg responses were uncommon unless viremia was reduced to levels persistently below 4 $\log_{10}$ copies/mL ***(22)***.
- While clinical efficacy responses were observable when HBV DNA levels were lowered to 6 $\log_{10}$ or less, HBV resistance (with YMDD-mutant HBV strains) commonly emerged eventually, except in those whose serum HBV DNA levels were brought below 2–3 $\log_{10}$ copies/mL in the first 6 mo of treatment ***(29)***.
- Lamivudine-resistant HBV strains were increasingly detectable by PCR methods in patients after the first 6–8 mo of treatment. After 3 or 4 yr of lamivudine, approx 50–65% of patients had PCR-detectable YMDD-mutant HBV strains, with or without evidence of virologic breakthrough ***(25,26)***.

- Therapeutic responses were variably diminished after the development of lamivudine-resistant HBV strains. Patients who developed YMDD mutants typically had return of HBV DNA levels > 6 $\log_{10}$ copies/mL and recrudescence of elevated ALT levels, although both parameters often remained partially improved compared to pretreatment values, for extended periods ***(19–23,25,26,30)***.
- In the combined Phase III data, patients who developed YMDD mutants reverted to an HBeAg loss/seroconversion rate that was indistinguishable from the HBeAg clearance rate observed in placebo recipients ***(30)***.
- In HBeAg-negative patients (with precore mutant HBV infection), virologic and clinical responses, that is, ALT normalization and histologic responses, were satisfactory in the first year of lamivudine treatment. Thereafter, diminished therapeutic responses were increasingly frequent with the development of YMDD-mutant HBV in many patients, so that a minority of HBeAg-negative patients exhibited continued clinical benefit after 3 yr of treatment ***(18,31)***.
- Lamivudine treatment of patients with decompensated cirrhosis appeared promising with regard to first-year HBV suppression and improvements in liver function in salvageable patients ***(32–35)***. Improvements in hepatic synthetic function (increases in serum albumin) and excretory function (decreases in serum bilirubin) were appreciable within 3–6 mo of initiation of lamivudine therapy. After a period of response, some patients later experienced viral breakthrough, which was occasionally associated with rapid or fatal hepatic disease progression ***(36)***.

The above observations from the clinical trials of interferon and lamivudine provide important background information relevant to clinical trial designs for new anti-HBV therapeutics. Additional important data will soon be available from publication of the Phase III data for adefovir dipivoxil. Clinical and virologic data from these previous trial programs, and other pertinent information in the literature regarding HBV epidemiology and natural history, should be carefully consulted when designing clinical trial programs for anti-HBV therapeutics. In the following discussion, HBV drug development and clinical trial design are organized topically, with selected reference to key publications and sources of data.

2. New HBV Therapeutics: A Changing Window of Opportunity

Before committing substantial resources to a clinical development program for a new anti-HBV agent, it is essential to define clearly the anticipated role for the new agent in the HBV therapeutic armamentarium. Several issues affect the long-term medical and commercial viability of a candidate anti-HBV agent. First, it is crucial to understand how the new agent might address unmet medical needs. The major deficiency of current antiviral therapy for hepatitis B, in both adults and children, is suboptimal sustained response rates. Lifelong suppressive therapy could prove to be beneficial in some patients, but is unrealistic in most regions of the world where HBV is endemic. Hence it would be highly desirable to be able to induce therapeutic responses in the vast majority of patients that could be shown to be durable posttreatment. Other deficiencies of current therapy include inadequate options for managing patients with advanced liver disease, that is, decompensated cirrhosis. Interferon is relatively contraindicated in this patient group, and the benefits of lamivudine are promising but sometimes transient in decompensated patients. Also, for both interferon and lamivudine, HBeAg-negative (precore mutant) hepatitis B has proved to be a special challenge, with suboptimal durable response rates and a clear need for additional options to allow long-term patient management. Other difficult subgroups include patients coinfected with HIV, HCV, or hepatitis delta virus (HDV). The potential role of a new HBV drug candidate for addressing these or other unmet medical needs should be clearly defined at the start of the clinical development program. A useful exercise in this regard is to define the desired product profile for the new agent with regard to efficacy and safety expectations for targeted HBV patient populations, and then to draft the key elements of the desired product label. This project team exercise provides a clear definition of the specific goals for the new agent and provides a framework for the design of the subsequent clinical development program, with relevance for both preclinical and clinical efforts going forward on the project.

In addition to the role of the new agent in addressing unmet medical needs, it is important to assess the commercial goals for the new product, to ensure its viability in the medical marketplace. At present, commercial forecasting for HBV therapeutics remains fraught with difficulty. Because there were no effective treatments for hepatitis B until recently, and because most hepatitis B patients reside in economically developing regions of the world, it is fair to say that the HBV marketplace is relatively unestablished at present. However, because of the presently large number of chronic HBV carriers (about 300–400 million, worldwide), it is apparent that the HBV pharmaceutic market will grow substantially over the next 10–15 yr, before leveling off and perhaps declining due to the eventual beneficial effects of global HBV vaccination programs in reducing the number of new patients with chronic hepatitis B. Market data suggest an approx 20-fold growth in hepatitis B related prescriptions in the first 4 yr following the global regulatory approvals for lamivudine, which bodes well for continued growth in the HBV antiviral marketplace in the next 10–20 yr as therapy gets better and better and world economies grow. It should therefore be apparent that the commercial viability of any new anti-HBV product is likely to depend on a global development and marketing approach, especially including Asia and other developing regions of the world. HBV clinical trial programs should be designed to prominently include patients from HBV-endemic regions with growing economies and adequate intellectual property laws.

Finally, before undertaking a detailed discussion of HBV drug development issues, a note of caution is warranted for the undertaking of new HBV research and development programs. In view of the HBV drug candidates currently in clinical trials, it is likely that by 2008 there will be three or four new regulatory-approved antiviral drugs (nucleosides/nucleotides, and possibly new interferons) for treating HBV infection, in addition to the current armamentarium of interferon-α (IFN-α), lamivudine, and adefovir. One or more of the new drugs may prove to be as safe and well tolerated as lamivudine, and by that time there may be supportive evidence for treatment regimens that are more effective than the current armamentarium—either monotherapy regimens or combination regimens. Consequently, any new drug candidates beyond those currently approved or in development will need to have well-defined expectations with regard to efficacy improvements. Conceivably, more profound antiviral effects from new nucleoside regimens will be sufficient to achieve substantially better HBV clearance than is currently feasible with interferon or lamivudine alone. It is worth noting that a recent retrospective analysis of clinical data suggested that reducing HBV viremia to nondetectable levels (by PCR) in the first 6–12 mo of treatment may be associated with early clearance of serum HBsAg, the ultimate predictor of probable long-term therapeutic benefit ***(37)***. However, it may also be the case that optimal HBV inhibition will require new drug candidates with unique mechanisms of action—for example, to provide more eradicative effects on cccDNA and better eradication of HBV-infected cells, through enhanced antiviral effects or through immunomodulatory mechanisms.

3. General Issues in Clinical Trial Design for HBV Drug Candidates

The following discussion primarily addresses issues related to the design of Phase II and III clinical trials of new HBV drug candidates, after a brief comment on Regulatory and Phase I (clinical pharmacology) issues. In this discussion, it is assumed that all future HBV clinical trials should be conducted to Good Clinical Practice (GCP) standards.

3.1. Regulatory Considerations

Because the majority of hepatitis B patients are in developing regions of the world, particularly Asian countries, a global approach is usually desirable for HBV clinical trial programs. Internationally agreed standards and guidelines for clinical development programs have been promulgated by the International Conference on Harmonization of Technical Requirements for Registration of Pharmaceuticals for Human Use, an international regulatory collaboration commonly known as "ICH." The ICH guidelines have clarified and partially standardized the scientific requirements for international drug development, and offer a chance for streamlining of clinical trial programs and multinational regulatory submissions through guidelines for clinical trial design and for a standardized submission format for clinical data known as the Common Technical Document (CTD). The original signatories to the ICH agreements (the United States, Europe, Japan) have fully committed to adhering to ICH recommendations. Also, many other (nonsignatory) countries have indicated their intent to recognize ICH standards and allow final data submissions in the CTD format, including several countries in Asia that are important for hepatitis B development programs. However, despite regulatory progress with the international adoption of ICH guidelines and standards, there can still be significant local variation in regulatory processes and requirements, both for clinical data submissions and for CMC (chemistry, manufacturing, and controls) issues. It is therefore essential that HBV pharmaceutic development teams include expertise in international regulatory affairs.

3.2. Phase I: Clinical Pharmacology Issues

Because hepatitis B is endemic in regions of the world where access to specialized medical care is often limited, it is highly desirable that HBV therapeutics have good oral bioavailability and good safety profiles, allowing simple outpatient management and minimal safety concerns for patients between clinic visits. If effective, safe, orally bioavailable alternatives are available, parenterally administered agents, especially those requiring frequent dosing and/or close patient monitoring for toxicities, are not likely to achieve widespread medical acceptance in areas of the world where chronic HBV infection is endemic.

To allow safe and effective use in all stages of liver disease, it is desirable that there be minimal or no hepatic metabolism of therapeutic agents for hepatitis B, and that they be primarily renally cleared rather than hepatically cleared. Also, because hepatorenal syndromes are common with decompensated liver disease, it is important to establish whether a renally cleared drug accumulates under conditions of renal insufficiency, and whether dose modifications may therefore be advisable in patients with renal insufficiency. These comments apply to many (but not all) nucleosides/nucleotides, which tend to be renally cleared, usually with minimal hepatic metabolism.

When designing dosing regimens for antiviral agents, it is desirable that systemic drug levels remain above the inhibitory concentrations (IC_{50} or IC_{90}) at which the agent has been demonstrated to inhibit virus replication in vitro. Many nucleoside or nucleotide agents have long intracellular half-lives (as triphosphates), and many have prolonged systemic elimination kinetics with a long terminal elimination half-life. Such agents can be conveniently used in once-daily dosing regimens while continuously maintaining viral-suppressive drug levels.

Other specific pharmacology issues include potential drug interaction issues, which are particularly important for HBV patient subgroups that may be treated with multiple concurrent medications, such as HIV-coinfected patients and liver transplant recipients. In the organ transplant setting and under other circumstances where glucocorticoid medications are routinely used (e.g., severe asthma and autoimmune disease), it is worth keeping in mind that the HBV genome has a steroid-responsive element, and commonly used glucocorticoids (such as prednisone and methylprednisolone) can induce higher levels of HBV replication. Finally, as the HBV therapeutic armamentarium expands, it will be important to conduct studies investigating potential drug interactions with other HBV antivirals, anticipating the possible use of new HBV drug candidates in combination regimens with other anti-HBV drugs. At present, for example, it would be appropriate to conduct drug interaction studies for new HBV drug candidates with IFN-α, lamivudine, adefovir, and possibly transplant-related immunosuppressive medicines such as cyclosporine and tacrolimus.

The following discussion addresses considerations in the design of Phase II and III trials for new candidate anti-HBV agents.

3.3. Patient Populations for Study

To date, HBV clinical development programs have primarily focused on assessing treatment in adults with chronic hepatitis B and compensated liver disease, a decades-long disease phase that precedes severe morbidity and mortality by many years, on average. Such patients have appreciable underlying necroinflammatory liver disease but are typically noncirrhotic, asymptomatic, or minimally (nonspecifically) symptomatic, and can safely be enrolled in long-term treatment studies (e.g., for trial periods of 1–2 yr, or possibly more), without substantial risk of severe morbidity or mortality during the study periods. For example, among more than 900 adult patients with compensated

HBeAg-seropositive chronic hepatitis B enrolled in four 1-yr Phase III lamivudine trials, there were no deaths and no episodes of hepatic decompensation during the 1-yr study periods for any of the subjects, including the 200 placebo recipients ***(19,20,23,30)***. In contrast, patients with more advanced disease stages (e.g., decompensated cirrhosis) can exhibit clinical disease progession, with severe morbidity or mortality, over relatively short time frames ***(4–7)***.

The pathogenesis of HBV-associated liver disease—that is, a progressive necroinflammatory response quantitatively related to the level of ongoing HBV replication in the liver—is similar in both HBeAg-positive and HBeAg-negative chronic hepatitis B, and the therapeutic goals are similar in both patient groups, that is, durable abrogation of HBV replication to ameliorate the necroinflammatory liver disease. Thus "combined" trial designs can be envisaged in which both HBeAg-positive and -negative patients with chronic hepatitis B are enrolled as a single trial population, prestratified for HBeAg status to facilitate secondary efficacy analyses of subgroup-specific efficacy endpoints. Traditionally, however, the two patient subgroups have been studied separately, for example, in the clinical trial programs for interferon, lamivudine, and adefovir.

A list of suggested entry criteria for Phase II–III trials, defining eligible adult patients with compensated chronic hepatitis B, is given in **Table 1**. Minor variations of these inclusion and criteria are apparent in the key controlled trials of interferon, lamivudine, and adefovir.

Note that entry criteria for Phase II trials do not necessarily require elevated serum aminotransferase levels, since the principal goals of Phase II antiviral trials are usually to assess dose-related antiviral effects (HBV DNA reductions) rather than clinical efficacy endpoints. Conversely, at the present time, Phase III trials should include only patients with elevated ALTs and substantial underlying liver disease, unless a new agent has preclinical data and Phase I–II clinical data supporting a novel HBV-eradicative effect that might be clinically beneficial in inactive HBV carriers.

Trial entry criteria for evidence of HBV replication typically require pretreatment serum HBV DNA levels of 5–6 $\log_{10}$ copies/mL. Results from numerous clinical studies indicate that patients with untreated HBeAg-seropositive chronic hepatitis B typically have HBV viremia levels in the range of 6–10 $\log_{10}$ copies/mL, averaging 8–9 $\log_{10}$ at study entry ***(13,19–23)***. Consequently, an inclusion criterion of serum HBV DNA $> 6 \log_{10}$ is most often used in current clinical trials for patients with HBeAg-positive chronic hepatitis B. Literature reports suggest somewhat lower average HBV DNA levels in untreated but histologically active HBeAg-negative chronic hepatitis B, averaging about 1 $\log_{10}$ lower than viremia levels in HBeAg-positive patients, perhaps related to the generally more advanced liver disease in HBeAg-negative patients ***(3,10,38)***. Consequently, an entry HBV DNA level of 5 or 6 $\log_{10}$ copies/mL is appropriate for clinical trials in HBeAg-negative patients. A cautionary note is that, at HBV DNA levels of about 5 $\log_{10}$ copies/mL, the patient population with histologically active, HBeAg-negative chronic hepatitis B can overlap with the inactive HBV carrier population, in whom HBV viremia is typically 2–5 $\log_{10}$ copies/mL. Therefore in such patients it is important to document, at study entry, elevated ALT levels and significant chronic inflammation on liver biopsies.

After establishing a preliminary safety profile and determining the preferred dose of a new anti-HBV agent in Phase I–II trials, the goals of Phase III trials are to provide adequate and well-controlled data regarding efficacy and safety of the new agent in the primary patient population targeted for product labeling. In designing Phase III trials for anti-HBV agents, the critical trial design dilemma is the imperfect correlation between antiviral effects (HBV DNA reductions) measured in Phase I–II trials and the clinically relevant endpoints to be measured in Phase III controlled trials. This issue is further addressed below in the efficacy endpoints discussion.

3.5. Observation Periods in Phase III Trials

As noted earlier, Phase III trials have typically been conducted in populations of chronic hepatitis B patients with compensated liver disease, in whom a prolonged period of treatment benefit should be demonstrated in light of the expected long period of minimally symptomatic disease prior to the development of decompensated cirrhosis or hepatocellular carcinoma. Early registration trials with interferons typically included treatment periods of 4–6 mo, with posttreatment observation periods of 6–12 mo. Phase III trials with lamivudine utilized a 1-yr treatment period with 3- to 4-mo follow-up periods, and Phase III trials with adefovir, currently ongoing, utilize a 2-yr study period with an interim analysis after 1 yr. Therefore, while ALT normalization and histologic improvements can be seen with effective antiviral treatments within 4–6 mo, previous antiviral registration programs for hepatitis B have set an important precedent, to the effect that, in patients with compensated liver disease, clinical benefit for new anti-HBV agents should be demonstrated for at least one year or more. Indeed, because of the previously demonstrated possibilities of diminished benefit due to viral resistance or post-treatment relapse of an HBV replicative state, it is currently desirable that pivotal trials for new agents demonstrate longer periods of clinical benefit, for example, 2 yr or more. For efficient registration, it may be desirable for the initial clinical dossier to be constructed on the basis of an analysis of first-year data, but the trial program should subsequently proceed to gather controlled efficacy and safety data for 2 yr or more. In addition, Phase IIIb–IV follow-on trials for lamivudine and adefovir are providing open-label extended-treatment data for reenrolled Phase III patients, to 5–6 yr of total treatment.

If controlled Phase III trials were to be conducted in patients with decompensated liver disease, trial observation periods in principal could be somewhat shorter (6–12 mo), as improvements in clinical endpoints (Child–Turcotte–Pugh scores, albumin and bilirubin levels, etc.) reflecting improved hepatic function are immediately beneficial to these patients. However, decompensated patients are more difficult to accrue in large numbers, and the high frequency of expected adverse events in these patients (related to their hepatic decompensation) can confound the safety profile of new anti-HBV drug candidates. Hence, trials in decompensated patients should be approached with caution, and should be initiated only after sufficient preliminary safety data have been gathered. More discussion of conducting clinical trials in hepatitis B patients with decompensated liver disease is offered below.

Table 1
Key Entry Criteria for Phase II and III Trials in Patients with Compensated Chronic Hepatitis B

Inclusion criteria
- Age: Typically 18–65 (or 70) yr
- Male or female
- Medical history compatible with chronic hepatitis B
- HBsAg seropositive at Screen
  - Some protocols require documented HBsAg+ more than 6 mo; not necessary if patient has recent liver biopsy compatible with chronic hepatitis B
- HBeAg seropositive at Screen (if this is the target population)
- Serum HBV DNA:
  - $> 6 \log_{10}$ copies/mL for HBeAg-positive patients
  - > 5 or $6 \log_{10}$ copies/mL for HBeAg-negative ("pre-core mutant") patients
- Serum ALT levels
  - $< 10\times$ ULN, for Phase II studies (normal ALTs allowed)
  - > 1.2, >1.3, >1.5, or $> 2\times$ ULN *and* $< 10\times$ ULN, for Phase III studies
- Pretreatment liver biopsy compatible with chronic hepatitis B
  - Desirable for Phase III studies
- Willing and able to give informed consent

Exclusion criteria
- Coinfection with hepatitis C virus (HCV), hepatitis D virus (HDV), or HIV
- Previous antiviral therapy for hepatitis B (if target population is treatment-naïve)
  - Previous failure to interferon therapy is OK if no interferon in past 12 mo
- Concurrent medical condition that requires prolonged or frequent systemic corticosteroids
- Concurrent medical condition that requires prolonged or frequent acyclovir or famciclovir (e.g., for recurrent herpes virus infections, etc.), which can be defined as treatment with these agents for periods exceeding 10 d every 3 mo, or chronic suppressive therapy.
- History of signs of hepatic insufficiency: ascites, variceal bleeding, hepatic encephalopathy, spontaneous bacterial peritonitis, or other signs of hepatic decompensation.
- History of clinical pancreatitis
- History of hepatocellular carcinoma (HCC) or findings suggestive of possible HCC
  - If patient has suspicious foci on imaging studies or elevated serum α-fetoprotein (AFP) level, HCC should be ruled out prior to consideration for study
  - Currently abusing alcohol or illicit drugs, or has a history of alcohol or substance abuse within the preceding 3 years

Patient has one or more additional known primary or secondary causes of liver disease.
  - Gilbert's syndrome and Dubin–Johnson syndrome, two benign disorders associated with low-grade hyberbilirubinemia, should not disqualify patients.
  - Any concurrent medical condition likely to preclude compliance with the schedule of evaluations in the protocol, or likely to confound efficacy or safety observations. History of treated malignancy (other than HCC) is allowable if the patient's malignancy has been in complete remission off chemotherapy and without additional surgical interventions during the preceding 3 yr.
- Abnormal laboratory values at Screen:
  - Hemoglobin < 11 g/dL for men or < 10 g/dL for women
  - Total WBC count $< 3000/\text{mm}^3$ or absolute neutrophil count (ANC) $< 1500/\text{mm}^3$

continued

Table 1 (continued)
Key Entry Criteria for Phase II and III Trials in Patients with Compensated Chronic Hepatitis B

Platelet count < 75,000/mm^3
Elevated serum creatinine
Serum amylase or lipase ⩾ 1.5 × ULN
Low serum albumin (e.g., < 3.5 g/dL)
Total bilirubin ⩾ 2.0 mg/dL
Prothrombin time prolonged by more than 3 s despite vitamin K administration

3.4. Phase II and III Trial Goals

Phase II trials typically focus on assessments of optimal dosing and the generation of preliminary efficacy and safety data, in the patient population(s) targeted for Phase III registration trials. It is therefore desirable that Phase II patient populations should be similar to the expected Phase III population, with minor exceptions in inclusion/exclusion criteria for expediencies. Depending on the amount of existing human exposure data prior to the first Phase I–II study in patients, dose-ranging trials can be conducted with a true dose-escalation study design if previous human data are minimal, or in parallel dosing cohorts if preliminary safety is established by earlier Phase I studies or use of the agent in other patient populations. In either case, it is highly desirable that Phase I–II dosing studies be conducted in a randomized fashion, including some placebo patients within each dosing cohort. In general, Phase I–II dose cohorts in HBV trials should each have at least 6–20 subjects. With nucleoside/nucleotide agents, observed HBV DNA reductions can exhibit significant interpatient variation and can appear somewhat truncated in patients with relatively low pretreatment HBV DNA levels (e.g., < 7 $\log_{10}$ copies/mL). Thus, reasonable-sized dose cohorts are required, to avoid misleading dose–response results resulting from baseline imbalances in viral load and interpatient variation in response within dose cohorts.

Because Phase I–II studies are usually of short duration, serologic responses are generally the primary efficacy assessments in such studies. Serum HBV DNA reductions are typically the primary efficacy assessment in Phase I–II studies, although serum ALT normalization can be assessed in a preliminary fashion in Phase II studies with treatment periods of 3 mo or more. A note of caution: spontaneous HBeAg responses can occur in the first 3–6 mo of treatment in Phase II–III trials and should not be assumed to be treatment related. Such patients typically have low quantitative levels of HBeAg and relatively high ALT levels on study entry. Further discussion of HBV DNA response patterns and HBeAg responses is given below. Safety assessments in Phase II trials enrolling compensated hepatitis B patients include routine monitoring of hematologic parameters, routine serum chemistries, urinalyses (at limited time points), and any assessments that may be appropriate parameters for monitoring with respect to known potential toxicities of the investigational agent. Recommendations for Phase II efficacy and safety assessments are summarized in **Table 2**, and further discussion of efficacy and safety parameters is offered in the Phase III-related discussion below.

Table 2
Phase II and III Efficacy Assessments in Patients with Compensated Chronic Hepatitis B

- Phase II (or Phase I/II) Efficacy Assessments
  - Serum HBV DNA levels
    - Treatment-period changes in mean/median values
    - Proportions of patients who achieve HBV DNA reductions to various levels
      - To HBV viremia levels of 5 $\log_{10}$, 4 $\log_{10}$, and 3 $\log_{10}$ copies/mL
      - To PCR-nondetectable levels
    - Posttreatment changes in mean/median values
    - Assessments of virologic breakthrough to "clinically significant" levels
      - For example, to levels $> 5 \log_{10}$ or $> 6 \log_{10}$ copies/mL
      - Usually not necessary if treatment < 6 mo
  - Serum HBeAg and HBeAb
    - Assess at Screen, Baseline, and serially after 2–3 mo of treatment
  - Serum HBsAg and HBsAb
    - Assess at Screen, Baseline, and serially after 3–6 mo of treatment
  - Serum ALT levels
    - Changes in mean/median values during treatment and posttreatment
    - Proportion of patients with "ALT normalization" at each study visit
      - patients with ALT $\leq$ ULN whose ALT was $>$ULN at Baseline
    - ALT normalization not common until at least 2–3 mo of treatment

- Phase III Efficacy Assessments
  - All of the above, plus histologic response if required
    - Assess histologic scoring changes in paired liver biopsies
      - For example, 2-point (or greater) reductions in Knodell necroinflammatory score (sum of first three components of Knodell HAI score)
      - Fibrosis changes assessed by slide-ranking method and/or by scoring
        - pretreatment biopsy should be within 12 mo prior to start of treatment, with no intervening additional treatment
      - Follow-up biopsy usually stipulated for 1 yr; longer if possible

4. Efficacy Endpoints for Phase II and III Trials

This section focuses on a discussion of the various efficacy endpoints that are appropriate for study in hepatitis B clinical trials, and methodologic issues for these efficacy assessments. A discussion of trial design issues, including the choice of primary vs secondary efficacy endpoints, is presented later in this chapter.

4.1. Antiviral Responses (HBV DNA Reductions)

Antiviral responses in HBV clinical trials are measured as reductions in serum HBV DNA from pretreatment (baseline) levels. Earlier trials typically used unamplified hybridization assays for HBV DNA, which detected HBV viremia levels greater than 5–6 $\log_{10}$ copies/mL. Current HBV trials generally utilize more sensitive HBV DNA assays, utilizing DNA amplification methods (e.g., PCR or branched-chain amplification). Earlier literature reports and recent expert consensus publications support the notion that, in most HBV carriers, serum HBV DNA levels below 5–6 $\log_{10}$ copies/mL or so may not be clinically significant, as such low levels are usually not associated with a risk for progressive liver disease, except perhaps in cirrhotic patients. Hence in clinical practice unamplified assays for HBV DNA may be adequate for diagnostic purposes and for most patient monitoring purposes. However, in clinical trials it is desirable to assess the full range of changes in HBV DNA levels by using sensitive methods (e.g., PCR-based assays), as analyses of the quantitative degree of HBV suppression may prove to have relevance to eventual clinical efficacy observations and to the evolution of drug-resistant HBV variants.

Analytically, serum HBV DNA reductions are usually assessed as mean and median changes for each treatment group, with variance measures. Comparative treatment effects can also be assessed as a difference in average means (DAVG) of HBV DNA levels (or HBV DNA reductions) over a defined treatment period, or a conceptually similar approach termed AUCMB (area under the curve minus baseline) in which, for a given treatment group, the time-related area under the viral load curve is approximated by the use of trapezoidal rules. The DAVG and AUCMB methods allow sensitive comparisons of time-weighted average antiviral effects between treatment groups, requiring relatively low cohort sizes for statistically significant comparisons in Phase II dosing-cohort studies. However, this approach is not advisable for comparison of antiviral effects in Phase III studies, where the clinical focus is on the depth and duration of HBV suppression for each treatment group, with the most important timepoints for intergroup comparisons being the end-of-treatment and end-of-study visits, rather than a comparison of time-weighted average effects.

In addition to quantitative analyses of HBV DNA reductions, in Phase II or III clinical trials a categorical HBV DNA response can be defined, using the "one-point" or "two-point" methods. A two-point categorical HBV DNA response definition was utilized in the lamivudine trials, by which a patient was said to have achieved HBV DNA response if he or she had a detectable HBV DNA value at baseline and had undetectable HBV DNA levels (in an unamplified hybridization assay) on at least two consecutive post-baseline study visits. In the present era of sensitive, quantitative PCR-based assays, using the two recent consensus publications cited above a definition of HBV DNA response could be adopted to require the achievement of two consecutive HBV DNA levels below 5 $\log_{10}$ in a patient who had a baseline level $> 6 \log_{10}$ copies/mL ***(2,3)***. However, categorical response definitions for HBV DNA alone are somewhat arbitrary and are not necessarily advisable. If a categorical HBV DNA response definition is elected, it is desirable to analyze the proportions of patients exhibiting that response to the end of treatment, termed "maintained" response, and the proportion of patients exhibiting the response to the last posttreatment visit, termed "sustained" response. Rather than extensive analyses of arbitrary categorical response definitions for HBV DNA changes, however, it may be wiser to simply assess treatment groups with regard to mean/median HBV DNA reductions at key time points, on-treatment and posttreatment. In addition, because there may be "threshold effects" with regard to the relationship between HBV DNA suppression and clinical efficacy endpoints, it is desir-

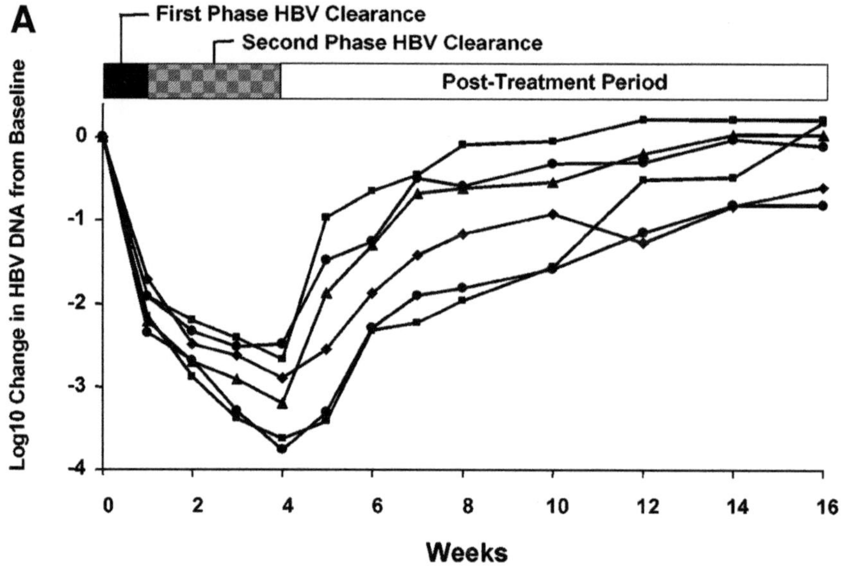

Fig. 1 HBV viral dynamics under antiviral therapy. **(A)** Typical pattern of early virologic response to potent anti-HBV therapy of short duration. Depicted here are results of a study with a 4-wk treatment period and a 12-wk posttreatment follow-up period. With highly active antivirals, serum HBV DNA reductions are rapid and steep during "first-phase" HBV clearance, that is, during the first week or two of treatment. HBV DNA reductions then become more gradual and more heterogeneous among different patients during "second-phase" HBV clearance. First-phase HBV clearance is thought to reflect the net result of catabolism of circulating HBV templates and inhibition of new HBV DNA replication from existing HBV templates. Slower second-phase clearance is thought to reflect the net result of continued inhibition of HBV replication and a gradual reduction in the number of HBV-infected cells. Consistent with this notion, as depicted in this figure, posttreatment return of HBV DNA levels is inversely proportional to the depth of observed second-phase HBV clearance, that is, patients with more profound second-phase clearance during treatment exhibit a slower post-treatment return to pretreatment HBV DNA levels.

able to analyze the proportions of patients achieving HBV DNA levels below 5 $\log_{10}$, below 4 $\log_{10}$, below 3 $\log_{10}$, and undetectable levels (by PCR) for each treatment group at key timepoints.

In hepatitis B patients, treatment-related changes in serum HBV DNA levels typically exhibit a biphasic pattern during the first 3–6 mo of treatment, illustrated in **Fig. 1**. After initiation of potent anti-HBV therapy there is usually an initial rapid drop in serum HBV DNA level in the first week or two, termed "first phase clearance," followed by a more gradual reduction in subsequent weeks, termed "second phase clearance." Second phase clearance can be quite heterogeneous. In this "viral dynamics" perspective, it is thought that the HBV DNA drop in the first phase reflects inhibition of HBV

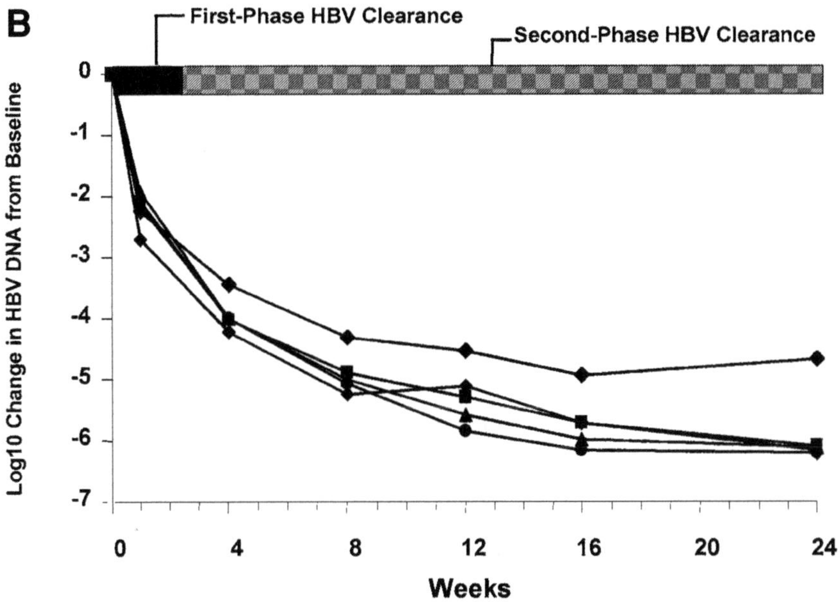

Fig. 1 *(continued)* **(B)** Typical pattern of virologic response to longer term anti-HBV therapy. Depicted here are results of 24 wk treatment. With potent nucleoside and nucleotide antivirals, approx 50–75% of the total 6-mo viral load reduction occurs in the first 4–8 wk of therapy, and the slope of second-phase HBV clearance becomes continuously more gradual during the first 6 mo of treatment, sometimes approaching a horizontal asymptote. One patient, exhibiting distinctly less virologic response during the early months of treatment, has started to show evidence of increasing viral load and may have developed drug-resistant HBV. Second-phase clearance is often more heterogeneous than is depicted here. Thus, improved second-phase HBV clearance remains a major goal for anti-HBV therapy.

replication from existing HBV genomic templates, while the continued drop in the second phase reflects a net reduction in the number of HBV-infected cells ***(39–41)***. With viral dynamics mathematical modeling, first-phase clearance is quantitatively reflected in the estimated half-life of HBV virions, and second-phase clearance is reflected in the estimated half-life of HBV-infected cells ***(39–41)***. For anti-HBV drugs that lack dose-limiting toxicities, both Emax modeling and analyses of serum HBV DNA changes using viral dynamics modeling can be helpful in Phase II dose-optimization, particularly when all tested doses are quite active ***(42,43)***. When all doses or treatment regimens tested are highly active in the first week or two of treatment, dose- or treatment-related increments in antiviral effect can be assessed further by comparisons of second-phase HBV DNA clearance, for example, during the period of time extending to 12–24 wk of treatment.

It is crucial that, in Phase I–II trials and particularly for Phase III registration trials, serum HBV DNA assays should be performed only at reliable central reference laboratories. At the time of this writing, commercially available diagnostic assays for

HBV DNA have varying amounts of supportive validation data, but the assays are poorly cross-standardized and none are FDA-approved. Also, none of the current HBV DNA assays is capable of the ideal 9- to 10-log linear performance range for quantitating HBV DNA levels—that is, levels in the range of 2–12 $\log_{10}$ copies/mL. Therefore, while the better assays are reasonably reliable for relative quantitation of HBV viremia within a given trial population, extreme caution is warranted when comparing results across different trials, particularly if a different assay or different laboratory is utilized in the trials being compared. Hopefully these issues of poor assay cross-standardization and suboptimal dynamic range will be alleviated in the next few years.

While serum HBV DNA reductions are usually the primary efficacy assessment in Phase I–II trials of anti-HBV agents, few regulatory bodies will accept HBV DNA reduction as a primary efficacy endpoint for Phase III registration trials, due to the imperfect (or inadequately established) correlation between serum HBV DNA changes and clinical benefit. Consequently, other efficacy endpoints with more established clinical relevance are generally utilized in Phase III hepatitis B trials—that is, HBeAg loss/seroconversion, HBsAg loss/seroconversion, ALT normalization, and histologic response. These clinically relevant Phase III endpoints are described below.

4.2. HBV e-Antigen Responses

As noted above, in patients with HBeAg-positive chronic hepatitis B, HBeAg loss and HBeAg seroconversion (loss of HBeAg with gain of detectable anti-HBe) are considered to be clinically beneficial, at least in precirrhotic patients, because they are usually associated with durable transition to a state of reduced HBV replication and subsequently reduced risk for progressive liver disease. Also, after documentation of persistent HBeAg loss/seroconversion, patients with compensated liver disease can often be discontinued from antiviral therapy and observed periodically thereafter for signs of virologic or clinical disease reactivation ***(1–3,20,21,27,28)***. Hence, in HBeAg-positive patients, HBeAg response (loss or seroconversion) is a key clinical efficacy endpoint, and is the only efficacy endpoint with a demonstrated predictive value for improved long-term patient outcomes ***(1–3,14–16)***. At present most clinical experts and regulatory bodies regard HBeAg responses and histologic responses as the two most important efficacy endpoints to measure in Phase III registration trials of new anti-HBV therapeutics in patients with compensated liver disease.

Experience with HBV antivirals indicates that, in a typical population of adults with HBeAg-positive chronic hepatitis B, treatment-related clearance of HBeAg does not begin to become readily appreciable until the second half of the first year of treatment ***(24)***. HBeAg loss in the first 6 mo of treatment is variable and often reflects spontaneous HBeAg clearance. Reliable intergroup assessment of HBeAg responses therefore requires Phase III treatment periods of at least 1 yr and substantial numbers of patients in each treatment group.

HBeAg responses can be measured in several ways: as HBeAg loss alone, as HBeAg seroconversion, and as HBeAg loss or seroconversion coupled with additional documentation of suppressed HBV DNA levels (e.g., HBeAg loss or seroconversion linked with serum HBV DNA < 5 $\log_{10}$ copies/mL). The featured HBeAg response endpoint in early interferon trials was simple HBeAg loss, while later interferon trials utilized a composite endpoint of HBeAg loss coupled with HBV DNA nondetectability in an unamplified hybridization assay ***(44,45)***. The Phase III lamivudine trials featured a three-component HBeAg response endpoint, comprising loss of HBeAg, gain of anti-HBe, and HBV DNA nondetectable by the unamplified hybridization assay ***(19–21)***. Recent adefovir trials have featured HBeAg seroconversion without a concurrent measure of HBV DNA suppression, which was assessed separately as a secondary endpoint ***(38,46)***.

The divergent approaches to defining HBeAg response have produced a muddled scientific literature on HBV therapeutics, resulting in quantitatively varying estimates for what should be the same biologic phenomenon, that is, the achievement of a therapeutic response that will potentially be durable posttreatment. What are the minimal parameters needed to define a potentially durable HBeAg response? Loss of detectable HBeAg may by itself be adequate, in patients at low risk for evolution of precore mutant HBV infection. In the Phase III lamivudine experience, at 1 yr 92% of patients with HBeAg loss also had nondetectable HBV DNA in the unamplified hybridization assay, and most of the rest had relatively low HBV DNA levels (e.g., several million copies/mL). Furthermore, during the protocol-mandated no-treatment follow-up periods of 12–16 wk, the posttreatment durability of such responses was similar regardless of whether patients had detectable anti-HBe antibody, that is, regardless of whether the patients had fully seroconverted ***(47)***. These data suggest that the documentation of detectable anti-HBe may not be clinically important with regard to posttreatment durability of HBeAg response. However, utilization of HBeAg loss alone as the primary HBeAg response assessment is probably not prudent in the era of global clinical trials, in which many patients (especially from southern Europe and Southeast Asia) will be at risk for the development of precore mutant HBV infection. Patients with precore mutant HBV infection can appear to have HBeAg-seroconverted, yet can have significant levels of ongoing HBV replication (generally with HBV DNA > 4–5 $\log_{10}$ copies/mL) and can experience progressive liver disease ***(8–10,18)***. Hence, probably the most prudent HBeAg response assessment for HBV registration trials is loss of HBeAg coupled with documentation of serum HBV DNA suppression to levels below 5 $\log_{10}$ copies/mL. This composite (two-component) HBeAg response definition has been recently endorsed by an NIH consensus panel and in a Practice Guideline promulgated by the American Association for the Study of Liver Diseases (AASLD) ***(2,3)***. In these publications, this recommended two-component HBeAg response definition has been termed "Virologic Response" and is qualitatively similar to the primary efficacy endpoint utilized in the earlier registration trials for IFN-α-2b ***(13,45)***. To remove the quandary of variable HBeAg response assessments across different clinical trial programs, this two-component "Virologic Response" definition can be recommended as the primary HBeAg response assessment for future clinical trial programs involving HBeAg-positive patients, although program sponsors and clinical investigators may want to continue to collect data regarding anti-HBe antibody detectability for further assessments of HBeAg loss vs HBeAg seroconversion, and to allow comparisons of new trial results with results from previous development programs.

4.3. HBsAg/Antibody (Ab) Responses

As chronic HBV carriers, all hepatitis B trial patients should be HBsAg seropositive at study entry. Some will also be concurrently seropositive for HBsAb, usually reflecting either (past or present) coinfection with heterotypic HBV species or assay artifact, that is, dissociation of HBsAg–Ab complexes under assay conditions. The concurrent serodetectability of HBsAg and HBsAb does not usually represent ongoing HBsAg seroconversion, and is highly unlikely to be so in patients who are seropositive for HBeAg or have high-level HBV viremia.

Some patients responding to antiviral therapy will eventually lose detectable HBsAg and may gain detectable HBeAb, usually months or years after HBeAg loss/seroconversion and after prolonged reduction in HBV replication. Low-level peripheral HBV viremia (i.e., PCR-detectable levels of serum HBV DNA) tends to persist after HBeAg clearance, but usually disappears after HBsAg loss/seroconversion ***(1–3,14)***. Of note, the liver may remain positive for PCR-detectable HBV DNA even after HBsAg seroconversion and disappearance of detectable HBV DNA from the peripheral blood ***(2,3,14)***. Some of this residual hepatic HBV DNA may comprise integrated HBV genomes, but in most patients this HBV DNA is likely to largely reflect residual hepatic cccDNA, with a potential for future reactivation of HBV infection under conditions of immunosuppression or debilitation. In the lamivudine and interferon trials, HBsAg loss was rare in Asian patients and was evident in only 3–10% of Western patients in the first year of treatment, but was observed months or years later in up to 40–70% of HBeAg-responders in follow-up studies. Therefore, it is not necessary to follow HBsAg serostatus closely at early study visits. Rather, HBsAg serostatus can be evaluated periodically beginning 3–12 mo after initiation of treatment, or it can be evaluated as a reflex assessment in patients who have exhibited HBeAg loss (wild-type HBV infection) or prolonged HBV DNA suppression (in patients with precore mutant HBV infection).

4.4. Serum ALT Normalization

Persistently (albeit variably) elevated serum aminotransferase levels are typically found in patients with chronic hepatitis B, reflecting the patients' underlying chronic necroinflammatory liver disease. Hepatitis B patients' ALT and AST levels will sometimes spontaneously dip into the normal range for awhile, a phenomenon that becomes increasingly common with advanced cirrhosis; and conversely, ALT levels can range very high during periods of disease "flare" activity. While liver biopsies provide better information regarding the grade and stage of HBV-associated histologic activity, serum aminotransferase levels are easily monitored in the clinic and provide a convenient means for indirectly assessing the patient's underlying hepatic necroinflammatory activity over time. Consequently, serum aminotransferase levels are an important monitoring tool in clinical trials. Serum ALT levels are a more specific indicator of hepatic disease activity, while AST levels include isoenzyme components contributed by other body tissues; hence ALT is usually chosen as the primary aminotransferase monitoring tool in hepatitis trials.

Elevated ALT levels reflect patients' ongoing immune responses to their HBV infection. The level of ALT abnormality chosen as the trial entry criterion is an important choice, as experience in multiple HBV clinical trials has repeatedly indicated that entry ALT level directly influences patients' propensity to achieve HBeAg loss/seroconversion with antiviral treatment ***(1–3,13,24)***. In patients with low or normal ALT levels, HBeAg response rates are low and can be similar in drug-treated patients and placebo recipients. Interferon trials have typically utilized an entry requirement that pretreatment ALT level should be at least 1.5–2.0 × ULN, while the lamivudine Phase III trials required entry ALT > 1.3 × ULN and the adefovir trials required entry ALT >1.2 × ULN. Recent expert consensus panels do not recommend antiviral treatment for patients with ALT levels below 1.5–2.0 × ULN unless there is histologic evidence of substantial disease activity. Hence at this time a reasonable choice for an ALT entry criterion would be 1.5–2.0 × ULN, although patients with lower ALT levels can be included for the purposes of study if their underlying liver disease is substantial and is histologically documented at study entry.

To avoid including patients with ongoing disease flare activity, who may confound study assessments due to decompensation events or spontaneous HBeAg seroconversion during the first few months of study participation, most trials have excluded patients with very high ALT levels at screening, for example, ALT levels >10× ULN. Such patients may be suitable for later study screening if their ALT levels subside into the qualifying range and they otherwise qualify for the study.

In clinical trials it is usually advisable to measure ALT/aspartate aminotransferase (AST) levels at entry (screen and baseline) and at each periodic clinic visit during the course of the trial. Efficacy data analyses primarily key on treatment-related improvements in ALT levels, while safety analyses should include assessments of ALT/AST elevations above patients' baseline levels. ALT normalization can be assessed by one-point or two-point methods similar to HBV DNA responses. A two-point definition was used in the lamivudine trials, by which a patient was said to have experienced ALT normalization if their baseline ALT level was elevated (> 1 × ULN) and ALT levels subsequently became normal on two successive study visits. Regardless of whether a one-point or two-point definition is used for ALT normalization, it is probably more important to assess ALT normalization that is maintained to the end of treatment (termed "maintained" ALT normalization), and responses that persist post-therapy to the end of study. Because ALT values can transiently fluctuate into the slightly elevated range even in healthy hosts, an acceptable analytic algorithm for "maintained" ALT normalization can allow occasional intervening abnormal values, but should not allow two consecutive abnormal ALT values between the achievement of initial ALT normalization and the time point defining end-of-treatment.

4.5. Histologic Responses

Clinical outcomes in patients with chronic hepatitis B are ultimately associated with the extent of necroinflammatory damage in the liver. Chronic immune-mediated necroinflammatory activity related to ongoing HBV replication is ultimately responsible for endstage cirrhosis and may be the principal promoting stimulus for neoproliferative activity leading to hepatocellular carcinoma. Hence, in clinical development programs for antiviral agents for hepatitis B, it is important to assess treatment effects on liver histology in at least one large trial, at least until the quantitative relationship between HBV suppression and hepatic disease progression is better understood.

Currently, at least three different histologic scoring systems have been used in large clinical trials involving viral hepatitis patients: the Knodell histologic activity index (HAI score), the French Metavir scoring system, and the Ishak scoring system ***(48–51)***. The Knodell HAI score is the oldest and has been widely used in registration trials, but this scoring system has been criticized for the discontinuous integer scores within its four component evaluations and for overweighting of one component of hepatic necroinflammatory activity, that is, periportal necrosis, which is assigned a score of up to 10 points while each of the other three scoring components range up to only 4 points. The Ishak scoring system derives from the Knodell approach but incorporates a continuous integer scoring system and other potential improvements. The Metavir system has interesting validation data with regard to reducing interobserver variability and has been used in several hepatitis C trials, but this scoring system has not been used in hepatitis B registration trials to date.

In addition to the three semi-quantitative scoring systems, a nonquantitative "global" or "ranking" evaluation has also been used for histologic evaluations in most Phase III hepatitis trials, usually as a confirmatory assessment ***(13,19,20,23)***. In this approach, paired slides (pretreatment and follow-up) from each patient are blindly evaluated by the hepatopathologists for the global severity of histologic findings, with one slide ranked as "better" or both slides ranked as "same." Such ranking evaluations are conducted separately for necroinflammatory vs fibrosis features, and the pathologists are again blinded to patient identifiers, treatment, date, and sequence of the paired biopsy slides being evaluated. After unblinding of patient identifiers and treatment codes, it can be determined what proportion of follow-up slides were designated as "better" for each treatment group—and whether there was indeed a finding, after unblinding, that follow-up biopsies usually appeared "better" than pretreatment biopsies.

Regardless of what scoring or slide evaluation system is used, protocol-mandated histologic assessments in hepatitis clinical trials should be conducted only by contracted independent expert hepatopathologists who are experienced in the scoring systems being used. Also, to ensure nonbiased evaluations, the slides should be scored or evaluated only under blinded conditions—that is, for each slide evaluation the central pathologist should be blinded with regard to patient identifiers, treatment, date, and sequence of the slides (pretreatment vs follow-up).

Hepatitis B trials with interferon incorporated relatively limited histologic evaluations. In the lamivudine Phase III trials in hepatitis B patients, similar to earlier interferon trials in hepatitis C patients, histologic responses were primarily assessed as 2-point or greater reductions in the Knodell HAI score ***(10–12)***. In addition to the results of Knodell HAI scoring, confirmatory histologic analyses in the lamivudine trials included separate slide "ranking" evaluations. For the evaluation of treatment-related changes in hepatic necroinflammatory activity, the lamivudine trials assessed the frequency of 2-point (or greater) changes in the so-called "Knodell necroinflammatory score," that is, the sum of the first three components of the Knodell HAI score, in line with recommendations promulgated from hepatitis C trials and the 1997 NIH

Consensus Conference on Hepatitis C ***(52,53)***. However, because fibrosis component scores in the Knodell system are limited and discontinuous, the slide "ranking" approach was felt to be potentially more reliable for evaluation of fibrosis changes. Therefore the primary evaluation of "worsening in fibrosis" (i.e., progression in fibrosis) in the lamivudine trials was through use of the slide ranking method. This approach proved to be useful, in that it became apparent after unblinding of the evaluations that placebo patients often had their follow-up biopsy blindly evaluated as "worse" for fibrosis (relative to the pretreatment biopsy slide), while this was an unusual finding for lamivudine recipients ***(19,20,23)***. In the adefovir Phase III trials, a conceptually similar but modified approach was utilized, in which the primary endpoint for histologic response was defined as a 2-point or greater improvement in the Knodell necroinflammatory score in the follow-up biopsy with no worsening in the fibrosis score ***(38,46,54)***.

5. Safety Assessments in Hepatitis B Trials

5.1. Routine Safety Assessments in Phase I–III Trials

Clinical adverse events and categorically graded laboratory abnormalities (e.g., grades 1–4) are routinely assessed in all clinical trials. Serious adverse events are regulatory defined as any untoward clinical event which meets one or more of the following criteria: (a) fatal; (b) immediately life-threatening; (c) permanently or significantly disabling; (d) requires or prolongs inpatient hospitalization; (e) comprises a congenital anomaly/birth defect; or (f) is a medically significant event that may otherwise jeopardize the patient or require medical or surgical intervention to prevent one of the outcomes listed (a–e). If a serious adverse event (SAE) occurs in a trial, is unexpected on the basis of what is known about the drug (as judged by information in the product label and/or investigator brochure), and is thought by the clinical investigator to be possibly or reasonably attributable to the study drug, then that SAE is likely to be subject to urgent reporting requirements by prevailing regulatory laws. In the United States and other ICH territories, drug-attributed SAEs are to be reported to the regulatory authorities within 15 calendar days of learning of the event. If the SAE is fatal or involves an immediately life-threatening event and is thought to be potentially attributable to the study drug, then the timeframe for regulatory reporting is shorter (7 calendar days).

Phase I and II trials of new anti-HBV agents should broadly assess the potential for toxicities attributable to the new agent, through close monitoring of clinical adverse events and through relatively broad monitoring of clinical laboratory parameters reflecting hematopoietic function and major organ functions. Hematologic monitoring should assess changes in red blood cells, leukocytes, and platelets. Serum chemistries reflecting visceral organ functions should be broadly monitored for most new drugs in early (Phase I–II) trials—for example, electrolytes, blood urea nitrogen (BUN)/creatinine, liver function tests (ALT, AST, albumin, bilirubin), amylase, lipase, creatine kinase, and calcium and phosphorus are usually appropriate for periodic monitoring in early trials, together with any other serum chemistry parameters suggested by preclinical toxicologic findings. Serial urinalyses, with assessments of hematuria, glycosuria, and proteinuria, are usually included in Phase I–II trials. Also, the Food and Drug Administration (FDA) and other regulatory bodies are placing increasing emphasis on electrocardiographic (ECG) assessments in early trials of new pharmaceutical candidates.

Once the early trials have delineated the preliminary human safety profile for the new anti-HBV agent, subsequent Phase IIb–III–IV trials generally can be accomplished with more limited laboratory monitoring than was utilized in the Phase I–IIa trials. In the Phase IIb–III–IV trials, monitoring of subjects' hematologic parameters, serum chemistries, urinalyses, ECGs, and so forth, is guided by the results of safety monitoring in the earlier trials, recognizing that continued monitoring of several routine laboratory parameters (e.g., blood counts, creatinine, liver function tests) is usually desirable in the larger Phase III trials even if the earlier findings regarding these essential parameters have been unremarkable.

The pharmacologic disposition and safety of new anti-HBV drugs should be assessed in subjects with varying degrees of hepatic and renal impairment, via specialized Phase I trials, as aberrant drug clearance could potentially be associated with safety and efficacy concerns. Also, the potential for drug–drug interactions, involving the new anti-HBV drug and medications commonly used in hepatitis patients, should be addressed in Phase I pharmacokinetic trials, as drug interactions could engender both safety and efficacy concerns.

Phase III registration trials require adequate and well-controlled data for safety determinations as well as efficacy. Therefore, a key aspect of Phase III safety evaluations is the choice of the comparator, that is, placebo or an active control agent. It is usually desirable that a new drug be more effective than standard treatment, with a similar (or better) safety profile. If superior safety is the most important goal of the new product, then the primary endpoint for Phase III trials can be a relevant safety endpoint, rather than the more customary practice of designating an efficacy endpoint as primary. However, under this circumstance, it is advisable that the Phase III development goal also include demonstration of noninferiority of the new product on key efficacy parameters, because inferior efficacy against a potentially life-threatening disease such as hepatitis B would be problematic with regard to clinical and regulatory acceptance.

5.2. Specialized Safety Evaluations in Hepatitis B Trials

As noted above, improvements in ALT levels in hepatitis patients usually reflect reduced inflammatory activity in the liver; hence, ALT normalization is usually an important efficacy endpoint in hepatitis trials. However, because disease exacerbations and "flare" activity (reflected by sudden ALT/AST elevations) are common in hepatitis B patients, safety assessments of worsening in ALT levels are also important, and are usually keyed to patients' baseline ALT level rather than to the upper limit of normal (ULN). WHO-type toxicity grading scales can be adapted for analytic purposes by substituting patients' baseline values in place of the ULN denominator. By this approach, grade 3 and 4 ALT elevations, as a multiple of the patient's pretreatment ALT level, can be targeted for attention in protocolled patient management schemes or in the data analyses ***(30,45,54)***.

Table 3
Categorical Analysis of ALT Flares[a]

1.	ALT elevation $\geqslant$ 2× Baseline and >ULN
2.	ALT elevation $\geqslant$ 3× Baseline and >ULN
3.	ALT elevation $\geqslant$ 500 IU/L and $\geqslant$ 2 × Baseline
4.	ALT elevation $\geqslant$ 2× Baseline with bilirubin $\geqslant$ 2× Baseline (and $\geqslant$ 2× ULN)

[a] Some would recommend also analysing ALT flares >5× Baseline and > 10× Baseline

In addition to standard "graded toxicity" tables for laboratory abnormalities, the lamivudine Phase III trials additionally incorporated a four-category analysis of ALT flare activity, as summarized in **Table 3**. This categorical scale of ALT flare phenomena was not used for patient management in the lamivudine trials, but proved useful in analytically identifying and meaningfully categorizing minor ALT flares vs ALT flares of potential clinical concern—for example, those in which patients' ALT levels exceeded 500 IU/L, or those in which an ALT elevation was associated with biochemical signs of hepatic decompensation [(i.e., a concurrent bilirubin elevation ***(30)***].

In hepatitis clinical trials, it is important to devise analytic means for identifying and characterizing hepatic decompensation events and adverse events related to worsening portal hypertension. Therefore, in addition to a categorical algorithm for assessing ALT flares elevations as, noted above, other composite analytic algorithms can be developed as needed, to capture the range of clinical events associated with worsening hepatic function. For example, the protocol and data analysis plan can include linked assessments of Child–Turcotte–Pugh scores, Model for End-stage Liver Disease (MELD) scores, or clinical decompensation manifestations such as variceal and gastrointestinal bleeding, spontaneous bacterial peritonitis and sepsis, hepatic encephalopathy, and so forth. Depending on the trial goals and the nature of the comparator treatment (active vs placebo), analyses of such "disease progression" events can be adopted as safety assessments, or reductions in such outcomes can be incorporated as efficacy assessments, particularly in trials in patients with decompensated cirrhosis.

6. Trial Design Issues

6.1. Active vs Placebo Controls: Medical and Ethical Considerations

For any pharmaceutic agent, well-designed, well-conducted placebo-controlled trials provide the most reliable assessment of true treatment effect. However, under circumstances in which regulatory-approved and clinically accepted treatment options are available, the conduct of placebo-controlled trials can be ethically problematic, particularly if the disease is severe enough that some patients may suffer mortality or significant morbidity while assigned to placebo treatment. Data from the recent Phase III lamivudine and adefovir trials indicate that, while no deaths occurred and clinical decompensation events were rarely observed during 1–2 yr of study in patients with compensated hepatitis B, the placebo cohorts consistently experienced modest but measurable progression in hepatic fibrosis during the trial periods. Therefore, with the current availability, in most countries, of two or three regulatory-approved antiviral treatments for hepatitis B, it is more desirable to conduct Phase III registration trials with active-comparator designs. In Phase I–II trials, new anti-HBV agents can be initially assessed in small, short placebo-controlled trials, to assess dose-related antiviral effects and preliminary safety. Later (Phase IIb–IV) trials should be primarily active-control studies, comparing the new agent to one or more of the existing agents. This approach has the additional advantage of offering potentially active treatment to all patients, and helps to define the role for the new agent in the evolving therapeutic armamentarium for hepatitis B, with the comparative data providing the basis for product differentiation post-marketing if the new agent or new treatment regimen demonstrates a significant efficacy or safety advantage.

6.2. Choice of Primary Endpoint for Phase III Registration Trials

The chosen primary endpoint for Phase III trials should be a clinically meaningful efficacy endpoint, assuming the new agent is targeted to improved efficacy, and it should be an acceptable endpoint from both the clinical and regulatory perspectives. In the Phase III programs for currently approved hepatitis B agents, in which the target Phase III patient populations comprised patients with compensated chronic hepatitis B, a measure of HBeAg clearance was used as the primary endpoint in the registration trials for IFN-α-2b, while histologic response was the primary efficacy endpoint in the lamivudine and adefovir registration trials ***(30,47,54)***.

Future hepatitis B registration trials will therefore primarily employ active-control designs, with the new agent compared to one or more of the existing regulatory-approved agents. The choice of primary efficacy endpoint in an active-controlled registration trial is a critically important choice for optimization of the clinical and scientific assessments in the study. In active-control trial designs, histologic response does not serve well as a primary efficacy endpoint for several reasons. First, all current histologic scoring systems comprise semiquantitative visual evaluations that have subjective aspects, resulting in significant intra- and interobserver variation and unpredictable degrees of intraobserver and interobserver variance. Even in large trials, it has been common for the observed quantitative variance in histologic score changes, expressed as a standard deviation or standard error of the mean, to be similar or greater in magnitude to the apparent treatment effect. Under these circumstances postulating response rates and treatment differences is fraught with uncertainties. Also, even in the most rigorously conducted trial there will be missing biopsy data for some patients, who may refuse the follow-up biopsy or whose baseline or follow-up biopsy slides may be found to be inadequate for the central pathologist's evaluation. In major Phase III trials to date for the various regulatory-approved anti-HBV agents, 9–36% of patients have had missing biopsy data. In an intention-to-treat data analysis, missing data are presumptively designated as failure data. Therefore, in active-control trials the intention-to-treat failure assumption, applied to missing biopsy data, can make the new agent look more similar to the active control agent than it really is. Because missing data contribute a bias toward similarity of two agents when the missing data are designated as failure data, most regulatory bodies have adopted a preference for efficacy subset analyses as the primary analysis for active-control registration studies. In this approach, patients with missing biopsy data are excluded from the primary analysis of histologic responses. This convention, which reduces the evaluable patient denominator, makes it even more difficult to demonstrate the potential superiority of a new agent, however, and is not ideal since the resultant efficacy subpopulation may not be truly representative of the randomized population. Other issues for histology as a primary endpoint include the objection that it is "only a snapshot in time," and the fact that histology does not necessarily reflect the degree of viral control at the time of the liver biopsy nor the probability of a durable response (in contrast to HBeAg clearance, for example).

Because of the problematic aspects of histology as a primary endpoint, especially in active-control study designs, there is a current movement to return to serologic measures as primary efficacy endpoints in hepatitis B clinical trials ***(2,3,55)***. Compared to histologic scoring, serologic parameters are measured by more precise laboratory tests, which exhibit less variance and are less likely to be associated with substantial degrees of missing data compared to histologic scoring techniques.

In trials involving HBeAg-positive patients, as noted above the composite Virologic Response endpoint recommended by the AASLD can be recommended as a good choice as primary efficacy endpoint—that is, HBeAg loss with HBV DNA suppression to levels below 5 $\log_{10}$ copies/mL ***(3)***. In HBeAg-negative patients, a composite serologic endpoint comprising ALT normalization and HBV DNA suppression has been used in some trials and can be recommended as a primary efficacy endpoint ***(17,18,56)***. Because HBeAg-negative patients can have active liver disease with lower average viremia levels, some experts believe that the viral suppression requirement for HBeAg-negative patients should be lower than the 5 $\log_{10}$ viremia criterion recommended for HBeAg-positive patients ***(3,10)***. At this time, it seems prudent to assess viral responses in HBeAg-negative patients at several different viremia levels, for example, $< 5 \log_{10}$ copies/mL, $< 4 \log_{10}$, $< 3 \log_{10}$, and PCR-undetectable.

An interesting three-component endpoint can be used to assess therapeutic responses in an overall population of hepatitis B patients, regardless of HBeAg status (i.e., a population comprising both HBeAg-positive and HBeAg-negative patients). This endpoint has been termed "therapeutic response" and comprises: HBeAg loss or ALT normalization, with HBV DNA viremia suppressed to levels below 5 $\log_{10}$ copies/mL. This composite serologic efficacy endpoint essentially operates as a hybrid of the two composite endpoints described above for HBeAg-positive and HBeAg-negative patients, and is attractive because it captures both kinds of clinical benefit achievable in hepatitis B patients (i.e., HBeAg clearance or ALT normalization) together with a requirement for a reasonable level of viral suppression. If this endpoint is chosen as primary, then patients should be prestratified by HBeAg status at entry to ensure the ability to also analyze the two patient subgroups separately in secondary analyses of the final dataset, using "traditional" endpoints for the HBeAg-positive and HBeAg-negative subgroups. Also, as noted above, in secondary analyses of responses in the HBeAg-negative subgroup it is advisable to analyze such a composite efficacy endpoint at several levels of HBV suppression, for example, $< 5 \log_{10}$ copies/mL, $< 4 \log_{10}$, $< 3 \log_{10}$, and nondetectable by PCR.

The best indicator of HBV clearance is, of course, clearance of detectable HBsAg from patients' sera. In the future, as HBV therapies improve and more patients are driven to profound states of HBV suppression, more patients will achieve PCR nondetectable serum HBV DNA levels and HBsAg clearance may then become a more tractable primary endpoint. With current anti-HBV therapeutic modalities, however, HBsAg clearance is too rare in the first 1–2 yr of treatment to allow its recommendation as a primary endpoint in registration trials.

Finally, it should be noted that it has recently been proposed that efficacy responses to anti-HBV agents should be assessed in three phases: "initial" responses (occurring in the first 6 mo of treatment, "end-of-treatment" responses (also termed "maintained" responses), and "sustained" responses (e.g., responses that are durable to last follow-up, at least 6–12 mo posttreatment) ***(2,3,55)***. Of note, in the absence of durable (posttreatment "sustained" responses), the clinical value of "maintained" therapeutic responses should not be underestimated. With current therapies, for unclear reasons many patients cannot achieve durable HBeAg clearance (or HBsAg clearance), yet there is considerable value in keeping such patients' liver disease under control through continued HBV suppression with maintained histologic improvement and ALT normalization.

6.3. Difference Assumptions and Statistical Conventions in Phase III Trials

In controlled trials, "delta 1" is the treatment effect of active drug vs placebo, while "delta 2" is the postulated difference between an investigational agent and an active control agent. Active-control trials are typically designed to show the superiority or noninferiority of a new agent to an approved active agent. True "equivalence" trials are typically not undertaken, as the sample sizes required for such trials are larger than the sample sizes required for superiority or noninferiority designs. In some instances, Phase III data may indicate the likelihood of substantial superiority in efficacy, sufficient to justify direct superiority designs for Phase III registration trials. In most cases, however, a more conservative approach is desirable for pharmaceutic sponsors, in which Phase III trials are statistically designed as noninferiority trials with a superiority reflex test if the trials' results meet prepostulated superiority criteria. This approach to Phase III trial design, that is, noninferiority with a superiority reflex, is specifically endorsed by the current ICH guidelines and is the preferred approach unless the sponsor is exceedingly confident that the new agent will achieve substantial superiority on the primary Phase III endpoint.

In the absence of placebo-controlled studies in the registration program, to ensure that a new agent is in fact active in a noninferiority trial design the new agent should demonstrate a response rate on the primary endpoint that is well within the confidence intervals of the differential response rate ascribed to the active control agent compared to placebo. In designing noninferiority trials it has become conventional to require a response rate for the new agent that is not less than half the delta 1 ascribed to the active control agent, or within 10–15% of the response rate of the active agent, whichever is smaller. Most importantly, the chosen primary endpoint and the postulated treatment difference for the new agent (vs the active control) should be reviewed with clinical experts and with key regulatory authorities, to help ensure future acceptance of the Phase III trial results and the criteria for noninferiority and superiority.

6.4. Treatment Discontinuation for Efficacy

Data from natural history studies, studies of interferon therapy, and the lamivudine trials have established that, in patients with HBeAg-positive chronic hepatitis B, clearance of detectable serum HBeAg is usually associated with beneficial effects that are durable in most patients if treatment is discontinued, for example, persistently lower HBV viremia levels (usually < 5–$6 \log_{10}$ copies/mL), continuing histologic improvements, and normalization of serum ALT levels ***(1–3,11,14–16,21,27,28,44,45)***. Therefore, in clinical trials employing prolonged treatment periods ($>$ 6–12 mo) for patients with compensated liver disease, it is appropriate to incorporate treatment discontinuation criteria into the study protocol for patients who achieve well-documented HBeAg clearance with low HBV DNA levels. Not all such responses will be durable posttreatment, however. It appears that, for HBeAg loss that has occurred spontaneously, with IFN treatment, or with nucleoside therapy, the 1- to 3-yr recurrence rate for active disease is as high as 30–35%, when assessed from the day of discontinuation of treatment ***(27,47)***. Retrospective analyses of lamivudine data suggest that this posttreatment disease relapse rate can be lower if patients are treated for a minimum of 1 yr and for at least 6 mo after initial HBeAg loss ***(28)***. Therefore, current trials design often employ some or all of the following treatment-discontinuation criteria: (1) antiviral treatment for at least 1 yr for nucleosides/nucleotides, and at least 4–6 mo for interferon; (2) HBeAg nondetectable for 6 mo or more; (3) low serum HBV DNA level (e.g., $< 5 \log_{10}$ copies/mL); and (4) no evidence of decompensated cirrhosis or immunodebilitation. Some protocols also require detectable serum anti-HBe; however, retrospective analyses of lamivudine data did not indicate a difference in posttreatment response durability for patients who exhibited only HBeAg loss vs HBeAg seroconversion ***(47)***.

For patients with HBeAg-negative chronic hepatitis B, and for hepatitis B patients with decompensated liver disease, treatment discontinuation criteria are not established. Some protocols have suggested HBsAg loss or HBsAg seroconversion as a treatment discontinuation criterion for such patients, which seems reasonable as HBsAg-seroconverted patients, who lack any remaining peripheral signs of HBV replication, would not be expected to gain any detectable benefit from continued antiviral therapy. However, as noted above, residual HBV DNA is detectable in the livers of HBsAg-seroconverted patients, and such patients have a theoretic risk for reactivation of HBV replication and recurrence of liver disease, which can be substantial under conditions of immunodebilitation. In light of these considerations, a closely monitored trial of treatment discontinuation may be appropriate for HBsAg-seroconverted patients with stable liver disease, as long as they are not posttransplant, not on immunosuppressive medications, and do not have other debilitating illnesses.

In clinical trials, patients who are discontinued from treatment for efficacy should be kept on-study whenever possible and should be followed on a regular visit schedule, to document the posttreatment durability of efficacy responses and to monitor for evidence of posttreatment disease reactivation, which can be retreated with the study drug regimen if recognized appropriately. Posttreatment disease reactivation should also be defined in the study protocol, and includes a requirement for detectable serum HBsAg with recrudescence of HBV viremia to levels $>$ 4–6 $\log_{10}$ copies/mL with return of elevated ALT levels, with or without return of detectable HBeAg.

6.5. Study Discontinuation for Treatment Failure

The three Achilles heels of IFN therapy are frequent nonresponse, a requirement for parenteral self-administration, and significant tolerance/safety issues. The Achilles heels of nucleoside/nucleotide therapy are the emergence of drug-resistant HBV strains and variable safety issues. Because the current anti-HBV armamentarium includes three regulatory-approved antiviral therapies, it is usually appropriate for trials of investigational anti-HBV agents to include treatment failure criteria, to allow patients failing study treatment to be discontinued from study to receive other treatment as available. The lamivudine experience suggests that viral resistance emerges relatively slowly in HBV infection compared to HIV infection. It appears that PCR-detectable drug-resistant HBV strains are uncommon in the first 6 mo of lamivudine therapy, but show a cumulative incidence after that, exceeding 50% of patients after 3 yr of treatment ***(25,26)***. Therefore, treatment failure criteria are particularly important for patients receiving lamivudine or investigational nucleoside/nucleotide therapies for longer than 6 mo (24 wk).

As long as the lamivudine experience remains the most relevant precedent, hepatitis B patients failing antiviral therapy because of the emergence of drug-resistant HBV strains will typically have the following features: (1) treatment $>$ 24 wk; (2) serum HBV DNA levels $>$ 5–6 $\log_{10}$ copies/mL (on a persistent or recrudescent basis); (3) persistently elevated serum ALT levels; and (4) persistently seropositive for HBeAg (if patient was HBeAg-positive pretreatment) ***(57)***. With the emergence of drug-resistant HBV strains, virologic breakthrough can trigger a severe disease flare (with large ALT elevations and sometimes with hepatic decompensation) or, more commonly, a prolonged period of mildly to moderately elevated ALT levels with serum HBV DNA levels continually exceeding 5–6 $\log_{10}$ copies/mL. Clinical trial protocols employing long treatment periods should therefore incorporate treatment failure criteria reflecting these observations from previous anti-HBV drug trials, with the protocol recommending discontinuation for patients meeting these criteria. Patients discontinued prematurely from study for treatment failure can seek other treatment off-study but are, of course, presumptively captured as treatment failures for all efficacy in the final study analysis.

7. Phase IIIb–IV Studies

7.1. Special Patient Populations

In drug development parlance the term "special populations" refers to recognized patient subgroups that may not be fully addressed in the core Phase III registration studies. It is common to begin clinical investigations of new antiviral agents in special populations prior to the initial New Drug Application (NDA), whenever possible, but such studies often continue into the post-approval period as Phase IIIb–IV trials. The issue of how to include special patient populations in the clinical development program should be discussed proactively with the FDA and other regulatory agencies. The regulatory perspective is that the new drug may well be used in such patient groups post-approval. Therefore, gaining relevant data in special patient subgroups is often a high-priority issue for regulatory agencies.

In hepatitis B therapeutics, most registration programs have prioritized Phase III data collection for adult patients with HBeAg-positive and HBeAg-negative chronic hepatitis B with compensated liver disease. The inclusion of additional patient subgroups in the clinical development program is discussed below.

7.1.1. Children with Chronic Hepatitis B

For antiviral drugs with no substantial safety issues, a common drug development practice is to complete a Phase II pediatric pharmacokinetic study during Phase II–III development (prior to initial regulatory submissions), affording a potential pediatric dosing recommendation at the time of regulatory approval. This pediatric dosing recommendation can sometimes be incorporated into the initial product label, usually with caveats for lack of controlled efficacy and safety data in children at the time of product registration. Thereafter, although there are relatively few children with active HBV-associated liver disease (compared to the large adult disease burden), a controlled pediatric efficacy study should be strongly considered, as a Phase IIIb–IV study. Fortunately, incentives for performing large-scale controlled trials in children have increased in recent years, especially with the prospect of gaining 6 mo of extra patent protection if an FDA-acceptable pediatric efficacy trial is conducted. Other considerations include competitive product strategy issues (e.g., competitor profiles and product differentiation), as large-scale pediatric trials have now been completed for interferon and lamivudine and such a trial is anticipated for adefovir.

HBV infection and HBV-associated liver disease have differences in nuance between adults and children. For example, children are more likely to be high-viremic carriers with minimal liver disease. Also, as might be expected, in children with chronic HBV infection and active liver disease, the cumulative liver damage is less, on average, with lower histologic scores for necroinflammatory activity and fibrosis. However, worldwide there are many children with active HBV-associated liver disease and, in principle, the fundamental pathogenesis of hepatitis B is similar in children and adults, that is, chronic necroinflammatory liver disease quantitatively associated with persistent HBV replication. In that light, there is no obvious reason why a pediatric efficacy trial could not be designated as a pivotal study for initial product registration, perhaps together with a second controlled trial involving adults with hepatitis B. However, medical and regulatory acceptance of such an approach would need to be proactively explored in a thorough manner.

7.1.2. Patients with Decompensated HBV-Related Cirrhosis

As noted above, due to safety issues interferon is considered to be relatively contraindicated in patients with clinically decompensated cirrhosis, but lamivudine and adefovir have shown promise in hepatitis B patients with decompensated cirrhosis. Management of this patient population is not yet optimal, however, because of frequent viral breakthrough during lamivudine therapy and a risk for renal toxicity with prolonged adefovir treatment. Another current issue is that substantial controlled efficacy and safety data are not yet available for either lamivudine or adefovir in this patient population; most of the data so far are derived from relatively short-term uncontrolled studies.

Because of unmet therapeutic needs in decompensated patients, there is a recognized medical and regulatory urgency toward performing controlled trials of new treatments for this patient population, which can speed marketing applications and help product differentiation. Several cautions apply to conducting trials in this population, however: (1) the new drug(s) should not have significant hepatic metabolism or clearance; (2) the preliminary safety profile of the new drug should first be established in other, less ill patient groups, as decompensated patients frequently have severe adverse events which can be somewhat unpredictable and may cloud the emerging safety profile of a new drug candidate; and (3) clinical care and support modalities for these patients can differ significantly by clinical center and by geographic locale, potentially confounding efficacy and safety observations in large multicenter, multinational trials.

Efficacy assessments in trials involving decompensated patients need to reflect not just improvements in viral markers and ALT levels, but also improvements in measures of hepatic synthetic function (e.g., albumin, prothrombin time) and excretory function (bilirubin levels), and improvements in clinical status. The latter are typically measured as changes in clinical status scoring systems such as Child–Turcotte–Pugh scores or, more recently, MELD scores ***(58,59)***. A reasonable approach for a primary efficacy endpoint in decompensated patients is to link clinical improvement or stabilization (assessed by CTP or MELD score) with ALT normalization and with a requirement for HBV suppression to a low level, for example, serum HBV DNA levels < 3 or $< 4 \log_{10}$ copies/mL. The latter is required because, in this patient group, historic studies have suggested that liver disease can continue to progress at lower levels of HBV viremia compared to patients with compensated liver disease.

7.1.3. Liver Transplant Patients

In the 1980s and early 1990s, end-stage chronic hepatitis B patients were considered to be poor candidates for liver transplantation, owing to high recurrence rate of HBV infection posttransplant and, subsequently, an often rapid course to recurrent liver failure and death. With the advent of combined anti-HBV prophylaxis with lamivudine and HBIg (hepatitis B immune globulin), rates of posttransplant HBV recurrence are presently very low, and hepatitis B patients are now considered to be excellent transplant candidates ***(2,3)***. The principal unmet need in this setting is for an agent or treatment regimen that would shorten the course and/or lower the costs of HBV prophylaxis posttransplant. Conceivably, a very potent new anti-HBV antiviral, or a combination regimen, could be devised that would clear any residual HBV infection during the first 1–2 yr posttransplant, without the discomforts and costs of prolonged HBIg treatment.

7.1.4. Acute Hepatitis B

It has not proved feasible to conduct large controlled trials in patients with acute hepatitis B, owing to the sporadic nature of clinically evident cases. Indeed, recognizable cases of acute hepatitis B appear to be waning in frequency in most countries, for a variety of reasons including better practices with blood products and increasingly widespread HBV vaccination. There are also scientific issues in firmly establishing the diagnosis of acute hepatitis B. It has been shown that, in countries where chronic HBV infection is endemic, a positive result for IgM antibody to HBV antigens could represent an acute flare in chronic disease activity rather than acute primary HBV infection. Finally, while open-label studies have been done with small patient series, interpretation of longitudinal improvements in patients with acute hepatitis B is difficult because primary HBV infection (and its associated acute liver disease) resolve spontaneously over 3–12 mo in more than 90% of cases.

8. Virologic Evaluations in HBV Clinical Trials

From the perspectives of clinical and basic science, as well as regulatory interpretability of clinical trial data, it has become increasingly desirable to provide supportive viral genotyping data for clinical development programs, for hepatitis B and C therapeutics. In hepatitis B development programs, the virologic scope has evolved to include detailed and comprehensive molecular genotyping efforts targeted to three purposes: (1) to characterize the array of mutant HBV strains that may be associated with evolution of resistance to a given antiviral drug candidate; (2) to characterize any variation in treatment response by patients' HBsAg genotypes; and (3) where relevant, to characterize the array of precore/core HBV mutant genotypes in HBeAg-negative patients' sera. These three endeavors receive further comment below. For pharmaceutic sponsors lacking strong internal virology research capabilities, an increasing number of HBV genotyping assays and virology contractors are available. For the linked analyses of viral genotype data with efficacy and safety endpoints in the clinical databases, it is essential that the virologic data be comprehensive and accurate.

8.1. Viral Resistance and Breakthrough Assessments

The Phase III–IV lamivudine data aptly illustrate the consequences of antiviral resistance in hepatitis B patients. With the emergence of lamivudine-resistant HBV strains containing mutations in the *YMDD* polymerase motif, patients experience variable diminution of therapeutic response, with a substantially reduced likelihood of HBeAg seroconversion and return of disease flares and hepatic inflammatory activity quantitatively related to the return of HBV replication ***(2,3,19–23,25,26,30)***. This scenario of HBV resistance emerging cumulatively, after 6 mo or more of therapy, is likely for any HBV antiviral agent if serum HBV DNA levels cannot be fully suppressed to very low levels ***(29)***.

Owing to structural homologies between the HIV reverse transcriptase and the HBV polymerase, for HBV antiviral candidates with activity against HIV the nature of potential HBV escape mutants can often be predicted from assessments of the in vitro resistance profile of the agent against serially propagated HIV strains. For example, generation of lamivudine-resistant HIV strains in vitro, exhibiting codon 184 mutations, resulted in a prediction that lamivudine-resistant HBV would harbor mutations in the *YMDD* motif, the structural homolog of codon 184 in HIV. When data from other viral systems suggest a pattern of mutations that are likely to predict the resistant HBV genotype for a given antiviral drug candidate, this preknowledge can be used to focus resistance-related virologic evaluations in clinical trials enrolling hepatitis B patients.

However some anti-HBV agents, such as LdT and LdC, have little or no activity against HIV or other viruses ***(60)***. In the absence of serial in vitro propagation systems for HBV, the potential drug-resistant HBV genotypes for such agents cannot be predicted from preclinical experiments.

Although predictive data from other viral systems can be helpful, in any case it is essential to thoroughly evaluate virologic "breakthrough" in trials of new anti-HBV agents, especially when trial treatment periods exceed 6 mo or so. Experience to date indicates that DNA sequence analyses of HBV DNA amplified from the sera of patients with virologic breakthrough remains the best way to identify clinically significant drug-resistant HBV genotypes ***(61–64)***. Therefore evaluations of virologic breakthrough phenomena should be prespecified in study protocols for each new anti-HBV agent, especially for clinical trials in which treatment periods exceed three months. However, there is no uniform or perfect approach to defining analytic algorithms for virologic breakthrough. As noted in the preceding, in the absence of truly eradicative therapy the treatment goal in hepatitis B is to at least maintain HBV DNA suppression at levels found in "inactive" HBV carriers, that is, below 4–5 $\log_{10}$ copies/mL. With potent anti-HBV nucleosides, most (but not all) patients can be expected to achieve good initial responses, with serum HBV DNA levels usually reduced below 5–6 $\log_{10}$ copies/mL after 3–6 mo of treatment. Evaluations of virologic breakthrough can therefore be targeted to identifying patients with recrudescent HBV viremia to levels persistently exceeding 5–6 $\log_{10}$ copies/mL after a good initial virologic response and after a treatment period of at least 6 mo; patients fitting this profile are most likely to have developed underlying drug-resistant HBV mutants ***(57)***. For data analysis purposes, and perhaps for patient management purposes, a second form of suboptimal virologic response can be termed "primary virologic nonresponse," in which serum HBV DNA levels never get consistently below 5–6 $\log_{10}$ copies/mL. For planning virologic genotyping analyses it is potentially important to distinguish between breakthrough viremia vs primary nonresponse, as the viral genotypes associated with these two phenomena could in principle show substantial differences.

Other approaches to analyses of virologic nonresponse and virologic breakthrough can also be taken. Regardless of the precise details of the analytic algorithms, the lamivudine and adefovir trial experiences indicate that clinically relevant HBV resistance can be assessed through identification of patients who, after 6 mo or more of treatment, exhibit substantial viremia levels. For each new agent, once the drug-resistant HBV genotypes have been identified and characterized, broad PCR-based assessments of the emergence of these HBV genotypes should be incorporated into Phase III–IV trials, to help regulators and clinicians gain a perspective on the likely resistance profile of the new agent in long-term clinical use.

8.2. HBV Surface Antigen Genotyping

The notion that HBV disease progression and treatment responses may vary by surface antigen genotype (A–G) has been gaining credence in recent years, although most literature reports in this regard still involve retrospective data analyses and datasets of varying adequacy. Therefore, although this area is still highly controversial, it is advisable to perform HBsAg genotyping on all patients' pretreatment sera in Phase III registration trials for new anti-HBV agents, to allow analyses of treatment effects by HBsAg genotype. At this time, in the absence of conclusive prospective evidence for an affect of HBsAg genotype on treatment outcomes, HBsAg genotyping does not need to be done real-time during a clinical trial. Instead, the collected sera can be run batched for these analyses toward the end of the trial.

8.3. Precore/Core Genotyping

In clinical studies involving patients with HBeAg-negative chronic hepatitis B, it is scientifically desirable (but not, at this time, essential from a regulatory standpoint) to conduct viral genotyping analyses for the common precore "stop" mutation as well as analyses of other precore/core gene mutations and deletions ***(2,3,10,18)***. Again, such analyses can be performed on stored pretreatment sera and can be run as batched analyses, rather than real-time.

A comprehensive approach to precore/core genotyping would also include genotyping of HBV DNA amplified from the sera of patients who appear to achieve HBeAg loss and seroconversion during investigational anti-HBV therapy, at least for trial populations at substantial risk for evolution of precore/core HBV variants, for example, patients enrolled from southern Europe and Asia. However, a caveat here is that, when a comprehensive precore/core genotyping approach is undertaken, the genotyping results can have confusing implications for HBeAg seroconversion assessments because in these locales, especially in older adult patients (beyond age 40–50 yr), mixed infections with wild-type HBV and precore/core HBV variants are quite common. Hence, for example, an HBeAg-positive patient could achieve HBeAg seroconversion due to control of their wild-type HBV infection, yet could also have PCR-detectable precore/core HBV variants present at low levels at the time of HBeAg clearance, that would make interpretation of the biology of the HBeAg clearance difficult. To cover this possibility, it is probably best to recommend that, if the patient's total serum HBV DNA level falls below protocol response criteria (e.g., below 4–5 $\log_{10}$ copies/mL), then such patients should be given a trial off-treatment after a suitable period of documenting HBeAg clearance (perhaps 6 mo), to determine whether they have achieved a durable response.

9. Conclusions

Much progress has been made in HBV therapeutics over the past 10–15 yr. The panoply of anti-HBV agents now commercially available or visible on the near horizon will likely render chronic hepatitis B a largely manageable disease within the next 10–20 yr. In contrast to antiviral therapy for HIV infection, it is now clear that some hepatitis B patients can achieve durable responses to antiviral therapies, that is, beneficial responses that will be durable for prolonged periods, possibly for life, after cessation of antiviral treatment. New anti-HBV therapeutics will need to offer improved efficacy, good tolerability and dosing convenience, and minimal treatment-limiting toxicities. And because chronic hepatitis B is most prevalent in developing countries, new anti-HBV drugs will need to achieve these efficacy and safety profiles while remaining relatively affordable. These are daunting goals, but current data suggest that they may be achievable if new agents afford prolonged HBV suppression at viremia levels below 4 $\log_{10}$ copies/mL and preferably below the level of PCR detectability, although the issue of whether immunomodulation will also be needed for optimal rates of durable HBV clearance remains an open question.

As HBV infection becomes increasingly manageable, and even eradicable in some patients, countries with high social costs from HBV-related morbidity and mortality are likely to commit increasing resources to identification and treatment of chronic HBV carriers at risk for progressive liver disease. Because of the large current global pool of HBV carriers, under these circumstances both the medical and commercial dimensions of HBV therapeutics will expand considerably. With continued social and pharmaceutic advances, the large global disease burden of chronic hepatitis B can finally be resolved.

Acknowledgments

The author is grateful to Ms. Jean Nuzzo for assistance with preparation of the chapter manuscript.

References

1. Lee, W. (1997) Hepatitis B virus infection. *N. Engl. J. Med.* **337**, 1733–1745.
2. Lok, A. S., Heathcote, E. J., and Hoofnagle, J. H. (2001) Management of hepatitis B 2000: summary of a workshop. *Gastroenterology* **120**, 1828–1853.
3. Lok, A. S. and McMahon, B. J. (2001) AASLD Practice Guidelines: chronic hepatitis B. *Hepatology* **34**, 1225–1241.
4. Weissberg, J. I, Andres, L. L., Smith, C. I., (1984) Survival in chronic hepatitis B: an analysis of 379 patients. *Ann. Intern. Med.* **101**, 613–616.
5. Realdi G., Fattovich, G., Hadziyannis, S., et al. (1994) Survival and prognostic factors in 366 patients with compensated cirrhosis type B: a multicenter study. *J. Hepatol.* **21**, 656–666.
6. Fattovich, G., Brollo, L., Giustina, G., et al. (1991) Natural history and prognostic factors for chronic hepatitis type B. *Gut* **32**, 294–298.
7. De Jongh, F. E., Janssen, H. L. A, DeMan, R. A., et al. (1992) Survival and prognostic indicators in hepatitis B surface antigen-positive cirrhosis of the liver. *Gastroenterology* **103**, 1630–1635.
8. Bonino, F., Rosina, F., Rizzetto, M., et al. (1986) Chronic hepatitis in HBsAg carriers with serum HBV-DNA and anti-HBe. *Gastroenterology* **90**, 1268–1273.
9. Carman, W. F. (1996) Molecular variants of hepatitis B virus. *Clin. Lab. Med.* **16**, 407–428.
10. Chu, C-J., Hussain, M., and Lok, A. S. F. (2002) Quantitative serum HBV DNA levels during different stages of chronic hepatitis B infection. *Hepatology* **36**, 1408–1415.
11. Hoofnagle, J. H., Dusheiko, G. M., Seef, L. B., Jones, E. A., Waggoner, J. G., and Bales, Z. B., (1981) Seroconversion from hepatitis B e antigen to antibody on chronic type B hepatitis. *Ann. Intern. Med.* **94**, 744–748.
12. Werle, B., Wursthorn, K., Petersen, J., et al. (2002) Quantitative analyses of hepatic HBV cccDNA during the natural history of chronic hepatitis B and adefovir dipivoxil therapy: an international multicenter study. *Hepatology* **36**, 102A (Abstr. 534).
13. Perrillo, R. P., Schiff, E. R, Davis, G. L., et al. (1990) A randomized, controlled trial of interferon alfa-2b alone and after prednisone withdrawal for the treatment of chronic hepatitis B. The Hepatitis Interventional Therapy Group. *N. Engl. J. Med.* **323**, 295–301.

14. Korenman, J., Baker, B., Waggoner, J., et al. (1991) Long-term remission of chronic hepatitis B after alpha-interferon therapy. *Ann. Intern. Med.* **114**, 629–634.
15. Niederau, C., Heintges, T., Lange, S., et al. (1996) Long-term follow-up of HBeAg-positive patients treated with interferon alfa for chronic hepatitis B. *N. Engl. J. Med.* **334**, 1422–1427.
16. Lau, D. T. Y, Everhart, J., Kleiner, D. E., et al. (1997) Long-term follow-up of patients with chronic hepatitis B treated with interferon alfa. *Gastroenterology* **113**, 1660–1667.
17. Lampertico, P., Del Ninno, E., Manzin, A., et al. (1997) A randomized controlled trial of a 24-month course of interferon alfa 2b in patients with chronic hepatitis B who had hepatitis B virus DNA without hepatitis B e antigen in serum. *Hepatology* **26**, 1621–1625.
18. Hadziyannis, S. J. and Vassilopoulos, D. (2001) Hepatitis B e antigen-negative chronic hepatitis B. *Hepatology* **34**, 617–624.
19. Lai, C. L., Chien, R. N., Leung, N. W., et al. (1998) A one-year trial of lamivudine for chronic hepatitis B. *N. Engl. J. Med.* **339**, 61–68.
20. Dienstag, J. L., Schiff, E. R., Wright, T. L., et al. (1999) A placebo-controlled trial of lamivudine in United States patients with chronic hepatitis B: efficacy, safety, and posttreatment observations. *N. Engl. J. Med.* **341**, 1256–1263.
21. Dienstag, J. L., Schiff, E. R., Mitchell, M., et al. (1999) Extended lamivudine retreatment for chronic hepatitis B: maintenance of viral suppression after discontinuation of therapy. *Hepatology* **30**, 1082–1087.
22. Gauthier, J., Bourne, E. J., Lutz, M. W., et al. (1999) Quantitation of HBV viremia and emergence of YMDD variants in chronic hepatitis B patients treated with lamivudine. *J. Infect. Dis.* **180**, 1757–1762.
23. Schalm, S. W., Heathcote, J., Cianciara, J., et al. (2000) Lamivudine and alpha interferon combination treatment of patients with chronic hepatitis B infection: a randomised trial. *Gut* **46**, 562–568.
24. Perrillo, R. P., Lai, C. L., Liaw, Y. F., et al. (2002) Predictors of HBeAg loss after lamivudine treatment for chronic hepatitis B. *Hepatology* **36**, 186–194.
25. Leung, N. W. Y, Lai, C. L., Chang, T. T., et al. (2001) Extended lamivudine treatment in patients with chronic hepatitis B enhances hepatitis B e antigen seroconversion rates: results after 3 years of therapy. *Hepatology* **33**, 1527–1532.
26. Chang, T. T., Lai, C. L., Liaw, Y. F., et al. (2000) Incremental increases in HBeAg seroconversion and continued ALT normalization in Asian Chronic hepatitis B patients treated with lamivudine for four years. *Antivir. Ther.* **5(Suppl 1)**, 44 (Abstr).
27. Schiff, E., Cianciara, J., Willems, B., et al. (2000) Durability of HBeAg responses to lamivudine and interferon in the early post-treatment period in adults with hepatitis B. *Hepatology* **32**, 377A (Abstr 872).
28. Pil, H. S., Kwang-Hyub, H., Hoon, A. S., et al. (2001) Additional lamivudine therapy after HBeAg seroconversion would prolong the durability of response in HBV endemic area. *Hepatology* **34**, 322A (Abstr. 600).
29. Yuen, M. F., Sablon, E., Hui, C. K., et al. (2001) Factors associated with hepatitis B virus DNA breakthrough in patients receiving prolonged lamivudine therapy. *Hepatology* **34**, 785–791.
30. Epivir-HBV™ (lamivudine 100 mg) product label (2000) *Physicians Desk Reference*, 54th edit.: Medical Economics, Montvale, NJ, pp. 1175–1178.
31. Hadziyannis, S. J., Dimou, E., and Papatheodoridis, G. V. (2002) Long-term lamivudine monotherapy in HBeAg-negative HBV chronic liver disease: maintenance of remission for more than three years. *Hepatology* **36**, 634A (Abstr. 1883).

32. Villeneuve, J. P., Condreay, L. D., Willems, B., et al. (2000) Lamivudine treatment for decompensated cirrhosis resulting from chronic hepatitis B. *Hepatology* **31**, 207–210.
33. Yao, F. Y., and Bass, N. M. (2000) Lamivudine treatment in patients with severely decompensated cirrhosis due to replicating hepatitis B infection. *J. Hepatol.* **33**, 301–307.
34. Fontana, R. J., Hann, H-W., Perrillo, R., et al. (2002) Determinants of survival in patients with decompensated chronic hepatitis B treated with antiviral therapy. *Gastroenterology* **123**, 719–727.
35. Hann, H. W. L., Fontana, R. J., Wright, T., et al. (2003) A United States compassionate use study of lamivudine treatment in non-transplantation candidates with decompensated hepatitis B virus-related cirrhosis. *Liver Transplant.* **9** 49–56.
36. Tillmann, H. L., Bock, T. C., Locarnini, S. A., et al. (2000) Risk factors for selection of YMDD mutants, their consequences in liver transplant recipients, ranging from sudden onset of liver failure to no disease. *Hepatology* **32**, 376A (Abstr. 867).
37. Zollner, B., Schafer, P., Feucht, H. H., Schroter, M., Petersen, J., and Laufs, R. (2001) Correlation of hepatitis B virus load with loss of e antigen and emerging drug-resistant variants during lamivudine therapy. *J. Med. Virol.* **65**, 659–663.
38. Hadziyannis, S., Tassopoulous, N., Heathcote, E., et al. (2002) GS-98-438, A double-blind, randomized, placebo-controlled study of adefovir dipivoxil (ADV) for presumed precore mutant chronic hepatitis B: 48 week results. *J. Hepatol.* **36 (suppl 1)**, 4 (Abstr. 5).
39. Nowak, M. A., Bonhoeffer, S., Hill, A. M., et al. (1996) Viral dynamics in hepatitis B virus infection. *Proc. Natl. Acad. Sci USA* **93**, 4398–4402.
40. Tsiang, M., Rooney, J. F., Toole, J. T., and Gibbs, C. S. (1999) Biphasic clearance kinetics of hepatitis B virus from patients during afefovir dipivoxil therapy. *Hepatology* **29**, 1863–1869.
41. Lau, G. K. K., Tsiang, M., Hou, J., et al. (2000) Combination therapy with lamivudine and famciclovir for chronic hepatitis B-infected Chinese patients: a viral dynamics study. *Hepatology* **32**, 395–399.
42. Johnson, M. A., Moore, K. H. P., Yuen, G. J., et al. (1999) Clinical pharmacokinetics of lamivudine. *Clin. Pharmacokinet.* **36**, 41–66.
43. Zhou, X-J., Lim, S. G., Brown, N. A., Myers, M. W., Pow, D. M., and Lai, C-L. (2001) Importance of second-phase HBV clearance and viral dynamic modeling for dose optimization of hepatitis B antiviral nucleosides. *Hepatology* **34** 324A (Abstr. 607).
44. Perrillo, R. P., Schiff, E. R., Davis, G. L., et al. (1990) A randomized, controlled trial of interferon alfa-2b alone and after prednisone withdrawal for the treatment of chronic hepatitis B. The Hepatitis Interventional Therapy Group. *N. Engl. J. Med.* **323**, 295–301.
45. Intron-A™ (interferon alfa-2b) product label (2000) *Physicians Desk Reference,* 54th edit. Medical Economics, Montvale, NJ, pp. 2808–2817.
46. Marcellin, P., Chang, T-T., Lim, S. G., et al. (2001) GS-98-437, a double-blind, randomized, placebo-controlled study of adefovir dipivoxil (ADV) for the treatment of patients with HBeAg+ chronic hepatitis B infection: 48 week results. *Hepatology* **34**, 340A (Abstr. 674).
47. Wright, T., Dienstag, J. L., Lai, C-L., et al. (2000) Lamivudine for HBeAg-positive chronic hepatitis B: serologic and histologic parameters associated with durable responses, in *Abstracts of the 40th International Conference on Antimicrobial Agents and Chemotherapy* (ICAAC); p. 272 (Abstr 1405).
48. Knodell, R. G., Ishak, K. G., Black, W. C., et al. (1981) Formulation and application of a numerical scoring system for assessing histological activity in asymptomatic chronic active hepatitis. *Hepatology* **1**, 431–435.
49. Desmet, V. J., Gerber, M., Hoofnagle, J. H., Manns, M; and Scheuer, P. J. (1994) Classification of chronic hepatitis: diagnosis, grading and staging. *Hepatology* **19**, 1513–1520.

50. The French Metavir Cooperative Study Group (1994) Intraobserver and interobserver variations in liver biopsy interpretation in patients with chronic hepatitis C. *Hepatology* **20**, 15–20.
51. Ishak, K., Baptista, A., Bianchi, L., et al. (1995) Histological grading and staging of chronic hepatitis. *J. Hepatol.* **22**, 696–699.
52. Farrell, G. C., Bacon, B. R., and Goldin, R. D. (1998) Lymphoblastoid interferon alfa-n1 improves the long-term response to a 6-month course of treatment in chronic hepatitis C compared with recombinant interferon alfa-2b: results of an international randomized controlled trial. *Hepatology* **27**, 1121–1127.
53. Lindsay, K. L. (1997) Therapy of hepatitis C: overview. *Hepatology* **26** (**Suppl 1**), 71S–77S.
54. Hepsera™ (adefovir dipivoxil 10 mg) product label (2002) Gilead Sciences, Foster City, CA.
55. Shaw, T., Bowden, S., and Locarnini, S. (2002) Chemotherapy for hepatitis B: new treatment options necessitate reappraisal of traditional endpoints. *Gastroenterology* **123**, 2135–2140.
56. Tassopoulos, N. C., Volpes, R., Pastore, G., et al. (1999) Efficacy of lamivudine in patients with hepatitis B e antigen-negative/hepatitis B virus DNA-positive (precore mutant) chronic hepatitis B. Lamivudine Precore Mutant Study Group. *Hepatology* **29**, 889–896.
57. Atkins, M., Hunt, C. M., Brown, N., et al. (1998) Clinical significance of YMDD mutant hepatitis B virus (HBV) in a large cohort of lamivudine-treated hepatitis B patients. *Hepatology* **28**, 319A (Abstr 625).
58. Child, C. G., and Turcotte, J. G. (1964) Surgery and portal hypertension, in *The Liver and Portal Hypertension* (Child, C. G., ed.), W. B. Saunders, Philadelphia, pp. 50–58.
59. Wiesner, R., Edwards, E., Freeman, R., et al., and the United Network for Organ Sharing Liver Disease Severity Score Committee (2003) Model for End-stage Liver Disease (MELD) and allocation of donor livers. *Gastroenterology* **124**, 91–96.
60. Bryant, M. L., Bridges, E. G., Placidi, L, et al. (2001) Antiviral L-nucleosides specific for hepatitis B virus infection. *Antimicrob. Agents Chemother.* **45**, 229–235.
61. Tipples, G. A., Ma MM, Fischer KP, Bain, V. G., Kneteman, N. M., and Tyrrell, D. I. J. (1996) Mutation in HBV RNA-dependent DNA polymerase confers resistance to lamivudine *in vivo*. *Hepatology* **24**, 714–717.
62. Ling, R., Mutimer, D., Ahmed, M., et al. (1996) Selection of mutations in the hepatitis B virus polymerase during therapy of transplant recipients with lamivudine. *Hepatology* **24**, 711–713.
63. Bartholomew, M. M., Jansen, R. W., Jeffers, L. J., et al. (1997) Hepatitis-B-virus resistance to lamivudine given for recurrent infection after orthotopic liver transplantation. *Lancet* **349**, 20–22.
64. Allen, M., Deslauriers, M., Andrews, C., et al. (1998) Identification and characterization of mutations in hepatitis B virus resistant to lamivudine. *Hepatology* **27**, 1670–1677.

36

Testing Antivirals Against Hepatitis Delta Virus

Farnesyl Transferase Inhibitors

Bruno B. Bordier and Jeffrey S. Glenn

1. Introduction

Since the discovery of hepatitis delta virus (HDV) about 25 yr ago *(1–3)*, no medical therapy has yet been developed to eradicate effectively this cause of acute and chronic liver disease. This small RNA virus is composed of three main elements: a 1.7-kb circular single-stranded RNA genome, two isoforms of an antigenome-encoded protein—the delta antigens—and a lipid envelope embedded with hepatitis B virus (HBV) surface antigens (HBsAgs) (**Fig. 1** *[4,5]*). These latter proteins are necessary for the production of infectious HDV particles, which explains why clinical infections with HDV occur only in the presence of an HBV infection. The presence of HDV can dramatically increase the severity of the underlying HBV infection *(6–8)*. Clearance of delta infections is refractory to interferon *(9)*, and recent improved therapies that clear HBV viremia but still fail to abolish HBsAg levels have no impact on HDV *(10)*. Thus other anti-HDV strategies need to be considered.

Once the HDV genomic RNA has entered the cell (**Fig. 2**), it migrates to the nucleus where it is replicated via a rolling circle mechanism catalyzed by an apparent combination of delta antigen and a recruited host cell RNA polymerase *(11–13)*. During this RNA-dependent RNA replication, an antigenomic form of the RNA is synthesized and serves as a template for more genomic RNA species. The antigenomic RNA also bears the open reading frame (ORF) for synthesis of delta antigen. In the course of replication, an RNA editing event occurs at the translational stop codon for small delta antigen, extending the ORF to the next downstream stop codon *(14–16)*. This generates the larger isoform of delta antigen—a protein 19 amino acids longer at the carboxyl (C)-terminus than the small form (**Fig. 3**). While both isoforms have in common nuclear localization, oligomerization, and RNA binding domains, the large delta antigen also displays activities completely different from its smaller counterpart: it inhibits HDV

From: *Methods in Molecular Medicine, vol. 96: Hepatitis B and D Protocols, volume 2*
Edited by: R. K. Hamatake and J. Y. N. Lau © Humana Press Inc., Totowa, NJ

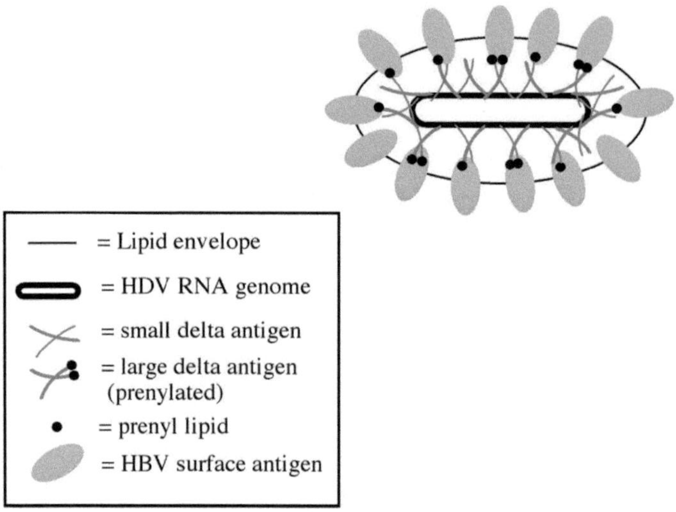

Fig. 1. Schematic overview showing the principal structural elements of a HDV particle: genomic circular RNA, complexed with delta antigen (large and small), is surrounded by a lipid envelope embedded with HBV surface antigen proteins. (The precise stoichiometry is not known and simplified here for illustrative purposes.)

genome replication and promotes virion formation through interaction with HBV small surface antigen ***(17–20)***. Essential to this latter function is a sequence motif located at the extreme C-terminus of the 19 amino acid extension unique to large delta antigen. This motif, termed a CXXX box (where C = cysteine and X is any amino acid), is the substrate for a posttranslational modification: prenylation ***(21–23)***. The latter consists of the covalent addition of the prenyl lipid farnesyl (a metabolite derived from mevalonic acid through the cholesterol biosynthesis pathway) to the CXXX box cysteine. If farnesylation of the cysteine is prevented by mutation of the CXXX box cysteine, HDV particle formation is abolished ***(24,25)***. The prospect of similarly preventing prenylation, but by *pharmacologic* means, thus represents an attractive potential strategy for disrupting the replication cycle of HDV.

Although a number of the multiple steps in prenyl lipid synthesis from mevalonate to farnesyl pyrophosphate could be considered for inhibition, we have chosen to target the last step in the formation of prenylated delta antigen, namely, the covalent addition of fully formed farnesyl to delta antigen. This bisubstrate reaction is catalyzed by a cellular enzyme: farnesyl transferase (FTase ***[26]***, **Fig. 4**). FTase belongs to a family of protein isoprenoid transfer enzymes, which includes geranylgeranyl transferases I and II, whose substrates bear a CXXX box or a variation thereof (e.g., CC or CXC), respectively ***(27)***. To date, many prenylated proteins have been identified. Geranylgeranylated proteins include the gamma subunit of G proteins ***(22)*** and members of the Rab family, involved in vesicular transport ***(28)***. Farnesylation modifies such proteins as lamin B ***(29)***, peroxisomal membrane protein PxF ***(30)*** and p21 ras ***(31,32)***. Farnesylation of H-

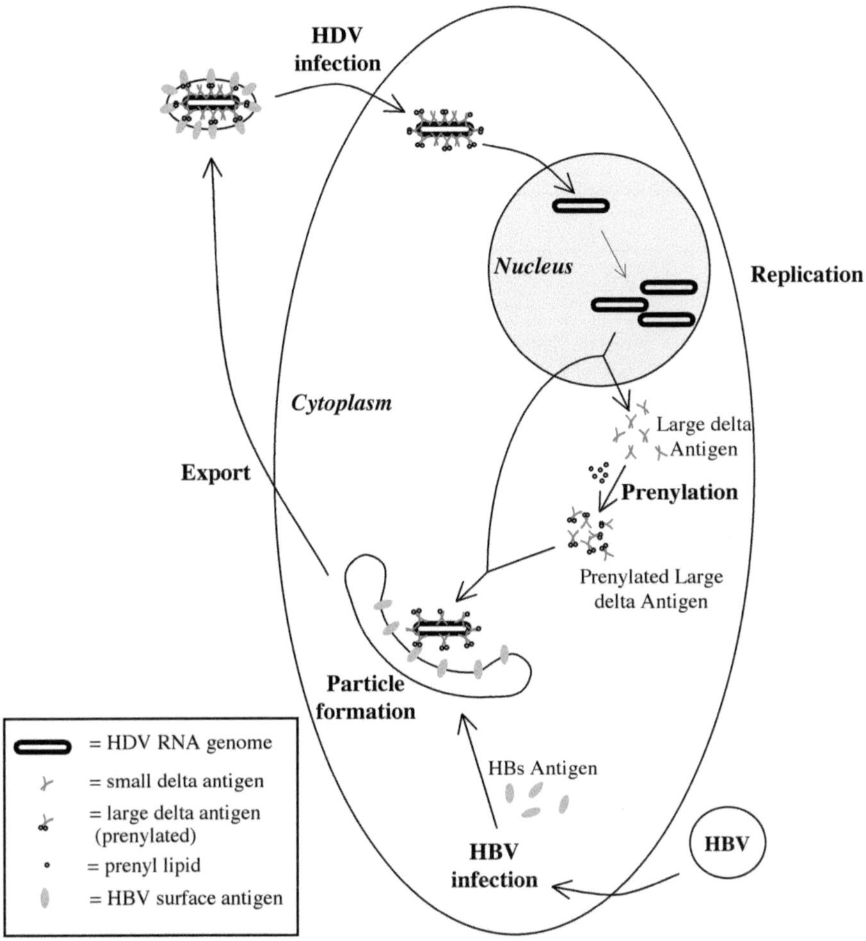

Fig. 2. Replication cycle of HDV. On infection of a hepatocyte, the HDV ribonucleoprotein complex migrates to the nucleus where replication is promoted by small delta antigen. Once an RNA editing event occurs at the end of the ORF encoding for delta antigen, the large form of this protein is synthesized (*see* **Fig. 3**). This large delta antigen undergoes prenylation and inhibits further genome replication while promoting virus particle formation. This last event also requires the presence of a coinfecting HBV that provides the surface proteins necessary for HDV to exit the cell and infect new targets.

ras is an essential step in cellular transformation by the oncogenic form of this protein. As a consequence, this reaction has been extensively studied and several inhibitors of FTase developed ***(33,34)***. These farnesyl transferase inhibitors (FTIs) include CXXX box peptidomimetics (molecules derived from the structure of a CXXX box tetrapeptide) ***(35,36)***, farnesyl diphosphate (FDP) analogs ***(37)***, bisubstrate inhibitors containing structural motifs of both CXXX box and FDP ***(38)***, and several other compounds

Fig. 3. Small and large delta antigens. At the C-terminus (*COOH*), a 19 amino acid extension *(shaded box)* differentiates large delta antigen from the small isoform. The last four amino acids of this extension represent a so-called "CXXX box" in which C is a cysteine and X any amino acid (HDV type I CXXX ***(24,44)*** box is shown: Cys, cysteine, Arg, arginine, Pro, proline, Gln, glutamine; not drawn to scale).

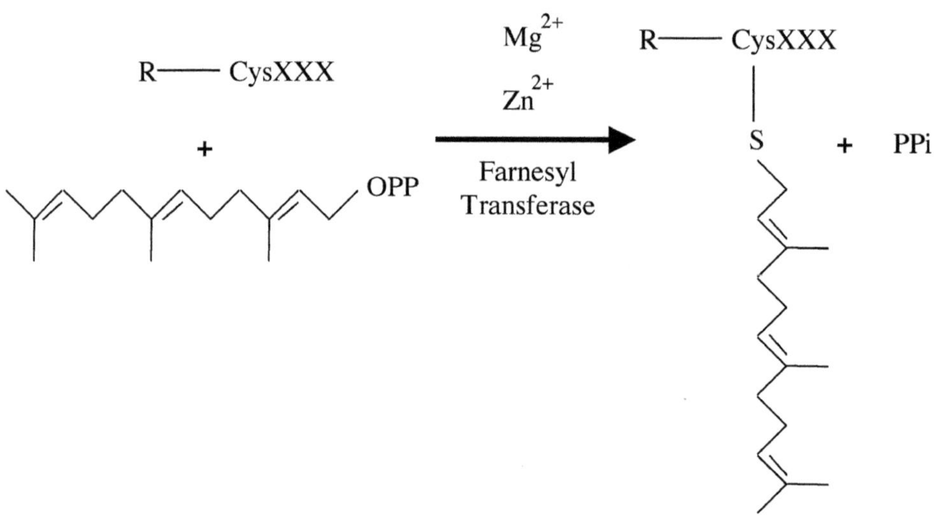

Fig. 4. Farnesyl transfer reaction. Farnesyl transferase catalyzes the covalent attachment of a farnesyl group (coming from a farnesyl pyrophosphate precursor) to a CXXX box-containing protein. R, Polypeptide; Cys, cysteine, X, any amino acid; OPP, pyrophosphoryl group, PPi, inorganic pyrophosphate. [According to Tamanoi ***(45)***.]

screened from random chemical libraries and not based on the structure of either FTase substrates ***(39)***. All of these types of compounds represent attractive potential inhibitors of HDV large antigen prenylation.

One should take into account that inhibitors developed to prevent ras prenylation may not inhibit large delta antigen prenylation with similar efficacy. The prenyl transfer reaction follows a random order sequential mechanism ***(40)***, with independent binding of both substrates (e.g., the protein undergoing prenylation and the prenyl pyrophosphate to be transferred) to the FTase. Moreover, the catalytic efficiencies of CXXX substrates seem to depend largely upon their relative binding affinity for FTase, which could be different for ras and large delta antigen. Such caveats, however, are readily addressed by our two-step screening procedure used to identify suitable candidates for an FTI-based antiviral therapy against HDV.

The first step involves a rapid assay to assess the efficacy of inhibiting large delta antigen prenylation in vitro ***(24)***. In the second step, the ability of the candidate compound to inhibit production of HDV particles is assessed (***[41]*** and *see* **Fig. 5**). For the first step, coupled in vitro transcription/translation reactions are performed with rabbit reticulocyte lysates programmed to express the large delta antigen in the presence of [^{3}H]mevalonate—the metabolic precursor of prenyl lipids—and the candidate compound (**Fig. 5A**). These lysates contain the enzymes required for synthesis of farnesyl from mevalonate as well as farnesyl transferase. Thus the covalent addition of labeled farnesyl to large delta antigen can be simply monitored by subjecting aliquots of the reactions to polyacrylamide gel electrophoresis (PAGE) and fluorography or phosphorimager analysis. Potential nonspecific effects on translation of the delta antigen substrate prior to its farnesylation can be independently monitored by Western blot analysis.

Candidate compounds identified in the first step are then subjected to a more lengthy and informative cell culture based assay of actual HDV particle production (**Fig. 5B**). Transient transfection of a liver-derived cell line with plasmids encoding the entire HDV and HBV genomes leads to the release into the medium of infectious particles that are detectable by assays for the HDV RNA that they contain. As preventing prenylation of large delta antigen abolishes production of mature virus particles, Northern blot analysis of pelleted media supernatants provides a convenient and sensitive method to monitor the effect of prenylation inhibitors on HDV particle formation. Given the time span of this kind of experiment (maximal virion production in the absence of inhibitors is not achieved until approx 1 wk in this system), it is best reserved for inhibitors passing the first screen.

2. Materials

1. Drugs to be tested
2. Dimethyl sulfoxide (DMSO), enzyme grade.
3. 1 *M* Dithiothreitol (DTT).

2.1. First Screening: In Vitro Prenylation Assay

1. TNT® Quick coupled transcription-translation for SP6 RNA polymerase (Promega).
2. A suitable plasmid containing the ORF for large delta antigen under the transcriptional control of a SP6 promoter ***(24)***.
3. 60 Ci/mmol of [5-^{3}H]mevalonate [*R, S*] (American Radiolabeled Chemicals).
4. 1.5-mL Microcentrifuge tubes, sterile autoclaved.

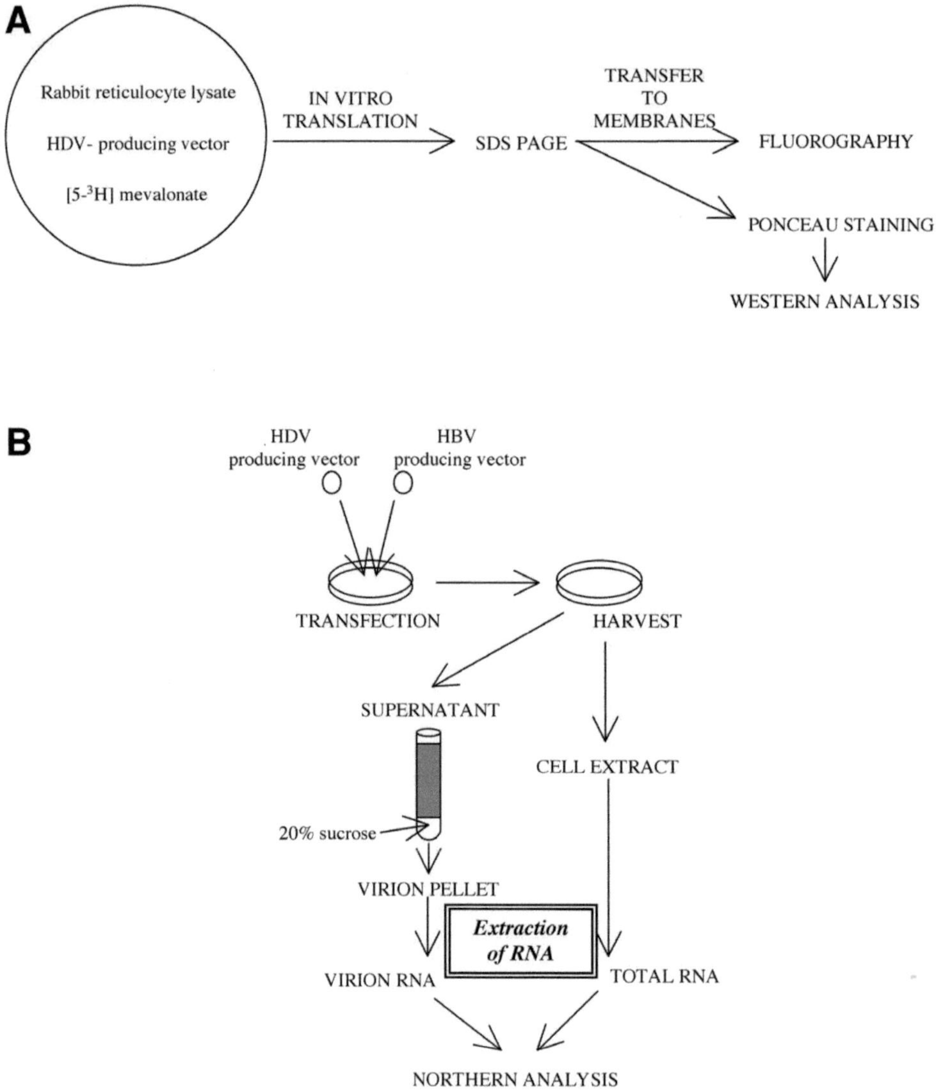

Fig. 5. Outline of the FTI screenings. **(A)** First step: in vitro prenylation assay. **(B)** Second step: virus particle formation assay (*see* text for details).

5. Reagents and equipment for sodium dodecyl sulfate-polyacrylamide gel electrophoresis (SDS-PAGE).
6. Nitrocellulose (0.45 μm, Bio-Rad).
7. Transfer buffer: 200 m*M* glycine, 250 m*M* Tris-HCl, 1% SDS, 20% methanol.
8. Semidry transfer apparatus (Semidry blotting unit, FisherBiotech).

9. Ponceau S solution: 0.2% (w/v) Ponceau S, 3% (w/v) trichloroacetic acid, and 3% sulfosalicylic acid.
10. Western wash buffer (WWB): 10 m*M* Tris-HCl pH 7.6, 150 m*M* NaCl, 0.1% (w/v) bovine serum albumin, 0.1% sodium azide, and 0.1% Tween-20.
11. Blocking solution: 5% (w/v) nonfat dry milk in water.
12. Primary antibody: Anti-delta antigen (e.g., serum from a patient chronically infected with HDV).
13. Secondary antibody: Alkaline phosphatase-conjugated rabbit anti-human antibody (Promega).
14. Alkaline phosphatase (AP) buffer: 100 Tris-HCl, pH 8.5, 100 m*M* NaCl, and 5 m*M* $MgCl_2$.
15. Nitroblue tetrazolium (NBT, Promega).
16. 5-Bromo-4-chloroindoxlyl phosphate (BCIP, Promega).
17. PhosphorImager (Molecular Dynamics).

2.2. Second Screening: Virus Particle Formation Assay

1. Huh7 cells.
2. CO_2 incubator (Nuaire).
3. 100-mm diameter plastic tissue culture plates (Falcon).
4. Huh7 medium: 45% Dulbecco's modified Eagle medium (DMEM) medium (Cellgro), 45% RPMI 1640 medium (Cellgro), 10% fetal bovine serum (FBS, GibcoBRL).
5. Antibiotics: Penicillin–streptomycin.
6. Lipofectamine 2000 (GibcoBRL).
7. OPTI-MEM (GibcoBRL).
8. Suitable plasmids encoding the HDV (pSVLD3 *[42]*) and HBV (pGEM4ayw.2x *[43]*) genomes.
9. Tabletop centrifuge.
10. 1X Phosphate-buffered saline (PBS) without magnesium or calcium (Cellgro).
11. Trizol reagent (GibcoBRL).
12. 15-mL culture tubes, sterile (Falcon).
13. Chloroform.
14. Isopropanol.
15. 30-mL tubes, SA600 rotor, and RC5B or equivalent centrifuge (Beckman).
16. 100% and 80% ethanol.
17. 1.5-mL tubes, sterile autoclaved.
18. Microcentrifuge (Eppendorf).
19. 100% Formamide.
20. Spectrophotometer (Beckman)
21. Cushion solution: 20% Sucrose in 1X PBS (Cellgro).
22. Ultracentrifuge tubes (15-mL tubes, Beckman cat. no. 344059 or 331372), SW41Ti rotor and ultracentrifuge (Beckman).
23. Pellet Paint™ NF (a nonfluorescent coprecipitant that does not interfere with subsequent enzymatic steps, Novagen).
24. 20X Gel running buffer: 200 m*M* sodium phosphate, pH 6.8.
25. Glyoxalation solution: 1.9 *M* glyoxal (Fisher Scientific, Fair Lawn, NJ), 7.1 m*M* sodium phosphate, pH 6.8, 4.5 m*M* EDTA, 35% DMSO.
26. 1000X Aurintricarboxylic acid (ATA) solution: 20 m*M* ATA.
27. 6X gel loading buffer: 0.25% w/v bromophenol blue, 0.25% (w/v) xylene cyanole FF, 40% (w/v) sucrose in water.
28. Agarose gel apparatus with recirculation capabilities (Hoefer).

29. 20X SSPE: 3 *M* NaCl, 0.2 *M* NaH_2PO_4, 20 m*M* EDTA, pH 7.0.
30. Zeta probe charged nylon membrane (Bio-Rad).
31. 3MM Whatman paper.
32. UV crosslinker (Stratalinker, Stratagene).
33. Tris-treat solution: 20 m*M* Tris-HCl, pH 7.5.
34. Methylene blue: 0.04% (w/v) in 0.5 *M* sodium acetate, pH 5.2.
35. Probe-producing plasmid: A suitable plasmid to allow synthesis of antigenomic RNA under the dependence of a T7 promoter and linearized with the appropriate enzyme (such as in Glenn and White *[18]*)
36. [α-^{32}P]UTP (3000 Ci/mmol, Amersham).
37. Riboprobe kit for T7 RNA polymerase (Promega).
38. Microspin G25 columns (Amersham Biosciences).
39. Hybridization oven and tubes (Hybaid).
40. Prehybridization/hybridization solution: 5X SSPE, 5X Denhardt's solution, 0.5% (w/v) SDS, and 20 μg/mL of denatured yeast tRNA (Sigma).
41. BioMax MR autoradiography film (Kodak).

3. Methods

Many FTIs are hydrophobic molecules with an active sulfhydryl group. These compounds are best dissolved first in an organic solvent and maintained in a reduced state. On final dilution into the screening assays, appreciable amounts of these carrier organic solvent and reducing agents remain. Therefore, it is necessary to account for any possible effects attributable to these agents alone by including the carrier composition in parallel control assays run with no drug. Typically, duplicate reactions of multiple drug concentrations are assessed in parallel.

1. Resuspend drugs in appropriate volume of DMSO containing DTT (as needed).
2. Store aliquots at –80°C.

3.1. First Screening: In Vitro Inhibition of Large Delta Antigen Farnesylation

3.1.1. Prenylation Reaction

1. Dry down the label in a SpeedVac.
2. Resuspend with 50 m*M* Tris-HCl, pH 8.5, and incubate at 37°C for 30 min to break the lactone ring.
3. In 1.5-mL tubes, assemble the reactions according to the manufacturer's instructions. In brief, mix 40 μL of TNT® Quick master mix, 1 μL of 1 m*M* methionine, 1 μg of plasmid DNA (*see* **Note 1**), 1 μL of [5-^{3}H]mevalonate (*see* **Note 2**), and H_2O to 50 μL.
4. Incubate at 30°C for 90 min.
5. Subject 1 μL equivalent to SDS-PAGE (12% separating, 4% stacking) acrylamide gels.
6. Transfer to a nitrocellulose membrane with a semidry transfer apparatus (2 mA/cm^2 of membrane for 75 min).
7. After transfer, wash the membrane briefly in distilled water to remove any adherent pieces of gel.

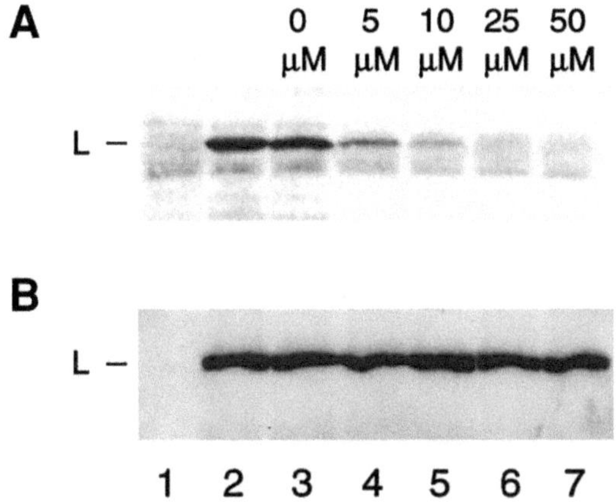

Fig. 6. Example of first screening assay. In vitro prenylation as a function of the concentration of a farnesyl transferase inhibitor. Combined in vitro transcription–translation reactions were performed with rabbit reticulocyte lysates programmed with water *(lanes 1)* or a plasmid encoding large delta antigen *(lanes 2–7)* in the presence of [5-^{3}H]mevalonate and either water *(lanes 2)*; carrier (0.5 m*M* DTT and 0.05% DMSO) *(lanes 3)*; or carrier with 5, 10, 25, or 50 µ*M* BZA-5B, a farnesyl transferase inhibitor ***(46)***, as indicated. Aliquots (1 µL) were subjected to SDS-PAGE and either fluorography (**A**) or immunoblot analysis (**B**). L, Large delta antigen. (Reprinted with permission from Glenn et al. ***[44]***.)

8. Air-dry completely and analyze by PhosphorImager, or
9. Impregnate with 20% 2,5-diphenyloxazole (PPO)–toluene.
10. Air-dry completely and analyze by fluorography with preflashed ^{3}H film.

3.1.2. Western Analysis

After PhosphorImager analysis (see **Subheading 3.1.1.**, **step 8**), the membrane can be used for Western blot analysis.

1. Stain with Ponceau S for 5 min. Destain with water until red bands appear on a white background and take a picture.
2. Block for 1 h in blocking solution (*see* **Note 3**).
3. Wash one time with WWB.
4. Incubate in WWB containing the primary antibody for at least 1 h at room temperature (or overnight at 4°C). (The dilution should be determined for each patient serum experimentally prior to using it in this analysis. The serum we use is typically diluted 1:250,000 in WWB.)
5. Wash briefly four times with WWB.
6. Incubate in WWB containing the secondary antibody (AP-conjugated, anti-human 1:7500 dilution) 1 h at room temperature (*see* **Note 4**).
7. Wash three times with WWB and one time with AP buffer.

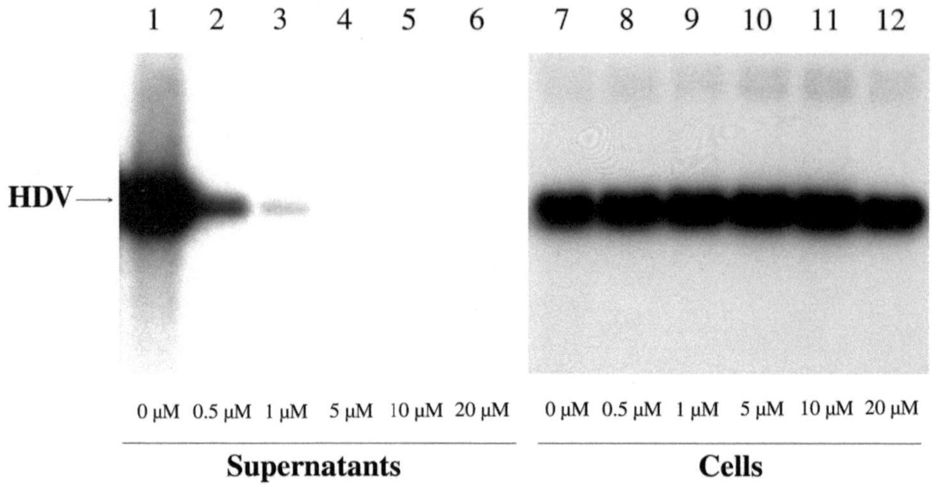

Fig. 7. Example of second screening assay. Northern analysis of HDV virion production as a function of the concentration of a farnesyl transferase inhibitor. Following transfection with both HDV and HBV genome-encoding constructs (*see* text), Huh7 cells were maintained in medium changed daily containing carrier (0.2% DMSO and 400 μ*M* DTT) alone (*lanes 1* and *7*) or carrier plus 0.5 μ*M* (*lanes 2* and *8*), 1 μ*M* (*lanes 3* and *9*), 5 μ*M* (*lanes 4* and *10*), 10 μ*M* (*lanes 5* and 11), or 20 μ*M* (*lanes 6* and *12*) of FTI-277, a farnesyl transferase inhibitor ***(47)***. On d 10 after transfection, supernatants *(lanes 1–6)* and cells *(lanes 7–11)* were processed for Northern analysis of HDV RNA, as described in the text.

8. During this latter wash: Prepare the developing solution: 10 mL of AP buffer in a 15-mL tube. Add 66 μL of NBT, mix, then add 33 μL of BCIP. Mix and use immediately by replacing the solution on the membrane with this developing solution.
9. Wait until development is satisfactory. Stop the reaction by replacing solution with distilled water for 10 min or more.
10. Transfer the membrane between two sheets of Whatman paper. Let it dry at least 1 h.

3.2. Second screening: Inhibition of HDV Particle Production (See Note 5*)*

1. The day before transfection, seed Huh7 cells at 90% confluency (about 8.5×10^6 cells per 100-mm diameter dish) in Huh7 medium (*see* **Note 6**).
2. On the day of transfection: Prepare lipofectamine 2000/DNA complexes according to the manufacturer's instructions. In brief, per plate: Dilute 24 μg of each plasmid DNA in 1.4 mL of OPTI-MEM. Dilute 60 μL of lipofectamine 2000 in 1.4 mL of OPTI-MEM. Mix both solutions together and let stand at room temperature for 20 min.
3. Remove the cell medium. Add complexes to the cells dropwise while rocking the plate gently. Add 12 mL of Huh7 medium with antibiotics. Keep the cells at 37°C, 5% CO_2.
4. Change the medium daily, replacing it with medium containing carrier (e.g., DMSO and DTT) without or with the desired concentration of drug to be tested. On d 9, collect the supernatants (**steps 5–6**) and cells (**steps 7–8**).
5. Collect the supernatants in 15-mL tubes (Falcon), preclear them at 3000*g* for 5 min at 4°C in a tabletop centrifuge and transfer supernatants to fresh 15-mL tubes. Load them onto a 2 mL

of 20% sucrose in PBS cushion in ultracentrifuge tubes. Balance with 1X PBS. Centrifuge for 17 h in an ultracentrifuge at 40,000 rpm, in a SW41Ti rotor, 4°C.

6. When ultracentrifugation is finished, carefully remove liquid including cushion either by pipeting or by suction with a tipped Pasteur pipet linked to a vacuumed flask (*see* **Note 7**). Resuspend pellets in 100 µL of 1X PBS (*see* **Note 8**). Transfer to 1.5-mL tubes. Add 1 µL of Pellet Paint™ NF coprecipitant.
7. Harvest the underlying cells as follows: Wash the cells with 1X PBS. Aspirate. Cover the cells with 7 mL of Trizol reagent. Roll the plate around in your palm until the lysate gets off the plate by itself. Transfer the mixture of lysed cells to a 15-mL tube. Incubate at least 15 min at room temperature. Add 1.4 mL of chloroform. Mix well by vortexing. Centrifuge at maximum speed in a tabletop centrifuge (about 5000*g*). Transfer aqueous phase to 30-mL tubes. Add 3.5 mL of isopropanol. Mix well. Pellet RNA by centrifugation in a SA600 rotor for 20 min at 4°C at 13,000*g*. Remove the supernatant. Resuspend the pellet in 400 µL of sterile double-distilled H_2O. Transfer to 1.5-mL tubes. Add 1 mL of 100% ethanol. Centrifuge in a microcentrifuge at top speed (about 14,000*g*) for 20 min. Remove the supernatant. Add 1 mL of 80% ethanol. Centrifuge at top speed for 10 min. Remove the supernatant. Air-dry for at least 5 min or until the pellet looks dry.
8. Resuspend the pellets in 140 µL of 100% formamide (*see* **Note 9**). Make dilutions at 1:200. Read the absorbance at 260 nm and 280 nm. Calculate ratios to determine purity (they should be close to 2) and concentrations of original solutions (A_{260} × dilution factor × 0.04 mg/mL). Transfer 5 µg to fresh 1.5-ml tubes and adjust the volume to 7 µL with 100% formamide. Samples can be stored at –80°C until the supernatant samples are ready to be glyoxalated.
9. Add 500 µL of Trizol reagent to the sample from **step 6**. Follow the same procedure as before for the cellular total RNA (**step 7**) by downsizing volumes (100 µL of chloroform, 250 µL of isopropanol). After isopropanol precipitation, wash directly with 0.5–1 mL of 80% ethanol. Resuspend the air-dried pellet in 7 µL of 100% formamide.
10. To all samples (including RNA markers and standards), add 8 µL of glyoxalation solution. Incubate for 50 min at 55°C. Quickly centrifuge the samples, then add 3 µL of 6X loading buffer (*see* **Note 10**).
11. Prepare a 1.5% agarose gel in 1X gel running buffer and 1X ATA. Load samples. Apply maximum voltage possible (typically approx 280 V). Begin recirculation of buffer after samples have begun to enter the gel (*see* **Note 11**). Stop migration when the level of bromophenol blue reaches 8–10 cm from the wells. Cut the gel and set up a capillary blotting system with 20X SSPE as the transfer buffer and Zeta-probe as the membrane. Transfer for at least 12 h.
12. When the transfer is completed, subject the membrane to UV crosslinking (Stratalinker, function "Autocrosslink"). Pour boiling Tris-treat solution over the membrane and let it shake slowly until the solution is at room temperature.
13. Stain with methylene blue for 5–10 min and destain with distilled water until bands appear. Take a picture, then incubate the membrane in 25 mL of prehybridization solution for at least 1 h at 70°C (*see* **Note 12**).
14. Prepare the riboprobe for detection of genomic HDV RNA according to the manufacturer's instructions. In brief, in a 1.5-mL tube, combine 4 µL of 5X transcription buffer; 2 µL of 100 m*M* DTT; 1 µL each of 10 m*M* ATP, GTP, and CTP; 1 µL of RNasin (20U/µL); 0.1–0.5 µg of linearized probe-producing plasmid, 5 µL of [α-^{32}P]UTP; and 1 µL of T7 RNA polymerase (40 U/µL). Incubate at 37°C for 1 h. Add 1 µL of RQ1 DNase. Incubate at 37°C for 15 min. Purify the probe on Microspin columns according to the manufacturer's instructions. (In brief, after snapping the bottom tip of the column, centrifuge in a 1.5-mL tube for 1 min

at 5000*g*. Load the labeling reaction onto resin, then centrifuge in a fresh 1.5-mL tube at 5000*g* for 2 min.)

15. When prehybridization is finished, remove 20 mL of prehybridization and use 1–2 mL to dilute the probe. Add the diluted probe to the 5 mL of prehybridization solution remaining in the tube. Incubate the membrane overnight (minimum 12 h) at 70°C.
16. Wash the membrane sequentially with 500 mL of 2X SSPE–0.1% SDS, 500 mL of 1X SSPE–0.1 % SDS, and 500 mL of 0.1X SSPE–0.1 % SDS at 70°C.
17. Remove the membrane from the tube. Wash with 6X SSPE. Briefly dry between two sheets of Whatman paper, then for 20 min in another pair of Whatman paper sheets at 70°C. Cover the membrane with Saran Wrap and expose to a film at –80°C in a cassette (starting with an overnight exposure, then adjusting exposure time according to the results from the first exposure). Alternatively, the membrane can be exposed on a PhosphorImager cassette followed by quantitative analysis of the data (*see* **Note 13**).

4. Notes

4.1. First Screening

1. It is not necessary to linearize the plasmid prior to the reaction. However, if no synthesis is detected, linearization should be performed and, if the product is still not detected, a separate in vitro transcription reaction should be set up to make sure that the expected RNA is synthesized
2. Although tritium has a weak energy, it has a very long half-life and is detectable only through swipes and scintillation counting. As with all experiments involving radioactive materials, care should be taken to avoid contamination of the work environment including the use of gloves, covering surfaces with a disposable bench paper, and using barrier pipet tips.
3. The blocking step is enough to remove the last remains of the Ponceau S stain. However, it is possible to remove the majority of Ponceau S by washing the blot with WWB 1–2 min prior to blocking.
4. AP/color development can be replaced by horseradish peroxidase/ECL. In this case, buffers should not contain sodium azide as it inhibits this enzyme.

4.2. Second Screening

5. Because this procedure aims to produce infectious HDV particles, all precautions pertaining to biohazardous material should be observed. These include BL2 containment conditions and workers being vaccinated against HBV (which provides protection against HDV as well).
6. The strain of Huh7 cells we use is fairly easy to work with, but one should pay attention to some details influencing the efficiency of transfection. For instance, if the cells display very bright dots in their bodies, it is a sign that they are stressed. In this case, expect transfection efficiencies of 30–40% or less.
7. When removing sucrose/precleared medium supernatants, remove first nine tenths of the liquid with a 10-mL pipet, then use a pipetman to remove the remainder.
8. When resuspending the pellet during supernatant concentrations, scrape the bottom of the tube with the tip of the pipetman containing the PBS. Simple pipeting may lead to a poor resuspension of the pellet.
9. When resuspending the cellular total RNA in formamide, it may be necessary to warm the samples at 65°C with regular shaking to ensure complete dissolution of the pellets.
10. After glyoxalation, RNA samples may be kept at –20°C or –80°C for several days.

11. Without recirculation of the buffer, ATA migrates toward the cathode, creating a front migrating in reverse of the nucleic acids, and eventually a zone where RNases can be active.
12. Ethidium bromide should be avoided during migration as it reacts with glyoxal and slows down migration. Moreover, methylene blue is safer to handle and gives very satisfactory images under our conditions.
13. Although not designed for ^{32}P autoradiography, BioMax MR films work very well with our level of signal, producing clean images with a very clear background.

References

1. Rizzetto, M., Canese, M. G., Aricò, S., et al. (1977) Immunofluorescence detection of new antigen-antibody system (delta/anti-delta) associated to hepatitis B virus in liver and in serum of HBsAg carriers. *Gut* **18**, 997–1003.
2. Rizzetto, M., Canese, M. G., Gerin, J. L., London, W. T., Sly, D. L., and Purcell, R. H. (1980) Transmission of the hepatitis B virus-associated delta antigen to chimpanzees. *J. Infect. Dis.* **141**, 590–602.
3. Rizzetto, M., Hoyer, B., Canese, M. G., Shih, J. W. K., Purcell, R. H., and Gerin, J. L. (1980) Delta agent: association of delta antigen with hepatitis B surface antigen and RNA in serum of delta-infected chimpanzees. *Proc. Natl. Acad. Sci. USA* **77**, 6124–6128.
4. Rizzetto, M. (1983) The delta agent. *Hepatology* **3**, 729–737.
5. Casey, J. L. (1998) Hepatitis delta virus: molecular biology, pathogenesis and immunology. *Antiviral Ther.* **3**, 37–42.
6. Buti, M., Estebán, R., Jardi, R., et al., (1987) Clinical and serological outcome of acute delta infection. *J. Hepatol.* **5**, 59–64.
7. Casey, J. L. (1996) Hepatitis delta virus. Genetics and pathogenesis. *Clin. Lab. Med.* **16**, 451–464.
8. de Man, R. A., Sprey, R. P., Niesters, H. G., et al. (1995) Survival and complications in a cohort of patients with anti-delta positive liver disease presenting in a tertiary referral clinic. *J. Hepatol.* **23**, 662–667.
9. Farci, P., Mandas, A., Coiana, A., et al. (1994) Treatment of chronic hepatitis D with interferon alfa-2a. *N. Engl. J. Med.* **330**, 88–94.
10. Lau, D., Doo, E., Park, Y., et al. (1999) Lamivudine for chronic delta hepatitis. *Hepatology* **30**, 546–549.
11. Modahl, L. E., Macnaughton, T. B., Zhu, N., Johnson, D. L., and Lai, M. M. (2000) RNA-dependent replication and transcription of hepatitis delta virus RNA involve distinct cellular RNA polymerases. *Mol. Cell. Biol.* **20**, 6030–6039.
12. Yamaguchi, Y., Filipovska, J., Yano, K., et al. (2001) Stimulation of RNA polymerase II elongation by hepatitis delta antigen. *Science* **293**, 124–127.
13. Moraleda, G. and Taylor, J. (2001) Host RNA polymerase requirements for transcription of the human hepatitis delta virus genome. *J. Virol.* **75**, 10161–10169.
14. Luo, G., Chao, M., Hsieh, S.-Y., Sureau, C., Nishikura, K., and Taylor, J. (1990) A specific base transition occurs on replicating hepatitis delta virus RNA. *J. Virol.* **64**, 1021–1027.
15. Casey, J. L. and Gerin, J. L. (1995) Hepatitis delta virus: RNA editing and genotype variations, in *The Unique Hepatitis Delta Virus* (Dinter-Gottlieb, G., ed.), R. C. Landes Austin, pp. 111–124.
16. Polson, A. G., Bass, B. L., and Casey, J. L. (1996) RNA editing of hepatitis delta virus antigenome by dsRNA-adenosine deaminase. *Nature* **380**, 454–456.
17. Chao, M., Hsieh, S.-Y., and Taylor, J. (1990) Role of two forms of hepatitis delta virus antigen: evidence for a mechanism of self-limiting genome replication. *J. Virol.* **64**, 5066–5069.

18. Glenn, J. S. and White, J. M. (1991) Trans-dominant inhibition of human hepatitis delta virus genome replication. *J. Virol.* **65**, 2357–2361.
19. Chang, F.-L., Chen, P.-J., Tu, S.-J., Wang, C.-J., and Chen, D.-S. (1991) The large form of hepatitis δ antigen is crucial for assembly of hepatitis δ virus. *Proc. Natl. Acad. Sci. USA* **88**, 8490–8494.
20. Lee, C.-Z., Chen, P.-J., and Chen, D.-S. (1995) Large hepatitis delta antigen in packaging and replication inhibition: role of the carboxyl-terminal 19 amino acids and amino-terminal sequences. *J. Virol.* **69**, 5332–5336.
21. Maltese, W. A. (1990) Posttranslational modification of proteins by isoprenoids in mammalian cells. *FASEB J.* **4**, 3319–3328.
22. Schafer, W. R. and Rine, J. (1992) Protein prenylation: genes, enzymes, targets, and functions. *Annu. Rev. Genet.* **30**, 209–237.
23. Zhang, F. L. and Casey, P. J. (1996) Protein prenylation: molecular mechanisms and functional consequences. *Annu. Rev. Biochem.* **65**, 241–269.
24. Glenn, J. S., Watson, J. A., Havel, C. M., and White, J. M. (1992) Identification of a prenylation site in delta virus large antigen. *Science* **256**, 1331–1333.
25. Hwang, S. B. and Lai, M. M. C. (1993) Isoprenylation mediates direct protein-protein interactions between hepatitis large delta antigen and hepatitis B virus surface antigen. *J. Virol.* **67**, 7659–7662.
26. Park, H. W. and Beese, L. S. (1997) Protein farnesyltransferase. *Curr. Opin. Struct. Biol.* **7**, 873–880.
27. Casey, P. J. and Seabra, M. C. (1996) Protein prenyltransferases. *J. Biol. Chem.* **271**, 5289–5292.
28. Seabra, M. C., Goldstein, J. L., Südhof, T. C., and Brown, M. S. (1992) Rab geranylgeranyl transferase. A multisubunit enzyme that prenylates GTP-binding proteins terminating in Cys-X-Cys or Cys-Cys. *J. Biol. Chem.* **267**, 14497–14503.
29. Farnsworth, C. C., Wolda, S. L., Gelb, M. H., and Glomset, J. A. (1989) Human lamin B contains a farnesylated cysteine residue. *J. Biol. Chem.* **264**, 20422–20429.
30. James, G. L., Goldstein, J. L., Pathak, R. K., Anderson, R. G., and Brown, M. S. (1994) PxF, a prenylated protein of peroxisomes. *J Biol. Chem.* **269**, 14182–14190.
31. Hancock, J. F., Magee, A. I., Childs, J. E., and Marshall, C. J. (1989) All ras proteins are polyisoprenylated but only some are palmitoylated. *Cell* **57**, 1167–1177.
32. Casey, P. J., Solski, P. A., Der, C. J., and Buss, J. E. (1989) p21ras is modified by a farnesyl isoprenoid. *Proc. Natl. Acad. Sci. USA.* **86**, 8323–8327.
33. Rowinsky, E. K., Windle, J. J., and Von Hoff, D. D. (1999) Ras protein farnesyltransferase: a strategic target for anticancer therapeutic development. *J. Clin. Oncol.* **17**, 3631–3652.
34. Sebti, S. M. and Hamilton, A. D. (2000) Farnesyltransferase and geranylgeranyltransferase I inhibitors and cancer therapy: lessons from mechanism and bench-to-bedside translational studies. *Oncogene* **19**, 6584–6593.
35. Brown, M. S., Goldstein, J. L., Paris, K. J., Burnier, J. P., and Jarsters, J. C., Jr. (1992) Tetrapeptide inhibitors of protein farnesyltransferase: amino-terminal substitution in phenylalanine-containing tetrapeptides restores farnesylation. *Proc. Natl. Acad Sci USA* **89**, 8313–8316.
36. Kohl, N. E., Mosser, S. D., deSolms, S. J., et al. (1993) Selective inhibition of ras-dependent transformation by a farnesyltransferase inhibitor. *Science* **260**, 1934–1937.
37. Patel, D. V., Schmidt, R. J., Biller, S. A., Gordon, E. M., Robinson, S. S., and Manne, V. (1995) Farnesyl diphosphate-based inhibitors of Ras farnesyl protein transferase. *Med. Chem.* **21**, 2906–2921.
38. Manne, V., Yan, N., Carboni, J. M., et al. (1995) Bisubstrate inhibitors of farnesyltransferase: a novel class of specific inhibitors of ras transformed cells. *Oncogene* **10**, 1763–1779.

39. Bishop, W. R., Bond, R., Petrin, J., et al. (1995) Novel tricyclic inhibitors of farnesyl protein transferase. *J. Biol. Chem.* **270**, 30611–30618.
40. Pompliano, D. L., Rands, E., Schaber, M. D., Mosser, S. D., Anthony, N. J., and Gibbs, J. B. (1992) Steady-state kinetic mechanism of Ras farnesyl:protein transferase. *Biochemistry* **31**, 3800–3807.
41. Bordier, B. B., Marion, P. L., Ohashi, K., et al. (2002) A prenylation inhibitor prevents production of HDV particles. *J. Virol.* **76**, 10465–10472.
42. Kuo, M. Y., Chao, M., and Taylor, J. (1989) Initiation of replication of the human hepatitis delta virus genome from cloned DNA: role of delta antigen. *J. Virol.* **63**, 1945–1950.
43. Ohashi, K., Marion, P. L., Nakai, H., et al. (2000) Sustained survival of human hepatocytes in mice: a model for in vivo infection with human hepatitis B and hepatitis delta viruses. *Nat. Med.* **6**, 327–331.
44. Glenn, J. S., Marsters, J. C., Jr., and Greenberg, H. B. (1998) Use of a prenylation inhibitor as a novel antiviral agent. *J. Virol.* **72**, 9303–9306.
45. Tamanoi, F. (1993) Inhibitors of Ras farnesyltransferases. *Trends Biochem. Sci.* **18**, 349–353.
46. Marsters, Jr., J. C., McDowell, R. S., Reynolds, M. E., et al. (1994) Benzodiazepine peptidomimetic inhibitors of farnesyltransferase. *Bioorg. Med. Chem.* **2**, 949–957.
47. Lerner, E. C., Qian, Y., Blaskovich, M. A., et al. (1995) Ras CAAX peptidomimetic FTI-277 selectively blocks oncogenic Ras signaling by inducing cytoplasmic accumulation of inactive Ras-Raf complexes. *J. Biol. Chem.* **270**, 26802–26806.

Index

A
Adefovir,
covalently closed circular DNA response, 501, 502
efficacy against hepatitis B virus, 427
liver transplant patients, hepatitis B virus prophylaxis and treatment, 325, 326, 431
prophylaxis in liver transplantation, 431
resistant hepatitis B virus management, 487
Adenoviral vectors, hepatitis B virus,
advantages, 209, 210
host specificity, 209, 210
preparation,
amplification of vectors in cell culture, 214, 215, 217
bacterial strains, 212
construct design, 210, 211
high-titer stock preparation, 216, 217
homologous recombination in *Escherichia coli*, 214, 217
materials, 213, 214
plasmids, 211, 212, 216, 217
vector quantification assays, 215–217
tupaia hepatocyte infection, 158
Alanine aminotransferase (ALT),
assay in transgenic mice, 279
clinical trials,
endpoints, 454, 457, 518, 519
patient selection, 447, 448
safety assessments, 521, 523
Alcoholics, risks in hepatitis B virus infection, 487
ALT, *see* Alanine aminotransferase
Antisense oligonucleotides,
asialoglycoprotein receptor targeting of hepatitis B virus antisense,
antisense-ligand complex preparation, 166
cell culture, 166
cell treatment, 168, 171
enzyme-linked immunosorbent assays,
HBeAg, 168
HBsAg, 168
gel retardation assay for antisense protein carrier determination, 166, 171
liver uptake assay, 166–168, 171
long polymerase chain reaction confirmation of antisense activity, 169, 170
materials, 164–166
overview, 163, 164
RNA analysis, 170, 171
virus replication assays, 168–171
hepatitis B virus treatment prospects, 429, 430, 478

ASGPR, *see* Asialoglycoprotein receptor
Asialoglycoprotein receptor (ASGPR),
hepatitis B virus antisense oligonucleotide targeting,
antisense-ligand complex preparation, 166
cell culture, 166
cell treatment, 168, 171
enzyme-linked immunosorbent assays,
HBeAg, 168
HBsAg, 168
gel retardation assay for antisense protein carrier determination, 166, 171
liver uptake assay, 166–168, 171
long polymerase chain reaction confirmation of antisense activity, 169, 170
materials, 164–166
overview, 163, 164
RNA analysis, 170, 171
virus replication assays, 168–171
ligands, 163, 164

B

Baculovirus vectors, hepatitis B virus,
advantages, 221, 223
applications, 223
construct design, 219, 220
hepatitis B virus DNA extraction,
covalently closed circular DNA, 234
extracellular DNA, 234–236
replicative intermediate DNA, 233, 234
infection of hepatocytes, 232, 233
preparation,
homologous recombination, 226, 227, 235
infection of spinner flask cultures, 230, 231, 235, 236
materials, 223–225
plaque purification assay, 227, 228, 232
recombinant virus isolation, 228, 229
transfer plasmid generation, 226
virus concentration and purification, 231, 232, 236
principles, 220, 221
radioactive probe generation for hepatitis B virus, 235, 236
requirements, 219, 220

C

Children,
clinical trials for hepatitis B virus treatment, 528, 529
hepatitis B virus infection and management, 485
Chimpanzee model, hepatitis B virus,
chimpanzee hepatitis B virus,
genome sequencing, 304, 305
natural infection, 289
relevance to human infection, 305–307
chronic infection, 309, 310
course of infection, 289, 290
hepatocyte infection, *see* Hepatocyte culture infection studies
history of study, 290–292

immune response comparison with humans, 307, 308
inoculation studies, 293–297
limitations, 302, 303, 305
prevalence of hepatitis B virus infection, 291, 292
prospects for study, 309, 310
reinfection, 297
sequelae of infection, 297, 298
vaccine safety testing, 292, 293, 298–302
viral envelope and host cell difference comparison with humans, 308, 309
Clevudine, efficacy against hepatitis B virus, 427, 428
Clinical trial design, anti-hepatitis B virus therapies,
active versus placebo controls, 523
Asian patient study design,
alanine aminotransferase levels, 458
decompensated liver disease patients, 461
HBeAg status, 458, 459
hepatitis B virus DNA levels, 459, 460
liver histology, 460, 461
long-term endpoints, 462
monitoring, 461, 462
comparator selection, 448
cost considerations, 445
discontinuation for treatment failure, 527, 528
drug development considerations, 504–506
drug interaction considerations, 507
endpoint selection,
alanine aminotransferase levels, 454, 457, 518, 519
HBeAg responses, 516, 517
HBsAg response, 517, 518
liver histology, 449–451, 519, 520
overview, 448, 449
phase III registration trials, 524–526
seroconversion, 451–453, 457, 512–517
viral load, 453, 454, 457, 512–515
ethics, 523
insights from past trials,
interferon, 502, 503
lamivudine, 503, 504
patient selection,
acute versus chronic infection, 446, 507, 508
alanine aminotransferase baseline level considerations, 447, 448
cirrhotic patients, 447
coinfection exclusion, 448
decompensated liver disease patients, 447
entry criteria for phase II and phase III trials, 508–510
failed therapy patients, 447
geographical diversity, 447
HBeAg status, 446, 508
treatment-naive patients, 446, 447
phase I trials, 506, 507
phase II trial goals, 510, 511
phase III trials,
difference assumptions and statistical conventions, 526
efficacy assessments, 511, 512
goals, 510, 511

observation periods, 511, 512
primary endpoints, 524–526
regulatory considerations, 506
safety assessments,
routine assessments, 521, 522
specialized assessments, 522, 523
special populations and phase IIIb–IV studies,
acute infection patients, 530
children, 528, 529
decompensated hepatitis B virus-related cirrhosis patients, 529, 530
liver transplant patients, 530
treatment discontinuation for efficacy, 526, 527
virologic evaluations,
HBsAg genotyping, 532
precore/core genotyping, 533
resistance and breakthrough assessments, 531, 532
Confocal microscopy, HBsAg in hepatocytes, 149
CpG DNA,
coadministration with hepatitis B virus vaccine, 433
vaccine, *see* DNA vaccine, hepatitis B virus

D

β-L-2'-Deoxythymidine, efficacy against hepatitis B virus, 427
DHBcAg,
antibody preparation, 19, 20
enzyme-linked immunosorbent assay,
antibodies, 21, 23
antigen, 20, 23
DHBsAg, enzyme-linked immunosorbent assay,
antibody detection, 21, 23
antibody preparation, 19, 20
antigen detection, 20, 23
DHBV, *see* Duck hepatitis B virus
DNA microarrays,
hepatitis B virus infection studies of gene expression,
expression profile analysis, 61, 62
high-density oligonucleotide microarrays, 59, 61
materials, 57, 58
membrane cDNA microarrays, 58, 59
prospects, 62, 63
RNA preparation, 58
validation of results, 62
hepatocellular carcinoma studies, 55, 56
principles, 56
DNA vaccine, hepatitis B virus,
advantages, 44
cytokine coadministration, 44
immune response, 44
mouse studies,
gene gun vaccination, 49–51
intramuscular injection, 48, 49, 51
materials, 44–48, 51
DNA vaccine, hepatitis D virus,
administration approaches, 112
components, 112
immune response studies in mice,
CD8+ T-cell activity assay, 125, 126
cellular immunity, 114, 115, 117
enzyme-linked immunosorbent assay of hepatitis D virus antibodies, 124

humoral immunity, 112–114
intramuscular injection, 123, 126
materials, 17, 118, 120, 121
plasmid purification, 122
recombinant S-HDVAg
expression and
purification, 122, 123
serum collection, 123, 124
spleen cell isolation, 124, 125
T-cell proliferation assay, 12, 126
Dose–response surface approach
(DRS),
advantages, 393
assay system selection and
validation, 394–396, 411
Bliss parameters, 388–390, 407
combination chemotherapy
rationale, 387, 388
dose–effect model selection, 396, 397
frugal experimental design, 405,
406, 408
Lowe parameters, 388–390, 407
null reference model, 388–390
overview, 390, 393
reference model selection, 406–408
software, 393, 411
summary protocol, 408, 410–412
TC3D analysis,
dose–effect models, 397
goodness-of-fit criteria, 397,
399, 402
numeric summary, 402
predictions, 402
weighting data effects, 402, 405
DRS, *see* Dose–response surface
approach
Duck hepatitis B virus (DHBV),
core antigen, *see* DHBcAg
duck model,
antiviral agent studies, 262, 263
carrier flock establishment,
266, 267
DHBV DNA detection,
dot-blot hybridization, 267
extraction, 267
Southern blot analysis, 263, 265
infection, 261, 262
materials, 265, 266
viremic serum pool
preparation, 266
hepatocyte culture infection
studies,
antiviral screening, 195
cytotoxicity assay, 196
infection, 194, 196
materials, 190–193, 196
overview, 189, 190
primary hepatocyte culture,
embryonic hepatocytes, 193, 194
liver perfusion, 193
long-term culture, 194
viral DNA analysis, 195
host immune response
characterization,
antigen detection in tissues,
Kupffer cell staining, 18
materials, 13, 14
overview, 6, 8, 9
sample preparation, 17, 22
T-cell immunostaining, 17,
18, 22
viral antigen staining, 18, 19
peripheral blood cell
characterization,
interleukin-2-like cytokine
measurement, 16, 17

materials, 12, 13
mononuclear cell culture, 16
mononuclear cell purification, 15, 22
overview, 4, 5
T-cell flow cytometry, 15, 16
thrombocyte flow cytometry, 16
serum antigens, antibodies, and viral DNA detection,
DHBcAg antibodies, enzyme-linked immunosorbent assay, 21, 23
DHBsAg antibodies, enzyme-linked immunosorbent assay, 21, 23
DHBsAg antibody preparation, 19, 20
DHBsAg, enzyme-linked immunosorbent assay, 20, 23
materials, 14, 15
overview, 9–12
polymerase chain reaction detection of viral DNA, 21
natural infection, 261
surface antigen, *see* DHBsAg
transmission, 261, 262
Dynamic modeling, hepatitis B virus,
antiviral therapy studies,
biphasic solution of virus clearance, 366, 367
clinical utility, 375, 376
curve fitting of viral load data, 367
inhibition efficacy, 367, 369
intracellular and pharmacological delays, 370
mechanism of inhibition, 366
partial inhibition of infection, 373, 374
regimen studies, 369
basic model,
basic reproductive ratio, 362
formulation, 362
solution, 363, 365, 366
data sources, 361
noncytolytic loss of infected cells, 374, 375
rate constant estimation,
cell number in normal liver, 365
death rate constant, 365
infected cell number, 365
infection rate constant, 365
uninfected cell growth rate constant, 365
viral production rate, 365
viral rebound,
basic reproductive ratio, 372
induction/maintenance therapy, 373
initial rebound solution, 370, 372

E

Elderly, hepatitis B virus infection and management, 485
ELISA, *see* Enzyme-linked immunosorbent assay
ELISPOT, *see* Enzyme-linked immunospot assay
Emtricitabine, efficacy against hepatitis B virus, 427
Entecavir,
efficacy against hepatitis B virus, 427
liver transplant patients, hepatitis B virus prophylaxis and

treatment, 325, 326
Enzyme-linked immunosorbent assay (ELISA),
duck hepatitis B virus immune response studies,
DHBsAg, 20, 23
DHBsAg antibodies, 21, 23
DHBcAg antibodies, 21, 23
hepatitis D virus antibodies, 124
transgenic mouse hepatitis B virus model,
HBeAg, 245
HBsAg, 245, 246
Enzyme-linked immunospot assay (ELISPOT), CD4+ T-cell cytokine response to hepatitis B virus,
development, 104, 108
materials, 98
plate preparation, 102, 108
stimulation, 102, 108

F

Famciclovir,
liver transplant patients, hepatitis B virus prophylaxis and treatment, 325
polymerase mutations in resistance, 487
Farnesyltransferase (FTase),
inhibitors in hepatitis D virus antiviral therapy,
screening,
drug preparation, 546
hepatitis D virus particle production inhibition, 548–551
L-HDVAg farnesylation inhibition in vitro, 546–548, 550
materials, 543–546
overview, 543
types, 541, 542
L-HDVAg prenylation, 540
substrates and functions, 540, 541
FCH, *see* Fibrosing cholestatic hepatitis
Fialuridine, efficacy against hepatitis B virus, 428, 429
Fibrosing cholestatic hepatitis (FCH), hepatitis B virus induction and management following liver transplantation, 326
Flow cytometry,
CD4+ T-cell cytokine response to hepatitis B virus, 99, 104, 105, 108, 109
CD8+ T-cells in hepatitis B virus infection,
quantification, 74
selection, 75, 76, 81
duck peripheral blood cells,
T-cells, 15, 16
thrombocytes, 16
interferon-γ staining in CD8+ T-cells, 94–96
FTase, *see* Farnesyltransferase

G

Ganciclovir, liver transplant patients, hepatitis B virus prophylaxis and treatment, 325

H

HAI, *see* Histological activity index
HBcAg,
mutations and clinical significance, 480–482

promoter mutants, clinical significance, 423, 424
transgenic mouse immunohistochemical staining, 246, 247, 249, 250
HBeAg,
clinical trial endpoints, 516, 517
precore/core genotyping in clinical trials, 533
HBeAg,
clinical course of expression, 420
enzyme-linked immunosorbent assay of hepatitis B virus transgenic mouse, 245
mutations and clinical significance, 480–482
patient status in clinical trial design, 446, 458, 459, 508
precore stop codon mutants, clinical significance, 423
seropositivity in disease classification and outcomes, 500, 501
HBIG, *see* Hepatitis B immune globulin
HBsAg,
clinical course of expression, 57, 420
clinical trial endpoints, 517, 518
confocal microscopy in hepatocytes, 149
detection in mice following human hepatocyte transplantation, 259
enzyme-linked immunosorbent assay of hepatitis B virus transgenic mouse, 245, 246
genotyping in clinical trials, 532
hepatocyte binding studies, 143, 144
purification from hepatitis B virus-infected patients,
cesium chloride flotation, 146
sucrose density gradient centrifugation, 145, 146
ultrafiltration, 146
variants and clinical significance, 478, 479
HBV, *see* Hepatitis B virus
HBxAg,
expression and function, 479
hepatocellular carcinoma role, 333, 334, 422
mutations, 479
HCC, *see* Hepatocellular carcinoma
HCV, *see* Hepatitis C virus
HDV, *see* Hepatitis D virus
Hemodialysis, hepatitis B virus management in patients, 487, 488
Hepatitis B immune globulin (HBIG), liver transplant patients, hepatitis B virus prophylaxis and treatment, 319, 321–323, 330, 430, 431, 488
Hepatitis B virus (HBV),
adenoviral vector infection, *see* Adenoviral vectors, hepatitis B virus
antiviral therapy, *see also specific agents*,
clinical trials, see Clinical trial design, anti-hepatitis B virus therapies
combinatorial therapy, see Dose–response surface approach
prospects, 434, 435
viral load modeling, *see* Dynamic modeling,

hepatitis B virus
asialoglycoprotein receptor
targeting of therapeutic agents, *see* Asialoglycoprotein receptor
baculovirus-mediated gene transfer, *see* Baculovirus vectors, hepatitis B virus
chimpanzee hepatocyte studies, 132
chimpanzee model, *see* Chimpanzee model, hepatitis B virus
core antigen, *see* HBcAg
duck virus, *see* Duck hepatitis B virus
e antigen, *see* HBeAg
economic impact, 465
epidemiology, 27, 387, 415, 417, 418, 465–467
gene expression profiling, *see* DNA microarrays
genome, 303
genome mutation rates, 478
genotypes, 423, 424, 469
genotyping, *see* Polymerase chain reaction,
hepatocyte culture studies, *see* Hepatocyte culture infection studies
human immunodeficiency virus therapy comparisons, 501
immunopathogenesis, 419, 420
immunodeficient mouse studies, *see* Immunodeficient mice
infection status,
carrier state, 269, 468, 499
chronic disease, 468, 500
reactivation, 468
resolved hepatitis B, 468
natural history of infection, 420, 421, 485, 486
particle types, 469
receptor, 131
replication cycle, 417
serotypes, 469, 470
surface antigen, *see* HBsAg
transcriptional control, overview, 470, 472
transgenic mouse models, *see* Transgenic mouse, hepatitis B virus
transmission, 417, 418
vaccine, *see* DNA vaccine, hepatitis B virus; Vaccine, hepatitis B virus
woodchuck hepatitis virus, *see* Woodchuck hepatitis virus
x antigen, *see* HBxAg
Hepatitis C virus (HCV), hepatitis B coinfection, 482, 483
Hepatitis D virus (HDV),
antigen
large antigen, *see* L-HDVAg
small antigen, *see* S-HDVAg
chimpanzee hepatocyte infection with recombinant particles,
inoculation of primary cultures, 137, 138
inoculum preparation, 136, 137, 139
materials, 133–135
Northern blot analysis of RNA replication, 138
recombinant particle production, 135, 136
clinical features of infection, 483, 484

DNA vaccine, *see* DNA vaccine, hepatitis D virus
farnesyltransferase inhibitor targeting, *see* Farnesyltransferase
genome, 539
hepatitis B coinfection, 111, 483, 484, 539
immune response, overview, 111
liver transplantation patient infection, 327, 328
mouse models,
hydrodynamics-based transfection,
applications, 346
characterization of mice, 347, 348
genome replication evidence, 344
injection of mice, 347, 348
intramuscular injection comparison, 345, 346
materials, 346, 347
principles, 343, 344
RNA transfection, 344, 345
particle injection, 343
RNA transfection of hepatocytes,
materials, 352, 353, 356
overview, 351, 352
RNA preparation, 355
transcription template preparation, 354, 355
transfection culture, 356, 357
transgenic mice, 343
replication cycle, 539, 540
Hepatocellular carcinoma (HCC),
cirrhosis association, 422
DNA microarray studies of gene expression, 55, 56
epidemiology, 421, 422
hepatitis B virus association risks, 484, 485
hepatitis B virus vaccine impact, 416, 422
Hepatocyte culture infection studies,
adenoviral vector infection, *see* Adenoviral vectors, hepatitis B virus
asialoglycoprotein receptor targeting of therapeutic agents, *see* Asialoglycoprotein receptor
baculovirus-mediated gene transfer, *see* Baculovirus vectors, hepatitis B virus
chimpanzee hepatocyte infection with recombinant hepatitis D virus particles,
inoculation of primary cultures, 137, 138
inoculum preparation, 136, 137, 139
materials, 133–135
Northern blot analysis of RNA replication, 138
recombinant particle production, 135, 136
duck hepatitis B virus in duck hepatocytes,
antiviral screening, 195
cytotoxicity assay, 196
infection, 194, 196
materials, 190–193, 196
overview, 189, 190
primary hepatocyte culture,

embryonic hepatocytes, 193, 194
liver perfusion, 193
long-term culture, 194
viral DNA analysis, 195
hepatitis D virus RNA transfection of hepatocytes,
hydrodynamics-based transfection,
genome replication evidence, 344
principles, 343, 344
RNA transfection, 344, 345
materials, 352, 353, 356
overview, 351, 352
RNA preparation, 355
transcription template preparation, 354, 355
transfection culture, 356, 357
human hepatocyte studies of hepatitis B virus endocytosis and intracellular localization of particles,
confocal microscopy, 149
hepatocyte isolation, 147, 148
materials, 144, 145
overview, 143, 144
subviral particle labeling with fluorophore, 146, 147
subviral particle purification from hepatitis B virus-infected patients,
cesium chloride flotation, 146
sucrose density gradient centrifugation, 145, 146
ultrafiltration, 146
tupaia hepatocyte infection with hepatitis B virus,
adenoviral vector infection, 158
animal care, 157, 159
covalently closed circular DNA isolation, 158–160
inoculum preparation and infection, 158, 160
materials, 155, 156, 159
overview of tupaia system, 153–155
primary hepatocyte preparation, 157, 159, 160
V8 protease treatment of human hepatitis B virus and woodchuck hepatitis virus to enhance infectivity,
digestion conditions, 203, 207
immunofluorescent staining of viral proteins, 205, 206
infection conditions, 203, 207
materials, 200–202
overview, 199, 200
progeny virus DNA detection, 203–206
virus isolation, 202
Western blotting of treated viruses, 203
woodchuck hepatitis virus in woodchuck hepatocytes,
cell line generation and maintenance, 182, 183, 185
freezing and thawing of hepatocytes, 183
hepatocyte isolation,
microperfusion, 181
whole liver perfusion, 179, 180
infection, 183

long-term hepatocyte culture, 181, 182, 185
materials, 176–179
overview, 175
primary hepatocyte culture, 181
viral DNA detection,
cell preparation, 183, 184, 186
dot-blot hybridization, 174
polymerase chain reaction, 184, 185
Hepatocyte transplantation, *see* Immunodeficient mice
Histological activity index (HAI), clinical trial endpoints, 450, 451, 459, 519, 520

I

IFN-α, *see* Interferon-α
IFN-γ, *see* Interferon-γ
IL-4, *see* Interleukin-4
IL-5, *see* Interleukin-5
IL-10, *see* Interleukin-10
IL-15, *see* Interleukin-15
Immunodeficient mice,
human hepatocyte transplantation,
engraftment analysis,
human genomic DNA detection, 258
human serum albumin detection, 258
genotyping,
RAG-2 knockout, 256, 257
urokinase-type plasminogen activator transgene, 257
graft survival and repopulation, 254, 255
hepatitis B virus infection studies,
DNA detection, 259
HBsAg detection, 259
infection, 258
hepatocyte isolation, 257, 259
materials, 255, 256, 259
rationale, 253
transplantation, 258
urokinase-type plasminogen activator transgenic mouse/RAG-2 knockout mouse features, 254
severe combined immunodeficient mouse hepatitis B virus model, *see* Transgenic mouse, hepatitis B virus
Immunofluorescent microscopy, viral proteins in hepatocyte culture, 205, 206
In situ hybridization (ISH), hepatitis B virus DNA in transgenic mouse model of chronic liver disease, 283
Interferon-α (IFN-α),
clinical trial insights in hepatitis B virus treatment, 502, 503
combination therapy,
nucleoside analogs, 429
steroids, 425
efficacy against hepatitis B virus, 424, 425
forms for therapy, 477
liver transplant patients, hepatitis B virus prophylaxis and treatment, 326, 327

Interferon-γ (IFN-γ),
CD4+ T-cell response to hepatitis B virus,
enzyme-linked immunospot assay,
development, 104, 108
materials, 98
plate preparation, 102, 108
stimulation, 102, 108
flow cytometry staining, 99, 104, 105, 108, 109
secretion assay,
cell labeling and detection, 106–109
materials, 99
sensitivity, 105
stimulation, 106, 108
CD8+ T-cell response to hepatitis B virus, 74, 75, 81, 94–96
woodchuck hepatitis virus cytokine response characterization, 37–42
Interleukin-4 (IL-4),
CD8+ T-cell response to hepatitis B virus, 75
woodchuck hepatitis virus cytokine response characterization, 39–41
Interleukin-5 (IL-5), CD8+ T-cell response to hepatitis B virus, 75
Interleukin-10 (IL-10),
CD8+ T-cell response to hepatitis B virus, 75
woodchuck hepatitis virus cytokine response characterization, 39–41
Interleukin-15 (IL-15), woodchuck hepatitis virus cytokine response characterization, 39–41
ISH, *see In situ* hybridization

K

Kupffer cell, staining in duck hepatitis B virus infection, 18

L

Lamivudine,
clinical trial insights in hepatitis B virus treatment, 503, 504
efficacy against hepatitis B virus, 425, 426, 477
interferon combination therapy, 429
liver transplant patients, hepatitis B virus prophylaxis and treatment, 323–325, 430, 431, 488
viral mutations in resistance, 379, 426, 427, 477, 478, 480, 481, 486, 487
L-HDVAg,
farnesyltransferase inhibitor targeting, *see* Farnesyltransferase
functions, 539, 540
prenylation, 540
Limiting dilution assay, *see* T-cell
Liver biopsy, staging and grading of hepatitis B virus infection, 467
Liver transplantation,
Asian patient outcomes, 328, 329
clinical trials for hepatitis B virus treatment, 530

fibrosing cholestatic hepatitis, hepatitis B virus induction and management, 326
hepatitis B virus infection recurrence, 319, 430, 488, 489
hepatitis D virus infection, 327, 328
high-risk donors, 328, 329
immune system dysfunction and hepatitis B virus infection, 319–321
immunosuppression therapy modification, 327
prophylaxis and treatment of hepatitis B virus infection recurrence,
adefovir, 325, 326
entecavir, 325, 326
famciclovir, 325
ganciclovir, 325
hepatitis B immune globulin, 319, 321–323, 330, 430, 431, 488
interferon therapy, 326, 327
lamivudine, 323–325, 430, 431, 488
prospects, 330
vaccination of recipients, 328, 329

M

Mouse models, *see* Immunodeficient mice; Transgenic mouse, hepatitis B virus

N

Northern blot,
hepatitis D virus RNA replication, 138
transgenic mouse hepatitis B virus RNA, 244, 245, 249

O

Organ transplantation,
hepatitis B virus reactivation, 489
liver, *see* Liver transplantation

P

PCR, *see* Polymerase chain reaction
Perforin, CD8+ T-cell response to hepatitis B virus, 75
Polymerase, hepatitis B virus,
activities, 479
antiviral therapy resistance mutations, 426, 427, 477, 478, 480, 481, 486, 487
structure, 416, 417, 480
Polymerase chain reaction (PCR),
duck hepatitis B virus DNA detection, 21
genotyping of hepatitis B virus drug resistant variants,
amplification reactions for sequencing, 382
DNA extraction, 382, 384
DNA sequencing, 382
INNO-LiPA assay, 384
materials, 380–382, 384
overview, 379, 380
restriction fragment length polymorphism analysis, 382–384
TaqMan assay, 383, 384
RNA, *see* Reverse transcriptase-polymerase chain reaction
transgenic mouse hepatitis B virus DNA detection, 247, 248, 250
woodchuck hepatitis virus DNA, 184, 185

R

RAG-2 knockout mouse, *see* Immunodeficient mice
Restriction fragment length polymorphism (RFLP) analysis, hepatitis B virus genotyping,
  DNA extraction, 382
  gel electrophoresis, 383
  materials, 380, 381
  overview, 379
  polymerase chain reaction, 382, 383
  restriction digestion, 383
Reverse transcriptase-polymerase chain reaction (RT-PCR), woodchuck hepatitis virus cytokine response characterization, 40, 42
RFLP analysis, *see* Restriction fragment length polymorphism analysis,
Ribonuclease protection assay,
  hepatitis B virus RNA in transgenic mouse model of chronic liver disease, 282, 283
  woodchuck hepatitis virus cytokine response characterization, 40–42
RT-PCR, *see* Reverse transcriptase-polymerase chain reaction

S

Severe combined immunodeficient mouse, *see* Transgenic mouse, hepatitis B virus
S-HDVAg,
  functions, 539, 540
  recombinant protein expression and purification, 122, 123
Southern blot,
  DHBV DNA in duck, 263, 265
    duck hepatitis B virus DNA, 195
  transgenic mouse hepatitis B virus DNA, 244, 249

T

TC3D, *see* Dose–response surface approach
T-cell,
  CD4+ T-cell response to hepatitis B virus,
    cytokine secretion assay,
      cell labeling and detection, 106–109
      materials, 99
      sensitivity, 105
      stimulation, 106, 108
    enzyme-linked immunospot assay of cytokines,
      development, 104, 108
      materials, 98
      plate preparation, 102, 108
      stimulation, 102, 108
    flow cytometry cytokine staining, 99, 104, 105, 108, 109
    overview, 97
    proliferation assay,
      blood collection, 100
      freezing and thawing of cells, 100, 101, 107
      materials, 97, 98
      peripheral blood mononuclear cell separation, 100, 107
      stimulation, 101, 107
      thymidine incorporation assay, 102, 108

trypan blue exclusion, 101
CD8+ T-cell response to hepatitis B virus,
antiviral activity, 65, 66
cell isolation from liver resections, 69, 70, 79
fine-needle liver biopsy studies,
chromium release cytotoxicity assay, 77–79
cytokine assays, 74, 75, 79, 81
expansion, 76, 77, 81
flow cytometry quantification, 74
flow cytometry selection, 75, 76, 81
lymphocyte isolation, 70, 81
materials, 67–69
viability assay, 71, 74, 81
limiting dilution assay of precursor frequency,
culture conditions and quantification, 87, 88
lymphocyte separation, 87
materials, 86, 87
overview, 85, 86
sensitivity, 92
liver injury role, 43, 65, 66
tetramer staining,
advantages, 91
interferon-γ assay, 94–96
liver infiltrating lymphocyte samples, 93–95
materials, 92, 93
peripheral blood mononuclear cell samples, 93–95
principles, 89–92
duck hepatitis B virus immune response studies,
flow cytometry, 15, 16
immunostaining, 17, 18, 22
hepatitis B virus response, overview, 43, 419
hepatitis D virus DNA vaccine response,
CD8+ T-cell activity assay, 125, 126
proliferation assay, 12, 126
induction strategies in vaccination, 434
woodchuck hepatitis virus immune response, 27, 28
TNF-α, *see* Tumor necrosis factor-a
Transgenic mouse, hepatitis B virus,
breeding, 242, 243, 249
characterization,
antiviral agent treatment, 243
enzyme-linked immunosorbent assays,
HBeAg, 245
HBsAg, 245, 246
HBcAg immunohistochemical staining, 246, 247, 249, 250
materials, 240–242, 248
necropsy and sample collection, 243, 244, 249
Northern blot of hepatitis B virus RNA, 244, 245, 249
polymerase chain reaction for hepatitis B virus DNA detection, 247, 248, 250
safety issues, 243, 249
selection of mice, 242, 243, 248, 249
Southern blot of hepatitis B virus DNA, 244, 249
mouse lines, 239, 240, 248
rationale for generation, 239, 270

severe combined immunodeficient mouse hepatitis B virus model,
alanine aminotransferase assay, 279
applications, 271
chronic liver disease, 269–271
enzyme-linked immunosorbent assay of circulating viral antigens and antibodies, 281
immune reconstitution assessment, 279, 281
immunofluorescence microscopy of hepatitis B virus antigens, 277, 278, 284
in situ hybridization of hepatitis B virus DNA, 283
liver pathology, 281, 282
materials, 271–274
partial hepatectomy, 278
polymerase chain reaction detection of hepatitis B virus DNA, 275, 276
ribonuclease protection assay for hepatitis B virus RNA, 282, 283
splenocytes,
adoptive transfer, 278, 279
preparation, 278, 284
transgene detection, 275
transgenic mouse construction,
hepatitis B virus dimer DNA isolation, 274
microinjection, 274, 275
viral replication detection in liver, 276
Tumor necrosis factor-α (TNF-α),
CD8+ T-cell response to hepatitis B virus, 75
woodchuck hepatitis virus cytokine response characterization, 37–42
Tupaia hepatocyte, *see* Hepatocyte culture infection studies

U

Urokinase-type plasminogen activator transgenic mouse, *see* Immunodeficient mice

V

V8 protease, treatment of human hepatitis B virus and woodchuck hepatitis virus to enhance infectivity,
digestion conditions, 203, 207
immunofluorescent staining of viral proteins, 205, 206
infection conditions, 203, 207
materials, 200–202
overview, 199, 200
progeny virus DNA detection, 203–206
virus isolation, 202
Western blotting of treated viruses, 203
Vaccine, hepatitis B virus ,
chimpanzee safety testing, 292, 293, 298–302
CpG DNA coadministration, 433
DNA vaccine, *see* DNA vaccine, hepatitis B virus
hepatocellular carcinoma impact, 416, 422
liver transplant recipients, 328, 329
recombinant vaccines, 433

regimens, 431, 432
T-cell induction strategies, 434

W

Western blot,
farnesyltransferase inhibitor screening, 547, 548, 550
V8 protease-treated viruses, 203
WHV, *see* Woodchuck hepatitis virus
WMHBV, *see* Woolly monkey hepatitis B virus
Woodchuck hepatitis virus (WHV),
cell-mediated immune response characterization,
materials, 31, 32
overview, 27–31
peripheral blood mononuclear cells,
isolation, 32–35
proliferation assay with radioactive labels, 34, 35
cytokine response characterization,
materials, 38–40
overview, 37, 38
reverse transcriptase-polymerase chain reaction, 40, 42
ribonuclease protection assay, 40–42
RNA preparation, 40, 41
hepatocyte culture infection studies,
cell line generation and maintenance, 182, 183, 185
freezing and thawing of hepatocytes, 183
hepatocyte isolation,
microperfusion, 181
whole liver perfusion, 179, 180
infection, 183
long-term hepatocyte culture, 181, 182, 185
materials, 176–179
overview, 175
primary hepatocyte culture, 181
V8 protease treatment of virus to enhance infectivity,
digestion conditions, 203, 207
immunofluorescent staining of viral proteins, 205, 206
infection conditions, 203, 207
materials, 200–202
overview, 199, 200
progeny virus DNA detection, 203–206
virus isolation, 202
Western blotting of treated viruses, 203
viral DNA detection,
cell preparation, 183, 184, 186
dot-blot hybridization, 174
polymerase chain reaction, 184, 185
Woolly monkey hepatitis B virus (WMHBV),
hepatitis D virus as model system, 133
host specificity, 133

MIX
Papier aus verantwortungsvollen Quellen
Paper from responsible sources
FSC® C105338
FSC
www.fsc.org

If you have any concerns about our products,
you can contact us on
ProductSafety@springernature.com

In case Publisher is established outside the EU,
the EU authorized representative is:
Springer Nature Customer Service Center GmbH
Europaplatz 3, 69115 Heidelberg, Germany

Printed by Libri Plureos GmbH
in Hamburg, Germany